OPHTHALMIC PATHOLOGY

An Atlas and Textbook

SECOND EDITION

Edited by

Michael J. Hogan, M.D.

Professor and Chairman, Department of Ophthalmology,
University of California School of Medicine, San Francisco

Lorenz E. Zimmerman, M.D.

Chief of the Ophthalmic Pathology Branch and Registrar
of the Registry of Ophthalmic Pathology,
The Armed Forces Institute of Pathology, Washington, D.C.

Published under the Sponsorship of

The American Academy of Ophthalmology and Otolaryngology

and The Armed Forces Institute of Pathology

W. B. SAUNDERS COMPANY

Philadelphia   London

W. B. Saunders Company: West Washington Square
Philadelphia, Pa. 19105

12 Dyott Street
London, WC1A 1DB

833 Oxford Street
Toronto 18, Ontario

Ophthalmic Pathology   ISBN 0-7216-4725-1

MADE IN THE UNITED STATES OF AMERICA

Press of W. B. Saunders Company

Library of Congress Catalog Card Number 60–13684

Print No.: 14 13 12 11

PRINCIPAL CONTRIBUTORS

FREDERICK C. BLODI, M.D.

Associate Professor of Ophthalmology,
State University of Iowa;
Chief of Ophthalmology,
Veterans Administration Hospital,
Iowa City.

ALSON E. BRALEY, M.D.

Professor and Head,
Department of Ophthalmology,
State University of Iowa College of
  Medicine,
Iowa City.

F. PHINIZY CALHOUN, Jr., M.D.

Professor and Chairman,
Department of Ophthalmology,
Emory University School of Medicine;
Director of the L. F. Montgomery Labo-
  ratory of Ocular Pathology,
Atlanta.

LEONARD CHRISTENSEN, M.S., M.D.

Associate Professor of Ophthalmology,
University of Oregon Medical School,
Portland.

WINDSOR S. DAVIES, M.D.

Professor of Clinical Ophthalmology,
Wayne State University College of
  Medicine;
Chief, Pathology Department,
Kresge Eye Institute,
Detroit.

ARNOLD W. FORREST, M.D.

Instructor in Ophthalmology,
Columbia University College of Physi-
  cians and Surgeons,
New York.

MICHAEL J. HOGAN, M.D.

Professor and Chairman,
Department of Ophthalmology,
University of California School of Medi-
  cine,
San Francisco.

A. RAY IRVINE, Jr., M.D.

Assistant Clinical Professor,
Department of Surgery (Ophthalmology)
University of California School of Medi-
  cine, Los Angeles;
Trustee, Co-Director and Pathologist,
Estelle Doheny Eye Foundation,
Los Angeles.

TORRENCE A. MAKLEY, JR., M.D.

> Professor of Ophthalmology,
> Ohio State University School of Medicine,
> Columbus.

JOHN S. McGAVIC, M.D.

> Professor of Ophthalmology,
> Temple University School of Medicine;
> Professor of Clinical Ophthalmology,
> Graduate School of Medicine, University of Pennsylvania,
> Philadelphia.

JOHN M. McLEAN, M.D.

> Professor of Clinical Surgery,
> Department of Ophthalmology,
> Cornell University Medical College,
> New York.

THEODORE E. SANDERS, M.D.

> Associate Professor of Clinical Ophthalmology,
> Washington University School of Medicine,
> St. Louis.

JOSEPH JACKSON STOKES, M.D.

> Assistant Professor of Ophthalmology,
> Emory University School of Medicine,
> Atlanta.

JOSEPH A. C. WADSWORTH, M.D.

> Associate Clinical Professor of Ophthalmology,
> Columbia University College of Physicians and Surgeons,
> New York.

LORENZ E. ZIMMERMAN, M.D.

> Chief of the Ophthalmic Pathology Branch and
> Registrar of the Registry of Ophthalmic Pathology,
> The Armed Forces Institute of Pathology,
> Washington, D.C.

Consultants

DAVID G. COGAN, M.D.

> Professor of Ophthalmology,
> Harvard Medical School.
> Boston.

HELENOR CAMPBELL FOERSTER

> Ophthalmic Pathologist,
> University of California School of Medicine,
> San Francisco.

LEVON K. GARRON, M.D.

> Assistant Clinical Professor of Ophthalmology,
> University of California School of Medicine,
> San Francisco.

ARTHUR M. SILVERSTEIN, PH.D.

> Chief of the Immunochemistry Branch,
> The Armed Forces Institute of Pathology,
> Washington, D.C.

GEORGIANA D. THEOBALD, M.D.

> Clinical Associate Professor of Ophthalmology and
> Clinical Pathologist, Emeritus,
> Consultant to Department of Pathology,
> University of Illinois College of Medicine,
> Chicago.

J. REIMER WOLTER, M.D.

> Associate Professor of Ophthalmology,
> University of Michigan Medical School,
> Ann Arbor.

FOREWORD

THE FIRST EDITION of this book was received with such appreciation that it was soon sold out. The publishers were confronted with the problem of reprinting or production of a revised edition. The matter was referred to the Academy and to the Academy Committee on Ophthalmic Pathology. As in any new work of the kind portrayed in the Atlas-Textbook of Ophthalmic Pathology, some portions were not acceptable in the light of present day concepts and subjects of great importance conceived since the preparation of the text were, of course, not included. Suggestions were received from teachers of pathology concerning the organization of the text and it was the opinion of the Committee on Pathology that a revision was necessary and could conceivably be done in approximately three years.

The Committee graciously accepted the assignment and early in 1956 work on revision was started. It soon became evident that besides some reorganization of the text, several parts had to be rewritten and new chapters added. It meant an increase in pagination of the text and the addition of a number of illustrations. An estimate of the cost to the Academy for underwriting the revision was submitted to the Council together with the contract terms of the publishers. The necessary funds were appropriated to cover the actual out of pocket expenses incurred by the Committee in preparation of the manuscript for the printer and the authors gave generously of their time without compensation. Thus, a second edition of Ophthalmic Pathology, An Atlas and Textbook was made possible.

Some of the illustrations and legends prepared for the first edition have been used in this new edition and many new ones added. It has been the aim of the Committee to preserve the form of the earlier edition, in order to indicate lineage and to acknowledge the debt owed to Dr. Jonas Friedenwald and his co-authors in producing a new textbook in ophthalmic pathology, and to Mrs. Helenor C. Foerster, who assembled the most remarkable Atlas of ophthalmic histopathologic reproductions ever produced. This heritage is a most valuable possession of the Academy and reflects the objectives proclaimed by the founders that, "The object of the Academy shall be to promote and advance the science and art of medicine appertaining to the eye, ear, nose and throat; and to encourage the study of the relationship of these specialties to surgery, general medicine, and hygiene" (Constitution. Art. II).

W. L. BENEDICT, M.D., LL.D.

FOREWORD

THIS SECOND EDITION of Ophthalmic Pathology, An Atlas and Textbook represents the continued close collaboration and cooperation of the American Academy of Ophthalmology and Otolaryngology and the Armed Forces Institute of Pathology. The remarkably complementary relationship of the Academy and the AFIP goes back more than four decades, having had its origin in the organization of the Museum of Ophthalmic Pathology at the old Army Medical Museum in 1921. This Registry, the pioneer component of the American Registry of Pathology, is unequaled and can justly claim to be the largest and most active registry of ophthalmic pathology in the world today.

The popularity of the first edition of this book (like that of the earlier Atlases of DeCoursey and Ash) and the preparation of the second edition are signal tributes to the many ophthalmologists and pathologists working in harmony to advance the field of ophthalmology and ophthalmic pathology.

In this edition the Atlas component has been integrated with the text as closely as possible so as to achieve maximum teaching value and continuity. A majority of the ex-cellent plates prepared for the first edition have been retained while many new illustrations have been added. Many of the inevitable advances that have taken place in the understanding of specific etiology, pathogenetic mechanisms and natural course of various diseases have been described. The result is a volume in which both the American Academy of Ophthalmology and Otolaryngology and the Armed Forces Institute of Pathology can be justly proud.

While this Atlas is basically a textbook designed for the graduate student of ophthalmology or pathology, at the same time it serves a reference need for the hospital pathologist who must be expected to cope with the many complexities of ophthalmic pathology.

The staff of the Armed Forces Institute of Pathology takes pride in having been able to assist the authors in the preparation and completion of this very fine contribution to the advancement of pathology.

FRANK M. TOWNSEND, M.D.
COL., U.S.A.F., M.C.

PREFACE TO
THE SECOND EDITION

MANY ADVANCES have occurred in ophthalmology and in pathology since the first edition was printed. Not only has knowledge of eye diseases changed, but many of the general concepts of disease and its effects on tissue have undergone considerable revision. Newer methods of investigation of the causes and types of inflammation by immunochemical methods have become available, and histochemical techniques have been originated for detection of chemical changes in tissues in disease states. Former concepts of the anatomy of the ocular structures have been revised as the result of advances in phase microscopy and electron microscopy. Some viruses producing disease of the outer eye have been identified and their pathogenicity has become well known. The biochemist has made great advances in the detection and study of inborn errors of metabolism involving amino acids and other body constituents, and progress has been made toward determining the relationship of lipid metabolism to vascular diseases.

Certain diseases, such as retrolental fibroplasia, have been explained on a rational etiologic basis, reproduced in experimental animals, and virtually extinguished by institution of prophylactic measures. Still other conditions have become apparent as a result of attempts to control disease with new therapeutic agents, e.g., fungal infections superimposed on long-term topical corticosteroid and antibiotic therapy for ulcerative corneal lesions.

All these advances warranted the writing of a second edition of this text. In addition it seemed necessary to develop more fully the presentation of the pathologic anatomy of certain tissues (e.g., retina, optic nerve, and vitreous) which were treated in a somewhat cursory fashion in the first edition.

In preparing the new edition it was decided to revert to the anatomic method of discussing and describing pathologic changes in the eye. This method has the disadvantage of a certain amount of repetition, and the student has to refer to several chapters in order to obtain a complete picture of a certain disease affecting the eye. An attempt to overcome this drawback has been made in the first chapter by presenting a discussion of certain principles of general pathology which would serve as a background for subsequent chapters. Also it was decided to have a discussion of pathologic entities which affect the entire eye, and a general discussion of ocular injuries before proceeding to individual tissues. A certain amount of repetition is not harmful, and we believe the reader will obtain a complete picture of a disease entity without too much cross reference.

Changing the format has necessitated a certain amount of chopping and reorganization of the plates from the first edition so that they could be integrated with the text. The main criticism of the first edition was the lack of correlation of plates with the text. A large number of new plates have been added to show advances in ocular histology as well as in histochemistry and ophthalmic pathology. Many of these were contributed by authors of articles or chapters on special subjects, and the present authors are grateful to them for permitting their use in this edition. Credit is given in the text for the illustrations.

This revision is so extensive that it could really be termed a new textbook. However, one of the finest parts of the first edition, the illustrations, which were so carefully selected and prepared by Mrs. Helenor Campbell Foerster, have been largely reused. The authors wish, also, to indicate their great appreciation to Miss Eleanor V. Paul who devoted so many hours to the preparation of the new plates for this edition and to reading and correcting manuscript, galleys, and page proof.

We wish to thank the following persons for reading and correcting copy, and furnishing valuable consultation in the preparation of the various chapters: Bernard Becker, M.D., St. Louis; Milton Boniuk, M.D., Houston; David G. Cogan, M.D., Boston; Wendell C. Irvine, M.D., Los Angeles; Samuel T. Jones, M.D., Chicago; A. Edward Maumenee, M.D., Baltimore; William K. McEwen, Ph.D., San Francisco; Edith Parkhill, M.D., Rochester, Minnesota; John F. Porterfield, M.D., Columbia, Missouri; Christian Elmore Radcliffe, M.D., Iowa City; Robert N. Shaffer, M.D., San Francisco; William H. Spencer, San Francisco; and Phillips Thygeson, M.D., San Francisco.

We also wish to thank the following persons for kindly furnishing photographs for some of the chapters: L. Allen, Iowa City; Professor Norman Ashton, London, England; C. H. Binford, M.D., Washington, D.C.; J. M. B. Bloodworth, Jr., M.D., Columbus, Ohio; W. M. Boles, M.D., New Orleans; A. Braley, M.D., Iowa City; H. Burian, M.D., Iowa City; L. L. Calkins, M.D., Kansas City, Missouri; D. G. Cogan, M.D., Boston; F. C. Cordes, M.D., San Francisco; J. M. Dixon, M.D., Birmingham; L. Feeney, San Francisco; B. S. Fine, M.D., Washington, D.C.; L. K. Garron, M.D., San Francisco; J. W. Henderson, M.D.,

Rochester, Minnesota; A. S. Holmberg, M.D., Sweden; S. T. Jones, M.D., Chicago; A. Kallos, M.D., New York; H. Q. Kirk, M.D., Oak Park, Illinois; B. A. Klien, M.D., Chicago; T. Kuwabara, M.D., Boston; H. Lund, M.D., Greensboro, North Carolina; A. E. Maumenee, M.D., Baltimore; E. Okun, M.D., St. Louis; A. B. Reese, M.D., New York; B. Rones, M.D., Washington, D.C.; R. N. Shaffer, M.D., San Francisco; G. D. Theobald, M.D., Oak Park, Illinois; P. Thygeson, M.D., San Francisco; A. J. Tousimis, Washington, D.C.; J. A. C. Wadsworth, M.D., New York; and J. R. Wolter, M.D., Ann Arbor.

We wish to thank the Council of the American Academy of Ophthalmology and Otolaryngology for their very earnest support of this revision, and Col. Frank M Townsend, Director of the Armed Forces Institute of Pathology for his assistance in providing the use of the outstanding Medical Illustration Service of the Institute for many of the illustrations. Mr. John Dusseau, of the Saunders Company, has rendered invaluable aid at many of the meetings of the committee and we are very grateful for his excellent advice.

Finally, we want to dedicate this book to the Armed Forces Institute of Pathology which this year is celebrating its centennial. Established during the Civil War as the Army Medical Museum, the organization developed into the Army Institute of Pathology during World War II. Following the War, the Institute became the central Laboratory of pathologic anatomy for all the Armed Forces and for the Veterans Administration. Appropriately, the name was changed to the Armed Forces Institute of Pathology. In addition to its primary purpose, to support the Armed Forces by providing consultation, education and research, the Institute maintains active relationships with civilian medicine through the American Registry of Pathology. Significantly, the American Academy of Ophthalmology and Otolaryngology was the organization responsible for initiating the program which subsequently led to the organization of the American Registry of Pathology. The oldest of the Registries at the AFIP is the Ophthalmic which dates back to 1921.

Michael J. Hogan
Lorenz E. Zimmerman

CONTENTS

Chapter 1

General Pathology

INFLAMMATION

Definition

Inflammation may be defined as a series of local tissue reactions which take place at the site of injury. According to Ehrich and to Selye, these reactions follow a repetitive pattern regardless of the specific agent responsible for the injury. They include (1) an initial shock phase characterized physiologically by a disturbance of equilibrium and pathologically by necrosis or degeneration produced by the injurious agent, (2) a reactive countershock phase in which the acute exudative inflammatory reaction attempts to overcome the irritant, (3) an adaptive phase of great variability marked by features of subacute or chronic inflammation, progressing ultimately to (4) a reparative phase in which homeostasis is restored or (4a) exhaustion of local defensive mechanisms, with uncontrolled necrosis or degeneration. Selye has grouped these reactions to local injury under the heading of "local adaptation syndrome" and he has described experiments which support his belief that the local and the general adaptation syndromes are closely interrelated.

Causes and Mechanisms

Inflammation is not synonymous with in-fection; in fact, most inju.ious agents are noninfectious. All types of trauma are capable of provoking the cardinal features of inflammation. Abrasions, lacerations, foreign bodies, heat, cold, acids, alkalis, radiant energy, hypersensitivity reactions, in fact any stimulus capable of irritating (overstimulating) cells may be considered etiologic factors. Moreover the stimulus need not be exogenous. Noxious substances liberated from dead or dying tissues are effective irritants. Thus occlusion of the local blood supply to a tissue leading to its destruction may be attended by systemic as well as local signs of inflammation.

In ophthalmology we see many excellent examples of noninfectious agents which set up an inflammatory reaction. Corneal ulcers, for example, often provoke an iritis and sterile pus accumulates in the anterior chamber (hypopyon). Virtually every ocular injury and every surgical procedure is complicated by some degree of inflammation. Those which are attended by great tissue destruction, hemorrhage, the presence of foreign bodies, or infection generally will be complicated by more severe degrees of inflammation. One of the most significant clinical examples of purely endogenous but noninfectious inflammation encountered by the ophthalmologist is produced by malignant melanomas (and less frequently retinoblastomas) which outgrow or obstruct their blood supply and become necrotic. Eyes containing such tumors frequently are treated with antibiotics in the belief that the endophthalmitis or panophthalmitis is of bacterial origin. Another example is lens-induced uveitis.

Vascular and Cellular Aspects

Initial changes in ground substance. According to McCutcheon, the series of events which take place when tissues are irritated generally are described as vascular and cellular, but these, as Zweifach has shown by micromanipulative procedures, are preceded by alterations in the ground substance at the site of injury. In the conjunctiva, for example, the connective tissue matrix is normally a gel which impedes the spread of particulate matter. The earliest alterations observed after micro-injury occur at the site of trauma. The state of the ground substance is converted from gel to sol and particulate matter now flows freely through the injured tissues. Comparable connective tissue changes can be reproduced by trypsin, hyaluronidase, a variety of bacterial toxins and snake venom, but significantly not by histamine or heparin.

Local vascular response. The vascular inflammatory response to minimal trauma begins several minutes later. The terminal arteriole dilates and the endothelium of capillaries and venules downstream from the site of micro-injury shows a greatly increased affinity (stickiness) for particulate matter and circulating cells. This is a transient reaction which cannot be reproduced by histamine. With more intense injury blood platelets and leukocytes adhere to the vessel wall in greater numbers and over larger areas. These same areas become much more permeable, leaking colloids as well as water. With even more severe degrees of local injury the capillary walls become pervious to red blood cells and thrombi tend to form.

Reflex vascular phenomena. The vascular phenomena just described were found by Zweifach to be purely localized and not associated with recognizable increase in regional blood flow. After the injection of such irritants as xylol or tissue extracts, there ensues a widespread axon reflex-type of vasodilatation mainly affecting the arteriolar vessels. This gives rise to an active hyperemia which is associated with a great increase in volume of the capillary bed. Microscopic examination reveals large numbers of dilated capillaries (Fig. 1). Normally only a small fraction of

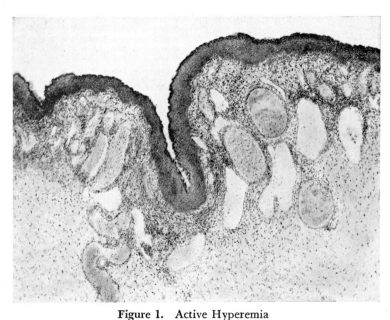

Figure 1. Active Hyperemia
There is an extreme degree of dilatation of the conjunctival blood and lymphatic capillaries. ×50. AFIP Acc. 484173.

the capillaries are functioning at a given moment, but in acutely inflamed tissues the majority of them are not only open but they are dilated. This change in function of capillaries can be studied easily in the conjunctival capillaries with the slit lamp. Active hyperemia thus accounts for two of the cardinal signs of inflammation, increased redness (rubor) and warmth (calor) of the tissue. These vascular phenomena, reflex arteriolar dilatation and endothelial damage, can be reproduced by histamine but they are not abolished by antihistaminics after microinjection of chemical irritants. Adrenal cortical extract diminishes the degree of reactive hyperemia of acute inflammation.

Inflammatory edema. In time or with severe degrees of injury, blood flow through this widely dilated capillary bed becomes sluggish and finally may cease in some vessels. The vessel walls become more permeable, first for water, then for blood proteins, and later for blood cells. Capillaries which normally would permit passage of only one or two cells at a time become widened to a diameter of 25 or more cells (Fig. 2). The interstitial spaces between vessels appear waterlogged. If much protein has escaped, this tissue juice will stain pink with eosin, the intensity of eosin-staining increasing with protein content. Because of its smaller molecular size albumin escapes first, later the globulins and fibrinogen (Fig. 3). The greater concentration of these plasma proteins in the tissue fluids constitutes one of the main differences between inflammatory exudates and other types of edema (transudates). The lymphatics soon enlarge because of this edema. Normal lymphatics are difficult to demonstrate by ordinary histology but in acutely inflamed tissues these vessels are easy to find because of their large numbers and great size.

The inflammatory edema causes the tissues to swell. This swelling accounts for the other two cardinal signs of inflammation, tumor and dolor. Zweifach found that adrenal cortical extract increased the vascular hyporeactivity during acute inflammation, and as a result of this effect there was loss of fluid from the damaged capillaries. The degree of edema depends partly on the amount of fluid leaking from the irritated vascular bed and partly on the efficiency of the lymphatic drain-

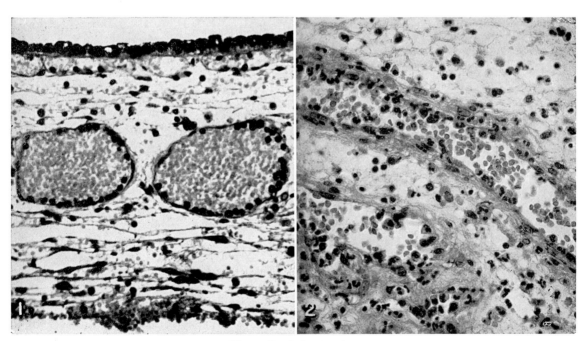

Figure 2. Inflammation
1. Dilatation and engorgement of choroidal vessels. Margination of leukocytes. Edema of surrounding tissue which contains red blood cells. × 145. AFIP Acc. 164016.
2. Polymorphonuclear leukocytes escaping through vessel wall. ×400. AFIP Acc. 291365.

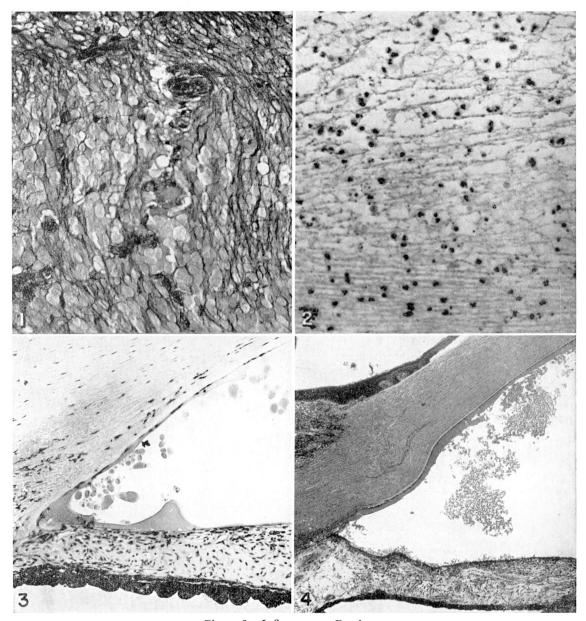

Figure 3. Inflammatory Exudates

1. Edema. Serous exudate between nerve fibers in papilledema. ×275. AFIP Acc. 185418.
2. Fibrin with enmeshed polymorphonuclear leukocytes. Note nodal points of fibrin. ×320. AFIP Acc. 48306.
3. Serous exudate with globular precipitate in anterior chamber. ×125. AFIP Acc. 167332.
4. Granular precipitated proteins in anterior chamber. ×48. AFIP Acc. 266650.

age. With the escape of fibrinogen there is a tendency for fibrin clots to form, not only in the interstitial spaces, but also within the lymphatics. Thus the initial inflammatory edema may become accentuated by a superimposed lymphedema resulting from obstructed lymph vessels.

All of the vascular aspects of inflammation just described are observed in the ocular tissues. In fact, hyperemia of the iris and the development of an "aqueous flare" without the presence of cells in the anterior chamber is one of our best examples of the purely vascular component of the inflammatory reaction.

For those who like to think teleologically

the vascular aspects of inflammation just described have a number of important functions. The exudation of fluid dilutes the irritant. Escaping blood proteins can bind certain irritants in a nonspecific manner and, in the case of antibody globulins, in a very specific reaction. Escaping fibrinogen can be precipitated as a fibrin network to prevent spread of the reaction and to serve as a scaffold upon which inflammatory and fibroblastic cells can function more effectively. In thinking teleologically, one must separate local and systemic manifestations; for example, precipitation of fibrin may produce deleterious local sequelae such as thrombosis of lymphatics and severe lymphedema. Yet were it not for these localizing effects of fibrin, it is possible many focal infections might otherwise become septicemic, as was demonstrated experimentally by Thuerer and Angevine in rabbits following administration of bishydroxycoumarin. Lastly the active hyperemia brings to the injured tissues an increased number of circulating leukocytes. This brings us to the cellular aspects of inflammation.

Cellular aspects. The cellular aspects of the inflammatory reaction begin soon after the vascular response is initiated. Leukocytes and endothelial cells in the capillaries and venules of the traumatized focus become sticky, and particulate matter within these vessels becomes deposited on them in amounts much greater than in vessels away from the irritated area. Leukocytes become adherent to the capillary endothelium. This margination of leukocytes can be demonstrated readily in routine histologic sections (Fig. 2-1). With more severe trauma blood platelets also adhere to the endothelial surface and to each other. By the time this occurs the vessel wall is sufficiently damaged that it is leaking much fluid, protein, and cells. The blood flow through the damaged capillaries is sluggish and there is a tendency for the agglutinated platelets and leukocytes to plug the vessel lumen (thrombosis).

Chemotaxis. The polymorphonuclear leukocytes which are adherent to the vessel walls emigrate into the injured tissues by ameboid movement. Instead of migrating in random fashion they move towards the site of injury under the specific influence of certain infectious agents, foreign bodies, and injured tissues. This directional type of ameboid locomotion, an important defense mechanism, is called chemotaxis. It should be of interest to ophthalmologists to note that the concept of chemotaxis was introduced into pathology by Leber in 1879 as a result of his studies of Aspergillus infection of the cornea. Chemotaxis may also be demonstrated in vitro. The substance present in sterile exudate that is responsible for attracting leukocytes has been identified as a polypeptide by Menkin and called "leukotaxin." This substance also has the property of increasing capillary permeability. While chemotaxis is characteristic of polymorphonuclear leukocytes, other blood elements, including erythrocytes, escape into the tissues as a result of the vascular damage.

We now have all the essential features of an *acute inflammatory reaction* which may be summarized as follows: (a) conversion of ground substance from gel to sol which permits more rapid diffusion of particulate matter, (b) active hyperemia giving rise to rubor and calor, (c) vascular damage resulting in escape of fluids and cells (inflammatory edema: tumor and dolor), (d) chemotaxis of polymorphonuclear leukocytes. Before proceeding to a description of subsequent stages and types of inflammatory reaction, a brief review of the morphology and function of the leukocytes and other related cells of inflammation will be given.

Morphology and Function of Inflammatory Cells

Neutrophils. Neutrophilic polymorphonuclear leukocytes (microphages of Metchnikoff) are the most numerous of the circulating leukocytes. They normally are produced by the bone marrow and carried by the circulating blood to sites of injury where they escape through injured vessels and are attracted to diseased areas. The level of circulating neutrophils is influenced by chemical substances liberated at sites of injury. Menkin has described leukocytosis-promoting and leukopenia-promoting factors. Neutrophils, as seen in ordinary histologic preparations, appear to be irregularly rounded cells about 50 per cent larger than erythrocytes

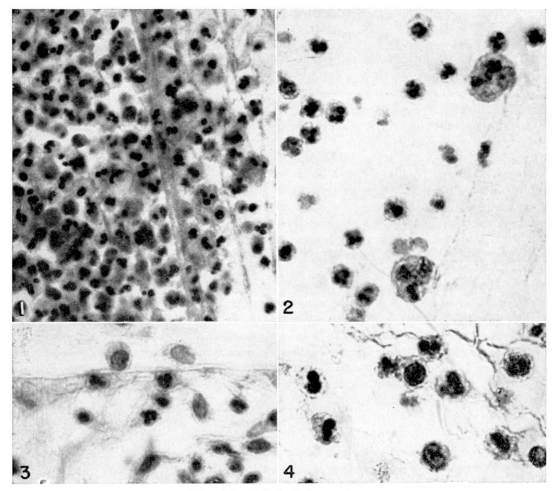

Figure 4.　Cells in Inflammation
1. Polymorphonuclear leukocytes in abscess. ×705. AFIP Acc. 89552.
2. Polymorphonuclear leukocytes. Two large macrophages have ingested polymorphonuclear leukocytes. ×1000. AFIP Acc. 121630.
3. Two monocytes on internal limiting membrane of retina. ×1000. AFIP Acc. 121630.
4. Monocytes and polymorphonuclear leukocytes clinging to strands of fibrin. ×1200. AFIP Acc. 105518.

(Fig. 4–1, 2). The ameboid pseudopods which these cells produce in vivo are not observed after fixation. There is a single multilobulated nucleus in the mature cell but more immature neutrophils may be observed with round to reniform nuclei. These, in tissue sections, may be readily confused with other inflammatory cells, especially monocytes (Fig. 4–3, 4). The moderately abundant cytoplasm contains granules which do not have a great affinity for either acid or basic dyes; hence the term neutrophilic leukocyte.

Leukocytes have the important functions of chemotaxis and phagocytosis during their life and proteolysis after their death. Because

they can be mobilized so rapidly from the circulating blood and attracted so effectively by chemotaxis, these cells constitute the most important first line of cellular defense. Their phagocytic ability is greatly enhanced by several changes which occur during the inflammatory process. Mention has already been made of the sticky surface which they acquire when still within the capillaries. Precipitated fibrin and certain antibodies also facilitate the phagocytic function of these cells. Although they are efficient in the phagocytosis of many bacteria and other small particles, neutrophils are far less effective than macrophages. Their life expectancy is short (a few days) and they cannot reproduce by cell division, but even after death they contribute to the inflammatory reaction by liberating proteolytic enzymes. The extensive necrosis which characterizes suppurative inflammatory reactions is largely attributable to these enzymes. The absence of such proteolysis in certain acute inflammatory reactions may be the result of substances, derived from the blood, which neutralize or destroy the leukocytic enzymes. Also the acidity of the tissue may be important, for the neutrophilic enzyme (in contrast with that of the macrophage) is effective only in alkaline media.

Eosinophils. Eosinophilic leukocytes normally constitute only one to two per cent of the circulating white blood cells. They may increase tremendously in the blood and may be found at sites of acute, subacute or chronic inflammation, particularly in patients with atopic types of hypersensitivity. Once thought

to be the main carrier of histamine, according to Riley eosinophils now appear to be more concerned with the detoxification and disposal of tissue histamine than with its elaboration. These leukocytes do share with neutrophils the properties of chemotaxis and phagocytosis. A sharp reduction in circulating eosinophils is produced by cortisone or by ACTH (providing the adrenals are capable of responding) or by stress (providing both the pituitary and adrenals can respond). As it is observed in tissue sections the eosinophil is a rounded cell about the size of a neutrophil but differing morphologically from the latter in two important respects. Its nucleus is bilobed rather than multilobed, and its cytoplasm stains intensely with acid dyes (Fig. 5–1). Even when the individual eosinophilic granules are difficult to distinguish because of necrobiotic or autolytic changes, the cytoplasm of these cells tends to maintain its

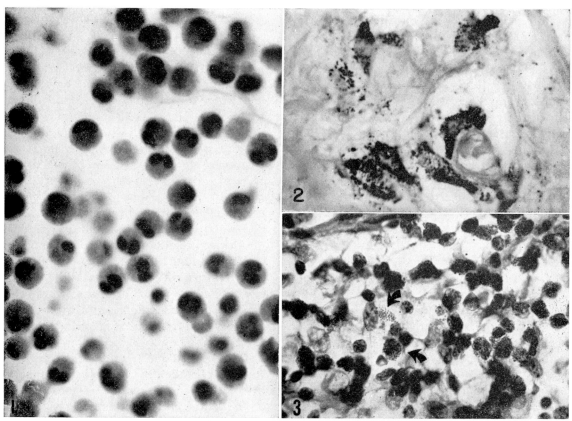

Figure 5. Cells in Inflammation
1. Eosinophils: bilobed nuclei. ×1000. AFIP Acc. 71811.
2. Mast cells. Giemsa stain. ×1000. AFIP Acc. 110883.
3. Eosinophils showing granules (arrows). ×540. AFIP Acc. 940346.

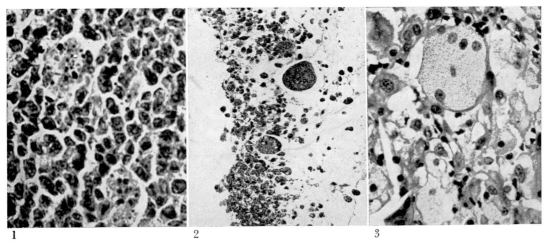

Figure 6. Cells in Inflammation

1. Two large macrophages in lymph follicle contain nuclear debris. ×355.

2. Absorbing hemorrhage. Macrophages ingesting red cells. ×145. AFIP Acc. 321668.

3. Macrophages (lipoidal histiocytes, foamy cells) which have ingested lipids. One giant macrophage in upper portion of field. ×355.

eosinophilia. The bilobed nucleus is an important feature which distinguishes the eosinophil from early stages of Russell's body formation in plasma cells (see p. 12).

Basophils and mast cells. Basophilic leukocytes, characterized morphologically by their coarse deeply basophilic cytoplasmic granules, are the fewest of the white blood cells in the peripheral blood. Their function remains obscure and, according to Michels (1938) and Riley (1954), an apparently related cell with similar basophilic granules, called the mast cell, is found in connective tissue (Fig. 5–2). The characteristic granules of these cells are water soluble but are well preserved by alcoholic fixatives. They exhibit metachromasia, are strongly Schiff-positive after treatment with periodic acid, stain intensely with Alcian blue, and possess a great affinity for radioactive sulfur. The granules disintegrate and lose their affinity for sulfur after cortisone therapy (Asboe-Hansen). These cells have been reported to be producers of heparin (Jorpes, 1946; Ehrich et al., 1949), histamine (Riley, 1954, 1955, 1959), serotonin (Benditt et al., 1955) and mucopolysaccharides of ground substance (Asboe-Hansen, 1954). According to Asboe-Hansen and Larsen there are numerous mast cells in the iris and ciliary body and their numbers are increased in iridocyclitis. Mast

cells normally are present in the synovial membranes of joints and in the skin and are greatly increased at these sites in certain mesenchymal diseases such as rheumatoid arthritis and lupus erythematosus.

Monocytes and histiocytes. There is a great family of large mononuclear phagocytic cells widely distributed throughout the blood and tissues. The circulating member is called a *monocyte* (Fig. 4), while those found in tissues have been given many names. Some are migrating cells (histiocytes, macrophages of Metchnikoff, clasmatocytes, etc.), while others are fixed in position, mainly within sinusoidal vessels of the liver, spleen, lymph nodes and bone marrow, and are called sessile histiocytes. Though macrophages are only weakly chemotactic and are mobilized slowly, they are the most efficient of all the phagocytic cells. They are capable of ingesting foreign particles and tissue debris which are not handled by neutrophils (Fig. 6). When confronted with larger particles they combine to form giant cells of the foreign body type (Figs. 7, 8). According to McCutcheon, these may liberate a protease which is active in spite of the acidity of the inflamed tissues, while the proteolytic enzyme of polymorphonuclears requires an alkaline medium. Another most important characteristic of macrophages is their extraordinary ability to proliferate

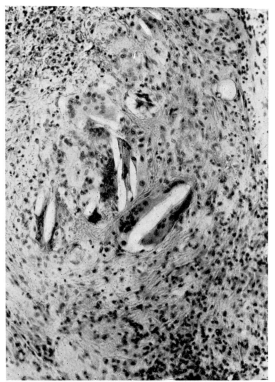

Figure 7. Cells in Granulomatous Inflammation Foreign body giant cells around cholesterol slits. ×185. AFIP Acc. 198761.

(reproduce) in various tissues; neutrophils, it will be recalled, must be mobilized from the bone marrow.

Formerly, it was believed that this family of cells was the main source of antibody formation, but, according to Ehrich (1954), phagocytic cells only degrade corpuscular antigen and release immunologically active molecules which then are available for exciting antibody production by plasma cells. There also is reason to believe these cells serve as precursors of plasma cells and fibroblasts. According to Jasmin and Robert, the macrophagic response to chemical, particulate, or infectious agents is stimulated by the "phlogistic" hormones which affect electrolyte and water metabolism (11-oxysteroids) but inhibited by the "antiphlogistic" hormones which affect carbohydrate and protein metabolism.

There is greater morphologic variation within this group of inflammatory cells than in any other cell type participating in the inflammatory response. As seen in tissue sections, the inactive large mononuclear cell appears round or ovoid and somewhat larger than a neutrophil. It has a variable amount

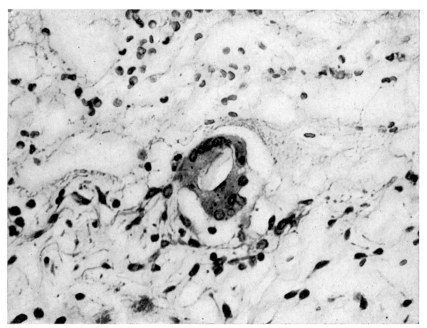

Figure 8. Giant cell containing cotton fiber in iris, following operation. ×500. AFIP Acc. 268403.

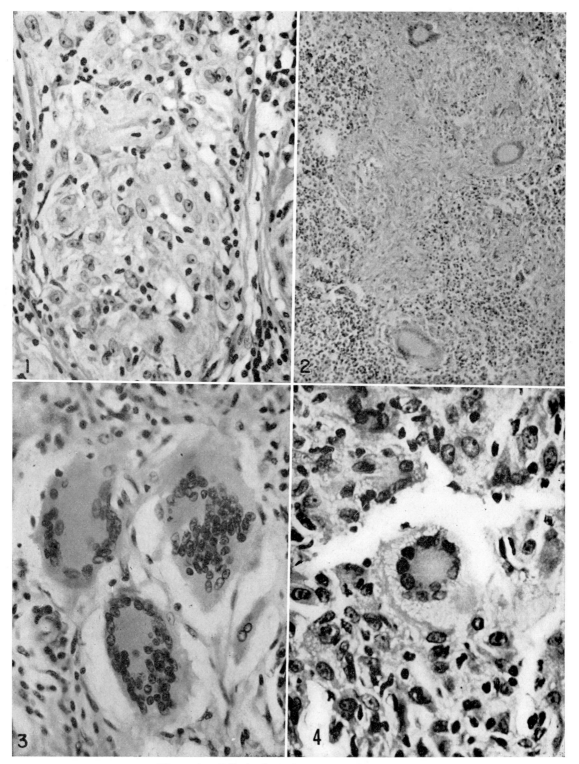

Figure 9.   Cells in Granulomatous Inflammation
1. Epithelioid cells. ×400. AFIP Acc. 71412.
2. Langhans' giant cells. ×150. AFIP Acc. 135649.
3. Langhans' giant cells. Cell at right was sectioned through peripheral nuclear rim. ×800. AFIP Acc. 79394.
4. Touton giant cell in juvenile xanthogranuloma of eyelid. ×500. AFIP Acc. 136738.

of pale-staining, often ill-defined cytoplasm and a reniform or ovoid nucleus (Fig. 4). Normally, it constitutes about five per cent of the circulating leukocytes and is found in the tissues only in small numbers. In diseased tissues innumerable variations in the size, shape and staining characteristics of macrophages are seen. This variation depends on the nature of the tissue injury and the character and amount of material being ingested by the phagocytes. For example, after consuming lipoidal matter, the cytoplasm of macrophages becomes distended by vacuoles which appear unstained unless special fat stains are used (Fig. 6–3). At the site of old hemorrhage the same cell might be stuffed with red, brown, or yellow pigment (Fig. 6–2) depending upon the degree of conversion of hemoglobin to hemosiderin and bilirubin. Bacteria, fungi, and other foreign material also may be identified within the cytoplasm of macrophages.

Epithelioid and giant cells. There are morphologic variations of macrophages known as "epithelioid cells" and "giant cells of the Langhans type" which deserve special consideration here. The presence of these cells in significant numbers establishes a diagnosis of granulomatous inflammation (see p. 15). Epithelioid cells are characterized by their abundant homogeneous, weakly eosinophilic cytoplasm. They have ill-defined cytoplasmic borders which tend to become fused in a sort of syncytium (Fig. 9–1). As a result of these morphologic alterations, these macrophages develop a resemblance to epithelial cells; hence the name epithelioid cell. As the cytoplasm increases in abundance, amitotic

nuclear division may occur, thus forming a giant cell containing a row of nuclei arranged along the periphery, the *Langhans' cell* (Fig. 9–2, 3). The center of this cell is typically homogeneous or finely granular, but its phagocytic ability may be evident by the presence of intracytoplasmic particulate matter (Figs. 10, 11, 12).

Although very little is known about the fundamental problem of epithelioid cell formation, Rich and his associates have presented evidence that the interaction of antigen and antibody, experimentally as well as in diseases of man, can cause the development of tuberculoid granulomatous lesions. *Giant cells* also may be formed by the fusion of macrophages about foreign bodies (Figs. 7, 8). Such giant cells are more pleomorphic than Langhans' cells and tend to exhibit more evidence of phagocytosis. The characteristic arrangements of epithelioid and giant cells as they are observed in different forms of granulomatous inflammations are described on pages 15–20.

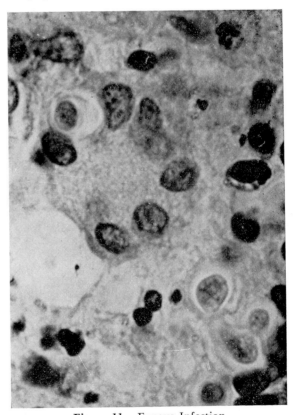

Figure 11. Fungus Infection
Blastomyces dermatitidis in giant cells; budding form in lower right corner. ×1670. AFIP Acc. 87260.

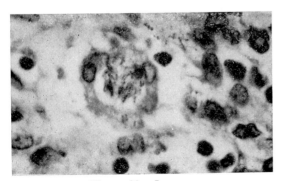

Figure 10. Leprosy
Leprous giant cell filled with bacilli (carbol-fuchsin stain). ×1000. AFIP Acc. 217656.

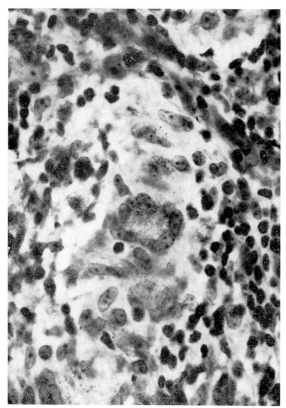

Figure 12. Sympathetic Uveitis
Fine melanin granules in epithelioid and giant cells.
×655. AFIP Acc. 37381.

Lymphocytes. Some 15 to 30 per cent of the circulating leukocytes are lymphocytes. These, like those which make up the bulk of such tissues as lymph nodes, spleen, and thymus, are round cells about the size of erythrocytes. In histologic preparations the small mature lymphocyte frequently appears to be only a dark blue staining nucleus without cytoplasm (Fig. 13–1). Larger less mature lymphocytes possess slightly more abundant basophilic cytoplasm which is often visible around only a portion of the nucleus (Fig. 6–1). Although lymphocytes are motile, they do not exhibit chemotaxis or phagocytosis. Acute infections, like many other forms of severe stress, will produce lymphocytolysis and a resultant lymphocytopenia. This can be reproduced experimentally by the administration of ACTH or cortisone. On the other hand, most chronically inflamed tissues are characterized by the presence of excessive numbers of lymphocytes. Although lymphocytes do emigrate from the blood, it is stated by Ehrich (1953) that they are also formed in situ from undifferentiated mesenchymal cells. The cell is very short-lived and its precise function remains obscure. The hyperplasia of regional lymph nodes which follows injection of antigenic material and the recovery of specific antibody from such nodes and their efferent lymph led to the supposition that lymphocytes produce antibody. Harris and Harris state, however, that it is far from being conclusive. Ehrich (1953), who believes antibodies are produced by plasma cells, has suggested that lymphocytes function as trephocytes. According to Wagner and Ehrich (1950), cortisone produces lymphocytolysis which is associated with increased adenosine diaminase but not in xanthine oxidase activity. Thus, after acute stress, lymphocytes may provide purine and pyrimidine building blocks from their rich store of nucleic acid, while in adaptation (chronic inflammation) the storehouse becomes restocked and overstocked.

Plasma cells. There is another cell which is typically present at sites of subacute and chronic inflammation. This is the plasma cell, but this cell, unlike the lymphocyte, is not normally present in the circulating blood. Although frequently lumped with lymphocytes as "small round cells of chronic inflammation," the plasma cell easily is distinguished on histopathologic study. It is larger and less evenly rounded than the lymphocyte (Fig. 13–2, 3, 4). Frequently the cell tapers toward one end and its single round nucleus will be found at this smaller end. The opposite end of the cell contains an abundant, rather homogeneous basophilic cytoplasm except near the center of the cell adjacent to the nucleus where there is a pale staining crescentic zone, the site of the Golgi apparatus. Sometimes the nucleus presents a cartwheel arrangement of its chromatin. Typical plasma cells in chronically inflamed tissues often are accompanied by "degenerated" forms, the so-called *plasmacytoid cells* and *Russell's bodies.* The former is characterized by the presence of many small refractile eosinophilic granules throughout its ordinarily basophilic cytoplasm (Fig. 13–5). These granules generally are more coarse and less intensely eosinophilic than those of eosinophilic leukocytes.

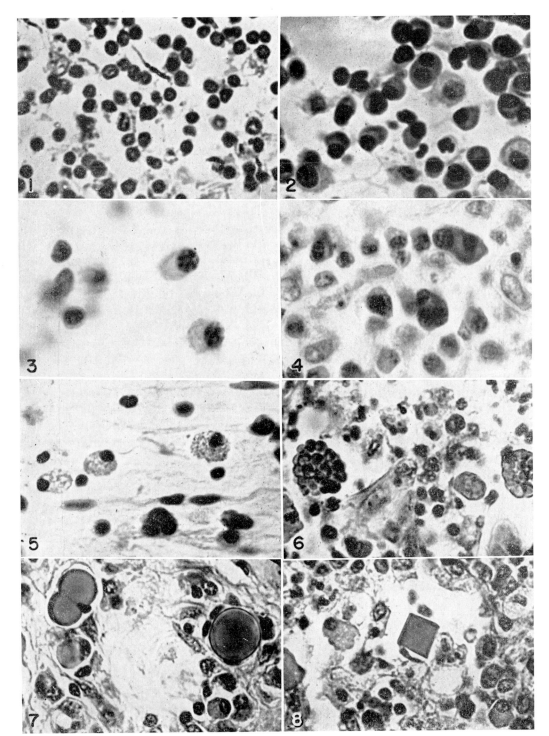

Figure 13. Cells in Chronic Inflammation

1. Lymphocytes. ×750. AFIP Acc. 219775.
2. Plasma cells, one binucleated. ×750. AFIP Acc. 219775.
3. Plasma cell showing cartwheel nucleus. ×1400. AFIP Acc. 78171.
4. Multinucleated plasma cells. ×750.
5. Plasmacytoid cells. Trinucleated plasma cell, lymphocytes and fibroblasts can also be identified in lower portion of field. ×750. AFIP Acc. 219775.
6. Russell's bodies at extreme left and right. Plasma cells and lymphocytes can also be identified. ×750. AFIP Acc. 219775.
7. Russell's bodies. Compare size to that of plasma cell and two lymphocytes in lower right corner. ×750. AFIP Acc. 219775.
8. Square Russell's body, center. Plasmacytoid cell, left. Plasma cell, lower right corner. ×750. AFIP Acc. 219775.

Plasmacytoid cells also are distinguished from eosinophils by their typically small round nucleus, since eosinophils have a characteristic bilobed nucleus. As the granules enlarge they apparently coalesce to form a few large globules. These may be several times larger than the original plasma cell and are called Russell's bodies (Fig. 13–6). In the process of forming such cytoplasmic structures the remainder of the cell becomes so atrophic that it no longer is visible unless the plane of section fortuitously demonstrates the nucleus crowded to one side (Fig. 13–7). Occasionally Russell's bodies may be mistaken for fungi or parasites.

Ehrich (1953) recently has summarized the reasons for believing the plasma cell to be *cellula sui generis,* totally unrelated to lymphocytes and derived, as was believed by its discoverers, Cajal and Unna, from the undifferentiated mesenchymal cell. He also has concisely summarized the evidence, especially the direct evidence made possible by newer immunohistochemical techniques, that the plasma cell is the site of antibody formation. Harris and Harris are not satisfied that all antibody protein is produced by plasma cells. It has been demonstrated that the intracytoplasmic granules and globules characteristic of "plasmacytoid cells" and Russell's bodies probably represent accumulated masses of antibody protein.

Classification of Inflammatory Reactions

It is customary to subdivide inflammatory processes into two main groups, acute and chronic, and then to further classify these into subgroups according to the character of the inflammatory exudate. The main types of acute inflammation are serous (exudation of serum), fibrinous (precipitation of fibrin), purulent or suppurative (pus-producing), hemorrhagic (bloody), sanguineopurulent (formation of bloody pus), serosanguineous (exudation of serum and red blood cells), catarrhal (hypersecretion of mucous), mucopurulent (formation of purulent mucous secretion), and putrefactive (formation of foul odoriferous exudate, usually by gas producing bacteria). Ordinarily the pathologist associates a polymorphonuclear response with acute inflammation and a mononuclear infiltrate with chronic reactions. In most instances this is true, but exceptions occur; for example, a remarkable mononuclear reaction may develop in a previously sensitized subject within a very few days after the injection of antigenic substances. If conditions are proper, there develops an acute, clinical reaction, characterized histologically by a proliferation of large and small mononuclear cells which after a few days includes a significant number of plasma cells. If the degree of sensitization is too great, a violent reaction develops, with suppuration and hemorrhage.

Chronic inflammation. Chronic inflammation takes place during the adaptive phase of reaction to injury. It varies tremendously in its duration, morphology, and clinical significance. If the injurious agent which initiated the inflammatory reaction is readily overcome, then the acute phase will predominate. In this event the chronic phase represents merely a transitional period during which mesenchymal cells are mobilized to clean up the debris and to repair the damage. Histopathologic examination reveals macrophages exhibiting their characteristic phagocytic functions, a scattering of lymphocytes and plasma cells, perhaps a few remaining polymorphonuclear leukocytes and early proliferation of fibroblasts and capillaries. Later the proliferation of fibroblasts and capillaries dominates the microscopic picture. Should there be a large surface area to be filled in by fibrovascular proliferation, tiny granulations representing proliferating blood vessels and connective tissue may become visible clinically (granulation tissue). The formation of granulation tissue is stimulated by the somatotropic hormone of the anterior pituitary and by desoxycorticosterone. According to Taubenhouse (1953), cortisone, compound F, estradiol, testosterone, and methyl androstenediol have an inhibitory effect. Jasmin and Robert (1953) and Asboe-Hansen (1954) have indicated that the ground substance, as well as fibroblasts, blood vessels, and collagen fibers, is altered by these hormones.

Granulomatous vs. nongranulomatous. When the injurious agent continues to stimulate the tissue or when the sequelae of the initial injury are such that equilibrium is not easily restored, a prolonged adaptive phase ensues. This we call chronic inflammation. Two main forms are recognized, granulomatous and nongranulomatous. Unfortunately, the criteria employed in making the distinction between these has been far from uniform—among pathologists as well as clinicians. There have been two main schools of thought. The older of the two applied the term "granuloma" to any tumor-like mass of chronic inflammatory tissue (granulation tissue + oma). Thus the distinction was useful mainly for clinicians in separating certain inflammatory processes from neoplasms. Today, however, the emphasis has been turned to microscopic differences observed within the group of chronic inflammatory lesions and no longer are the clinical or macroscopic features considered most significant in differentiating granulomatous from nongranulomatous inflammation. Those lesions which are characterized by a significant proliferation of large mononuclear cells, particularly their modified forms, the epithelioid and giant cells (see p. 11), are called granulomatous. Such lesions usually contain varying admixtures of other inflammatory cells, particularly plasma cells and lymphocytes, but the modified macrophages constitute the *sine qua non*.

Granulomatous inflammation. According to Rich (1959), we still have a very fragmentary understanding of the biologic significance of the transformation of histiocytes into epithelioid cells and giant cells. The practical reason for studying granulomas is that frequently the reaction pattern found in granulomatous lesions will suggest certain specific etiologic factors. Not infrequently, with the aid of a variety of histopathologic techniques now available, the causative agents (animate and inanimate) may be demonstrated within granulomatous lesions. This seldom is the case with nongranulomatous inflammation. Even when the granulomatous process does not suggest a definite etiology, its character may nevertheless suggest a particular diagnosis. Good examples are Boeck's sarcoidosis and sympathetic uveitis. Each of these is typified by its own almost pathognomonic, granulomatous reaction pattern even though the

precise etiology is not known in either condition. Because granulomatous inflammations so often suggest specific diagnoses, they are often termed "specific inflammations" in contrast with the "nonspecific" character of nongranulomatous types. Such glib terminology is objectionable for three reasons: (1) granulomas do not always suggest a specific diagnosis; (2) the pattern may suggest one diagnosis to one observer and other diagnoses to other observers; and (3) time may prove our impressions fallacious as we have found in the case of toxoplasmic chorioretinitis

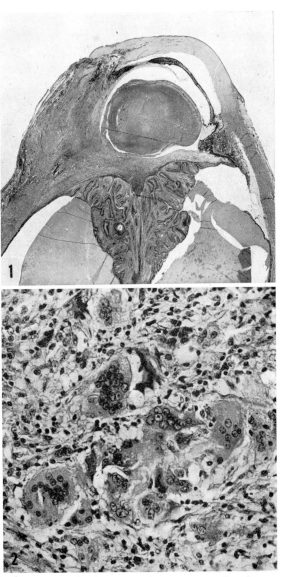

Figure 14. Diffuse granulomatous reaction due to multiple minute intraocular foreign bodies. 1. ×8. 2. ×275. AFIP Acc. 737587.

which formerly was considered a tuberculous lesion (Wilder, 1952), and as was also true in the case of so-called tuberculomas of the lung, many of which are now known to be due to histoplasmosis and coccidioidomycosis (Zimmerman, 1954).

DIFFUSE TYPE. Granulomatous inflammatory lesions may be subdivided into at least three main reaction patterns: (1) diffuse, (2) discrete or tuberculoid and (3) zonal. These, however, are frequently mixed, one portion of the tissue revealing one pattern while an-

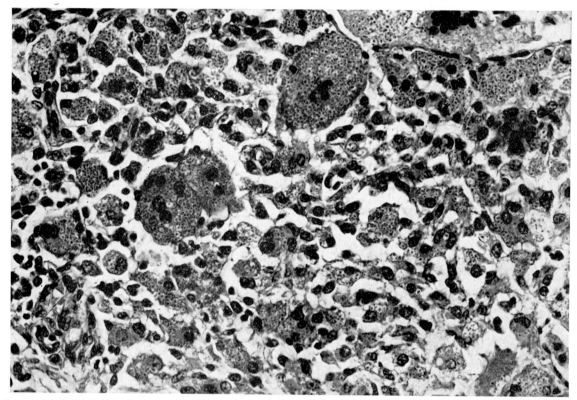

Figure 15. Diffuse granulomatous reaction pattern in histoplasmosis. There is a profuse proliferation of the fungi within the cytoplasm of macrophages and giant cells. ×500. AFIP Acc. 60841.

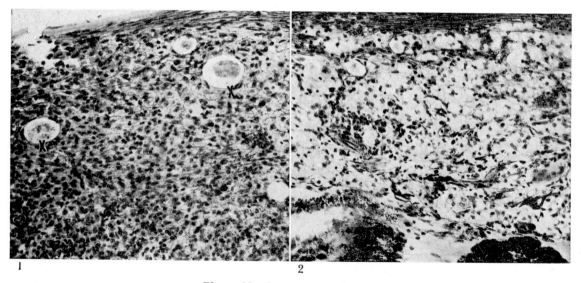

Figure 16. Lepromatous Leprosy
Diffuse proliferation of histiocytic cells including leprous giant cells called globi (x) in ciliary body. AFIP Acc. 123164.

other area exhibits a different reaction. The diffuse granulomatous reaction is characterized by a more-or-less widespread proliferation of macrophages, epithelioid cells and giant cells against a background of equally diffuse lymphocytic and plasmacytic infiltration. One may see focal accumulations of epithelioid cells but these lack the discrete delineation of true tubercles. This pattern is observed when rather fine particles of foreign

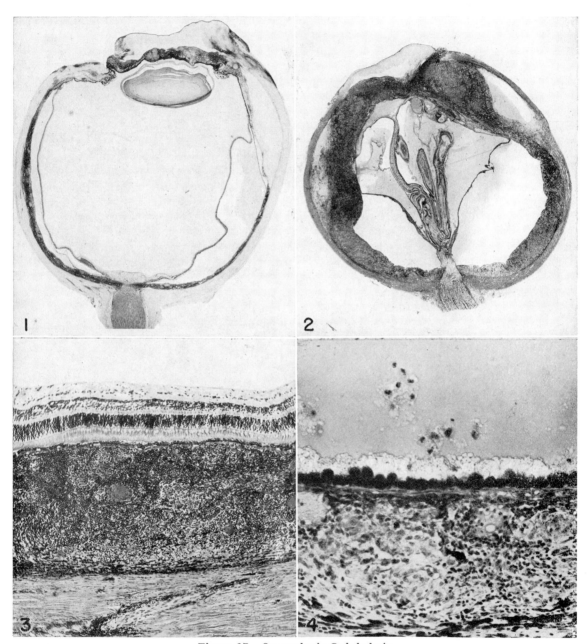

Figure 17. Sympathetic Ophthalmia

1. Penetrating wound of eye at limbus with prolapse of iris and ciliary body. Granulomatous uveitis. Serous separation of retina. ×4. AFIP Acc. 53904.

2. Penetrating wound of eye at limbus with injury to iris, ciliary body and lens. Massive granulomatous uveitis. Separation of retina. ×3. AFIP Acc. 105961.

3. Diffuse thickening of choroid by inflammatory cell infiltration. No involvement of retina. ×75. AFIP Acc. 37381.

4. Noncaseating aggregations of epithelioid cells in choroid. Diffuse lymphocytic infiltration. Choriocapillaris involved only slightly, if at all. ×75. AFIP Acc. 329514.

matter (Fig. 14) are widely scattered in the tissues. It also is observed characteristically in certain infections, e.g., disseminated histoplasmosis (Fig. 15) and lepromatous leprosy (Fig. 16), and it is typical of sympathetic uveitis (Fig. 17). In all of these examples of diffuse granulomatous inflammation necrosis is exceptional. As Selye (1953) has pointed out, granulomatous inflammation and necrosis seem to be two related but fundamentally

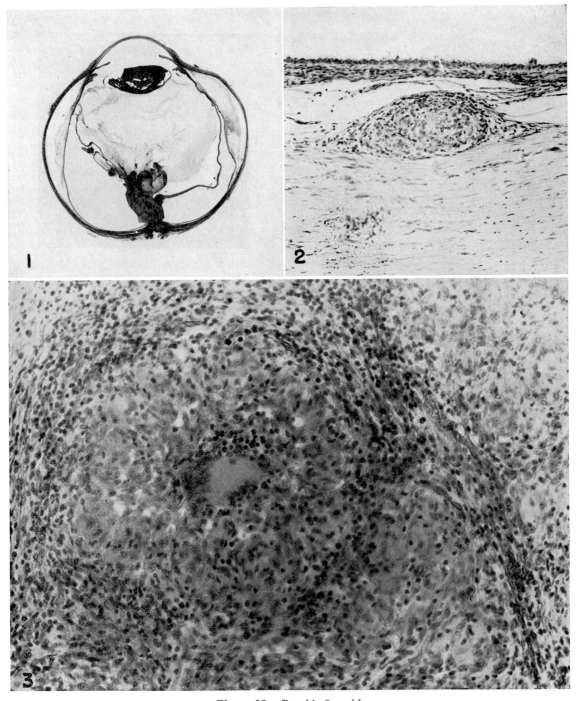

Figure 18. Boeck's Sarcoid

1. Granulomatous retinitis. Separation of retina, ciliary body and choroid. AFIP Acc. 90189.
2. Discrete nodule of epithelioid cells in choroid of same eye. ×185. AFIP Acc. 90189.
3. Epithelioid cells with central giant cell in retina of same eye. ×425. AFIP Acc. 90189.

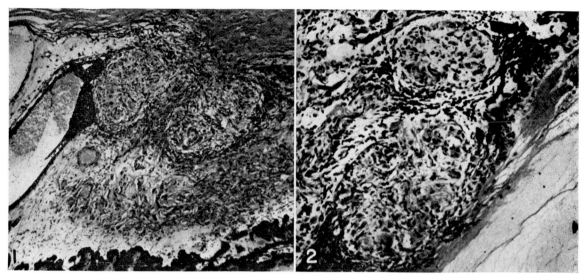

Figure 19. Tuberculosis
1. Miliary tubercles in ciliary body. ×73. AFIP Acc. 28137.
2. Miliary tubercles in vascular layer of ciliary body, breaking through into vitreous. ×175. AFIP Acc. 28137.

opposed tissue reactions. The antiphlogistic corticoids inhibit the former while stimulating the latter; the phlogistic corticoids operate in the reverse direction.

DISCRETE TYPE. Discrete or tuberculoid granulomatous lesions are characterized by the formation of compact, sharply outlined accumulations of epithelioid and giant cells, the so-called epithelioid tubercle (Figs. 18, 19). Sometimes there is a small focus of necrosis in the center of these tubercles, but characteristically these are pure cellular nodules. Many minute tubercles may become tightly packed and conglomerate. Tuberculoid granulomas often are encountered in association with the necrotizing zonal lesions to be described. Sarcoidosis, however, is the important exception for in this disease one sees only the typical non-necrotic epithelioid tubercle. In sarcoidosis the tubercles are all about the same size (Figs. 20, 21) although they may coalesce to form conglomerate masses which typically involve the iris and ciliary body (Fig. 21). Similar lesions may fill the posterior chamber, but elsewhere in the eye one usually sees only isolated epithelioid tubercles (Fig. 22).

ZONAL TYPE. Granulomatous lesions exhibiting a zonal pattern are characteristic of a number of inflammatory processes of differing etiology (Figs. 23 to 32). The center of the lesion is usually composed of more or less necrotic tissue and it is here that the causative agents are most likely to be found. Thus we may find fungi, bacteria (Fig. 23), parasites (Figs. 25, 26, 27, 32) or their eggs, masses of altered collagen (Fig. 28), lens protein (Fig. 29), or foreign bodies (Fig. 30) forming the nucleus about which the zonal reaction pattern develops. This central necrotic area which varies tremendously in size frequently contains disintegrating polymorphonuclear leukocytes. Next to the necrotic zone is a wall of palisaded epithelioid and giant cells and also macrophages which are not yet altered sufficiently to be termed epithelioid cells. Peripheral to this is a mantle of lympho-

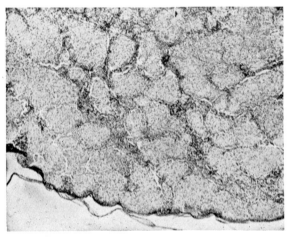

Figure 20. Sarcoidosis of Lymph Node
The tissue is almost completely replaced by discrete noncaseating epithelioid cell tubercles of relatively uniform size. ×53. AFIP Acc. 316231.

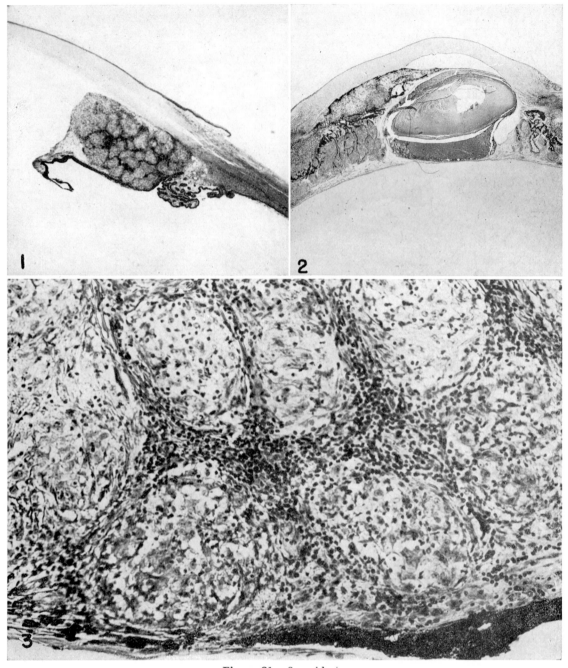

Figure 21.   Sarcoidosis
1. Involvement of iris. ×20. AFIP Acc. 71412.
2. The granulomas fill the posterior chamber. ×9. AFIP Acc. 165628.
3. Same iris shown in 1. Noncaseating, discrete aggregations of epithelioid cells, surrounded by moderate lymphocytic infiltration. ×350. AFIP Acc. 71412.

cytes and plasma cells and finally a zone of granulation tissue. In certain older lesions the granulation tissue will have been converted into an encapsulating band of collagenized connective tissue.

The typical granuloma with zonal pattern as just described is an irregularly spheroidal mass, but in certain situations this is modified by the architecture and reactivity of the affected tissues. One of the best examples is the typical segmental lesion of ocular toxoplasmosis (Figs. 25–3, 31). The retina is the seat of the infectious process. In the involved segment of the globe, the retina shows ex-

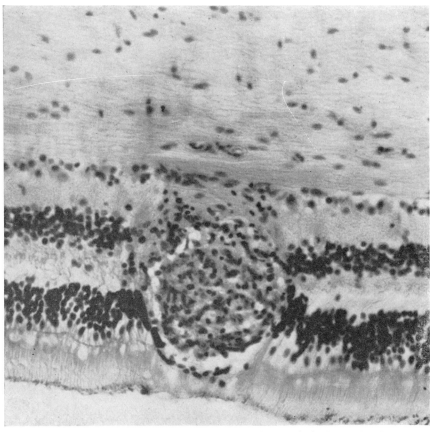

Figure 22. Epithelioid cell tubercle in retina from same case of sarcoidosis shown in Figs. 21–1 and 21–3. ✕330.

tensive coagulation necrosis and within this necrotic retinal tissue one finds the proliferative forms and cysts of the parasite (Figs. 25, 32). But in this situation, one does not see a complete spheroidal reaction pattern. Only the uveal and scleral sides react; the vitreous adjacent to the affected retina is altered, of course, but it does not respond by forming a wall of granulomatous inflammatory tissue. Thus a disk or plaque-like lesion, rather than a spheroidal mass, is formed.

Nongranulomatous chronic inflammation. Those inflammatory processes which are characterized microscopically by the proliferation of lymphocytes, plasma cells, fibroblasts, and capillaries and by the relative paucity of macrophages (especially their epithelioid and giant cell variants) commonly are termed chronic "nonspecific" or "nongranulomatous." It already has been indicated that reactions which clinically (or experimentally) are acute may be characterized microscopi-

cally by a predominantly mononuclear response. It is, therefore, entirely proper to question the common practice of labelling as "chronic" those tissue reactions characterized by a predominance of lymphocytes and plasma cells and containing few polymorphonuclears. Other signs of chronicity should be required. In the iris, for example, chronic nongranulomatous inflammation is attended by stromal atrophy, degeneration of the pigment epithelium, and proliferation of capillaries, fibroblasts, and pigment epithelium, often with the formation of dense adhesions to the cornea or lens (Figs. 33 to 36)—all of this in addition to a conspicuous infiltration of plasma cells and lymphocytes. Seldom is it possible for the pathologist to identify by ordinary histopathologic techniques the causative factors in nongranulomatous chronic inflammations. This is especially true in ophthalmic pathology where the utter futility of establishing the etiology of nongranulomatous uveitis stands in contrast to the less

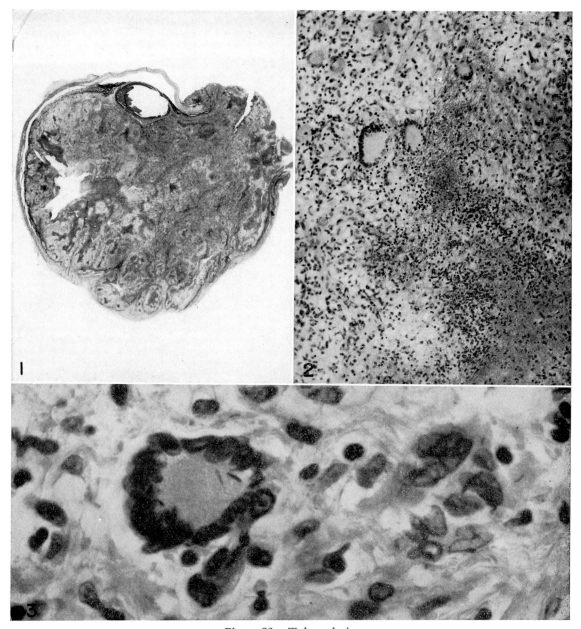

Figure 23. Tuberculosis

1. Tuberculous panophthalmitis with rupture of sclera, from 17-year-old girl with caseating pulmonary tuberculosis. Tubercle bacilli were demonstrated in eye. ×3. AFIP Acc. 84599.

2. Caseating tubercle with Langhans' giant cells, same eye. ×125. AFIP Acc. 84599.

3. Tubercle bacilli in Langhans' giant cell and in epithelioid cells (carbol-fuchsin stain). ×1000. AFIP Acc. 51026.

dismal prospects of determining the cause of granulomatous inflammations.

We should, however, anticipate success in the future, for the application of immunohistochemical procedures such as Coons' fluorescent antibody technique has provided a very promising breakthrough. By such methods it should be possible, by identification of the specific antibody being formed by these cells, ultimately to determine the reason for the intense plasmacytic activity and formation of Russell's bodies in the iris which characterize so many cases of nongranulomatous uveitis. (Continued on p. 36.)

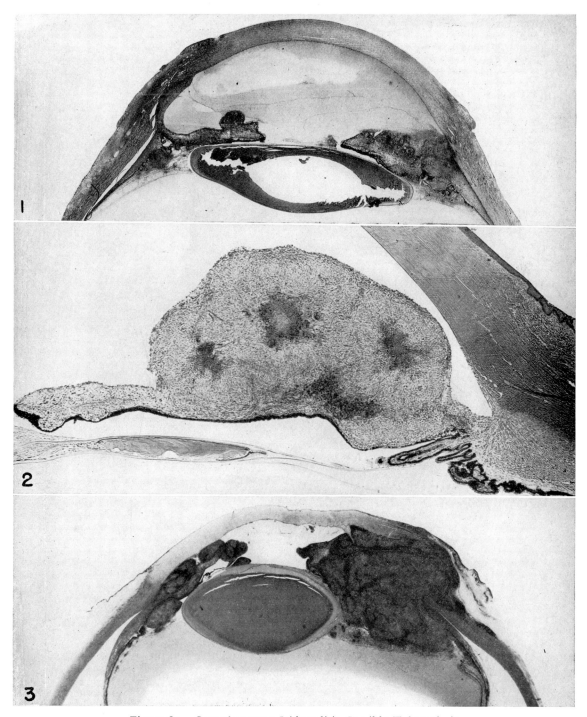

Figure 24. Granulomatous Iridocyclitis, Possibly Tuberculosis

1. Granulomatous iridocyclitis. AFIP Acc. 36877.

2. Granulomatous iritis with areas of caseation. Extension of lesion into anterior chamber. ×30. AFIP Acc. 119782.

3. Granulomatous iridocyclitis. Limbal rupture. AFIP Acc. 28896.

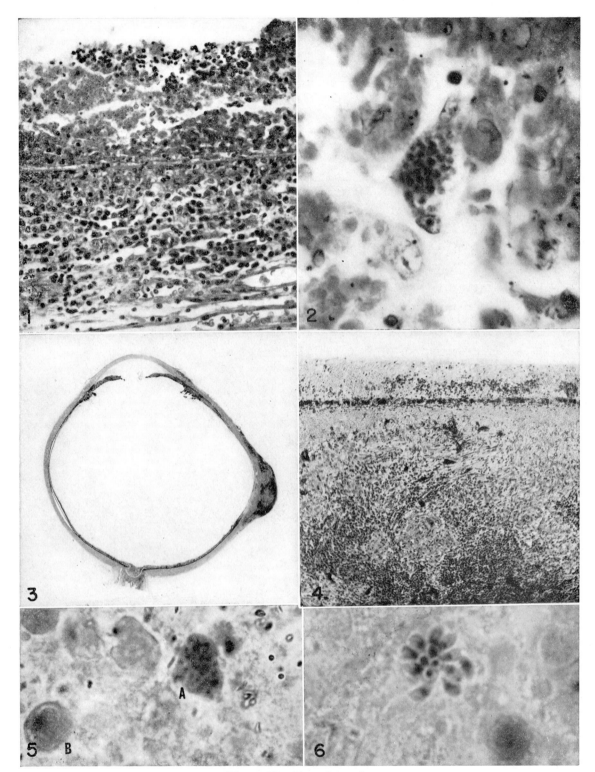

Figure 25. Toxoplasmosis

1. Chorioretinitis in an infant that died of toxoplasmosis. ×275. AFIP Acc. 197524.

2. Organisms in cyst, same eye. ×1100. AFIP Acc. 197524.

3. Granulomatous chorioretinitis and scleritis, giving rise to nodular lesion at equator, in adult without other symptoms. ×2. AFIP Acc. 70313.

4. Granulomatous choroiditis with necrosis of overlying retina, from similar case in adult. ×90. AFIP Acc. 482589.

5. Toxoplasma in cyst (A) in retina. Same eye as in Fig. 3. B, necrotic cyst. ×1260. AFIP Acc. 70313.

6. Rosette-like cluster of crescentic organisms in necrotic retina of adult. Necrotic cyst at lower margin of photomicrograph. ×1260. AFIP Acc. 165904.

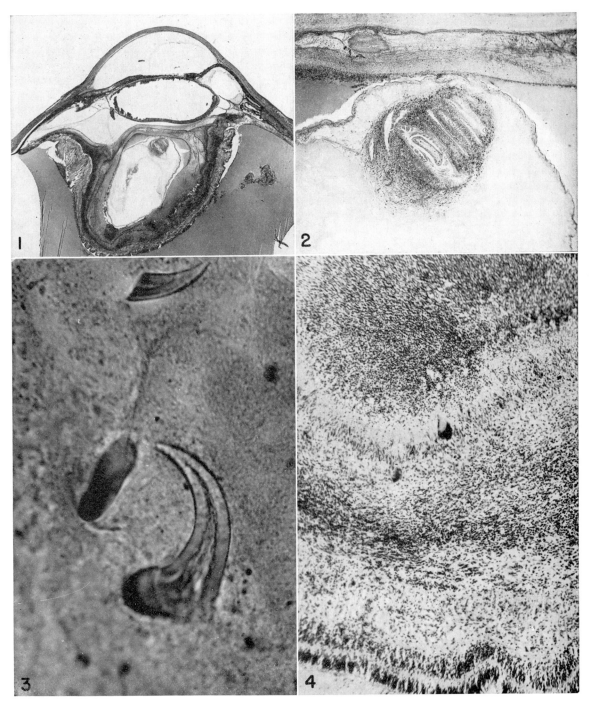

Figure 26.   Cysticercus Cellulosae (Taenia Solium), Intraocular
1. Cysticercus in vitreous chamber. ×6. AFIP Acc. 198704.
2. Cysticercus in vitreous chamber. ×48. AFIP Acc. 198704.
3. Cysticercus hooklets. AFIP Acc. 198704.
4. Abscess and granulomatous reaction around cysticercus in vitreous chamber. AFIP Acc. 198704.

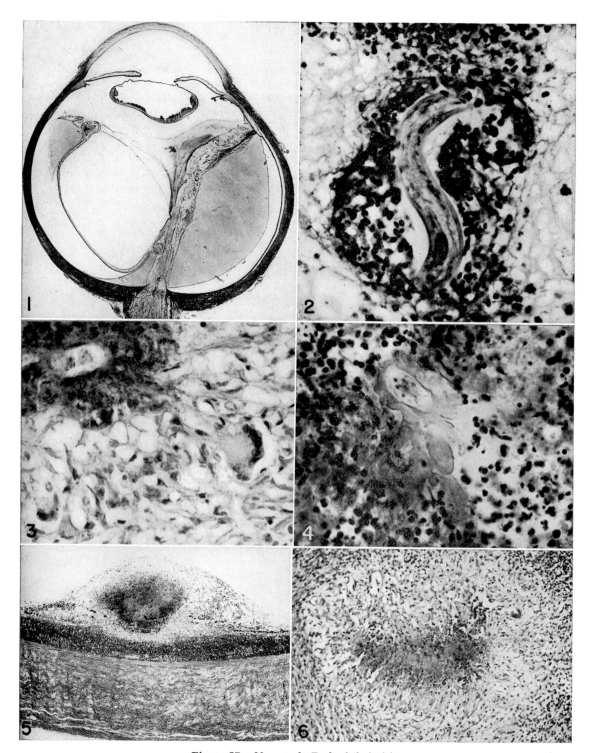

Figure 27. Nematode Endophthalmitis

1. Eosinophilic abscess containing larva in inflammatory membrane in vitreous. Retinal separation. ×4. AFIP Acc. 198761.

2. Nematode larva in eosinophilic abscess. ×220. AFIP Acc. 298563.

3. Degenerated larva in necrotic eosinophilic abscess surrounded by epithelioid and giant cells. ×400. AFIP Acc. 202593.

4. Hyaline material surrounding larva in eosinophilic abscess. ×450. AFIP Acc. 285189.

5. Necrotic eosinophilic abscess surrounded by epithelioid cells at site of entrance of larva from choroid. Lymphocytic and plasma cell infiltration of choroid. ×48. AFIP Acc. 132401.

6. Necrotic eosinophilic abscess surrounded by epithelioid cells and fibroblasts; older lesion. Hyaline fragment peripherally. ×125. AFIP Acc. 79868

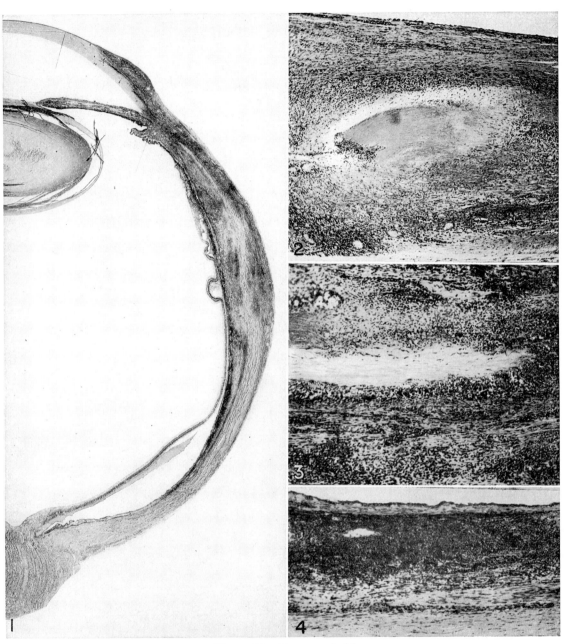

Figure 28. Brawny scleritis
1. Inflammatory thickening of anterior portion of sclera. ×5. AFIP Acc. 50814.
2. Inflammatory response to necrobiosis of collagenous fibers in sclera. ×75. AFIP Acc. 213570.
3. Granulomatous reaction to necrobiosis of scleral fibers. ×75. AFIP Acc. 50814.
4. Plasma cell infiltration of underlying choroid. ×75. AFIP Acc. 50814.

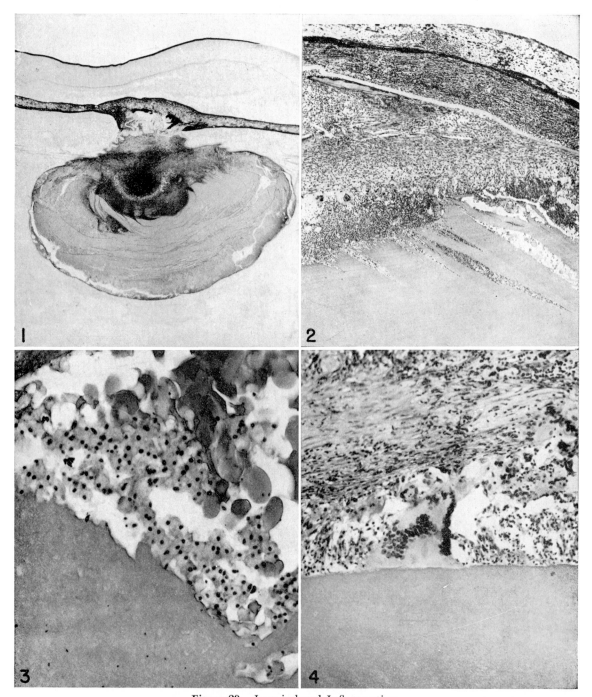

Figure 29. Lens-induced Inflammation

1. Abscess in lens following penetrating wound. ×25. AFIP Neg. 84730.

2. The lens in phaco-anaphylactic endophthalmitis. Inflammatory adhesion between iris and lens. Rupture of lens capsule. Inflammatory tissue containing mononuclear and giant cells invading lens. Deep infiltration by necrotic purulent exudate. ×48. AFIP Acc. 62572.

3. Mononuclear cells invading lens substance. Morgagnian globules. ×250. AFIP Acc. 17990.

4. Macrophage and foreign body giant cell reaction to degenerating lens substance. ×160. AFIP Acc. 62572.

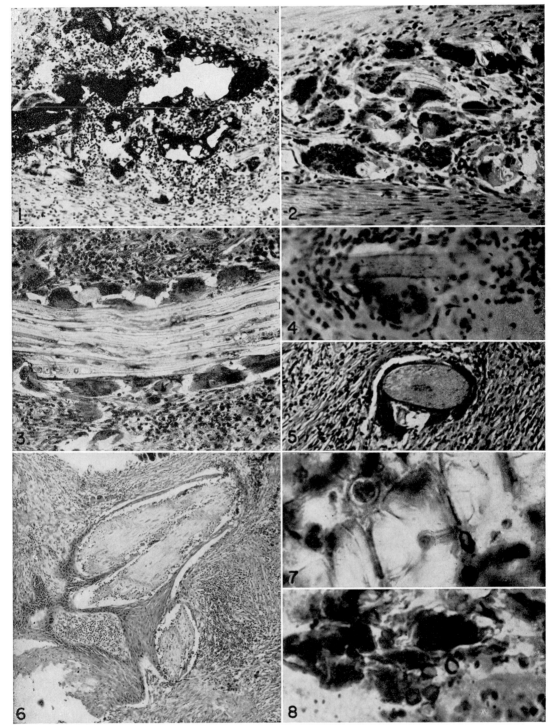

Figure 30.   Intraocular Foreign Bodies

1. Carbon particles in cyclitic membrane. Enucleation six weeks after injury. No giant cell reaction. **AFIP** Acc. 99767.

2. Marked giant cell reaction to cotton particles in cyclitic membrane of same eye. AFIP Acc. 99767.

3. Giant cell reaction to vegetable matter. ×160. AFIP Acc. 116867.

4. Giant cell reaction to cilium. Longitudinal section. ×355. AFIP Acc. 17990.

5. Giant cell reaction to cilium. Cross section. ×175. AFIP Acc. 88330.

6. Epithelial implant around thorn in inflammatory cyclitic membrane. ×50. AFIP Acc. 107052.

7. Saprophytic fungi associated with wood particle in vitreous abscess. ×1600. AFIP Acc. 96747.

8. Saprophytic yeastlike organisms associated with wood particle in vitreous abscess. ×900. AFIP Acc. **96747**

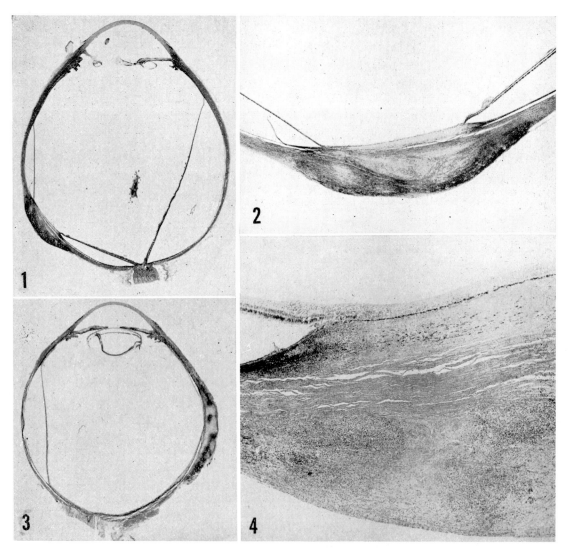

Figure 31. Toxoplasma Chorioretinitis

There is a segmental lesion characterized by complete necrosis of the retina and pigment epithelium, partial necrosis of the choroid, and granulomatous thickening of the choroid, sclera, and episclera.   1 and 2. AFIP Acc. 211318.   3. AFIP Acc. 171510.   4. AFIP Acc. 165904.

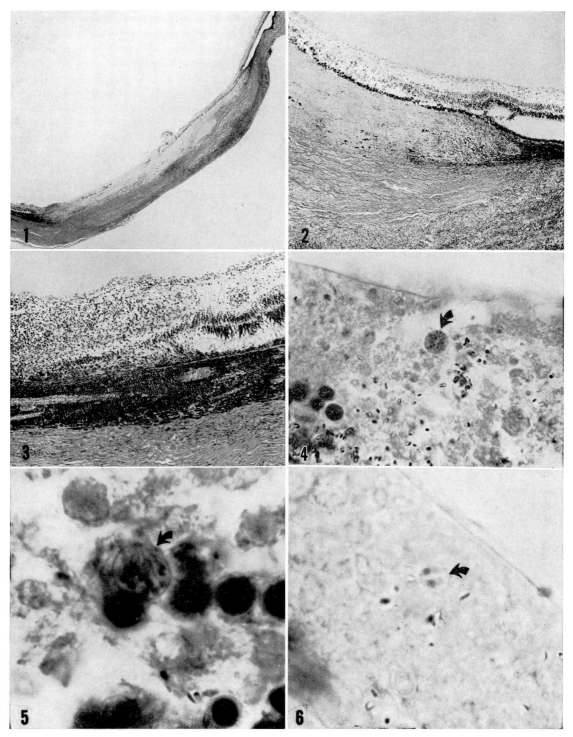

Figure 32. The first five illustrations are all from the same case of toxoplasmosis. AFIP Acc. 754058.
1, 2, and 3. The typical segmental lesion.
4 and 5. Cysts (arrows) containing multiple parasites contained in the necrotic retina.
6. Two proliferative forms (arrow) of the parasite in the necrotic retina of another case. AFIP Acc. 211318.

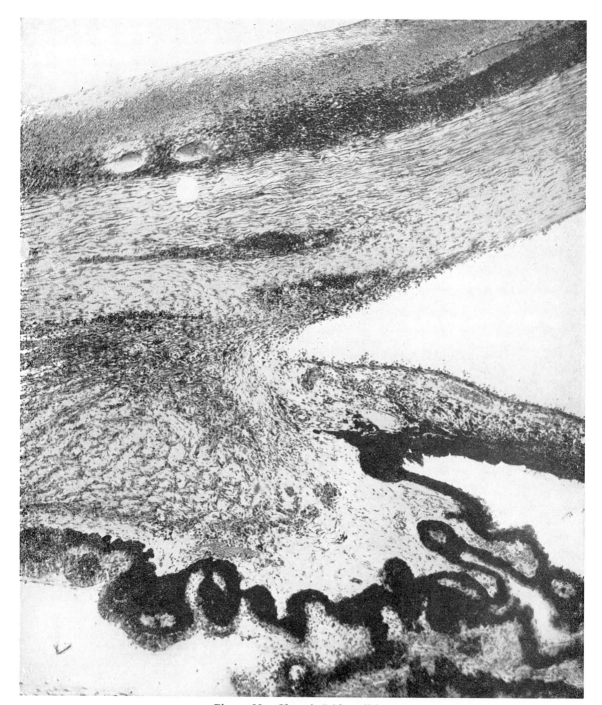

Figure 33. Chronic Iridocyclitis

Lymphocytic and plasma cell infiltration of iris, ciliary body, corneoscleral meshwork, conjunctiva and around vessels of intrascleral plexus. Chronic inflammatory cells adherent to anterior surface of iris, and ciliary epithelium. ×76. AFIP Acc. 19926.

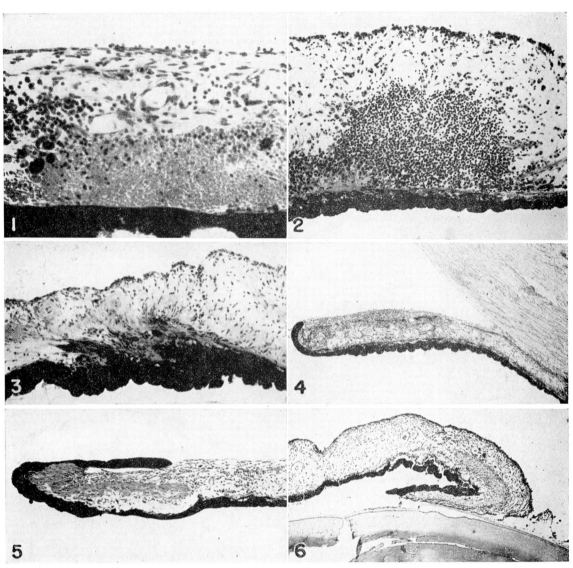

Figure 34. Chronic Iridocyclitis
1. Hemorrhage, and cells from pigment epithelium in iris stroma. ×220. AFIP Acc. 174709.
2. Chronic focal iritis. ×100. AFIP Acc. 186127.
3. Scar of chronic focal iritis. ×100. AFIP Acc. 327993.
4. Peripheral anterior synechia. Vascularization of anterior surface of iris. Early ectropion uveae. ×75. **AFIP** Acc. 309654.
5. Atrophy of iris. Marked ectropion uveae. ×75. AFIP Acc. 78871.
6. Entropion uveae. Posterior synechia. ×48. AFIP Acc. 337227.

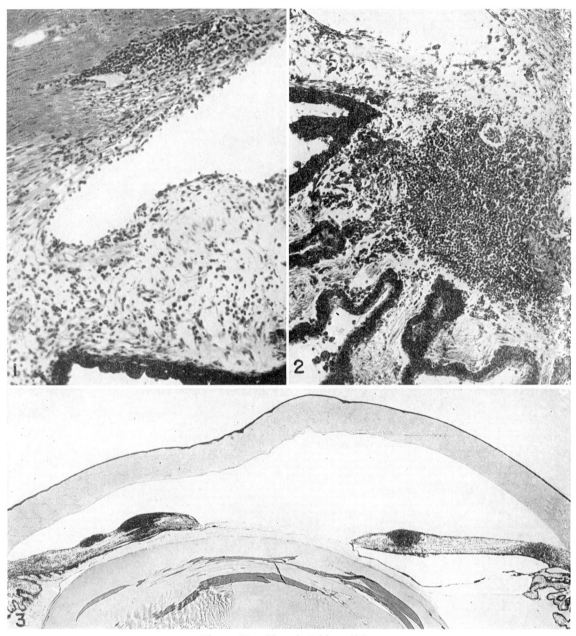

Figure 35. Chronic Iridocyclitis

1. Lymphocytic and plasma cell infiltration of iris and corneoscleral meshwork. Lymphocytes around canal of Schlemm. A few chronic inflammatory cells adhering to anterior surface of iris and to filtration angle. ×160. AFIP Acc. 86403.

2. Endogenous cyclitis, chronic. Dense lymphocytic infiltration around circulus arteriosus major (X). ×115 AFIP Acc. 29762.

3. Nodular iritis. Nodules of lymphocytes in iris bulging forward from the surface. ×15. AFIP Acc. 50983.

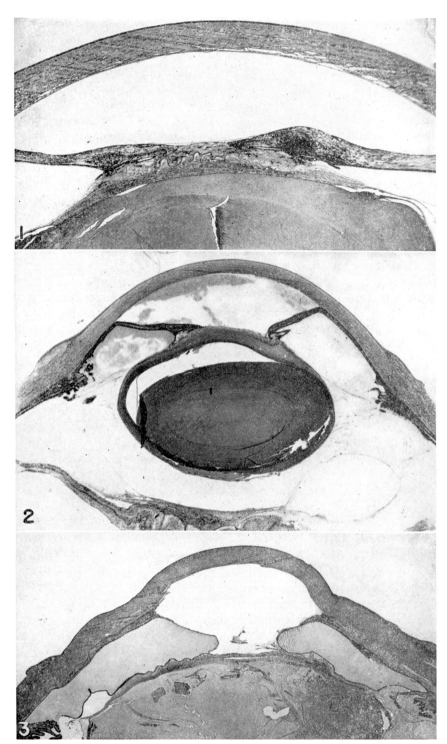

Figure 36. Chronic Iridocyclitis

1. Posterior synechia causing seclusio pupillae and inflammatory pupillary membrane causing occlusio pupillae. Anterior subcapsular cataract. ×24. AFIP Acc. 318622.

2. Iris bombé. ×15. AFIP Acc. 28381.

3. Iris bombé with cystoid serous separation of iris pigment epithelium. × 14. AFIP Acc. 122046.

INFECTION

Parasitism and Disease

At the beginning of this chapter, it was emphasized that inflammation and infection are not synonymous. Many irritants are capable of producing local inflammatory reactions which mimic those occuring at sites of inoculation of virulent bacteria. Infectious diseases, however, depend upon certain special characteristics of the infectious irritants which set them apart from inanimate irritants. In fact, not all infectious agents are injurious and certain microbes can live within the tissues, even within cells, without damaging their host. Infectious disease, therefore, is merely a part of the broader biologic phenomenon of parasitism.

The infectious agent subsists by deriving from its host nutrients required for growth and reproduction. In its pursuit of these requirements, the organism may manifest different types of behavior. Thus we have the frank predator which attacks and destroys its host, the commensal which merely survives without damaging the host, and the symbiotic agent which contributes beneficially to its host.

The first requirement of the infectious agent is that it gain entry into the host. The principal portals of entry are the natural orifices. Few organisms can actually pierce the intact skin, but the conjunctival sac, the glandular ducts, hair follicles, and wounds are potential portals of entry. It is not sufficient, however, that the organism enter the body. It must often find its way to a tissue in which there is an environment suitable for its survival.

In its effort to survive and multiply, the microbe engages its host in a biologic contest, accompanied frequently by the clinical manifestations we call "disease." If it causes injury to the host it is pathogenic. If the parasite can establish itself without damaging the host, it becomes part of the normal flora. An organism may be nonpathogenic in one site but pathogenic in another. The host has a number of specific and nonspecific mechanisms, discussed below, which it may employ to combat the invading organism. The parasite also has its own mechanisms of resistance against the attack of the host. The interplay of offensive and defensive forces of both host and parasite continue until the outcome is decided. This may consist in forcing the parasite to give up its aggressive activities or in the neutralization of its noxious products. At other times the parasite may become highly resistant to the unfavorable medium (e.g., the bacterium which "learns" to tolerate antibiotic preparations by modifying its enzyme systems). If the invading organism is not tolerated by the host, the interaction of the two may be brief eventuating in a violent acute disease, with death to one or both parties. In other instances the struggle may be prolonged, and include a series of skirmishes with intervening quiet periods, i.e., chronic disease with periodic exacerbations.

Bacteria generally tend to take up residence in specific tissue environments most suitable to their needs. In numerous instances they remain outside of the tissue cells and feed upon the secretions and excretions in the area. Some bacteria, fungi and protozoa (e.g., tubercle bacillus, Brucella, Toxoplasma and Histoplasma capsulatum) may enter the cells and maintain an intracellular residence as an important feature of the disease process. In its intracellular position, the parasite is more difficult to eradicate. It no longer behaves merely as a competitor for the general food supply but actually lives at the expense of the host cell.

The importance of the intracellular state becomes greater as one progresses downward phylogenetically. The rickettsiae and viruses are obligate intracellular parasites which can live and reproduce only in living cells. Their energy requirements are met by the diversion of the cell's metabolism to the purposes of the virus, but since all cells of the host do not furnish optimum conditions, these infectious agents frequently exhibit specific cytotropism.

Pathogenicity of Infectious Agents

The term pathogenicity as it is generally used refers to the capacity of microorganisms to cause disease. Virulence implies a measurement of pathogenicity, but this term is often used interchangeably with pathogenicity.

Infectious agents employ one or both of two main pathogenetic mechanisms: invasiveness and formation of toxins. Anthrax spores and cytotropic viruses are examples of agents which act mainly by their invasive characteristics. The Clostridia which are responsible for tetanus and gas gangrene infections are good examples of pathogenic agents which have virtually no invasiveness but which produce an extremely noxious toxin. Thus if washed tetanus spores are introduced into the normal healthy tissues of experimental animals, they fail to germinate and are engulfed and eliminated by the phagocytic cells. No disease occurs in this case. If, on the other hand, the spores are introduced into a wound, together with some agent capable of causing local tissue necrosis, germination of the spores takes place. During growth a highly poisonous and freely diffusible toxic protein, tetanus toxin, is elaborated. The bacteria themselves are present only at the original site of inoculation, but the fatal disease which follows is due to dissemination of the bacterial toxin. Many infectious agents employ both invasiveness and toxin-formation in varying proportions to produce their pathogenic effects.

Bacterial toxins are of two main types. *Exotoxins* are produced by actively growing, Gram-positive bacteria. *Endotoxins,* produced especially by Gram-negative bacteria, are intimately associated with the structural integrity of the cells and are not liberated until the bacterium has died. Bacteria also produce a number of other biologically active substances which play a role in the infectious process. Foremost among these are a group of enzymes which act either to convert normally occurring substances into toxins or else to enhance the ability of the organism to invade the tissue. *Clostridium welchii* elaborates lecithinase. Its effect is to split lecithin into a very highly hemolytic substance, lysolecithin, which lyses red blood cells and also kills other cells. Certain strains of staphylococci

produce a coagulase, which apparently causes a deposition of fibrin on the surface of the organism, thereby forming a sort of capsule which protects it from phagocytosis.

Hyaluronic acid, a viscous, polysaccharide acid of high molecular weight, is present as a constituent of the intercellular ground substance of many tissues. A great many bacteria produce enzymes which hydrolyze or depolymerize hyaluronic acid. Consequently, the ground substance becomes more fluid and bacteria and toxins diffuse throughout the tissues with greater ease.

Since viruses multiply within susceptible cells it is not surprising that they may produce rather distinctive pathologic pictures. Intracellular changes, including the formation of inclusion bodies and balloon degeneration are frequently seen in viral disease. Some viral inclusions are found only in the cytoplasm, others only in the nucleus, and still others in both locations. For example, Guarnieri's bodies of vaccinia and Negri bodies of rabies are found only in the cytoplasm. The inclusion bodies of herpes simplex and chicken pox occur only in nuclei; those of smallpox and paravaccinia are situated in both locations. Inflammation also occurs in many viral diseases and is usually characterized by the infiltration of mononuclear cells. The question of whether the inflammation is a primary or secondary phenomenon has puzzled many people.

It is often impossible, because of a complexity of tissues involved, to ascertain the nature of primary changes induced by viral infections. In some instances, however, this information is available. In vaccinal lesions of the rabbit cornea definite and characteristic changes are observed in epithelial cells before any evidence of inflammation in the form of cellular infiltrate is seen. Goodpasture found that the first evidence of injury caused by rabies virus is observed within ganglion cells and not in surrounding tissue; the infected cells may undergo complete necrosis before an inflammatory exudate forms about them.

Rivers has suggested that the primary changes produced in cells by viral infections are either proliferative or degenerative. In many viral infections, both hyperplasia and necrosis are observed. According to Rivers,

syphilis) despite the presence of viable organisms, should suddenly lose their ability to restrain the treponemas remains a profound mystery. Thus native resistance should not be considered a stable characteristic even among apparently healthy young adults.

Still other factors which influence resistance deal with the ability of the body to manufacture globulin. Patients with congenital agammaglobulinemia or hypogammaglobulinemia have such a defect and are poorly able to resist infections or respond to antigens. Such defects also may be acquired as a result of disease.

Finally, there exists a number of nonspecific blood and tissue factors which operate as mechanisms of immunity. Normal serum complement appears to play some role in the mediation of bactericidal activity by antibacterial antibodies and may, perhaps, have some protective capacity in its own right. Pillemer has recently made a discovery which contributes importantly to our knowledge of natural immunity. He described a new protein constituent of normal serum, named by him *properdin,* which apparently plays a major role as a bactericidal and antiviral agent. In conjunction with complement, the naturally occurring properdin exerts a nonspecific action leading to the destruction of certain bacteria and to the neutralization of certain viruses.

There also exists in most individuals, a set of so-called "normal antibodies" which have an affinity for certain microorganisms and enable them to combine with these organisms to lead either to their immediate death or to an intensification of normal phagocytosis. Finally, a great number of other substances and active factors have been suggested as participants in the body's defense against infection. Among these are lysozyme, a mucolytic enzyme present in tears which attacks bacterial capsules, antivasin which inactivates hyaluronidase, and many others.

Acquired Immunity

Nonspecific acquired resistance. Acquired resistance includes specific and nonspecific factors. As Selye has emphasized, there are general body reactions to stress; these he groups in the "general adaptation syndrome."

These have a general as well as a specific effect in enabling the individual to tolerate a variety of injurious agents. Thus the experimental animal that has been acclimated to a cold environment also develops increased resistance to infection. As the individual grows from infancy through childhood into adult life he is continuously being subjected to many forms of stress and presumably as a consequence of his adaptation to these, he develops increasing resistance to infection.

Specific immunity. Specific resistance to infectious agents implicates the action of immune bodies which may be produced by the individual or transferred passively. Passive transfer is mainly by the gamma globulin fraction of serum protein, but also by other substances such as colostrum. Such passively acquired immunity explains the greater resistance to infectious diseases of newborn infants as compared with older babies. Passive immunity always depends upon the active production of an immune state in another individual. This, in turn, requires contact with the infectious agent—in the form of: (a) clinical infection, (b) subclinical (unapparent) infection, or (c) artificial immunization. As a result of such specific immunity, a profound difference is observed when bacteria are introduced into the tissues. In the nonimmune animal the organisms proliferate and spread diffusely through the tissues in spite of an intense acute inflammatory response. Relatively few of the leukocytes exhibit their phagocytic potentialities. In the immune animal, the injected bacteria show little tendency to multiply and spread. They become agglutinated and adhere to tissue elements. Leukocytes become much more actively phagocytic. Such increased efficiency of phagocytosis, stimulated at least in part by the presence of specific antibodies (opsonins), can also be demonstrated in vitro. It is of the utmost importance in protecting the host, for the prompt immobilization and destruction of bacteria not only will prevent multiplication, invasion and dissemination, but also will minimize the formation of toxins. It should not be concluded, however, that all of the protection afforded by specific immunity is antibody-mediated. In tuberculosis, for example, the efficacy of BCG is not the result of any detectable circulating antibody.

Typhoid fever may not be prevented in spite of the presence of large amounts of circulating antibody against the typhoid organisms. The individual with agammaglobulinemia, incapable of developing an antibody response and thus unable to call upon these antibody-mediated mechanisms of resistance, yet may develop an immunity to certain viral diseases after once having suffered an attack by these viruses. Little is known at present about such mechanisms as "tissue immunity" which do not depend upon circulating antibody.

In summary, we may cite the contrast made by Wilson and Miles between the host-parasite relationship of normal and immune animals: "An immunized animal behaves towards a virulent strain of a particular pathogenic bacterium in the same way as a normal animal behaves towards an avirulent, or slightly virulent strain of the same bacterial species."

Effect of Therapeutic Agents

Chemotherapy, antibiotics, and hormones. Bacteriostatic agents depress the rate of microbial growth, thereby making easier the phagocytic task required of the mesenchymal cells. In order to do this it is necessary that the therapeutic agent employed reach the infectious agent in effective concentration. This may vary greatly from tissue to tissue and also may become significantly modified by the stage of infection, position of the infectious agent, and character of the tissue reaction. Intracellular parasites, for example, may be protected from antimicrobial agents present in the blood stream in concentrations that would be lethal in vitro. Likewise, the administration of adequate dosage of antibiotic might be ineffectual once the organisms have become encapsulated by a wall of dense inflammatory tissue, either because the antimicrobial can not penetrate to the organisms or because the inflammatory cells destroy or otherwise neutralize its effectiveness. Antimicrobial agents may penetrate poorly into some tissues, such as the vitreous, and therefore have little effect on the infection. Certain hormones as hydrocortisone, however, possess a remarkable ability to diffuse through sites of tissue damage and exert an inhibitory effect upon the proliferation of mesenchymal structures. According to Menkin (1953) not only do these hormones affect the local cellular reaction but they also inhibit other important reactions to injury such as antibody formation, though these, too, undoubtedly operate at the level of the mesenchymal cell. It has been demonstrated repeatedly that hyperconcentrations of cortisone and related antiphlogistic compounds lower the resistance of tissues to infectious agents while at the same time they potentiate the necrotizing effects of the organisms (Jasmin and Robert). An excellent clinical example of this has been the increasing number of perforated corneal ulcers produced by such relatively avirulent fungi as species of Aspergillus and Cephalosporium since the advent of widespread use of corticosteroids by ophthalmologists (Ley and Sanders; Haggerty and Zimmerman). Ley and Sanders have shown the enhanced pathogenicity of fungi inoculated into the cornea of cortisone-treated rabbits as compared with untreated controls.

Immunity vs. Hypersensitivity

The formation of immune bodies in response to an infection is beneficial since it may enable the host to combat the infection and to develop resistance to subsequent infections by the same agent. Immune body production, however, is such a general biologic phenomenon that many antigenic substances other than infectious agents are equally capable of initiating the process. Killed microorganisms, certain chemical constituents of these bacteria, and even such harmless substances as egg albumin stimulate the immune process. Thus not all immune bodies (i.e., antibodies) are concerned with protection against infection. The "pseudodefense" which the host elaborates in response to noninfectious substances may set up a sequence of reactions which are actually harmful to the host. The same immune mechanisms which may enable an animal to survive a severe infection and to protect itself from a second attack may also cause that animal to develop serum sickness, hay fever, urticaria, or die in anaphylactic shock. Collectively, the various immune reactions which are not beneficial to the individual are called hypersensitivity reactions. The different forms of hypersensitivity will be discussed in some detail later in this chapter.

Antigens

Any substance which stimulates formation of immune bodies (i.e., antibodies) upon parenteral introduction may be called an antigen. Most strong antigens are proteins, ranging from rather simple compounds such as egg albumin and diphtheria toxin to immunochemically complex living agents. The latter are characterized by a complex mosaic of antigenic determinants located upon their surfaces and often a complex of antigens located within the cells. Therefore, microorganisms may stimulate production of antibodies against a large number of different antigenic constituents. For example, Salmonella infections give rise to antibodies against somatic, flagellar and Vi antigens.

There seem to be no absolute criteria by which one can judge whether or not a substance is likely to be antigenic. It is believed that complex substances of relatively high molecular weight are required to serve as true antigens. In general, antigens must be foreign to the recipient in order to function immunologically. The more genetically dissimilar, the more antigenic a protein will be. However, differences in relative antigenicity exist among proteins from the same species. Horse hemoglobin, for example, is a weak antigen for rabbits although horse serum albumin is a strong antigen in the rabbit. There are instances in which proteins of the animal's own body can stimulate antibody production. A classical example of this is provided by the crystalline lens, the proteins of which may be autoantigenic. More recently, one or more components of thyroid, testis, nervous tissue, and erythrocytes have been shown capable of inducing an autoimmune response.

Burnet has postulated that common to all reactions of the body to foreign substances is a remarkable ability of the tissues to distinguish between "self" and "nonself." The process of cataloguing indigenous vs. foreign antigens is assumed to take place sometime during fetal development. Only after this cataloguing has taken place and the animal has developed immunologic competence will introduction of a foreign antigen allow the animal to recognize it as "nonself" and thus react to it by forming specific antibodies. Burnet's theory provides some insight as to the mechanism of autosensitization against such antigens as lens protein. Embryologically the lens protein becomes isolated from the rest of the body by the lens capsule at an exceptionally early period, long before the fetus has begun to catalogue its own antigens. Thus it never has an opportunity to recognize its own lens protein as "self." If, then, at a later date the lens capsule is ruptured and there is release of lens proteins into the circulation, the animal may react by forming antibodies. It is such a sequence of events that is believed to be responsible for the occurrence of certain cases of lens-induced uveitis, hence the term phaco-anaphylactic endophthalmitis. Fortunately, lens proteins are only weakly antigenic and the incidence of clinically significant autosensitization is much smaller than might be anticipated from the frequency of injury to the lens.

There are a number of substances called haptenes which have only limited immunologic activity. Landsteiner classified antigenic substances as (1) simple haptenes which will combine with specific antibodies but which will neither form a precipitate in vitro nor stimulate antibody production in vivo; (2) complex haptenes which will combine with specific antibodies and form a precipitate in vitro but which are unable to stimulate antibody production in vivo; (3) complete antigens which will combine with specific antibodies to form a precipitate in vitro and which may serve to stimulate antibody production in vivo. Some drugs and simple chemicals which demonstrate immunologic activity, such as atropine, sulfonamides and dinitrochlorobenzine are examples of simple haptenes. Typical of the complex haptenes are the polysaccharides of many bacteria, e.g., the pneumococcal polysaccharides. In purified form these are unable to stimulate antibody production but will react with the specific antibody. Examples of complete antigens are the proteins found in serum, tissues, and bacteria.

Antibodies

Antibodies are serum proteins which have been formed in such a way that they react selectively with the antigens that induced their formation. Biophysical analysis of antibody-containing sera have established the fact that antibodies are indistinguishable from certain "normal" serum globulins except for their immunologic specificity. Most antibodies have been found to be gamma globulins, but beta and alpha globulins possessing antibody activity also have been recognized.

The antibodies which are produced during a response to an antigenic stimulus are generally capable of reacting only with the stimulating antigen or a very closely related substance. A very high degree of specificity is a prerequisite for assigning an immunologic basis to a given reaction. Immunologic specificity is so great that antibodies may distinguish proteins of different species and different proteins of the same species. There is, however, a limit to the astonishing precision of serologic specificity when homologous proteins or carbohydrates of related species are used. For example, rabbit antibodies against beef lens will also precipitate antigens prepared from lenses of other animals. Rarely, antibodies may react with substances of quite a different biologic origin. Use of such a cross-reaction is made in the Weil-Felix test for typhus. Patients with this rickettsial disease develop high titers of agglutinins against certain strains of Bacillus proteus.

The reaction between antibody and antigen is chemical. However, depending upon the environment in which the antigen-antibody reaction is carried out there may be observed a great variety of secondary effects. At first sight it might appear that different substances were reacting to produce each of the observable phenomena. The primary immunologic reaction is believed to be the chemical interaction of antigen with antibody. Once this interaction has taken place, the presence of an ancillary substance or the nature of the antigen itself will modify the subsequent course of the reaction leading to seemingly different serologic phenomena. In saline solution the interaction of many soluble antigens with their specific antibodies will lead to precipitation of the antigen-antibody complex. If the antigen is a red blood cell or a bacterium, then the visible effect may be one of agglutination. Should complement be present in these latter tests, the observable effects might be hemolysis or bacteriolysis. In the case of certain toxic or infectious antigens the observable effect of the interaction of these with their specific antibodies might be the neutralization of their respective biologic activities. At one time it was thought that distinctive antibodies were involved in the several immunologic reactions such as precipitation, agglutination, opsonic activity, lysis, etc., but the unitarian hypothesis of Zinsser is now quite generally accepted.

There are antibodies produced in certain situations which do not exhibit the entirely characteristic behavior of ordinary antibodies. Relatively little is known about these special types of antibodies. Among them are the atopic antibodies (reagins) associated with asthma, hay fever, and angioneurotic edema. Such antibodies are "atypical," in fact they do not precipitate with their homologous antigens even though they do react with their respective antigens to produce the typical sequence of events leading to clinical disease. Another unusual antibody is found in erythroblastosis fetalis, in which case the mother produces an "incomplete" antibody. This antibody is incapable of producing agglutination of Rh positive cells in saline solution, but upon transplacental passage will interact with and damage erythrocytes of the fetus. In certain blood dyscrasias the antibodies elaborated by the patient possess the peculiar ability of reacting with their antigenic substrates, usually erythrocytes, only at low temperatures; these are termed "cold agglutinins" or "cold hemolysins."

An appreciation of the mechanisms by which antibodies are produced together with a knowledge of the sites where this production takes place are fundamental to a study of the pathogenesis of immunogenic inflammatory conditions. It was once thought that the cells responsible for the removal of antigen from the circulation were also primarily concerned in the production of specific antibodies. Using antigens labeled with colored dyes or with radioactivity, careful studies have been made on the localization of these substances after injection into the animal. A more precise technique has been devised by Coons and his associates for localization of injected antigenic materials. This technique takes advantage of the fact that antibodies, being proteins, may be labeled chemically with fluorescent dyes. The fluorescein-labeled antibodies may then be used as specific immunohistochemical stains for the respective antigens. The distribution of antigen injected into an animal may be studied by treating fresh frozen sections of the tissues with the fluorescein-labeled antibody specific for the the antigen injected. The labeled antibody will interact, even intracellularly, with its antigen wherever the latter has localized. Then, after washing the section free of excess labeled antibody, the section may be mounted in glycerin and examined with the ultraviolet microscope. Wherever antigen was present, the labeled antibody will have reacted and become fixed. By virtue of the very intense fluorescence of the dye label upon ultraviolet excitation, the antigen may be visualized in a highly specific and extremely sensitive manner.

Using these techniques, it has been found that injected antigen is cleared quite rapidly from the circulation, principally by the phagocytic cells of the reticuloendothelial system. The Kupffer cells of the liver, the sinusoidal cells in the bone marrow, and phagocytic cells in the spleen and regional lymph nodes take up large amounts of the antigen. In these cells the antigen is degraded and metabolized, rapidly for proteins, often quite slowly for some polysaccharides. These phagocytic cells probably play only a supporting role in antibody synthesis. They seem to break down antigenic proteins into smaller units to which the antibody-producing cells may then be able to respond.

Coons and co-workers have developed a modification of their fluorescent antibody technique whereby not only antigen, but also antibody may be stained specifically in tissue sections. This notable advance has made it possible for the first time to definitely identify some of the cells responsible for antibody production. Antibody has been visualized in the immature and mature plasma cells generally found in the spleen, the regional lymph nodes and around the periphery of granulomas after antigenic stimulation. This demonstration of antibody in immature plasma cells, together with much circumstantial evidence, has convinced most investigators that the plasma cell is the principal source of antibodies. Significantly, the individual with hypogammaglobulinemia who is able to produce little or no antibody is also unable to elaborate plasma cells.

Most of the study of antibody production has been concerned with the response of the whole body to antigenic stimulation. It must be emphasized, however, that such antibody production is not restricted to the lymph nodes and spleen but may occur locally within a single organ. This is, perhaps, especially significant in ophthalmic pathology because of the conspicuous plasma cell infiltration that may be seen in nongranulomatous uveitis. It has been shown that in response to intravitreal injection of antigen in the rabbit there develops within a week to ten days a remarkable plasmacytosis in the iris and ciliary body and about the retinal blood vessels. These observations are indicative of local production of antibody within the eye. Indeed Witmer has demonstrated a higher titer of antibody in the aqueous of the horse infected with leptospirosis than in its serum, suggesting local antibody production. Similarly, O'Connor has demonstrated higher titers of antibody in the aqueous of patients with ocular toxoplasmosis than was found in their sera. The role of local ocular antibody production and its relationship to ocular hypersensitivity mechanisms is discussed on pages 47 and 48.

One of the characteristic features of an immunologic response is the lag period of five to ten days between injection of an antigen and the appearance of antibodies. This represents the time required by the body to mobilize its antibody-forming mechanism. Once the antibody-producing cells have been stimulated, antibody is released into the blood stream. Antibody production may then proceed for variable periods of time, depending on the nature and duration of the antigenic stimulus. When the same or a closely related antigenic substance is introduced into the body at a later date, there is often a characteristic fall in the antibody titer (negative phase) for several days, and then a marked rise in the antibody content of the blood to even higher levels than before. The response of the body to an antigen to which it had previously responded is called the anamnestic reaction. It is typical of such secondary responses that antibody is produced much more rapidly and in greater amounts than after the initial antigenic stimulus. Repeated injections of the same antigen will, if suitably timed, provoke increasing production of antibodies until a peak is reached.

In most tissues the earliest response to both primary and secondary challenge is a proliferation of immature mononuclear cells. The histologic picture then changes into one which the pathologist has customarily called nonspecific chronic inflammation, character-ized by the presence of immature and mature plasma cells along with other mononuclear cells.

The mechanisms by which the antibody may mediate immunity include: (a) neutralization of toxins and other biologic products of infectious agents; (b) cytotoxic and other direct effects upon various microorganisms; (c) potentiation of the normal phagocytic powers of polymorphonuclear leukocytes; and (d) production of inflammatory exudates as a consequence of antigen-antibody interaction in various hypersensitivity states. These mechanisms may play a role (along with delayed hypersensitivity mechanisms) in inciting granuloma formation and the setting up of physical barriers to wall off the infectious process.

HYPERSENSITIVITY

Introduction

It is generally assumed that immunologic mechanisms are protective and therefore beneficial. It is necessary, however, to introduce an extension of the word "immune" to cover such situations as the immunologic response to substances like egg albumin. Although egg albumin is not inherently toxic for the normal guinea pig, the animal does respond to it, just as it would respond to a bacterial toxin, with the production of antibody. This serves no useful protective purpose. Indeed, quite the opposite; an animal which has been injected with such a harmless protein may become so highly susceptible to a subsequent injection of this protein that it may die soon after injection. Such an altered reactivity induced by antigenic stimuli is called a hypersensitivity state. The manifestations of hypersensitivity are so protean that antigenic insults may lead to many different clinical syndromes.

Many confusing terms are encountered in the literature relating to hypersensitivity. The problem is covered well by Rich who points out that the term allergy and its derivatives hypoergy (reduced reactivity), anergy (lack of reactivity), and hyperergy (heightened reactivity) have been robbed of their potential value by the indiscriminate way in which they have been employed. It is easier to drop these particular terms from our vocabulary than it is to define and use them in a consistent and meaningful way.

A great variety of antigenic substances may sensitize an animal and initiate an immunogenic inflammatory response. For convenience, such materials are called allergens.

The term hypersensitivity implies that the processes under discussion are immunogenic in nature, i.e., that they generally satisfy certain requirements: (1) previous exposure to the allergen (or passive transfer from a donor so exposed); (2) an induction period (usually about five days to two weeks) before the response may be elicited; and (3) initiation of the response only upon subsequent exposure to the same or a closely related allergen. Additional characteristics include the ability to passively transfer the hypersensitivity state from the sensitive individual to a normal recipient either by the transfer of serum or by certain cell suspensions, and the ability to desensitize, to some extent at least, the hypersensitive individual.

Just as it is impossible to discuss resistance to infectious agents without considering the nature of the agent itself, the way in which it enters the body, and the type of reaction which it provokes, so it is necessary in discussing hypersensitivity states to consider the nature of the allergen, the way in which it is introduced, and the clinical and histologic appearance of the resulting lesion. By so doing, it has been found that hypersensitivity reactions are separable into two main types, the *immediate* and *delayed*. These adjectives refer to the time required for the clinical appearance of an inflammatory response to an antigen, which is injected into the skin. These terms, while not entirely satisfactory, are so widely employed that we must, for the present, live with them; but it must always be realized that they imply nothing about basic pathogenetic mechanisms, and occasionally they are actually misleading for they do not accurately indicate the temporal sequence of events. It may be more advantageous in the present discussion to define the several hypersensitivity states in terms of pathogenetic factors, indicating as we proceed their main differences and similarities.

Immediate Hypersensitivity

At the beginning of the century, Portier and Richet reported their observations on a curious phenomenon which seemed opposite to that of prophylaxis. They found that dogs which had survived an initial injection of highly toxic derivatives of sea anemones, instead of becoming protected against a subsequent dose, were actually thrown into a state of profound and lethal shock. This phenomenon they termed *anaphylaxis*. In this condition specific antibodies are usually demonstrable in the circulation and they may be transferred passively to normal individuals with the induction of a temporary state of hypersensitivity. Only small amounts of antigen are required to evoke profound reactions in the host; these reactions are characterized by spasmodic contraction of smooth muscle. The organ systems exhibiting the most marked response vary with the animal species being tested, e.g., the bronchopulmonary in the guinea pig, the liver and gastrointestinal tract in the dog. Doses of antigen insufficient to kill the animal with anaphylactic shock may, nevertheless, produce symptoms of serum sickness with generalized urticaria. The intracutaneous analogue of generalized anaphylaxis is the typical "wheal and erythema" reaction. Intracutaneous administration of

antigen leads to a series of events resembling those which follow the injection of histamine. First, there is a flare, a local reddening at the injection site produced by an axon reflex vasodilatation. The capillaries become more permeable, leaking fluid into the tissue and producing a wheal.

Subsequent investigations have shown that a number of clinical syndromes are related pathogenetically to anaphylaxis: *urticaria, angioneurotic edema, hayfever,* and *asthma*. It does not seem to be useful to separate completely atopic allergic reactions in man from the foregoing, although there are some superficial differences such as genetic predisposition and peculiarities of the antibody (called reagin). The clinical, physiologic and histopathologic features are almost identical with those observed in the rest of this group and, therefore, it seems reasonable to treat them together.

The conditions classed as immediate hypersensitivity are grouped together on the basis of a number of convincing similarities in mechanism and sequence of events. First (and the reason for the term immediate hypersensitivity), the reaction in the sensitized subject usually appears in from seconds to minutes after challenge with the offending allergen, runs a fairly rapid course, and then quickly subsides. More important, however, they all seem to be related to the initial interaction of antigen with some type of circulating antibody. The reaction between antigen and antibody may take place in the blood or on tissue cells. The pathogenesis of the lesion is not completely understood but it is generally thought that the antigen-antibody reaction (perhaps mediated by complement) leads to the most significant event, damage to certain types of cells with the subsequent liberation from them of pharmacologically active substances such as histamine, serotonin, heparin and perhaps others. The symptomatology associated with this group of conditions is produced by the action of these pharmacologic agents on certain shock organs.

In further support of the pathogenetic unity of these immediate hypersensitivity reactions, it may be pointed out that: (1) histamine can reproduce most of the symptoms and antihistamines can protect against most of them; (2) the hypersensitivity state usually can be transferred passively to normal individuals by means of serum containing specific antibody; (3) both precipitating and non-precipitating antibodies can mediate these responses; (4) the reactions will not take place using antigen-antibody systems which do not fix complement; (5) the very small amounts of antigen generally required for local immediate hypersensitivity reaction do not mediate such reactions in the normal avascular cornea but will do so if the cornea has been vascularized by a previous disease or injury (Rich and Follis).

The cornea can, however, be used both for sensitization and challenge. Long ago Wessely demonstrated that intracorneal injection of protein antigens into the normal rabbit will produce a keratitis after a lag of some 12 to 14 days. The "Wessely phenomenon" was studied further by von Szily who showed that after intracorneal injection of antigen, re-injection of the same antigen into the cornea gives rise to a recurrence of the keratitis. Even an intravenous injection of the same antigen provokes a recurrence of the keratitis, but only in the eye previously injected. More recently, Germuth, Maumenee, and co-workers have obtained similar results with passively sensitized rabbits. These investigators have provided an even more convincing demonstration of the effect of antigen-antibody interaction in the cornea by injecting one side of the corneal stroma with antigen and the other side with antibody. When this is done the injected proteins diffuse through the corneal stroma toward one another. Where they meet, there develops a line of antigen-antibody precipitate similar to that obtained by the Ouchterlony agar diffusion analysis of antigens and antibodies. Microscopically, this zone of antigen-antibody reaction shows damage to the corneal cells and an intense infiltration by inflammatory cells. These investigations indicate that antigen-antibody mediated inflammation can occur in the avascular cornea, and they show that this antigen-antibody interaction damages the parenchymal cells. These observations must be reconciled with the older belief, expressed by Rich and Follis, that the cornea must be vascularized to support an immediate hypersensitivity reaction. It may be simply a matter of concentration of antigen and antibody. If the concentration of circulating antibody, for example, is very low, there may be insufficient diffusion from the limbal vessels to support a reaction with small doses of antigen injected into the clear cornea. If the cornea is vascularized, small concentrations of circulating antibody can diffuse into the corneal stroma more readily.

Nongranulomatous uveitis has also been produced repeatedly in the past by similar methods. Starting with the work of Sattler at the beginning of this century, an extensive literature has developed on the experimental production of inflammation of the uveal tract by immunologic methods. This recently has been reviewed in a monograph by Foss. In brief, the most noteworthy points are: (1) intravitreal or anterior chamber challenge with homologous antigen of a parenterally sensitized animal provokes an immediate ocular hypersensitivity reaction; (2) injection of antigen into the vitreous of a normal rabbit will give rise to a spontaneous inflammatory reaction in the inoculated eye after seven to ten days but a similar response is not obtained when antigen is injected only in the anterior chamber; (3) after having once received intraocular antigen, the injected eye will generally be more highly sensitized than the rest of the body and will respond to antigenic challenge with an immunogenic uveitis for long periods thereafter. Seegal and Seegal and others have shown that subcutaneous injections, or even ingestion of the allergen and its absorption through the gastrointestinal mucosa, may produce a uveitis in the previously sensitized eye. The implications of this work with respect to recurrent nongranulomatous uveitis in man is obvious.

Such experimental inflammations of the uvea are similar clinically and pathologically to those observed in human nongranulomatous uveitis. Acute inflammations characterized almost entirely by polymorphonuclear cell infiltration are encountered in the passive ocular Arthus reaction; this resolves into the plasmacytic-lymphocytic picture characteristic of "chronic inflammation." Severe iridocyclitis, characterized from the start by a round cell infiltrate consisting mainly of lymphocytes and monocytes, which gradually evolves into a predominantly plasmacytic reaction, is also observed. In view of the demonstration of the plasma cell as an active producer of antibody, it is not surprising that this cell type is found following stimulation with antigen. Since in human nongranulomatous uveitis, plasma cells are characteristically present and often the principal cell type in the iris and ciliary body, one must on this basis, if on no other, consider the possibility of a pathogenetic mechanism involving immediate hypersensitivity as contributing to nongranulomatous uveitis in man.

The Arthus Phenomenon

It was found by Arthus and Breton that if an animal were to receive, instead of a single injection of antigen, repeated injections of the same antigen at intervals of several days, an exaggerated cutaneous re-activity would result. Instead of the rapidly subsiding wheal and erythema characteristic of local cutaneous anaphylaxis, the Arthus reaction proceeds to hemorrhagic necrosis at the injection site. Since the reaction commences within a very short time after antigenic challenge and since circulating antibody has been shown to play a role in the response, the Arthus phenomenon usually is classed as an immediate hypersensitivity reaction. More recent work, however, has shown that the Arthus reaction is not identical with the wheal and erythema or the generalized anaphylactic response, nor with those allergies of man called atopy.

The main event in the Arthus phenomenon seems to be the interaction of large amounts of antigen and antibody to form immune precipitates which, in the presence of blood vessels, lead to cell clumping, thrombosis, damage to vascular endothelium, hemorrhage and necrosis. Infiltration by polymorphonuclear leukocytes is a conspicuous feature. The Arthus reaction differs from cutaneous anaphylaxis also in that: (1) histamine does not duplicate the response and antihistaminics are ineffective for protection; (2) precipitating antibody is required; (3) the amount of antibody required for the Arthus response is about 1000 times that needed for anaphylactic responses; and (4) complement fixing antibodies are apparently not required as they appear to be in anaphylactic reactions.

Delayed Hypersensitivity

There exist two groups of conditions which are classified together as delayed hypersensitivity responses, since they have much in common. These are the bacterial or tuberculin-type reactions and contact dermatitis (of which poison ivy is the prototype). Here we seem to be dealing with a pathogenetic mechanism completely different from those responsible for immediate hypersensitivity and the Arthus phenomenon. They are distinct, not only because the cutaneous reaction to antigen develops much later than in immediate hypersensitivity, reaching a maximum only after 24 to 72 hours, but for other more compelling reasons. In the tuberculin-type skin reaction, the inflammatory response is less vascular and edematous, consisting of an infiltration primarily by mononuclear cells, but not including plasma cells. Clinically, these responses are characterized by firm induration rather than by the wheal and flare characteristic of the immediate hypersensitivity reaction. It was once thought that all parenchymal cells of the delayed hypersensitive individual were sensitive to antigenic insult, but more recently the cells of the mononuclear series have been implicated as the seat of delayed hypersensitivity.

Delayed hypersensitivity was originally observed in tuberculosis, and was subsequently found to be characteristic of many other infectious processes caused by viruses and fungi as well as bacteria. For this reason it is also called allergy of infection or microbial allergy. Raffel has demonstrated that certain waxy fractions of mycobacteria modify the antigenic effect of bland proteins which ordinarily evoke an immediate hypersensitivity response. Thus when egg albumin is administered with such waxy adjuvants a delayed hypersensitivity state is obtained. More recently, Uhr and co-workers and Salvin have found that the intradermal injection of antigen-antibody aggregates, or even of minute amounts of simple proteins themselves, may induce a transient state of delayed hypersensitivity. Subsequently the immediate hypersensitivity state supervenes and either replaces or obscures the initial state of delayed hypersensitivity.

The hypersensitivity responsible for contact dermatitis appears to be identical with microbiologic forms of delayed hypersensitivity, except that the cytotoxicity appears to be restricted to the skin.

The term "drug allergy" should not be used synonymously with contact dermatitis for there are other types, for example atopic hypersensitivity, which are based on immediate hypersensitivity.

Characteristically the delayed hypersensitivity reactions to chemicals and drugs, called *contact dermatitis*, involve sensitization and subsequent insult through the skin. Once sensitization has been effected, the subsequent hypersensitivity is not limited to the original site of contact, but rather is generalized over the entire skin surface. The lesions are predominantly in the epidermis, but with perivascular accumulations of lymphocytes in the dermis. The causative agents are not antigens in the strict sense, but are haptenes in that they induce their effects by combination with certain of the tissue proteins of the host. These "conjugated antigens" then serve to sensitize the individual and at a later time to stimulate the hypersensitivity response. It has been postulated that only certain proteins of the skin are capable of combining with the active drug to form the antigen required for sensitization and challenge. Thus allergens which might cause severe skin reactions in sensitized people may often be ingested or administered intravenously without provoking a hypersensitivity response.

The characteristics which serve to differentiate delayed hypersensitivity from the immediate and Arthus responses, and in a sense operationally define the entity are: (1) the lack of participation of conventional antibody in the response; (2) the inability to transfer the delayed hypersensitivity state with serum containing specific antibodies; (3) the occurrence of delayed hypersensitivity states in agammaglobulinemic individuals who are incapable of developing antibodies and therefore cannot develop immediate hypersensitivity states; (4) the apparent lack of participation of histamine and other pharmacologic agents; (5) the transferability by mononuclear inflammatory cells, of delayed hypersensitivity, which can not be accomplished in immediate hypersensitivity; and (6) the ability to induce a keratitis in the avascular cornea upon intracorneal challenge with minute amounts of antigen. (There is still some question about the value of injecting antigen into the avascular cornea as a means of distinguishing immediate hypersensitivity from delayed hypersensitivity as was proposed by Rich and Follis. However, the delayed hypersensitivity lesions may be obtained with amounts of antigen that are far less than those required to produce corneal inflammation on the basis of immediate hypersensitivity.)

Homograft Reactions

The transplantation of living tissue from one individual to another of the same species (homograft) generally results in a slough (rejection) of the graft. The "homograft reaction" is an immunologic response to antigenic substances present in the graft which are foreign to the recipient. Only when the donor and recipient tissues are genetically identical do they have the same set of antigens. Thus in the case of identical twins tissue transplantation is often successful just as it is when tissue is grafted from one part of the body to another of the same individual (autograft). With a few important exceptions, homografts are otherwise rarely successful.

The immunologic nature of homograft rejection seems to be well established. The graft remains viable and for a while transplantation appears to be successful. After a variable lag period during which immunologic processes are mobilized, signs of incompatibility begin to appear. The grafted tissue loses its viability and is sloughed. After having once sloughed a graft, the recipient then becomes sensitized to further grafts from the same donor; this causes a more accelerated rejection of subsequent grafts. Immunity against normal tissues may be transferred by lymphocytes from a previously sensitized individual to a normal recipient, and there are other good reasons for regarding homograft rejection as a manifestation of delayed hypersensitivity.

The homograft-rejection response is of interest to ophthalmologists because it is one of the most important causes for failure in corneal transplantation. The immunologic factors affecting corneal grafts have recently been reviewed by Maumenee. He discusses the reason for the comparative infrequency of reactions to corneal homografts and points out that for certain reasons the cornea is a "privileged" tissue. It appears to be the nuclei which contain the antigenic substances responsible for the immunologic reactions to grafted tissues. The cornea is an exceedingly weak antigen, possibly because of the relative paucity of cells and their wide separation by the stromal ground substance. A second factor is the apparent necessity for the antigenic material to come into actual contact with the vascular bed of the host in order to initiate the sensitization response. Thus if the corneal button is placed centrally in the avascular cornea of the recipient and if subsequent vascularization of the cornea does not occur, sensitization to the graft is not likely to occur. A third requirement is that once sensitization has been effected, it is necessary for the sensitized cells of the host (probably lymphocytes) to invade the transplanted tissue before the graft becomes damaged and sloughs.

The Shwartzman Phenomenon

A phenomenon first described by Sanarelli and studied extensively by Shwartzman is often confused with some of the previously described hypersensitivity reactions. This, however, is not a specific manifestation of antigen-antibody interaction. If any one of a number of bacterial filtrates is injected into the skin and 24 hours later the same or an-

other material is injected intravenously, then hemorrhagic necrosis may occur at the initial cutaneous injection site. It is believed that local vascular damage produced by the initial injection makes the tissue highly susceptible to further nonspecific injury from circulating toxin. It seems not unlikely that this type of nonspecific vascular injury might be operative in some of the clinical syndromes encountered by ophthalmologists, e.g., the vitreous hemorrhages in retinal perivasculitis which apparently can be induced by tuberculin treatment, menstruation or ascariasis. Just as the Shwartzman phenomenon has been suggested as a possible mechanism for the exacerbation of pulmonary tuberculosis provoked by unrelated intercurrent infections, so it might explain some of the episodic bouts of uveitis precipitated by a variety of factors. On the other hand, the typically hemorrhagic character of the Shwartzman lesion should be kept in mind while trying to relate this phenomenon to those observed in clinical practice.

The Shwartzman phenomenon differs from specific hypersensitivity reactions in several ways: (1) the time interval between injections differs from that of any known immunologic process. Sensitization appears too quickly and disappears too soon; (2) there is apparently a lack of specificity in the response, i.e., no antigenic relationship between sensitizing and challenging substances. Pathologically this reaction, reaching a peak after several hours and including thrombosis, vasculitis, and hemorrhage may simulate to a very high degree the Arthus reaction.

CELLS, CELL GROWTH AND NEOPLASIA

Kinds of Cells

All tissue cells of the adult organism either have been present since the time of embryologic development or they represent the progeny of cells which were being formed at that time. In the life cycle of each tissue cell two important stages may be recognized: the period of cell division, and that of cell growth and function, also called the "mitotic" and "intermitotic periods," respectively. For the adult organism this concept is not entirely accurate since we know that certain cells have

become so highly differentiated that they have lost the ability to reproduce their kind. For such cells, examples of which are the neurons, erythrocytes, polymorphonuclear leukocytes and lens fibers, the term "postmitotic" is more precise. Among the intermitotic cells we may distinguish two broad categories. The most undifferentiated cells which exist only to serve as a reservoir for more cell production are called the "vegetative intermitotics." Examples are the "blast" cells of the bone marrow, the basal cells of the epidermis, and spermatogonia. Cells derived from these, but which have begun to differentiate though retaining their capacity for cell division, are called "differentiating intermitotics." Examples are promyelocytes, prickle cells of the epidermis, and spermatocytes.

Appearance and Function of Nuclei

In the study of cells it is most important to pay special attention to the appearance and staining characteristics of the nucleus, the nucleolus, and the cytoplasm for these structures will provide information as to what the cell is doing or is capable of doing. In the adult, certain cells such as erythrocytes and the older lens fibers have lost their nuclei; from this information we can surmise they are no longer capable of cell division.

In a very general way it may be said that the cell nucleus has two main functions: (1) reproduction and the passing of special characteristics to subsequent generations of cells by augmentation of its gene protein; and (2) control of the formation of cytoplasmic proteins by the nucleolus. The following summary of some of these aspects of cell growth and cell function is condensed from Caspersson's monograph.

During mitosis there is a progressive increase in nucleic acid and a loss of nuclear protein so that the ratio of nucleic acid to protein which is approximately 1:30 during early prophase shifts to 1:3 in the metaphase. During metaphase the chromosomes alone represent the total detectable nuclear material. All other substances have disappeared or cannot be identified in the cell. A reversal of the process takes place during telophase.

Not only is there evidence that the quantity of nucleic acid within the chromosomes is maximal during cell division but there is also reason for believing that disturbances in gene reproduction are related to disordered nucleic acid metabolism. It has, therefore, been concluded that the nucleic acids are necessary prerequisites for the reproduction of genes and that they are probably necessary for the multiplication of self-reproducing protein molecules in general.

Between mitoses the cell enlarges and carries out its special functions. During these periods there is a great increase in the total protein, which either is concentrated in the cytoplasm or is secreted out of the cell. In those cells which normally form a great deal of cytoplasmic protein, there is a chromatin mass associated with the nucleolus. This nucleolus associated chromatin produces proteinaceous substances rich in diamino acids which accumulate and form the main bulk of the nucleolus. These proteins diffuse out through the cytoplasm from the perinuclear area. A great variety of cells which produce much cytoplasmic protein are characterized by having large nucleoli and nucleic acid rich cytoplasm. Thus in contrast with the disappearance of nucleoli in dividing cells is the prominence of nucleoli in cells exhibiting cytoplasmic protein synthesis. So consistent are these observations under a wide variety of physiologic and pathologic situations that one may deduce much about the functions of a cell by paying close attention to the character of its nucleus, the size of its nucleolus and the staining characteristics of its cytoplasm.

The nuclear changes and chromatin arrangements characteristic of the various phases of the mitotic process are well known and will not be described here. Cells which are not only dividing rapidly but are also busily engaged in protein synthesis are characterized by having large nucleoli and prominent chromatin masses associated with the nucleolus, but when the cell is preparing to divide its nucleolus shrinks and finally disappears. Cells which are neither reproducing rapidly nor forming much protein are characterized by having rather small nuclei, rare mitotic figures and inconspicuous nucleoli.

These general principles have long been applied to the study and classification of neoplastic tissues. Uveal melanomas, for example, were classified by Callender according to their cytologic characteristics and the prognostic significance of Callender's schema has stood the test of time. Tumors composed of cells possessing small nuclei, absent nucleoli, and rare mitotic figures (Spindle A melanomas for example) carry a very much more favorable prognosis than do those in which the cells reveal large nuclei with prominent chromatin masses, huge nucleoli and numerous mitoses.

Another important piece of information

that can be derived from cytologic study relates to sex-determination. Barr and his associates discovered that a peculiar chromatin mass, now believed to represent the combined X chromosomes, is present in the intermitotic nuclei of the majority of cells in the female, both human and animal. This "sex chromatin" usually is a single planoconvex body attached to the nuclear membrane, but it may be found free in the nucleoplasm or adjacent to the nucleolus. It is demonstrable by a variety of staining techniques but, according to Guard, only a combination of Biebrich scarlet and fast green FCF differentiates the sex chromatin from other heterochromatin granules. The sex chromatin stains red while the remainder of the nuclear chromatin is stained green. Pedler and Ashton have described structures in the eye identified as the female sex chromatin which have been found in conjunctival, ciliary, and corneal epithelium, in stromal cells of the iris and ciliary body, in the nuclear layers of the retina, and in the ganglion cells where the chromatin masses were particularly well defined.

Terminology

A number of descriptive terms are available to enable us to categorize a wide variety of abnormalities of cell growth and differentiation. These are extremely useful but only when they are employed in a consistent manner. Cells can only grow and mature if their embryologic precursors have made their appearance. Failure of the anlage of an organ to appear and develop leads to *agenesis*. Anophthalmos is an example of agenesis. When specific cell groups fail to develop, this leads to *aplasia*. If, for example, the ganglion cells of the retina fail to develop, the nerve fibers do not form and an aplasia of the optic nerve occurs. *Hypoplasia* is merely a lesser degree of malformation than aplasia, i.e., all precursor cells have not failed to develop. Most of the reports in the literature pertaining to aplasia of the optic nerve are in reality reports of cases of hypoplasia. Although the word hypoplasia simply implies a diminished number of cells, by convention the term is applied only to embryologic or developmental anomalies, not to acquired lesions.

When the anlage of an organ makes its appearance but only to develop in a faulty manner, this is called *dysgenesis*. The many variations of severe microphthalmus are examples of ocular dysgenesis. *Dysplasia* is a closely related abnormality but one occurring at the tissue level after the primordial cells have appeared and begun to differentiate, e.g., retinal dysplasia. *Hyperplasia* is the increase in tissue bulk which results from an increased number of cells. It is almost always an acquired process, but is differentiated from *hypertrophy* which is the increased tissue mass that results from increased size of cells. Often these occur as associated phenomena. For example, in the early stages of anterior polar cataract formation, epithelial cells of the lens are increased in size as well as in number. *Atrophy* is a loss of tissue mass resulting mainly from the diminution in size of individual cells. The shrinkage of skeletal muscle observed in advancing age or disuse is the prototype. In certain relatively acellular tissues such as the iris, atrophy is the result of a loss of intercellular ground substance. When cells become so altered in form and function that they produce a differentiated tissue which is no longer characteristic for the anatomical site in which they are located, the process is called *metaplasia*. Bone formation between the choroid and retina is an excellent example.

Terms used in dermal pathology. Another group of descriptive terms employed mainly in dermal pathology must be introduced here. The epidermis consists of four main layers of cells which represent different stages of maturation (Fig. 37–1). The youngest and least differentiated are in the basal layer. Next are the squamous or prickle cells which form the bulk of normal skin. Near the surface there is a stratum of cells containing basophilic cytoplasmic granules, the granular layer. Finally at the surface the cells have lost their nuclei and have become keratinized. Mucous membranes composed of stratified squamous epithelium differ mainly in the absence of the keratinized surface and of the granular layers (Fig. 37–2). When a tissue like the bulbar conjunctiva becomes keratinized and begins to resemble skin, the process is called *epidermidalization* (Fig. 38–1). The keratin layer varies in thickness in different parts of the skin. It is normally very thin in the eyelids. When increased keratin formation is observed, we speak of *hyperkeratosis* (Fig. 38–2). Accompanying this is a thickening of the granular layer. In certain dermatoses, such as psoriasis, there is a characteristic persistence of nuclei up into the keratinized layer (Fig. 38–3). This is known as *parakeratosis*. It is typically associated with a disappearance of the granular layer. An increased thickness of the prickle cell layer is called *acanthosis*. It presents many different patterns and may be directed outward as in verrucal lesions (Fig. 39–1), or downward into the dermis as in the majority of dermatoses (Fig. 39–2). Chronic inflam-

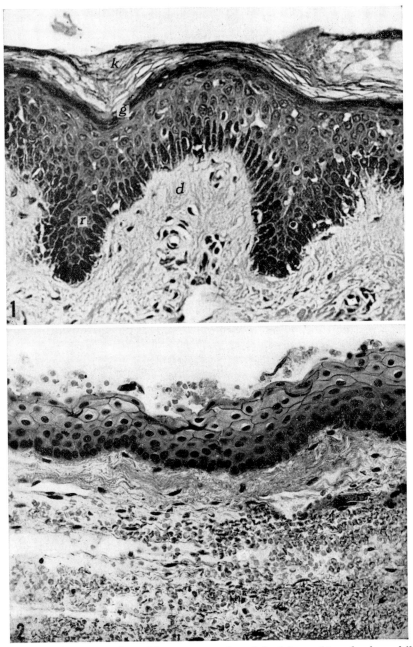

Figure 37. The epidermis (upper picture) has an outer keratinized layer (k) and a basophilic granular layer (g) as well as rete pegs (r) and dermal papillae (d) which are not observed in normal mucous membranes such as the conjunctiva (lower picture). 1. ×390. AFIP Acc. 177191. 2. ×305. AFIP Acc. 720856.

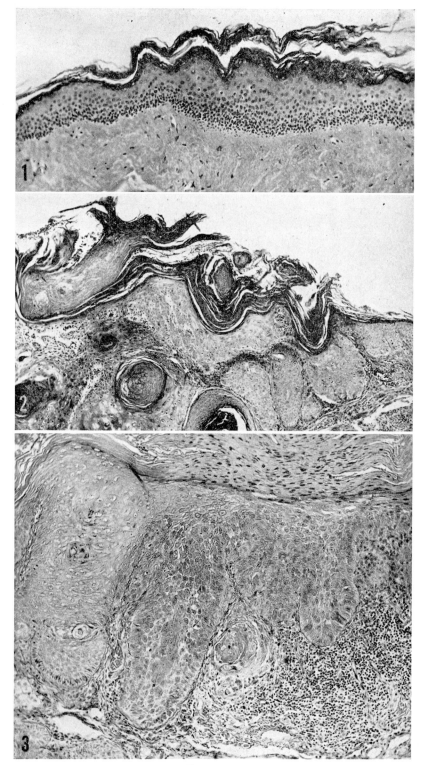

Figure 38.
1. Epidermidalization of conjunctiva: a thick keratin layer and a prominent granular layer are present. ×125. AFIP Acc. 338247.

2. Hyperkeratosis in senile keratosis: the keratin and granular layers have become greatly thickened in places. ×55. AFIP Acc. 933270.

3. Parakeratosis in senile keratosis: retention of nuclei in the keratinizing layer is striking in the upper right corner and the granular layer is poorly developed. ×115. AFIP Acc. 933270. Downward acanthosis is evident in 2 and 3.

matory processes sometimes stimulate excessive acanthosis, giving rise to lesions which simulate squamous cell carcinoma. Such non-neoplastic proliferations are called *pseudo-epitheliomatous hyperplasia* (Fig. 40). Alterations in the normal orderly differentiation of cells from the basal layer through the prickle cell layer into the granular and keratinized layers are collectively called *dyskeratosis*. Some dyskeratotic changes have a very distinctive appearance, for example those of molluscum contagiosum. Others, especially those seen in neoplastic lesions, are much more variable and consist of varying degrees of pleomorphism, irregularity in staining, loss of polarity, keratin formation by individual

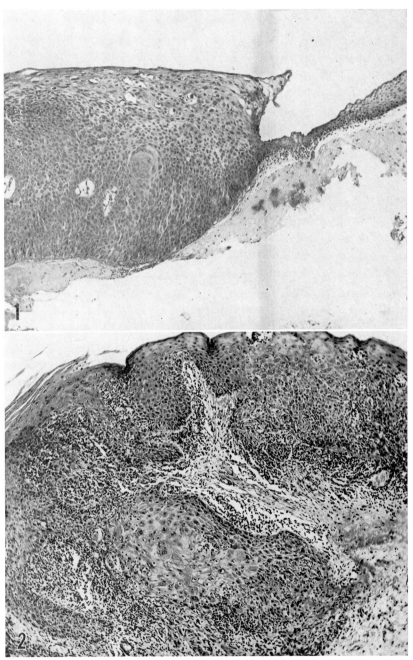

Figure 39. Acanthosis
The thickening of the limbal epithelium is mainly outwards (away from the surface) in 1 while in 2 it is principally downward into the subconjunctival tissues. 1. ×80. AFIP Acc. 873376. 2. ×75. AFIP Acc. 710769.

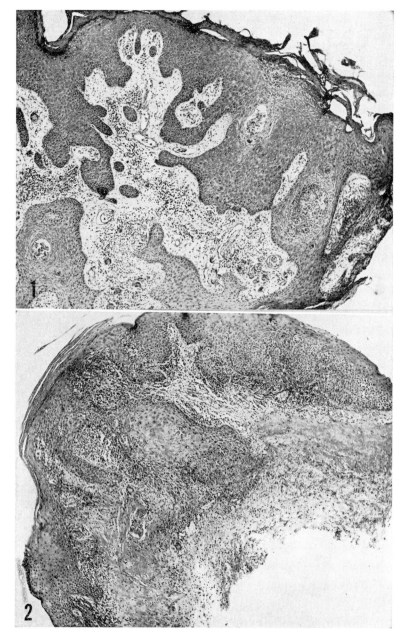

Figure 40.   Pseudoepitheliomatous Hyperplasia
1. Blastomycosis of the skin. ×46. AFIP Acc. 67322.
2. Chronic inflammation, etiology undetermined, of the bulbar conjunctiva. ×48. AFIP Acc. 710769.

cells within the prickle cell layer and mitotic division near the skin surface.

Neoplasia

The formation of new tissue which no longer responds to the normal growth-controlling mechanisms of the body is called neoplasia. By many people the term "tumor" is used synonymously with "neoplasm," but this is unfortunate for two reasons. The former term implies a mass of tissue, a pathologic enlargement. Many neoplasms, particularly the "in-situ carcinomas," do not produce large masses. On the other hand, many tumefactions are the result of non-neoplastic proliferations. For this reason, we shall avoid using the word "tumor" when we mean "neoplasm."

Benign neoplasms.   Benign neoplasms are

usually slow-growing lesions composed of well differentiated mature cells which resemble those of the tissues from which they have arisen. Therefore, great pleomorphism is unusual and mitotic figures are not numerous. The benign neoplasm grows expansively rather than by infiltration. Its cells maintain a cohesiveness which tends to prevent dispersion. A nevus of the iris, for example, even though situated on the anterior surface in contact with aqueous, will not seed cells into the anterior chamber, but such seeding is a characteristic feature of many malignant melanomas of the iris. Because of their slow growth by expansion, benign neoplasms compress the adjacent tissues and tend to become encapsulated. The most important characteristic of benign neoplasms is their inability to metastasize.

Malignant neoplasms. Malignant neoplasms, though they show very great variations in behavior, tend to be composed of more rapidly growing cells which generally are less well differentiated than those of benign lesions. Mitotic figures are more numerous and there is a tendency towards pleomorphism. Many pathologists like to grade malignant tumors, either by applying such descriptive terms as "well differentiated" and "undifferentiated" or by a number scheme, "grade one," etc. Such grading is based upon the degree of similarity or dissimilarity to normal tissue exhibited by the neoplasm. Undifferentiated (grade four) cancers, when they are first seen in a metastatic site, frequently reveal so few recognizable characteristics of the tissue from which they developed that the pathologist is often at a complete loss to suggest a primary site. A malignant melanoma may be so poorly differentiated that it fails to produce pigment and its growth pattern simulates that of a carcinoma or a sarcoma. On the other hand, highly differentiated neoplasms will not only grow in a fashion characteristic of the parent tissue but will also produce special structures or products such as fat (in meibomian gland carcinomas), striated muscle fibers (in rhabdomyosarcomas), melanin (in melanomas), keratin pearls (in squamous cell carcinomas), or mucin (in adenocarcinomas).

Malignant neoplasms grow in many different ways. Though they share with benign tumors the feature of expansile growth (char-acteristic of many uveal melanomas), they possess the more important ability to infiltrate, permeate, and disseminate. About the periphery of malignant neoplasms one observes cords or nests of cells which have broken away from the main mass. The cells lose their cohesiveness for one another and are carried away by tissue fluids, lymphatics and blood vessels. Spread to regional or distant tissues takes place as a result of one or another of several mechanisms exhibited to varying degrees by different types of cancer. Basal cell carcinomas, for example, grow by direct extension through bone as well as soft tissues, yet they rarely spread by way of lymphatics or blood vessels. Uveal melanomas, on the other hand, are usually well contained by the sclera but they tend to invade blood vessels and disseminate hematogenously. Most carcinomas have a propensity for lymphatic invasion.

Precancerous lesions and etiologic factors. Benign neoplasms seldom become malignant. Though this is a sound generalization, an important exception is encountered in ophthalmology. There is good reason to believe that many, if not most, malignant melanomas of the uvea and conjunctiva arise from pre-existing benign nevi. During recent years much has been learned about etiologic factors in the causation of cancer (Mellors, 1957). Chronic trauma in one form or another is an important predisposing factor. The trauma may be chemical (naphthylamine carcinomas of the bladder and polycyclic hydrocarbon carcinomas of the skin and mucous membranes), solar radiations (carcinoma of exposed skin and mucous membranes in seamen and farmers), ionizing radiations (osteosarcoma and leukemia after exposure to x-rays), or mixtures of these with other factors such as chronic mechanical irritation (carcinoma of lip in pipe smokers and bronchogenic carcinoma in cigarette smokers). Hereditary factors are important in certain instances and again we find one of the best examples in ophthalmology. Patients who have survived to adult life after treatment of retinoblastoma in infancy and who have children are almost certain to produce some offspring with retinoblastoma. Environmental factors may aggravate precancerous conditions which in themselves are hereditary. A good example is found in xeroderma pigmentosum, which becomes a more disabling disease and, more frequently, is complicated by a variety of skin cancers in patients who are not protected from solar radiation.

Hamartomas and choristomas.   There are a number of tumors which differ from true neoplasms in that they seem to represent anomalies in tissue formation rather than cellular proliferation arising in previously normal tissues. Such tumors fall into two main groups depending upon the types of tissue forming the lesion. An anomaly which involves only tissue elements normally found at the involved site is called a *hamartia,* and when a tumor mass arises from such a lesion it is called a *hamartoma.* Other anomalies in tissues which contain elements not normally present at the involved site are termed *choristas,* and when a mass is formed it is called a *choristoma.* Hemangiomas and the hairy nevi are good examples of isolated hamartomas. There are several syndromes characterized by the formation of hamartias and hamartomas involving multiple tissues. These could be called disseminated hamartioses but they are collectively referred to by ophthalmologists as the *phakomatoses.* Individually they are generally given eponymic designations—von Recklinghausen's neurofibromatosis, the Sturge-Weber syndrome, Bourneville's disease, and the von Hippel-Lindau syndrome. The characteristic pathologic features of these disseminated hamartioses are described in other chapters. Choristomas are also well known to ophthalmologists in the form of solid dermolipomas of the limbus and cystic dermoids of the orbit.

PIGMENT AND DISTURBANCES OF PIGMENTATION

Melanin and Melanocytes

Alterations of pigmentation involve pigments which are endogenous and exogenous. Among the endogenous, melanin is most important but hemoglobin, hemosiderin, acid hematin, lipochromes, and certain compounds of copper must also concern the ophthalmic pathologist. Soluble salts of iron released from intraocular foreign bodies are the most common exogenous cause of a focalized or generalized increase in ocular pigmentation. Mercurial salts and tattoos are much less common.

Melanin is the pigment which is responsible for most of the variations in normal and pathologic coloration of the dermal and ocular tissues. Cells which contain melanin have been called by a variety of names and there is much confusion in the classification of pigment cells. In order to minimize this difficulty the authors of this text have agreed to follow the nomenclature recommended at the conference on the Biology of the Normal and Atypical Pigment Cell sponsored by the National Research Council in 1951. *Melanocytes* are mature and *melanoblasts* immature melanin-forming cells found in man and in higher vertebrates. *Melanophages* are macrophages that have phagocytized melanin. *Melanophores* are contractile cells found in lower animals. It is this last term that has been used most indiscriminately, especially in the ophthalmic literature. Since it is inappropriate and totally unnecessary, its use will be avoided in this book. The term *chromatophore* also has been used indiscriminately in connection with a number of pigmented cells, and of recent years is considered the same as a macrophage. This term will not be used in this book. One other type of pigmented cell should be mentioned here, though it is not given a special name. Normal basal cells and some of the more deeply situated squamous cells of the skin may be pigmented, but these are not pigment-forming cells. They receive their pigment from the melanocytes which are insinuated between the epithelial cells along the dermo-epidermal junction. It is curious that more pigment often is observed in the epithelial cells than in the melanocytes of the skin. Because cutaneous melanocytes have this tendency to give up their secretory product to other cells, Masson has suggested calling them "cytocrine cells" and since they may retain or promptly discharge their pigment, melanocytes may be further characterized as "continent" or "incontinent." In the uvea, the melanocytes are continent and so they are easily recognized by their branching cytoplasmic processes that are so heavily laden with pigment. But in the skin and mucous membranes, melanocytes are usually unrecognizable unless they are identified by histochemical procedures which test for their specific enzyme (DOPA-oxidase*) or by silver stains which demonstrate minute, finely dispersed melanin granules.

Ocular melanocytes. In the eye there are melanin-producing cells in three main tissues: the surface epithelium, the uvea, and the pigment epithelium of the retina, ciliary body, and iris. The embryology of the first two remains an unsettled issue, though the proponents of the theory of neural crest origin seem to have the largest and most enthusiastic following. By contrast there is no controversy as to the development of the pigmented epithelium of the retina, ciliary body, and iris which differentiates from the cells of the optic vesicle. These pigmented tissues should be set apart from those of the uvea, skin, and conjunctiva because of their embryologic, morphologic and oncologic differences. Embryologically these cells are distinctive because they differentiate in situ and their pigment formation takes place very early (about the fifth to sixth week of gestation). According to Rawles (1947) and Bartelmez (1954) the melanocytes of the skin and uvea differentiate in their respective locations only after having migrated from the neural crest, and their production of pigment begins late, shortly before birth. Furthermore, according to Mann, cutaneous and uveal pigmentation increases after birth while that of the pigment epithelium remains stationary. Morphologically the pigment epithelium is characterized by cells which appear cuboidal in meridional sections and by pigment granules which are considerably larger than those of the uvea. Under low power microscopy the epithelial melanocytes appear considerably darker than those of the uvea. The most distinctive feature of the retinal pigment gran-

ule is its shape as seen by oil immersion microscopy. In the human, they are ovoid with somewhat pointed ends (like footballs), while in many lower animals they are even more elongated, sometimes needle-like. The much more finely granular pigment of uveal and cutaneous melanocytes is so tightly packed that the cells appear homogeneous or stippled.* Finally there is a striking difference in the proliferative capacities of these pigmented tissues. Benign proliferations with and without metaplastic features frequently are observed in the retinal and ciliary epithelium. In fact, most of the hyperpigmented lesions of the ocular fundus observed after trauma or inflammatory processes are the result of proliferations of the pigment epithelium, not of the uveal melanocytes. In striking contrast with the great tendency to reactive proliferation is the seeming inability of the pigment epithelium to give rise to malignant tumors. Melanotic neoplasms arise from all parts of the uvea, the conjunctiva, eyelids, caruncle, and even the cornea, but only with great rarity from the pigment epithelium.

Variations in melanotic pigmentation. Variations in pigmentation due to genetic, hormonal, environmental, and other influences are observed in the uvea but rarely in the pigment epithelium. An exception to this is observed in complete albinism wherein there may be a total lack of melanin formation. More often in human albinos there is some melanin in the pigment epithelium even though the skin and the uvea are completely free. In hyperpigmented individuals a great increase in uveal melanin may be evident, yet the pigment epithelium, which seemingly possesses all the pigment it can hold, even in blondes, reveals no increase.

Many forms of increased melanotic pigmentation are observed in the skin, conjunctiva and uvea. Microscopically, these can usually be lumped into two main categories: (1) increased pigmentation without other obvious cytologic or architectural alterations of the affected tissues, and (2) increased pigmentation associated with hypertrophy and/or hyperplasia of melanin-forming cells.

---

* DOPA is an abbreviation for 3,4–dihydroxy–phenylalanine. The enzyme, tyrosinase, which produces DOPA from tyrosine, is now believed to also have the second function of DOPA–oxidase.

* This refers only to man; in many animal species the uveal pigment granules are elongated.

A simple increase in the content of melanin, accompanied by an inconspicuous increase in melanoblastic "clear cells," but without more noteworthy cellular activity, accounts for the variations commonly observed between persons of different races, after sun-tanning, in such discrete lesions as freckles and café-au-lait spots, and with endocrine alterations such as occur in Addison's disease and pregnancy. In contrast with these are the cellular nevi and melanomas. Nevi are characterized by the presence of an increased number of melanocytic cells which usually are also of increased size. Thus one should distinguish between nevi and freckles of the skin or iris. Freckles are merely acellular pigmented spots which are not elevated, and which do not affect the architecture of the tissue as determined either by clinical examination or by histologic study. On the other hand, nevi of the iris usually project into the anterior chamber and alter the iris architecture.

Nevi, Melanosis Oculi and Precancerous Melanosis

Nevi. The common nevi of the skin and conjunctiva are classified mainly according to the position of the nevus cells. If they are confined to the epithelium they are called *intraepithelial* or *junctional* since the cell clusters are usually seen along the junction of epithelium with subepithelial tissues. Those confined to the subepithelial tissues are called *dermal*. This term is inappropriate for the conjunctiva but it makes little difference, since nevi of this type are most uncommon on the conjunctiva. The most frequently encountered nevi have both intraepithelial and subepithelial components; these are called *compound* nevi. Frequently, in compound nevi, there is an associated Schwannian proliferation about the terminal filaments of the dermal nerves beneath the more superficial components of the nevus. These cells, which are closely related to the nevus cells arising in the melanocytes of the epithelium, stream upward to intermingle with them. When this Schwannian element is unusually prominent, the nevus is sometimes called a "neuronevus." Since pure dermal nevi are believed never to become malignant,

much attention is paid to the intraepithelial component of nevi. It is in these cell clusters, particularly as they pass from the epithelium down into the dermis, that malignant change occurs.

Mongolian spots and related nevi. A totally different group of pigmented nevi are to be distinguished from those just described. These are the result of deeply situated melanocytes that are not associated with nevus cells in the epithelium or superficial layers of the dermis. The ill-defined, non-elevated, blue-gray spots produced by these cells are observed most often in non-Caucasians, and in certain locations such as the sacral area, where they are called "Mongolian spots." Another site of predilection is about the orbit where not only the skin, but also the conjunctiva, sclera, and other ocular and orbital tissues may be involved. A variety of names are given to this lesion but the most frequently used are "extrasacral Mongolian spot," "nevus of Ota," and "oculodermal melanocytosis." Another pigmented lesion closely related to Mongolian spots is the "blue nevus." This is a bluish nodule composed of deeply pigmented elongated and branched melanocytes similar to those found in Mongolian spots. Often there is also a proliferation of larger, plumper, spindle-shaped cells among which are very discrete fascicles of nonpigmented spindle cells. Such tumors, which are called "cellular blue nevi," may closely resemble melanomas of the uvea, but they differ from uveal melanomas in that they almost never metastasize.

Melanosis oculi. The term melanosis in itself is not very meaningful and it must be further qualified. Two forms of diffuse melanosis of the eye are recognized, the congenital and the acquired. Congenital melanosis oculi may involve either the uveal or more superficial ocular tissues. One example has already been described—the nevus of Ota. Congenital melanosis oculi may involve all or only a portion of the uvea. In exaggerated forms the sclera, episclera, optic nerve, meninges and orbital tissues may contain large numbers of perfectly normal-appearing dendritic melanocytes similar to those usually confined to the uvea. These pigmented cells are observed readily through the transparent conjunctiva. Malignant change rarely occurs in congenital melanosis. This is in distinct contrast with the frequency of malignant melanoma arising from acquired melanosis.

Precancerous melanosis. Because of its many important distinguishing features and because of the significant incidence of malignant change, Reese has set apart acquired melanosis under the designation of "precancerous melanosis." This is characteristically an ill-defined, nonelevated hyperpigmentation of the conjunctival epithelium which is first observed in middle or late adult life. There is great variation in the extent to which the bulbar and palpebral conjunctiva may be involved. The skin of the lids and adjacent face also may participate, but intraocular involvement typically is absent. Histologically this process is observed to be a very diffuse junctional type of nevus and there usually is an associated chronic inflammatory reaction. This may account for the waxing and waning that is observed (in contrast with the stationary or slowly progressive course of congenital melanosis) and possibly for the regression obtained with radiation therapy.

Blood Pigments

When red blood cells escape into the tissues, they usually are phagocytized by macrophages which convert their hemoglobin to hemosiderin, identified by its irregular granularity, yellow-brown color, and positive histochemical reaction for iron, and to hematoidin, an iron-free pigment which is rather rapidly absorbed and excreted as bilirubin. After repeated or massive hemorrhage, the accumulated hemosiderin may be sufficient to give the tissues a rusty appearance. A blue iris may become brown after much hemorrhage into the anterior chamber and when it

is examined microscopically large hemosiderin deposits are seen throughout the stroma and epithelium. Similarly, after posterior segment hemorrhages, the usually transparent retina may become opaque and yellow-brown from its contained hemosiderin. While hemosiderin is probably the only blood pigment of importance to the clinical ophthalmologist, the pathologist frequently encounters two others, hemoglobin and acid hematin. Free hemoglobin, not yet converted into hemosiderin, is observed most often in the vitreous. Possibly because of its avascularity and relative freedom of mesenchymal cells, the vitreous does not seem to absorb and remove large collections of disintegrating erythrocytes as promptly as other tissues. Globules of hemoglobin may be mistaken for red blood cells because they both stain similarly; their morphologic differences serve to distinguish one from the other. Acid hematin, commonly referred to as "formalin pigment," is really an artifact produced by the action of acid fixatives on hemoglobin. It is of practical importance to the ophthalmic pathologist who encounters it frequently and must avoid the error of misinterpreting it as melanin or iron. Acid hematin is differentiated by its negative reaction to tests for iron and by its ability to polarize light. Sorting out different pigments histologically can be made relatively easy with the aid of a few simple tests. Table 1, which summarizes their differential characteristics, shows that hematogenous iron pigment (hemosiderin) cannot be distinguished from exogenous iron absorbed from a foreign body. Siderosis bulbi is discussed further in Chapter III. Special ocular pigmentations such as the deposition of copper compounds in corneal tissues of patients with Wilson's disease are taken up elsewhere.

Table 1. Recognition of Melanin and Other Brown Pigments

	Morphology of granules	*Color**	*Iron†*	*Bleaches*	*Birefringence*
Uveal melanin	Uniformly fine	Yellow-brown	Neg.	Yes	No
Pigment epithelial melanin	Uniformly coarse, ovoid to round	Brown-black	Neg.	Yes	No
Hemosiderin	Irregular in size and shape	Yellow-brown	Pos.	No	No
Exogenous iron	Irregular in size and shape	Yellow-brown	Pos.	No	No
Hemoglobin	Rounded, much variation in size	Orange-red to Orange-brown	Neg.	No	No
Acid hematin	Fine, short needle-like crystals	Brown-black	Neg.	No	Yes

*Asseen in sections stained with hemotoxylin and eosin.
† Prussian blue reaction.

RETROGRADE PROCESSES

Definitions

It is desirable, though often difficult, to use properly three terms which distinguish different categories of retrograde processes: atrophy, degeneration, and necrosis. *Atrophy* is a loss of tissue mass, usually the result of diminution in the size of the constituent cells. In certain tissues atrophy may also result from the loss of intercellular ground substance. Atrophy typically is a reversible process, exemplified by the wasting of skeletal muscle that occurs with disuse or starvation. *Degeneration* encompasses a much broader group of alterations which generally are more complex and often irreversible. The affected tissues are viable but their metabolism is disturbed. Distinctive morphologic changes are observed and it is upon these alterations that the group is subdivided (e.g., fatty, hyaline, mucinous).

There are two terms encountered in the ophthalmic literature which are intended to designate particular types of degeneration. One is "dystrophy," the other "abiotrophy." However, both terms have been used so indiscriminately and with such different meanings that they have become more confusing than helpful. In the chapter on corneal pathology the term, "heredofamilial dystrophy" will be used to designate a group of highly specific, genetically determined degenerations of the cornea. The term abiotrophy was used by Sir William Gowers to indicate a sort of presenile tissue degeneration. This term was first applied in ophthalmic pathology by Treacher Collins. The familial primary pigmentary retinal degenerations are examples of the types of processes that have been labelled as abiotrophies. It should be evident from these two examples that there is no clear cut distinction between a dystrophy and an abiotrophy.

Whereas atrophy and degeneration are processes involving viable tissue, *necrosis* implies death of cells or tissues. A variety of adjectives are used to indicate morphologic and pathogenetic differences (e.g., ischemic, coagulative, and hemorrhagic necrosis).

Degenerations

Degenerative changes occurring in cells and tissues usually are characterized morphologically by: (1) the presence of substances which are not normally present (e.g., amyloid, fat, calcium, etc.); (2) the loss of substances normally present (e.g., depigmentation of retinal pigment epithelium); or (3) physicochemical modification of substances that are normally present (e.g., cloudy swelling or hydropic degeneration). Thus the various degenerations are generally named according to their morphologic characteristics.

Cloudy swelling usually is a very mild reversible process affecting parenchymatous tissues. It is characterized grossly by diminished transluscency and histologically by the formation of fine to coarse granules in the swollen cytoplasm and loss of good nuclear staining. *Hydropic degeneration* is a relatively mild type which is characterized by great imbibition of water, causing the affected cells to stain very poorly, sometimes with vacuolated appearance.

Hyaline degeneration refers to the deposition of acellular homogeneous eosinophilic material of various types, either within cells or in the interstitial spaces. Thus we speak of intracytoplasmic hyaline droplets or granules, hyalinization of connective tissue, etc. A relatively specific type of hyaline degeneration is known as *amyloidosis* because in this condition the hyaline deposits give certain chemical reactions, which are similar to those given by starches. Amyloidosis is given further discussion later in this chapter.

Several types of fat deposition are recognized, but all are not, strictly speaking, degenerations. In true *lipid degeneration* (also called fatty metamorphosis) fat globules appear in the cytoplasm of cells or in other structures which normally do not contain histologically demonstrable fat. Since fat solvents are used in the preparation of ordinary paraffin sections, fat deposits in such preparations appear as unstained empty spaces. In order to demonstrate the fat globules it is necessary to use frozen sections and special dyes. A good example of fatty degeneration commonly seen in the eye is arcus senilis. In this condition the fatty deposits are so very finely dispersed that ordinary preparations even fail to reveal unstained vacuoles in the affected corneal tissues, but fat stains of frozen sections readily demonstrate the marked fatty change.

Fatty infiltration differs from fatty metamorphosis. In this condition true adipose tissue develops in the stroma of parenchymatous organs, or in such mesodermal structures as the sclera and extraocular muscles which normally contain little or no fat.

The types of fatty deposit which are most important in ophthalmic pathology are different from both fatty degeneration and fatty infiltration. They are accumulations of fatty substances in areas of tissue damage. In some, the fat is derived from the damaged tissue itself while in others the altered tissue appears to take up lipids from the blood. According to Cogan and Kuwabara the latter phenomenon is responsible for the accumulation of fatty substances in *atheromas* of blood vessels and in certain lipid keratopathies.

When normal fat-containing cells such as those of the meibomian gland or adipose tissue are damaged by disease or trauma and their fatty contents are liberated into adjacent tissues, they may provoke an intense inflammatory response; often it is granulomatous in character. Such a *lipogranulomatous reaction* is characteristic of the chalazion.

Degenerations characterized by the abnormal accumulation of carbohydrates in ocular tissues are mainly concerned with mucopolysaccharides. The only important example of *glycogen* storage is observed in certain cases of diabetes mellitus in which the cells of the iris pigment epithelium become markedly enlarged and vacuolated. Glycogen may be demonstrated within these vacuoles. *Mucoid degeneration* is observed in a number of ocular tissues. A form of microcystoid degeneration occurs in the peripheral retina and in the ciliary epithelium of the pars plana. The mucoid deposits in these lesions appear to be accumulations of hyaluronic acid. A similar condition in which hyaluronidase-sensitive acid mucopolysaccharide accumulates in cystoid spaces is Schnabel's cavernous degeneration of the optic nerve (Zimmerman, 1958). In the cornea a type of mucoid degeneration characterizes the lesions of macular dystrophy but in this condition the deposits are not sensitive to hyaluronidase (Jones and Zimmerman).

Degeneration may be associated with accumulation of minerals. Hemosiderosis and exogenous siderosis and chalcosis are discussed elsewhere. Pathologic calcification is of two types: (1) primary or metastatic calcification, and (2) secondary or dystrophic calcification. The former is the deposition of calcium salts in previously undamaged tissue as a consequence of markedly elevated blood levels of calcium and/or phosphate. Such deposits may be seen in the region of Bowman's membrane in patients who have either primary or secondary hyperparathyroidism. Dystrophic calcification is the deposition of calcium salts in pathologic tissues occurring in the absence of abnormal elevations of circulating calcium and phosphate. This type of calcific degeneration is observed very commonly in many of the ocular tissues.

Calcification and *ossification* are not synonymous. Calcification is merely the precipitation of calcium salts—usually apatite, rarely oxalate or sulfate (Cogan et al.; Zimmerman and Johnson). Such deposits always seem to occur in foci where there is an abnormal accumulation of acid mucopolysaccharide but there is no special organization of the ground substance comparable to what is seen in ossification. The latter process results from the metaplastic formation of osteoblasts which lay down an organized matrix of collagen and mucopolysaccharide called osteoid. Calcium salts are deposited in the osteoid; the resultant product is bone. Ossification in the eye is observed mainly in a plane between the choroid and retina, occasionally also in cyclitic membranes, rarely in other tissues.

Necrosis

Certain cells in the process of normal physiologic death *(necrobiosis)* continue to function. Examples are the circulating erythrocytes and the keratin layer of the epidermis. The pathologic death of cells or tissues is called necrosis. The histologic appearance of necrotic tissue varies with the cause and duration of the process. Often the microscopic appearance is sufficiently distinctive to provide evidence as to the cause.

Ischemic necrosis is produced by the occlusion of the arterial supply to a tissue. It is characterized by a protoplasmic coagulative process in which the general architecture of the tissue is preserved and cytologic detail, particularly nuclear staining, is lost. The affected tissues stain faintly with eosin but virtually not at all with hematoxylin (e.g., iris sphincter necrosis in acute glaucoma). Leukocytic infiltration is minimal or absent.

Hemorrhagic necrosis is produced by obstruction of the venous return best typified in the eye in central retinal vein obstruction. The affected tissues become extremely edematous and hemorrhagic. The massive disruption of engorged blood vessels and dissection by blood cells leads to considerable architectural disorganization.

Suppurative necrosis is produced by infectious agents and chemical substances which cause tissue damage and at the same time attract polymorphonuclear leukocytes in large numbers. Often it is the disintegration of leukocytes with the accumulation of their proteolytic enzymes that is responsible for most of the tissue necrosis. In other instances the noxious agent first damages the tissue and it is the altered tissue that attracts the white blood cells. In either case the resultant picture is that of an abscess in which the tissue architecture is largely destroyed and the whole area is heavily infiltrated by leukocytes.

Caseation necrosis is a term that was coined to describe the cheesy macroscopic appearance of the necrosis observed in large tuberculous lesions. It is not specific for tuberculosis and should not be used as a descriptive term in histopathology. Gummatous necrosis is another old term used to describe the rubbery macroscopic consistency of syphilitic granulomas. It, too, should not be used in histopathologic descriptions.

Putrefactive necrosis implies the formation of putrid products of partially split proteins by certain gas-forming bacteria. It is usually the result of infection of devitalized tissues by relatively nonpathogenic bacteria, and is characteristic of gas gangrene. Dry gangrene is a form of ischemic necrosis in which a peripheral artery supplying a digit, an extremity or segment of skin is involved.

There are several terms used to describe nuclear changes observed in dead or dying cells. If the nucleus shrinks into a small structureless hyperchromatic mass of nucleoprotein the process is called *pyknosis*. If the disintegrating nucleus becomes fragmented it is called *karyorrhexis*. If the nucleus swells with water and becomes pale-staining the change is called *karyolysis*.

VASCULAR DISEASES

Arteriosclerosis

Arteriosclerosis is a term used to include a variety of arterial lesions of diverse etiology and pathogenesis, the most important of which are atherosclerosis and arteriolar sclerosis.

Atherosclerosis. Atherosclerosis is the most common vascular disease; because of its great frequency in the older age groups it often has been assumed to be related specifically to the aging process. Now it is generally believed to be a complex systemic disease in which the larger blood vessels in particular are damaged. Etiologic and pathogenetic factors include hereditary predisposition, disturbed lipid metabolism, preference for a high fat diet, local vascular trauma produced by hemodynamic forces, and degenerative changes in the vessel walls related to senescence.

The characteristic arterial lesion is the atheroma, which begins as a sharply circumscribed accumulation of fat-laden cells clustered together between the internal elastic lamella and the endothelium of the artery wall (Figs. 41–1 and 41–2). The source of these cells is not entirely clear. They may be wandering cells or they may be derived from proliferation of the endothelial cells. They have rather large, pale-staining, vesicular nuclei and an abundant foamy cytoplasm. The empty cytoplasmic vacuolar spaces seen in paraffin sections represent the previous location of fat droplets.

As the disease progresses the atheroma grows. It may ulcerate and thereby stimulate thrombosis (Fig. 41–3). In small vessels an atheroma may occlude the lumen, even without ulceration and thrombosis. In time the underlying elastic lamella becomes thickened, sometimes fragmented, and often split into several separated layers. In large lesions, such as occur in large vessels, calcification of the

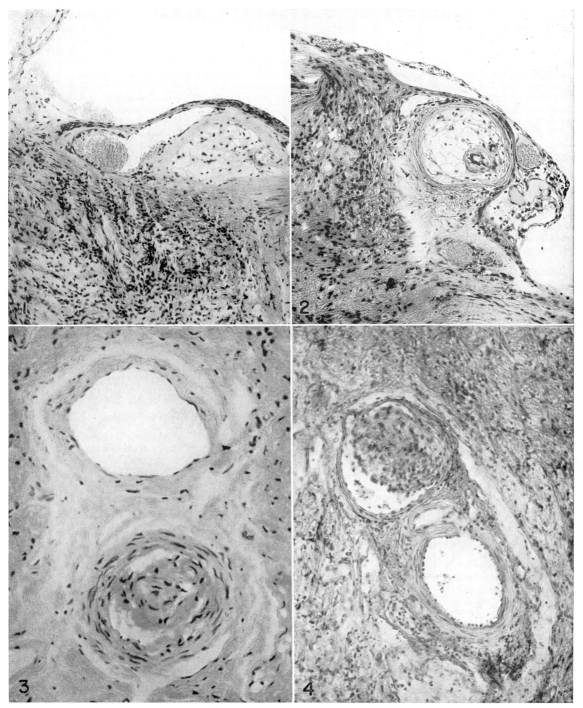

Figure 41. Arteriosclerosis

1. Atheromatous plaque in branch of central artery in optic disk. Lumen of artery is small and at right. Plaque, composed of foamy cells (lipoidal histiocytes), occupies and greatly enlarges subintimal space. ×125. AFIP Acc. 271711.

2. Atheromatous plaque in branch of central artery in optic disk, compressing overlying vein. Narrow and eccentrically placed lumen. Newly formed vessels protruding into cupped disk. ×125. AFIP Acc. 101143.

3. Thrombosis of central artery. ×240. AFIP Acc. 32287.

4. Thrombosis of central vein. ×125. AFIP Acc. 60190.

atheroma is frequent. The adjacent muscular coat becomes fibrotic and sclerosed. In large vessels necrosis and calcification of the muscular coat also may occur. After a long time the subendothelial fatty plaque tends to be replaced by fibrous tissue, and this change generally is most prominent in the smaller vessels. The resulting subendothelial fibrotic patch is usually much thinner than the fatty plaque which it replaces, and the vascular lumen tends to regain its normal contours. Complete healing of very small atheromas also may take place without subendothelial fibrosis.

Atheromatous plaques may occur anywhere in the arterial tree, but certain points of predilection almost always characterize the distribution of the lesions. The same pattern is seen in the spontaneous disease in man and in the experimental disease in animals. The points of predilection in the aorta, for instance, surround the origins of the intercostal arteries and other arterial branches. Points of predilection in the retinal artery are to be found where the artery penetrates the dural sheath of the optic nerve and the cribriform lamella. The whole vessel between these two points may, in fact, be diffusely involved. Atheromatous plaques in the intraocular portions of the retinal vessels are, on the other hand, much less frequent, and are much smaller and less extensive than in the neural portion of the artery. Friedenwald has demonstrated, however, that typical atheromatous plaques can be found even in those portions of the retinal arterial tree that are truly arteriolar in character, that is, in vessels that have no internal elastic lamina and no continuous muscular coat. This observation is of some importance because of the persistently recurrent and erroneous notion that arteriolar hyaline degeneration, the characteristic lesion of malignant hypertension, may be merely the manifestation of the atherosclerotic process in arterioles. In the small retinal arteries calcification of atheromas rarely if ever occurs, but fibrosis of the plaque and of the overlying muscular and even adventitial coats is common. This fibrotic change may reach sufficient thickness to be ophthalmoscopically visible as a localized irregular whitish sheath surrounding the arterial blood column. On histologic examination the subendothelial fibrotic plaques are much more frequently found than the fatty plaques, suggesting that the time between onset and healing of these minute lesions may be relatively short. In the course of the atherosclerotic process in the retinal arteries, lesions may also occur in the retinal veins. They consist in proliferated masses of cells in and under the venous endothelium and lead to venous occlusion (Fig. 41–4). Verhoeff has concluded that these are endothelial proliferations. Friedenwald pointed out their close similarity to atheromatous plaques in the arterial walls. They occur at the points of arteriovenous crossing where the artery and vein have a common wall, and also where the artery and vein in close approximation pass through the cribriform lamella.

These localized thickenings of the venous wall lead, in the first instance, to a narrowing of the venous lumen extending both up and down stream from the point of arteriovenous crossing. They may be recognized readily on ophthalmoscopic examination. Progressive development of these lesions can lead to venous occlusion. Verhoeff is of the opinion that this usually occurs without thrombosis, but it would appear difficult to exclude the possibility that small thromboses also may play a part in the production and spread of the occlusion; in fact, in the earliest lesions fine shreds of fibrin are sometimes included in the occlusive patch.

Arteriosclerosis obliterans. An important subgroup of atherosclerosis which definitely appears to be related to aging is called arteriosclerosis obliterans or endarteritis obliterans. This disease of older people is characterized by an extreme degree of hyaline fibrous thickening of the intima, interrupted here and there by atheromas, and consequent eccentric narrowing of the lumen. The iliac, femoral, and popliteal arteries are frequently most involved but other large arteries including the carotids may also be affected (Fig. 42). According to Hollenhorst this disease is an important cause of ocular symptoms.

Arteriolosclerosis. Arteriolar sclerosis (arteriolosclerosis) differs from atherosclerosis clinically by its relationship to systemic vascular hypertension and anatomically by the character and distribution of the vascular lesions. This disorder appears to be related pathogenetically to increased blood pressure (particularly benign essential hypertension) and vasospastic influences. The vessels affected are those that respond most actively to nervous influences and those that regulate the blood supply to important viscera. Although the intraocular vessels are involved, the early changes are not recognizable ophthalmoscopically because either the retinal vessels as a whole share less than the general average increase in tone, or the most intense retinal vasospasm occurs in terminal arterioles, beyond the range of ophthalmoscopic vision.

Microscopically, arteriolosclerosis is characterized by a combination of intimal hyalinization, medial hypertrophy, and endothelial hyperplasia (Fig. 43). Subintimal deposition of hyalin is most common in the retinal and choroidal vessels, as well as in other parts of the body. In the normal retina terminal arterioles are so delicate that microscopically they are often difficult to demonstrate. With arteriolosclerosis, however, the diffuse hyaline thickening that occurs throughout these vessels make them exceedingly prominent. Often, in advanced cases, these vessels appear to be thick hyalinized cords without lumens. Medial hypertrophy is rarely observed in the ocular blood vessels but some degree of intimal proliferation is not uncommon.

Necrotizing arteriolitis. Arteriolar necrosis or "necrotizing arteriolitis" is the characteristic vascular lesion observed in malignant hypertension. It usually is associated with extensive arteriolosclerosis but is not related to atherosclerosis. Typically it is also associated with severe azotemia and fatal renal insufficiency. The affected arterioles and small arteries exhibit a more intensely stained amorphous smudgy appearance than in

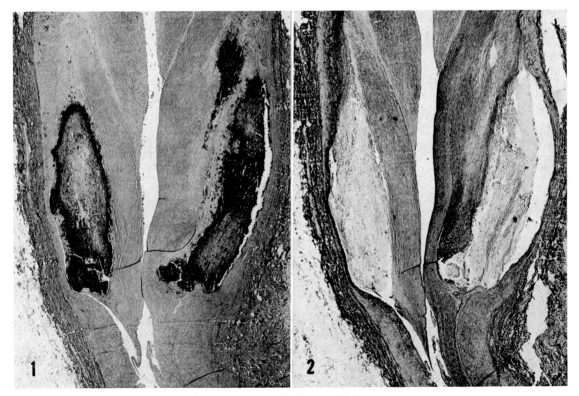

Figure 42. Arteriosclerosis Obliterans

The advanced atherosclerosis has led to extensive calcification, extreme fibrous intimal thickening, and marked narrowing of the lumen of the common carotid artery.

1. H and E.
2. Elastic tissue stain, ×18. AFIP Acc. 913758.

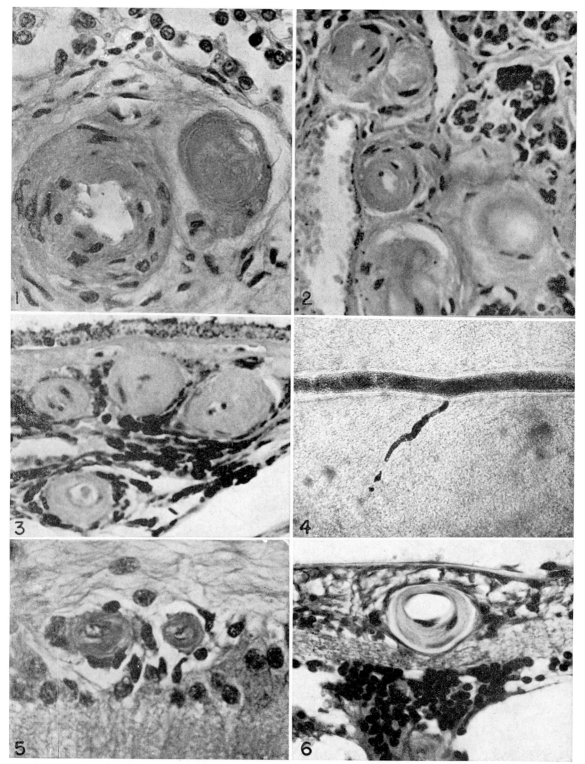

Figure 43. Hypertensive Vascular Disease

1. Kidney. Medial thickening of small artery. Hyalinization and occlusion of arteriole. ×700. AFIP Acc. 65132.
2. Pancreas. Hyalinization and occlusion of arterioles. ×475. AFIP Acc. 65132.
3. Choroid. Hyalinization and occlusion of arterioles. ×500. AFIP Acc. 62937.
4. Lipoid infiltration in arteriolar wall. Diffusely thickened and refractile wall of larger vessel. Fat stain of flat preparation of retina. AFIP Acc. 219548 (Friedenwald, J. S.: Arch. Ophth. *37:*403–427, 1947.)
5. Retina. Hyalinization of arteriole in ganglion cell layer. ×810. AFIP Acc. 64445.
6. Retina. Hyalinization of arteriole in ganglion cell layer. ×1000 AFIP Acc. 58322.

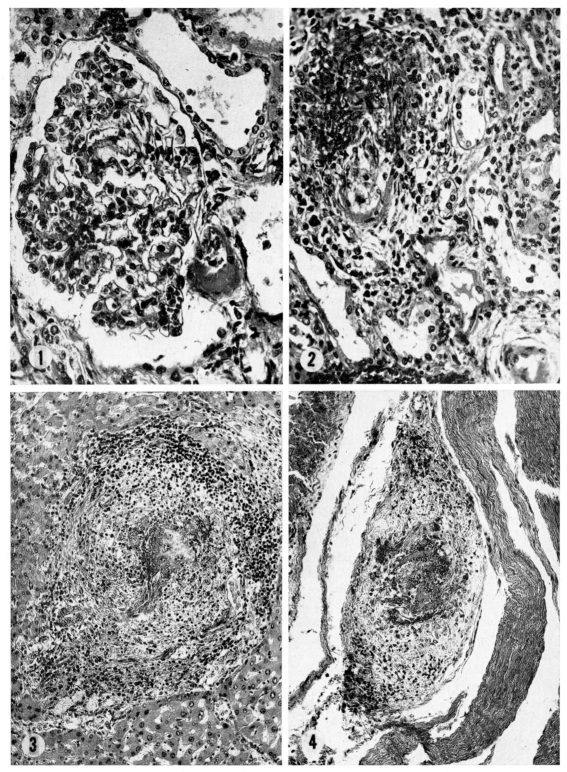

Figure 44. Arteriolar Lesions in Malignant Hypertension
1. Renal glomerulus. ×300.
2. Boundary zone between renal cortex and medulla, ×265.
3. Portal area of liver. ×130.
4. Muscularis of stomach. ×130.
All from AFIP Acc. 806087.

simple hyalinization. There is a complete loss of the architecture of the vessel wall and the necrosis may lead to microscopic hemorrhages (Fig. 44).

Vasculitis

Vasculitis includes inflammatory diseases of arteries, veins, and capillaries. Some are merely part of a known specific infectious disease (e.g., syphilis). Here, however, we are concerned mainly with several diseases of unknown etiology and uncertain pathogenesis which often may be differentiated on morphologic grounds. Some of the more important examples are thromboangiitis obliterans (Buerger's disease), hypersensitivity angiitis, periarteritis nodosa, cranial (temporal) arteritis, and pulseless disease (Takayasu's disease).

Thromboangiitis obliterans. Buerger's disease is a syndrome observed particularly in young men who typically are heavy smokers. It is characterized pathologically by panarteritis and panphlebitis of the medium-sized vessels of the extremities, associated with thrombosis and organization (Fig. 45–1, 2). Visceral involvement is rare.

Hypersensitivity angiitis. An acute necrotizing inflammation of the smallest arterioles and venules may be observed as a result of sensitivity to serum, drugs, etc. Cardiac and pulmonary lesions are most characteristic, but lesions also may be observed in other viscera, connective tissue, and the dermis. Subendothelial necrosis progresses to involve the entire vessel wall (Fig. 45–3). An intense neutrophilic and eosinophilic polymorphonuclear reaction may be observed.

Periarteritis nodosa. Periarteritis nodosa is a recurrent progressive necrotizing inflammatory process affecting small arteries where they bifurcate or give off smaller branches. Segmental necrosis produces aneurysmal dilatations measuring 2 to 4 mm. in diameter (Fig. 46–1, 2). The lesions initially contain many eosinophils. Later, lymphocytes, plasma cells, and macrophages appear, and considerable fibrous healing takes place. Complications include perforation and thrombotic occlusion.

Cranial arteritis. Cranial arteritis is a chronic granulomatous inflammatory process

which has a striking tendency to involve the temporal arteries of elderly adults. Generalized involvement of cranial vessels occurs in about one-fifth of the cases. According to

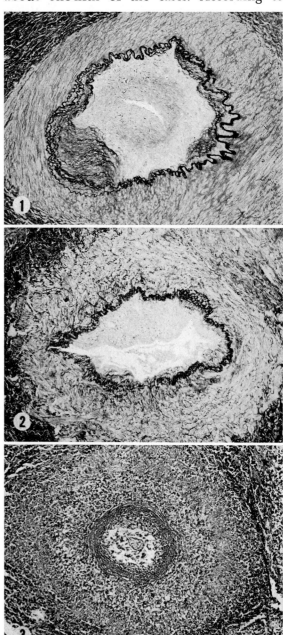

Figure 45.

1. Panarteritis with marked intimal thickening and virtual obliteration of lumen in Buerger's disease. Elastic tissue stain. ×85. AFIP Acc. 913694.

2. Panphlebitis is typically seen in association with the arteritis of Buerger's disease. Elastic tissue stain. ×65. AFIP Acc. 913694.

3. Panvasculitis of small blood vessels (hypersensitivity angiitis). ×130. AFIP Acc. 963511.

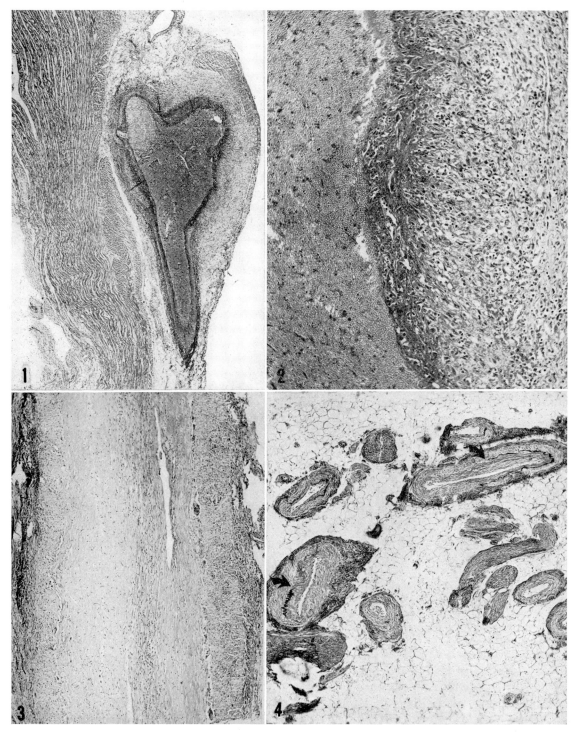

Figure 46.

1. Periarteritis nodosa of coronary artery. There is an acute necrotizing inflammatory process that has involved all coats of the vessel wall in the upper half of the field. A neurysmal dilatation and perivascular reaction have led to nodular thickening of the epicardium along the vessel. H and E, ×16. AFIP Acc. 781522.

2. A portion of the necrotic arterial wall from upper right corner of vessel shown in 1. H and E, ×115.

3. Cranial arteritis. There is a chronic granulomatous inflammatory process which has involved all coats of the temporal artery; the lumen is obliterated by a hyalinized thrombus. H and E, ×50. AFIP Acc. 747505.

4. Small arteries in orbital fat from same case as 3. Arrows indicate areas of marked destruction of internal elastic lamina and fibrosis of intima. Verhoeff-Van Gieson stain, ×50.

Wagener and Hollenhorst, and Harrison, this vascular disease is of special importance to ophthalmologists because visual impairment occurs in almost half of the cases and severe ischemic optic neuritis leading to blindness in about 30 per cent. Histopathologic examination reveals patchy areas of necrosis in the media with fragmentation of the internal elastic lamina (Fig. 46–4). A large number of multinucleated giant cells are found in the necrotic areas, particularly along the outer (medial) aspect of the internal elastic lamina, while marked fibrosis occurs on the intimal side. This diffuse chronic inflammatory process produces such an intimal reaction that the vessel lumen becomes occluded (Fig. 46–3).

Pulseless disease. Takayasu's disease (aortic arch syndrome) is a syndrome probably of diverse etiology characterized by such widespread obliterative endarteritis of the major vessels of the aortic arch that the pulse and blood pressures may be unobtainable in the upper extremities. A variety of ocular symptoms including blindness are characteristic.

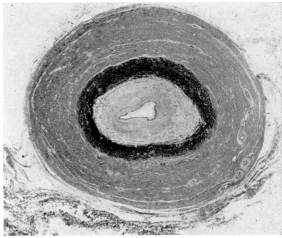

Figure 47. Pulseless Disease

All coats of this carotid artery are involved: dense sclerosis of the adventitia, partial destruction of the media, an extreme degree of connective tissue proliferation between the intima and the media, intimal hyperplasia, and marked narrowing of the lumen. Elastic tissue stain. ×10. AFIP Acc. 773000.

Microscopic examination reveals a nonspecific chronic inflammatory reaction involving all coats and an intense fibroplasia which results in obliteration of the lumen (Fig. 47).

CONNECTIVE TISSUES AND THEIR DISORDERS

Nature of Connective Tissue

Appreciation of the importance of the connective tissues in normal physiology as well as in pathologic states has grown progressively since the days of Virchow. During recent years a vast effort has been made on the part of chemists and physicists, as well as anatomists and biologists, in an attempt to fill in some of the great voids in our knowledge of these important structures. Despite an immense amount of investigation, the precise origin and physiochemical nature of the connective tissues remains to be revealed. Much information has been gathered, nevertheless, and some of this will now be summarized. Those desiring more detailed information are referred to the ever-growing lists of texts, symposia, and review articles which are trying to keep pace with the advances made in laboratories throughout the world.

Although the connective tissues of different sites are quite distinctive, e.g., bone and iris, each consists of three essential elements: mesenchymal cells, a variety of fibrils, and an interstitial colloidal substance. The principal cells are fibroblasts, histiocytes, mast cells, plasma cells, and lymphocytes. These have been described earlier in this chapter. The fibrillar elements include collagens, reticulins, and elastins. The colloidal ground substance is largely composed of hydrated mucopolysaccharides.

Fibrillar Components

Collagen. *Collagen* is the most abundant and ubiquitous of the connective tissue fibers. It is a protein, but in comparison with other body proteins it is distinguished chemically by its high content of proline and hydroxyproline and an absence of tryptophan. It is hydrolyzed enzymatically by collagenase. Collagen from certain sources (e.g., rat tail tendon) may be solubilized and reprecipitated as fibers in vitro. The formation of gelatin upon solubilization in hot water is one of the oldest ways of characterizing collagen.

At the level of light microscopy collagen appears as wavy, birefringent bundles of eosinophilic fibers cemented together in a polysaccharide matrix. These fibers, when examined in the electron microscope, are found to be composed of fibrils so delicate that they can not be seen with the light microscope. Examination of these fibrils of "mature" collagen fibers with the electron microscope (Fig. 48–1) has revealed a distinctive repeated pattern of cross-striations along the fibril with an average distance of 640 A between the "macroperiods." According to Banfield finer cross-patterns may be seen within these "macroperiods" and these are referred to as "microperiods." The periodicity of electron microscopy compares well with similar repeating units found by x-ray diffraction.

Very fine filaments which possess a much shorter periodicity ranging from 170 to 270 A have been found in embryonic tissues and about young growing fibroblasts in tissue culture. These filaments have been called "immature" collagen, for, as the tissue ages and more conventional collagen fibers appear, these "immature" filaments tend to decrease in number. The special staining characteristics of these filaments of immature collagen are similar to those of reticulin.

Reticulin Reticular fibers are fine, argyrophilic deposits in the basement membranes of epithelial tissues, the framework of lymphoid organs, and the boundary tissue about muscle fibers, fat cells, and blood vessels. In the eye, these argyrophilic fibers are most abundant in the vitreous and uvea; in the latter site they may be greatly increased by the presence of slow-growing nevi and certain melanomas. Reticular fibers are not birefrigent but are stained intensely by the periodic acid–Schiff procedure. A good place to compare the staining characteristics of reticulin and collagen is in the cornea. The basement membrane between the epithelium and Bowman's membrane contains typical argyrophilic reticulin which is bright red with

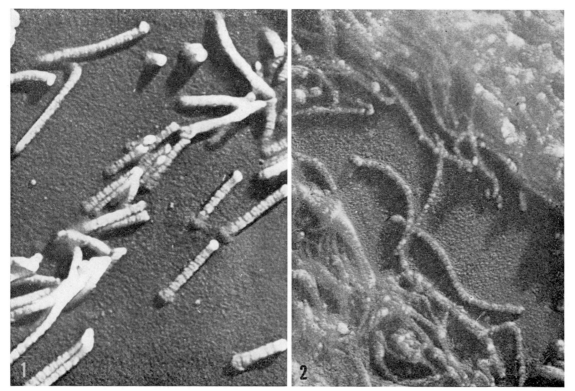

Figure 48. Electron micrographs of collagen in tissue sections cut at approximately 1/12 micron thickness and shadow cast with uranium.

1. So-called mature collagen fibrils from the iris stroma characterized by an average axial macroperiodicity of 640 A (from Tousimis and Fine, 1959). ×27,000.

2. Immature collagen filaments (or reticulin) from the vitreous body characterized by an average axial periodicity of 220 A (from Fine and Tousimis, 1961). ×47,000.

the periodic acid–Schiff procedure while the stromal collagen becomes brown with silver and pink with PAS. According to Kramer and Little, after treatment with sulfuric acid, reticulin becomes metachromatic while collagen remains orthochromatic.

Apparently reticulin is not significantly distinctive to be differentiated morphologically from "immature" collagen. Furthermore, histoenzymatic studies by Kramer and Little reveal identical reactions of collagen and reticulin, both are lysed by pepsin and collagenase but resist trypsin, alphachymotrypsin and testicular hyaluronidase. Nevertheless, there is reason to believe that an important chemical difference exists between reticulin and collagen, for immunologic studies have revealed them to be distinct. With the aid of fluorescent antiglomerulus globulin, Cruickshank and Hill found a common antigen in the basement membranes and reticulin of man and rat, but never was it found in collagen. It has been concluded that while the fibrillar component of reticulin almost certainly is a variety of collagen, the important histologic, chemical, and immunologic dissimilarities between reticular and collagen fibers are related to differences in the character and amount of ground substance and to the relationship of fibers to polysaccharides within the ground substance (Banfield, 1954; Cruickshank and Hill, 1953; Ehrich, 1952; Jacobson, 1953; Kramer and Little, 1953; Robb-Smith, 1952, 1953, 1954).

The terms reticulin and reticulum are often confused and improperly used. Reticulin, as just defined and described, is a type of connective tissue fiber. Many tissues (lymph nodes, spleen, and the uvea for example) have a very well-developed framework of reticulin fibers; such a reticular structure is called a reticulum.

While most of the ocular tissues contain fibers which are characteristic of "mature" collagen and reticulin, there are two noteworthy exceptions. The lens contains neither reticulin nor collagen. The vitreous body is peculiar in that its framework appears to be composed entirely of the "immature" type of filament with a 200 to 250 A periodicity (Fig. 48–2). According to Fine and Tousimis, these filaments stain in a manner characteristic of reticulin.

Elastin. Elastic fibers are refractile branching structures which vary in size, shape, distribution, and staining characteristics according to their anatomical site. Poorly stained by most dyes, elastin has an affinity for resorcin-fuchsin and orcein, and also for Schiff's reagent after treatment with periodic acid. Elastic fibers are remarkably insoluble, remaining after all other tissue elements have been removed by dilute acid or alkali. The amino acid content of elastin differs from that of collagen and it is not the same in the young as in the old. Lansing has suggested that the increased amounts of aspartic and glutamic acids in the aortas of older persons may account for the calcium-affinity of aging elastic tissue. Elastin resists pure trypsin and pepsin, but it is lysed by a pancreatic enzyme, elastase. Physically the elastic fiber is believed to be made up of an infinite number of generations of paired helically-coiled fibrils. A fiber visible with the ordinary light microscope treated with elastase splits into two coiled fibrils, each of which gives rise to two more coiled fibrils, and so on until the limits of resolution prohibit continued observation of the unravelling process. Results obtained by electron microscopy have been subject to question according to Lansing since preparations were not pure and since helically-coiled fibrils almost identical with those of elastic fibrils may be observed in phage-treated bacteria and in calcium soaps. In the eye, elastic fibers are found in the walls of the larger blood vessels and throughout the sclera and cornea. They are, of course, much less abundant than collagen and reticular fibers.

Ground Substance

The interstitial mucoid material, which fills the spaces between tissue cells and fibers and which we call ground substance, was studied extensively by embryologists long before it excited much attention among those interested in histology and pathology. From these early studies by Duran-Reynals and McCrea it was appreciated that ground substance of the mesenchyme (1) is a gel-like material exhibiting the general staining reactions of mucin; (2) provides anatomic and presumably physiologic support for the proliferating embryonic cells; and (3) furnishes a powerfully cohesive force which tends to keep the various tissue layers in place. During more recent years, this ground substance has been subjected to exhaustive study by chemists, physiologists, and electron microscopists, as well as histologists and pathologists. As a result we now conceive this viscid matrix to be a continuous gel completely filling all the so-called interstitial spaces. Chemically it is composed of water, electrolytes, protein and mucopolysaccharides. Mainly through the efforts of Karl Meyer and his associates we have considerable information about the acid mucopolysaccharides of ground substances; these include hyaluronic acid, the chondroitin sulfates (A, B, and C), and keratosulfate. There are two main groups, the sulfated and nonsulfated acid mucopolysaccharides. The latter are highly hydrated spacefillers which tend to serve as lubricants and shock-absorbers, but they are certainly not metabolically inert. The sulfated acid mucopolysaccharides are concentrated in less hydrated, more densely fibrillated connective tissues where they serve as cementing media and probably function as ion-exchange materials for the binding of important cations. Though the precise origin of these acellular elements of connective tissue is not established, it is generally assumed that they are secreted by mesenchymal cells.

Hyaluronic acid. Hyaluronic acid deserves special mention here, not only because of the current interest in the role it plays in controlling the resistance to aqueous outflow, but also because it was its very abundance in the vitreous that led to its isolation. Meyer, who first recovered the substance from the vitreous and found it to be a polymer of disaccharide composed of N-acetyl glucosamine and glucuronic acid, named it after the hyaloid body (hyaloid + uronic acid). Subsequently, it was found in many other tissues, notably the umbilical cord, synovial fluid, and cockscomb, as well as in certain bacterial cultures. In the eye it is most abundant in the vitreous, but its concentration there varies greatly among different animal species, and

also with the stage of development of the vitreous in a given species. According to Barany and to Zimmerman (1958) it also is normally present in the cornea, the aqueous, and within the trabecular meshwork, especially in the pore-tissue forming the inner wall of the canal of Schlemm where its presence is believed to account for a portion of the normal resistance to aqueous outflow. Strangely, hyaluronic acid does not occur in nature in sulfated form, according to Meyer, nor does there exist among the sulfated acid mucopolysaccharides a nonsulfated analogue, namely chondroitin.

Other acid mucopolysaccharides. Most of the other acid mucopolysaccharides that have been isolated and studied are sulfated. Chondroitin sulfate A, obtained from hyaline cartilage, and chondroitin sulfate C, from blood vessels and heart valves, may be confused with hyaluronic acid since they are said to be responsive to bovine testicular hyaluronidase. Bacterial hyaluronidases, however, do not depolymerize these chondroitin sulfates, and they are therefore more specific for hyaluronic acid. Although a mixture of acid mucopolysaccharides is present in the cornea and sclera, one in particular deserves special comment since it has been recovered only from the cornea. Again Meyer, who isolated this material, named it after the tissue from which he obtained it, keratosulfate. It is distinctive mainly because it is free of uronic acid. Recently the presence of an abundant interstitial substance which appears to be an acid mucopolysaccharide has been found about the rods and cones and between them and the retinal pigment epithelium. According to Zimmerman and Eastham, the chemical composition of this substance remains to be determined, but one fact is certain: this acid mucopolysaccharide resists the prolonged action of bovine testicular hyaluronidase. Although the function of this newly discovered mucoid material remains to be determined, a number of possibilities come to mind. It may serve as a cement substance, tending to keep the two layers of the optic cup in contact. It may somehow be concerned with the physiology of melanin since the outer (pigmented) layer of the optic cup seems to elaborate the substance. Finally, the material between the sensory retina and pigment epithelium might facilitate transportation of metabolites between the choriocapillaris and the retina or possibly furnish a suitable optical environment for the rods and cones.

Depolymerization of ground substance. Many factors are known to influence the physical state of ground substance in health and disease. Earlier in this chapter in the discussion of tissue reaction to irritants, for example, it was observed that among the very earliest changes observed in the immediate vicinity of an irritant is a change from gel to sol state of the ground substance. A variety of hormones are known to affect the ground substance, some increasing its amount and viscosity, others having an opposite effect. Associated with changes in viscosity of the ground substance are alterations in its barrier value; that is, the normal resistance to the spreading of particulate matter through the tissues is affected. Agents which promote more rapid diffusion by changing the state of the ground substance from a gel to a sol are therefore known as spreading factors. Certain bacteria which produce spreading factors (e.g., streptococci and clostridia) will therefore tend to become more widely and rapidly dispersed through the interstitial tissues and to produce such infections as erysipelas and gas gangrene. The best known and most active of these spreading factors are the hyaluronidases obtained from the bovine testis and from a variety of bacteria. The latter are more specific for the one substance, hyaluronic acid, while the bovine testicular enzyme exhibits chondromucinase activity, promoting depolymerization of chondroitin sulfate A and C as well. The potency of hyaluronidase may be measured by: (1) the degree to which it promotes spreading of particulate matter through tissue, (2) its effectiveness in reducing viscosity of a known substrate in vitro, (3) its ability to diminish the turbidity of solutions of the mucopolysaccharide, and (4) by determinations of an increasing concentration of hexosamine and/or uronic acid after treatment with the enzyme.

Mention must also be made here that mast cells are present throughout the uvea and that some workers believe these cells play an important role in the physiology of ground substance. According to Wagner, cortisone causes a loss of mast cell granules, but it is also said to affect ground substance profoundly by inhibiting the fibroblastic component of fibrillogenesis and the activity of hyaluronidase.

Degeneration and Proliferation

Pathology of connective tissue. A variety of degenerative and proliferative changes are observed in the connective tissues. The principal degenerative changes are mucoid, fibrinoid, amyloid, and paramyloid. *Mucoid degeneration* refers to an accumulation of acid mucopolysaccharides which, with ordinary staining methods, imparts a pale basophilic fibrillar appearance to the affected tissue. *Fibrinoid,* as defined by Neumann, is a form of connective tissue degeneration characterized by the development of bands or clumps of hyaline masses which resemble fibrin in their staining properties. Many subsequent workers have modified this definition in one way or another and some have tried to give undue pathogenetic meaning to the process. Today, however, it is generally recognized that fibrinoid degeneration occurs as a result of a rather broad assortment of pathologic situations, experimental as well as naturally occurring, and that there is no longer any reason for considering the lesion to be the direct morphologic expression of a specific hypersensitivity reaction. Moreover, as Wagner has emphasized, there are even distinctive histochemical differences among the fibrinoids which are present in the so-called diffuse collagen diseases. He observed that the fibrinoids of disseminated lupus erythematosus and scleroderma appear to be the result of fundamental metabolic disturbances in DNA and scleroprotein chemistry, respectively, while those of rheumatic fever and polyarteritis are more likely to be related to a hypersensitivity reaction. On the other hand, Vasquez and Dixon, utilizing immunohistochemical analysis, have shown that areas of fibrinoid necrosis in serum sickness, the Arthus reaction, amyloidosis, disseminated lupus erythematosus, rheumatic fever, and rheumatoid arthritis show an increased concentration of gamma globulin while in the generalized Shwartzman reaction, thrombotic thrombocytopenic purpura, and bilateral renal cortical necrosis accompanying premature separation of the placenta, lesions with fibrinoid necrosis exhibit a preferential concentration of fibrinogen or fibrin.

Amyloid and *paramyloid* are homogeneous structureless hyaline deposits in the ground substance and basement membranes. These are composed of mucopolysaccharide-protein complexes differing somewhat in physical and chemical characteristics from case to case. With the aid of Coons' fluorescent antibody technique, Vasquez and Dixon have demonstrated the preferential concentration of gamma globulin in human and experimental amyloidosis. Electrophoretic analyses of amyloid, on the other hand, have shown in some cases the presence of alpha-1 globulin and mucopolysaccharide moving as a complex, while in other instances the protein mucopolysaccharide complex contained alpha-2 and beta globulins. It has been suggested that amyloid and paramyloid represent connective tissue deposits which are derived from abnormal circulating protein mucopolysaccharide complexes (dysproteinemia) produced by dysfunctioning mesenchymal cells, mainly plasma cells. The cause for the abnormal plasmacytosis is often a specific antigenic stimulus, but this need not always be the case. The amyloidosis associated with multiple myeloma, for example, would seem to be the consequence of dysproteinemia produced by neoplastic plasma cells. The initial stimulus here remains unknown, of course, but it could be a virus, a chemical, or a genetic factor, as well as a specific antigenic substance.

Besides these degenerative changes, there are also a number of proliferative processes to be seen in the diffuse connective tissue diseases. These begin with mesenchymal cells, fibroblasts and their undifferentiated precursors, endothelial and perithelial cells, lymphocytes, plasma cells, etc. After excessive fibroblastic activity, much collagen may be deposited, a process called fibrosis. When this collagen is transformed into thick hyaline bands we speak of hyalinization or hyalinosis.

Collagen Diseases

Classification of connective tissue disorders.

The ever increasing use and abuse of the term "collagen diseases" has degraded it to the point that it is now about as nonspecific and meaningless as "uveitis." It should be recalled that Klemperer and his associates in coining the term, "diffuse collagen diseases," left no doubt that they were referring to the complete intercellular substance, but they employed the word "collagen" in a nonspecific sense for brevity's sake. Furthermore, they emphasized two essential features of disseminated lupus erythematosus and generalized scleroderma: (1) the conspicuous morphologic and physiologic alterations of the colloidal intercellular components of the connective tissues, and (2) the participation of the entire connective tissue system in these alterations. In recent years the group has been expanded (with justification) to include rheumatic fever, rheumatoid arthritis, disseminated lupus erythematosus, generalized scleroderma, dermatomyositis, polyarteritis (periarteritis nodosa), and serum sickness as well as many others which for one reason or another do not seem to belong, and therefore are not listed.

What, then, are the reasons for keeping the foregoing together as a group? Besides the original morphologic criteria, there are now certain biochemical and serologic features which tend to keep these disorders associated in our thinking. Ehrich has suggested an interesting working hypothesis to explain their pathogenesis, even though the specific etiologic factors in each may differ greatly. His idea is that the basic sequence in each of these is first the production of abnormal gamma globulins by plasma cells, and then the diffuse injury to connective tissues produced by these abnormal circulating proteins. Thus the so-called diffuse collagen diseases could be renamed "dysgammaglobulinemias," in order to separate them from other unrelated diffuse diseases of connective tissue, such as scurvy, myxedema, or arachnodactyly which have different pathogenetic mechanisms. It is possible that dysproteinosis or paraproteinosis might be more appropriate terms.

Connective tissue changes may therefore be subdivided, first, into localized and systemic disorders, and then according to etiologic or pathogenetic factors. Localized connective tissue lesions can be produced by physical trauma (e.g., keloids and pterygia), senescence (e.g., pingueculas), infection (e.g., erysipelas), hypersensitivity (e.g., urticaria), genetic factors (e.g., corneal dystrophies), etc. Systemic connective tissue diseases can result from avitaminoses (e.g., scurvy), metabolic defects (e.g., gout), hormonal disturbances (e.g., myxedema), genetic factors (e.g., arachnodactyly), dysgammaglobulinemia (e.g., lupus erythematosus), etc.

NEUROPATHOLOGY

Elements of Nervous Tissues

The retina and optic nerve, being modified parts of the central nervous system, are characterized by distinctive histologic details and pathologic reactions which deserve comment. Specialized histologic techniques must be employed in conjunction with the conventional methods of ophthalmic histology in order to recognize and differentiate the important cells and cell processes of the central nervous system, and to appreciate their pathologic morphology. Studies utilizing the methods of Cajal, Hortega, and their disciples have shown that the retina and optic nerve are composed of four main elements: neurons, neuroglia, microglia, and vascular connective tissue. The general form, function, and alterations of these will be considered here, but the reader is referred to Chapters VIII and IX for the special applications of this knowledge to pathology of the retina and optic nerve. Neurons and neuroglia are derived from the primitive medullary epithelium while the microglia and blood vessels are generally regarded as mesenchymal.

Neurons and Their Pathologic Changes

Neurons include all of the various specialized nerve cells which convey impulses from one area to another. Typical neurons have large cell bodies, huge nuclei and distinct nucleoli but there is much variation between the different types of neurons. Those of the ganglion cell layer, for example, are larger and more conspicuous than those of the inner and outer nuclear layers. Neurons possess two different kinds of cell processes, dendrites which conduct impulses towards the cell body and neurites (axons or axiscylinders) which transmit impulses away from it. The size, length and branching pattern of dendrites and neurites varies even more than does the appearance of the cell bodies. With routine histologic techniques individual cell processes cannot be distinguished with any degree of clarity. The plexiform layers of the retina, for example, appear as reticular zones of non-nucleated, nondescript tissue, whereas in reality this represents a meshwork of cell processes and their synapses. Many of the long axons of the central nervous system are sheathed in myelin but they are not invested by neurilemma as are the peripheral nerves. Axons together with whatever sheaths they might possess often are called nerve fibers. There are four classes of nerve fibers: (1) myelinated fibers with neurilemma, characteristic of the peripheral nerves; (2) myelinated fibers without neurilemma, found in the central nervous system, including the optic nerves; (3) unmyelinated (Remak) fibers of the sympathetic nervous system, and (4) naked axons found especially in gray matter and in the retina.

Acute neuronal degeneration. Neurons are highly specialized cells which have almost no ability to regenerate and none to proliferate. Any morphologic alterations observed are the result of degeneration or necrosis. A variety of such changes are recognized. These depend more upon differences in the severity and duration of insult than on the specific nature of the causative factors. Severe acute insults produce immediate damage which invariably leads to destruction of the cell. Bizarre swelling, fragmentation and dissolution of cell bodies and processes may be observed (Fig. 49). Such necrosis may be seen over large areas, as in cases of sudden occlusion of the central retinal artery and in acute panophthalmitis. When, in cases such as these, there is widespread destruction, other tissue elements will also be eliminated, and there is minimal reactive proliferation. The tissue at first appears edematous or cystic (status spongiosis), but later it collapses and appears

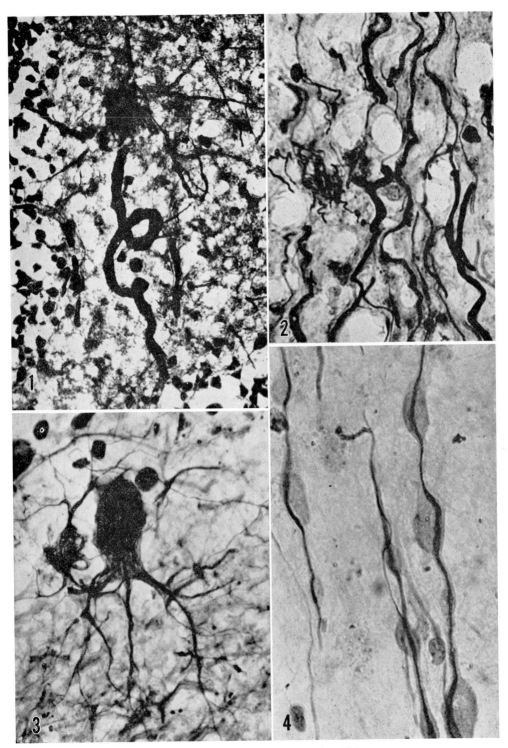

Figure 49. Degeneration and Necrosis of Neurons

1. Early dissolution of retinal ganglion cell in secondary glaucoma.
2. Fragmentation of optic nerve fibers secondary to craniopharyngioma.
3. Shrinkage of retinal ganglion cells in chronic primary glaucoma.
4. Irregular swelling of axons and myelin sheaths of nerve fibers in primary optic atrophy.
(Wolter's modification of Hortega's silver carbonate method.)

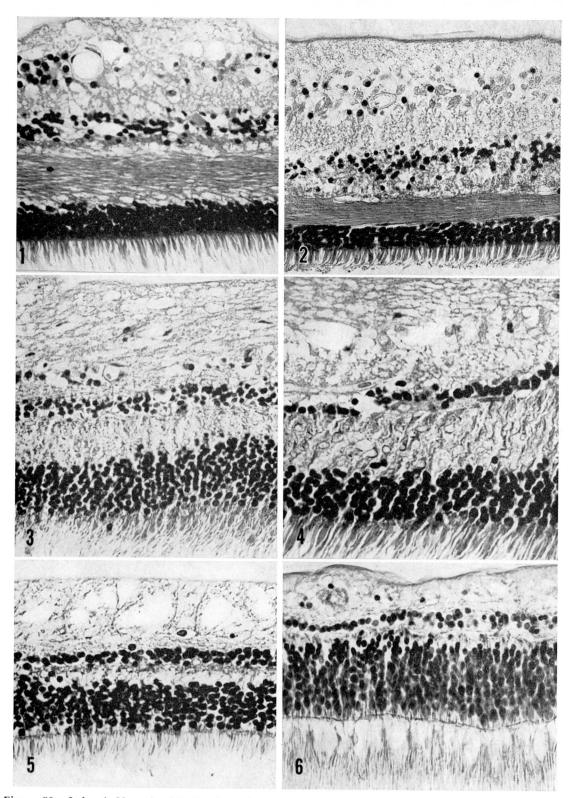

Figure 50. Ischemic Necrosis of Retina Secondary to Occlusion of Cenrtal Retinal Artery

1 and 2. Marked edematous swelling and incomplete destruction of ganglion cell layer of retina. ×305. AFIP Acc. 284675 and 679385, respectively.

3 and 4. More advanced destruction of ganglion cells and great depletion of nuclei in inner nuclear layer. ×305. AFIP Acc. 868622.

5. The edematous degenerated nerve fiber layer appears spongy and ganglion cells have disappeared. ×400. AFIP Acc. 679385.

6. The inner retinal layers have shrunk while the outer layers are well preserved. ×350. AFIP Acc. 650240. From Perraut and Zimmerman (1959).

shrunken (Fig. 50). More often there is selective damage to neurons because they are more vulnerable, and other cellular elements survive and react. Remnants of disintegrating ganglion cells are phagocytized by microglia, the scavengers of the central nervous system, and the defect is filled in by glial cells and fibers. This leads to a type of scarring generally referred to simply as "gliosis."

Chronic neuronal degeneration. In more chronic situations (e.g., chronic simple glaucoma) the neuronal changes are less striking, but a greater variety of stages may be discernible from one area to another. Some neurons appear swollen, and lipoidal vacuoles are present in their cytoplasm. Others, in later stages of degeneration, appear shrunken and ill-defined. Frequently only the pyknotic nuclei can be identified; cell bodies and processes are lost. Proliferated glial cells accumulate about the degenerative nerve cells. Some neurons appear to fade away, becoming progressively less well-stained and ultimately vanishing completely. Others seem to become hyalinized and are converted into laminated, non-nucleated spheroidal structures (Fig. 51–1, 2).

Degeneration of neurites. Pathologic processes leading to neuronal degeneration frequently begin in the long neurites at a considerable distance from their cell bodies. The eye furnishes an excellent example since the optic nerve is nothing more than an isolated bundle of such neurites and a great variety of lesions are known to produce alterations in these neurites, long before changes can be observed in the retinal ganglion cells. Similarly, the nerve fiber layer of the retina may be the site of changes which later will progress to involve the ganglion cells. In these neurites, the same variety of acute necrotizing and chronic degenerative changes as were described in the cell bodies may be observed. Special staining methods are imperative if one is to fully appreciate the irregular swelling, fragmentation, and dissolution that reflect the irreparable functional damage that has happened when a neurite is interrupted (Figs. 51, 52). Segments distal to the site of injury shrink and fade away rather quickly. Proximal segments still attached to their cell bodies survive longer, and characteristic ganglioform or varicose swellings develop at the free ends of the neurites at the site of injury. When this occurs focally in the nerve fiber layer of the retina, where it can be visualized directly, a soft fluffy-white superficial opacity often called a "cotton-wool exudate" is produced (see Chapter VIII). If only ordinary staining methods are used to examine such a lesion, the markedly swollen proximal end of the interrupted nerve fiber presents a superficial resemblance to a fading cell, hence the term "cytoid body" that has been applied to such lesions. These varicose swellings do not persist long for the severed neurite continues to degenerate. Ultimately the entire neuron disappears. It is well known, for example, that after longstanding atrophy of the optic nerve produced by lesions in the orbital or intracranial segments of the nerve the retinal architecture generally remains well preserved but there is a profound degeneration of the nerve fiber and ganglion cell layers. The microglial reaction that follows acute injury and the associated reactive proliferation of astrocytes (both of which will be more fully described later) are observed in nerve fiber bundles as well as in the regions occupied by cell bodies.

Regeneration after Wallerian degeneration. The type of neuronal degeneration just described, wherein there occurs a prompt dissolution of the distal segment which has been separated from the cell body, and a more gradual deterioration of the proximal segment and cell body, is known as *Wallerian degeneration.* Complete disintegration of the distal segment is observed after injuries of peripheral nerves as well as in the central nervous system. Ordinarily there is little or no trans-synaptic degeneration. Hence, examination of the retina of an eye with profound optic atrophy will reveal the inner and outer nuclear layers to be intact, even though there may have been a virtual disappearance of ganglion cells. Wallerian degeneration of the proximal segment of peripheral nerves usually is not very extensive and the demyelinizing process stops short of the cell body, usually at the next node of Ranvier. The neurilemmal cells which form a sheath investing the peripheral neurites possess a remarkable capacity for regeneration. These cells migrate from both the proximal and the distal segments towards each other to bridge

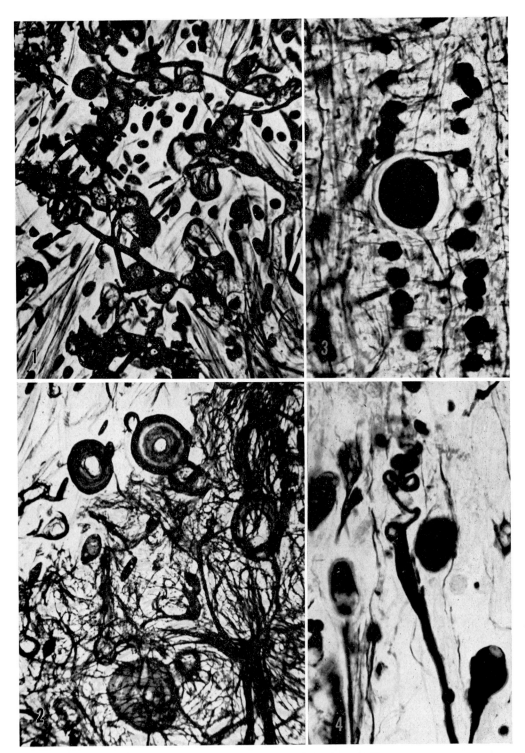

Figure 51. Degeneration with Hyalinization of Neurons

1 and 2. Numerous hyaline bodies derived from degenerated ganglion cells of peripheral retina in chronic secondary glaucoma.

3. Hyaline body formed in degenerated optic nerve fiber in senescence.

4. Terminal swellings of interrupted nerve fibers in retinal detachment; from the stump of one of these there has "regenerated" an irregular, partially coiled axis cylinder.

(Wolter's modification of Hortega's silver carbonate method.)

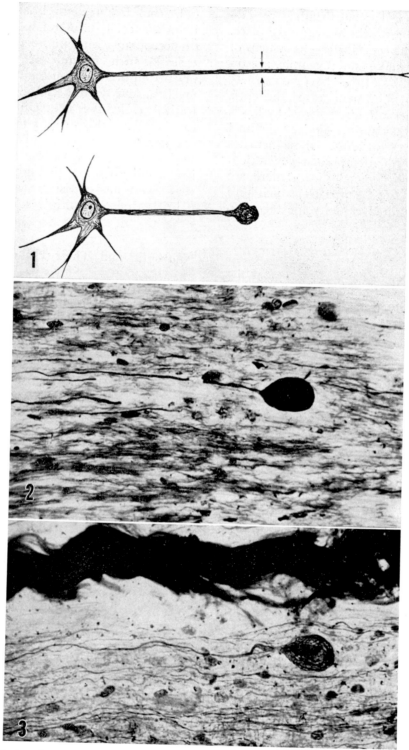

Figure 52. Wallerian degeneration of optic nerve fibers with ganglioform swelling of that part of interrupted axon still attached to cell body and dissolution of distal segment.
1. Schematic representation.
2. Nerve fiber layer of retina.
3. Optic nerve.
(Wolter's modification of Hortega's silver carbonate method.)

Production in the Rabbit Eye. J. Exp. Med. *54*:249–263, 1931.

Seegal, D., and Seegal, B. C.: Local Organ Hypersensitiveness; Inflammation Produced in the Actively Sensitized Rabbit Eye by the Introduction of Homologous Antigen into the Gastrointestinal Tract. J. Exp. Med. *54*:265–269, 1931.

Selye, H.: The Story of the Adaptation Syndrome. Montreal, Acta, Inc., 1952.

Selye, H.: The Part of Inflammation in the Local Adaptation Syndrome. In Jasmin and Robert: The Mechanism of Inflammation. Montreal, Acta, Inc., 1953, pp. 53–74.

Shwartzman, G.: Phenomenon of Local Tissue Reactivity and Its Immunological, Pathological, and Clinical Significance. New York, Paul B. Hoeber, 1937.

Silverstein, A. M., and Zimmerman, L. E.: Immunogenic Endophthalmitis Produced in the Guinea Pig by Different Pathogenetic Mechanisms. Amer. J. Ophthal. *48*:435–447, (Part II), 1959.

Silverstein, A. M., Welter, S., and Zimmerman, L. E.: A Progressive Immunization Reaction in the Actively Sensitized Rabbit Eye. J. Immunol. In press.

Speirs, R. S.: Physiological Approaches to an Understanding of the Function of Eosinophils and Basophils. Ann. N. Y. Acad. Sci. *59*:706–731, 1955.

Taubenhaus, M.: Further Studies of the Hormonal Regulation of Granulation Tissue Formation. In Jasmin and Robert: The Mechanism of Inflammation. Montreal, Acta, Inc., 1953, pp. 97–102.

Thuerer, G. R., and Angevine, D. M.: Influence of Dicumarol on Streptococcic Infection in Rabbits. A.M.A. Arch. Path. *48*:274, 1949.

Tompkins, E. H.: The Monocyte. Ann. N. Y. Acad. Sci. *59*:732–745, 1955.

Uhr, J. W., Pappenheimer, A. M., Jr., and Yoneda, M.: Delayed Hypersensitivity. I. Induction of Hypersensitivity to Diphtheria Toxin in Guinea Pigs by Infection with Corynebacterium Diphtheriae. J. Exp. Med. *105*:1–9, 1957.

Uhr, J. W., Salvin, S. B., and Pappenheimer, A. M., Jr.: Delayed Hypersensitivity: II. Induction of Hypersensitivity in Guinea Pigs by Means of Antigen-Antibody Complexes. J. Exp. Med. *105*:11–24, 1957.

Vasquez, J. J., and Dixon, F. J.: Immunohistochemical Analysis of Lesions Associated with "Fibrinoid Change." A.M.A. Arch. Path. *66*:504–517, 1958.

Verhoeff, F. H.: Obstruction of the Central Retinal Vein. A.M.A. Arch. Ophthal. *36*:1–36, 1907.

Verhoeff, F. H.: The Effect of Chronic Glaucoma on the Central Retinal Vessels. A.M.A. Arch. Ophthal. *42*:145–155, 1913.

von Szily, A.: Die Anaphylaxie in der Augenheilkunde-Experimenteller. Ferdinand Enke, Stuttgart, 1941.

Wagener, H. P., and Hollenhorst, R. W.: The Ocular Lesions of Temporal Arteritis. Trans. Amer. Ophthal. Soc. *55*:249–273, 1957.

Wagner, B. M., and Ehrich, W. E.: Adenosinase, Adenase and Xanthine Oxidase of Lymphoid Tissues. Fed. Proc. *9*:347–348, 1950.

Wagner, B. M.: Hypersensitivity: The Role of the Connective Tissue. In Mellors: Analytical Pathology. New York, McGraw-Hill, 1957, Chapter 7, pp. 429–470.

Waksman, B. H., and Bullington, S. J.: Quantitative Study of the Passive Arthus in the Rabbit Eye. J. Immun. *76*:441–453, 1956.

Wedgewood, R. J.: The Properdin System and Immunity: A Review. In Najjar, V. A., ed.: Immunity and Virus Infection, New York, Wiley, 1959, pp. 56–70.

Wessely, K.: Zur Frage der Anaphylaktischen Erscheinungen an der Hornhaut. Klin. Monatsbl. f. Augenh. *15*:508, 1913.

Wilder, H. C.: Toxoplasma Chorioretinitis in Adults. A.M.A. Arch. Ophthal. *48*:127–136, 1952.

Wilson, G. S., and Miles, A. A.: Topley and Wilson's Principles of Bacteriology and Immunity. 4th ed., Baltimore, Williams & Wilkins Company, 1955.

Witmer, R.: Experimental Leptospiral Uveitis in Rabbits. A.M.A. Arch. Ophthal. *53*:547–559, 1955.

Witmer, R.: Antibody Formation in Rabbit Eyes Studied with Fluorescein-labeled Antibody. A.M.A. Arch. Ophthal. *53*:811–816, 1955.

Wolter, J. R.: Astroglia of the Human Retina and Other Glial Elements of the Retina Under Normal and Pathologic Conditions. Amer. J. Ophthal. *40*:88–100, (Part II), 1955.

Wolter, J. R.: Über besondere Astroglia an der Innenfläche der Retina. Klin. Monatsbl. Augenh. *129*:224–230, 1956.

Wolter, J. R.: Reactions of Elements of Retina and Optic Nerve in Common Morbid Entities of the Human Eye. Amer. J. Ophthal. *42*:10–27 (Part II), 1956.

Wolter, J. R.: The Human Optic Papilla; A Demonstration of New Anatomic and Pathologic Findings. Amer. J. Ophthal. *44*:48–65, (Part II), 1957.

Wolter, J. R.: Das Verhalten der Astroglia bei fortgeschrittener Degeneration der Netzhaut; eine histopathologische Studie an phthisischen Augen mit sekundärer Netzhautablösung. Klin. Monatsbl. Augenh. *130*:498–511, 1957.

Wolter, J. R.: Perivascular Glia of the Blood Vessels of the Human Retina. Amer. J. Ophthal. *44*:766–773, 1957.

Wolter, J. R.: Hyaline Bodies of Ganglion-cell Origin in the Human Retina. A.M.A. Arch. Ophthal. *61*:127–134, 1959.

Wolter, J. R.: Glia of the Human Retina. Amer. J. Ophthal. *48*:370–393, (Part II), 1959.

Wolter, J. R.: Pathology of a Cotton-Wool Spot. Amer. J. Ophthal. *48*:473–485, 1959.

Wolter, J. R., and Butler, R. G.: Zur Pathologie des Papillenödems des menschlichen Auges. Klin. Monatsbl. Augenh. *130*:154–163, 1957.

Wolter, J. R., and Liss, L.: Hyaline Bodies of the Human Optic Nerve; Histopathologic Study of a Case of Advanced Syphilitic Optic Atrophy. A.M.A. Arch. Ophthal. *61*:780–788, 1959.

Wolter, J. R., Goldsmith, R. I., and Phillips, R. L.: Histopathology of the Star-Figure of the Macular Area in Diabetic and Angiospastic Retinopathy. A.M.A. Arch. Ophthal. *57*:376–385, 1957.

Wright, H. D.: Experimental Pneumococcal Septicaemia and Anti-Pneumococcal Immunity. J. Path. Bact. *30*:185–252, 1927.

Zimmerman, A. A., and Becker, S. W., Jr.: Precursors of Epidermal Melanocytes in the Negro Fetus. In Gordon, M.: Pigment Cell Biology, New York, Academic Press, 1959, pp. 159–170.

Zimmerman, L. E.: Demonstration of Histoplasma and Coccidioides in So-called Tuberculomas of Lung; Preliminary Report of 35 Cases. A.M.A. Arch. Intern. Med. *94*:690–699, 1954.

Zimmerman, L. E.: Fatal Fungus Infections Complicating Other Diseases. Amer. J. Clin. Path. *25*:46–65, 1955.

Zimmerman, L. E.: Demonstration of Hyaluronidase-Sensitive Acid Mucopolysaccharide in Trabecula and Iris in Routine Paraffin Sections of Adult Human Eyes; a Preliminary Report. Amer. J. Ophthal. *44*: 1–4, 1957.

Zimmerman, L. E.: Application of Histochemical Methods for the Demonstration of Acid Mucopolysaccharides to Ophthalmic Pathology. Trans. Amer. Acad. Ophthal. Otolaryng. *62*:697–703, 1958.

Zimmerman, L. E.: First Sloan Foundation Symposium on Uveitis. Survey Ophthal. *4*:370–375 (Part II), 1959.

Zimmerman, L. E., and Eastham, A. B.: Acid Mucopolysaccharide in the Retinal Pigment Epithelium and Visual Cell Layer of the Developing Mouse Eye. Amer. J. Ophthal. *47*:488–499, (Part II), 1959.

Zimmerman, L. E., and Johnson, F. B.: Calcium Oxalate Crystals within Ocular Tissues; A Clinicopathologic and Histochemical Study. A.M.A. Arch. Ophthal. *60*:372–383, 1958.

Zimmerman, L. E., and Rappaport, H.: Occurrence of Cryptococcosis in Patients with Malignant Disease of the Reticuloendothelial System. Amer. J. Clin. Path. *24*:1050–1072, 1954.

Zimmerman, L. E., and Silverstein, A. M.: Experimental Ocular Hypersensitivity; Histopathologic Changes Observed in Rabbits Receiving a Single Injection of Antigen into the Vitreous. Amer. J. Ophthal. *48*:447–465, (Part II), 1959.

Zinsser, H.: On the Essential Identity of the Antibodies. J. Immun. *6*:289–299, 1921.

Zweifach, B. W.: An Analysis of the Inflammatory Reaction Through the Response of the Terminal Vascular Bed to Microtrauma. In Jasmin and Robert: The Mechanism of Inflammation. Montreal, Acta, Inc., 1953, pp. 77–86.

Zweifach, B. W.: The Exchange of Materials Between Blood Vessels and Lymph Compartments. In Ragan, C.: Transactions of the Fifth Conference on Connective Tissue. New York, Josiah Macy, Jr. Foundation, 1954, pp. 38–77.

Chapter II

Diffuse Ocular

Disease and Its Sequelae

The tissue responses to injurious agents have been described in some detail in Chapter I to provide a background for the understanding of the gross and microscopic changes produced by disease in the human eye.

Those conditions which produce widespread changes in the eye will be discussed in this chapter. They include a variety of congenital and acquired diseases. The detailed changes produced by some of these diseases in individual tissues of the eye will be described in subsequent chapters.

ANATOMY AND HISTOLOGY

The enucleated human eye has a spherical shape. Its average dimensions are approximately 25 mm. anteroposteriorly, 24 mm. transversely and 24 mm. vertically.

The cornea changes the shape of this sphere, being somewhat more sharply curved than the sclera. It has a horizontal diameter of 12 mm. and a vertical diameter of 11 mm. in the adult. A shallow groove, known as the external scleral furrow, is seen in the limbal region at the juncture of cornea and sclera. If one views the eye from its superior aspect it can be seen that the temporal side has a longer arc from cornea to optic nerve than the nasal side. The optic nerve thus is placed toward the nasal side.

It may be desirable to distinguish the right from the left eye in enucleated specimens in order to identify the various quadrants. This helps orient the eye so that microscopic sections can be prepared in the proper plane to demonstrate pathologic processes. The following method seems best. The eye is held so that its posterior half can be seen. The entrances of the ciliary nerves on either side of the optic nerve serve to identify the horizontal meridian. The inferior oblique muscle attachment is seen near the horizontal meridian at the temporal side of the optic nerve. It is easy to identify because its muscle fibers extend up to the actual point of insertion. The thin tendinous superior oblique muscle

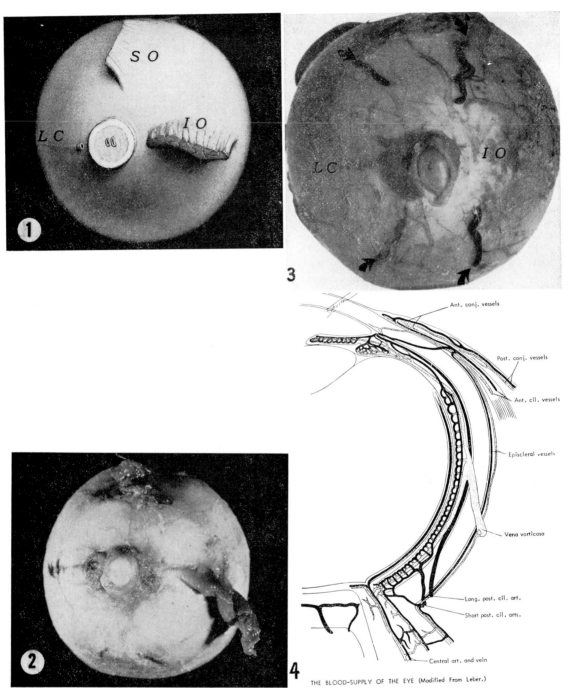

Figure 58.

1. Schematic drawing of posterior surface of right eye to show position of oblique muscle insertions in relation to optic nerve.

2. Posterior surface of right eye photographed and enlarged 2½ ×.

The enucleated eye is oriented most easily by examination of its posterior surface and identification of the attached oblique muscles. The inferior oblique (I.O.), which is a fleshy muscle even at its insertion into the sclera, is situated on the temporal side of the optic nerve in a position which corresponds with the macula. The superior oblique (S.O.) is almost completely tendinous and inserts above the nerve; its fibers are directed nasally. The long posterior ciliary vessels and nerves (L.C.) are always most conspicuous on the nasal side.

3. Right eyeball viewed from behind. Severed optic nerve with its dural sheath occupies the center of the field. Arrows point to sites of emergence of the four vortex veins. The extraocular muscles have been cut so close to the globe that they are not identifiable except for portions of the inferior oblique (I.O.). The long posterior ciliary vessels and nerves (L.C.) are seen on the nasal side.

4. Schematic representation of blood supply to the eye.

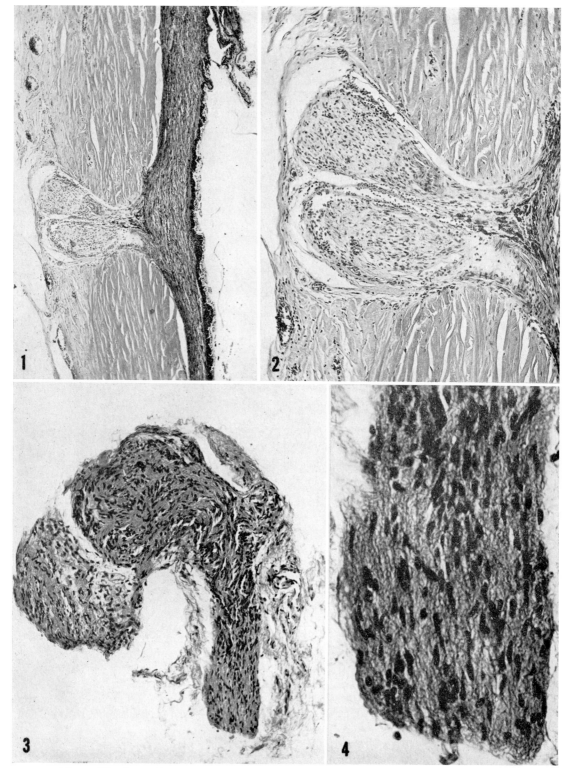

Figure 59. Intrascleral loops of ciliary nerves and blood vessels in region of pars plana.

1. ×50. 2. ×115. AFIP Acc. 840608.

3 and 4. An episcleral nerve loop that was excised with a clinical diagnosis of conjunctival cyst. ×145 and 525, respectively. AFIP Acc. 966456.

insertion is identified in the upper temporal quadrant. Once the horizontal meridian and the superior and inferior oblique muscles are identified the observer knows which is the temporal side, and which are the upper and lower halves of the eye (Fig. 58).

Further identification is obtained from the position of the rectus muscles. The medial rectus muscle attaches to the eye approximately 5.5 mm. from the cornea, the inferior rectus 6.5 mm., the lateral rectus approximately 7 mm., and the superior rectus 7.7 mm. The superior oblique muscle tendon terminates in the upper temporal portion of the posterior sclera in a rather broad insertion which is somewhat curved, with the convexity posterior. The oblique fibers then pass nasalward to the trochlea. The anterior insertion of this muscle lies in about the same meridian as the temporal edge of the insertion of the superior rectus muscle. The inferior oblique muscle inserts on the temporal side of the eye near the horizontal meridian and fairly close to the optic nerve, the nasal end of the insertion usually lying within 5 to 7 mm. of the optic nerve sheaths. The insertion line is somewhat curved, with the convexity upward. From its attachment the muscle passes downward. The direction of the superior and inferior oblique muscle fibers also assists in orienting the enucleated eye.

The upper vortex veins emerge from the sclera approximately 7 mm. (nasal), and 8 mm. (temporal) posterior to the equator. The lower vortex veins emerge on either side of the vertical meridian approximately 6 mm. posterior to the equator (Fig. 58). The an-

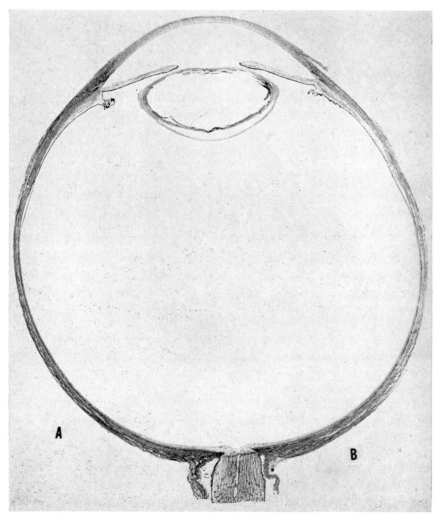

Figure 60. Anteroposterior section through pupil and optic disk. Lens nucleus lost during technical procedures. A, temporal side. B, nasal side. ×5. AFIP Acc. 165732.

terior ciliary arteries enter the sclera just in front of the insertion of the rectus muscles, and pass to the suprachoroidea, where they become continuous with the major circle of the iris. In some normal eyes, branches of the long posterior ciliary nerves loop externally through the sclera over the pars plana of the ciliary body and appear subconjunctivally as *intrascleral nerve loops* (Fig. 59). Frequently these are surrounded by pigmented uveal cells.

It may be desirable to determine whether a particular *microscopic section* being studied represents a vertical or horizontal plane (Fig. 60). If the nerve head and the macular region are present in the same section, it must have been cut approximately in the horizontal plane. The retina on each side of the optic nerve should be observed. If the ganglion cell layer is found to contain three or more layers it indicates the region of the macula, and therefore, the temporal side. If muscle fibers are attached to the sclera near the optic nerve, they represent the temporal insertion of the inferior oblique muscle. In horizontal sections the long ciliary arteries and nerves may be seen passing through the sclera to the suprachoroidea. The physiologic excavation of the optic nerve head usually is displaced somewhat temporally, while the major vessels are placed more to the nasal side of the disk. The ciliary body is better developed (more like the hyperopic eye) on the nasal side, and less developed (more like the myopic eye) on the temporal side, and the ciliary epithelial cells (particularly the pigmented layer) in the pars plana are larger on the temporal than on the nasal side. Cystoid degeneration (Blessig; Iwanoff) (see Chapter VIII) usually is more prominent on the temporal side.

GROWTH AND AGING

The growth and aging of the various parts of the eye will be discussed in some detail in subsequent chapters. Reference will be made here to changes occurring during general development of the eye.

Prenatal growth. The subject of *prenatal growth and differentiation* belongs in the field of embryology and will not be discussed here in detail. It has been shown that one part of an organism may exert an influence on another part, causing it to differentiate in a specific manner, and also that a disorderly pattern of growth results if one part of an organism is removed during development. This was demonstrated by Spemann, who produced neural plate formation in amphibia, using crushed tissue from the region of the dorsal lip. His work has been confirmed by many other investigators. Many of the basic experiments illustrative of this phenomenon of induction have been performed on embryonic ocular tissues in amphibia. The development of the optic vesicle is followed by an invagination of the overlying surface epithelium forming the lens vesicle. If the optic vesicle is removed, this invagination of the surface epithelium does not occur. If the surface over the optic vesicle is removed and replaced by a graft of surface epithelium taken from another portion of the embryo, the lens bud will develop in the grafted epithelium. Thus Boell has shown that the optic vesicle induces lens formation and that the surface epithelium from many parts of the embryo has the potency to produce a lens when subjected to the proper inductive influence.

In spite of a generation of intense study the mechanism of induction remains obscure. Needham and others have shown that tissue extracts obtained from the embryo, and indeed many substances taken from the chemist's bottles, have a partial inductive influence. Needham suggested that a particular inducing agent exists for each type of induction and suggested the name "organizer" for such agents. His experiments indicated that the organizers may be hydrocarbons of the steroid group.

Studies by Spiegelman and others have shown that the enzyme content of cells is greatly influenced by the presence of various substrates. It is their impression that the phenomena of induction and differentiation may rest on a much more complex set of metabolic interactions of adjacent tissue than one tissue and an inductive response to such a hormone-like substance by the neighboring tissue. An excellent discussion of the present knowledge in this complex field is to be found in the report of Danielli and Brown in the Cambridge University Symposium on Growth.

For a brief but excellent review of the subject the student is referred to *Human Embryology* by Hamilton, Boyd and Mossman.

Postnatal growth. As far as the eye is concerned, it seems probable that the influence of organizers of the type suggested by Needham is no longer exerted when differentiation of the tissues has been accomplished. In man this differentiation is essentially completed at birth, but there are certain animals in which differentiation of the ocular tissues continues for some time postnatally. In rats and rabbits the rods and cones do not develop until after birth. However, though the influence of the supposed organizers ceases when differentiation is completed, the mutual influence of the metabolic interaction of adjacent tissues must continue as long as the tissues survive, and hence, must play a role in postnatal growth and aging.

The maximum size of the body is usually attained toward the beginning of the third decade, whereas that of the eye is reached somewhat earlier. According to Drualt and Drualt, the average length of the eyeball of a *newborn* is approximately 16.5 mm., and the horizontal and vertical diameters measure approximately 19–20 mm. The word *size* is used here to connote size resulting from true growth, which, once attained, does not vary except through the atrophy of old age. The fat and water content of the body may increase under the influence of faulty habits and metabolism, but this cannot be interpreted as true growth.

Multiplication of cells does occur during growth, but increase in body size is accomplished for the most part by the maturation of individual cells rather than by increase in their number. It would be expected, then, that the least conspicuous postnatal change would be found in tissues composed largely of cells which are highly differentiated, or adult in type, at birth. Such tissue is represented in the eye by the sensory retina, the largest component of which is highly differentiated neurons, and by the retinal pigment epithelium. The process of maturation is particularly apparent in the supporting structures of the body—connective tissue and glial elements. The mesenchymal cells lay down collagen and elastic tissue (in their more differentiated forms, cartilage, bone, and muscle fibers), which together with an increase in intercellular ground substance add to the length and bulk of the body. Glial fibers are the greatest contributors to the enlarging mass of the central nervous system. As the fibrous element increases, the nuclear element becomes less conspicuous, and in the mature cell the nucleus may atrophy and disappear. This is demonstrated in the formation of scar tissue where young cellular tissue with delicate fibrils is converted into a hyaline, collagenous, anuclear mass.

Surface epithelium continues to grow throughout life, but after full growth is attained this is largely a matter of replacement of old desquamating cells by new. Such growth proceeds by mitosis and, as long as normal balance is maintained, does not disturb the proportional relationships between the cell types. The replacement process is most active in the small intestine and the epiderm. In the ocular tissues, it is most active in the lids, less so in the epithelium of the cornea and conjunctiva, and almost absent in the glandular structures.

In the growing eye, as elsewhere, some structures which attain their full growth and fulfill their functions during fetal life atrophy before birth; an example of this is the hyaloid system of vessels. In the fetal eye, strands of fibrous tissue bridge the filtration angle. They persist for a year or two after birth, but eventually atrophy and disappear. During growth little change is seen in the corneal epithelium and endothelium, in the retinal epithelium, the sensory retina, or in the epithelium of the ciliary body and iris. The lens retains its congenital pattern, although over a long time it increases from 7 up to 9 mm. (equatorial) in size by the laying down of more fibers. Its general form, however, changes very little with growth. In the corneal substantia propria and sclera where a certain maturity is evidenced at birth by the presence of collagenous and elastic fibers, there is moderate thickening and increased density of stromal fibers with a proportionate decrease in nuclei.

The newborn sclera is thinner, less condensed and more transparent than in the adult eye and the underlying vascular uveal tissues are more visible, giving it a bluish hue.

Rapid growth occurs in the cornea during the first year of life so that the approximate diameter of the adult cornea is attained.

Considerable growth occurs in the anterior segment of the eye during the first six or seven years of life. Minimal changes occur up to the age of fourteen, following which growth is more rapid up to the age of twenty-five. These changes would seem to account for the progress of myopia in established cases and the onset of the disease in others during these growth periods.

The most striking changes are in the uveal tract and optic nerve where the entire substantia becomes thicker and more fibers are seen in relation to the number of nuclei. Crypts in the anterior iris surface, resulting from a patchy atrophy related to atrophy of the pupillary membrane, may not be evident at birth but become prominent during the first year or two of life. Melanin granules are not numerous in the melanoblasts of the iris until a few days or more after birth. Their subsequent increase in density accounts for the deepening color of the iris. In the ciliary body of the young eye the corona is flat. The prominent corona of the adult results from thickening of muscle fibers combined with an increase in the surrounding connective tissue. It is the increase of connective tissue in the vascular layer that explains the difference between the narrow processes of the young eye and the broad processes of the adult eye. Ciliary processes on the posterior surface of the peripheral portion of the iris, present in fetal life and seen in many animals, normally move backward at, or soon after, birth in man and simians. In the young choroid, pigment is so sparse and its nuclei so numerous that the neophyte in eye pathology may interpret them as infiltrating inflammatory cells. In the optic nerve, the dural and pial sheaths and the septa all become thicker and more prominent during growth. The arachnoid villi, which are cellular and filamentous at birth, become greatly thickened and comparatively anuclear. In the nerve itself, where glial elements are more abundant than in the retina, the fibrillar content increases as it does in fibroblastic tissue. Myelination of the axis cylinders probably is not complete until after birth.

Aging. The changes associated with growth merge so gradually into those associated with aging that no sharp line of demarcation distinguishes one from the other. In principle, there would appear to be no difference between the process of atresia that leads to the disappearance of the hyaloid vascular system or the pupillary membrane of the embryo and the atresia that leads to peripapillary choroidal atrophy in the aging adult. Similarly, there would appear to be no difference in principle between the increasing accumulation of collagenous material that characterizes much of postnatal growth, and the hyalinization or other "degenerative" changes that occur in this collagenous material in the aged.

Though differences in principle between what we call development, growth, aging and degeneration are hard, or perhaps impossible, to establish, the fact remains that in the human eye there is a prolonged period from adolescence to middle age during which there is relatively little change. Finally, however, certain histologic features become manifest which, although by no means consistent either in the order or universality of their appearance, are more common in old eyes. It has been suggested that the body changes usually associated with advancing years may not be an inevitable aging process, but an aging disease of unknown etiology. In the absence of convincing evidence, it is generally accepted that although the ultimate degenerative process common to all living things is inevitable, it often is hastened and intensified by such factors as local or systemic disease and the buffeting of an unfavorable environment. In support of this, evidence of degeneration, similar to that found almost routinely in the eyes of the old, may be seen in young eyes enucleated because of local disease process, but only rarely in eyes removed from young persons at autopsy following traumatic death.

The so-called senile changes which affect

the eye include sclerosis of blood vessels, fatty infiltration, hyalinization of connective tissue, calcareous degeneration, and other degenerative and proliferative changes which seem unrelated to any specific general or local disease.

CONGENITAL AND DEVELOPMENTAL ABNORMALITIES

The concept of the etiology of congenital and developmental abnormalities has undergone considerable change in recent years. Advances in medical genetics, cytochemistry and physiology have been of such a character that interpretation of the cause of many types of congenital and developmental diseases is easier.

It is not completely understood how changes in the genes produce abnormal effects on tissues, but the biochemical changes in some diseases suggest that each gene controls a specific enzyme system. For example in albinism, there is an inability to convert intermediate products along the chain of reactions leading to synthesis of melanin.

It is now recognized that a number of degenerative or vascular diseases most likely are due to a genetic disturbance. Formerly it was believed that genetic disturbances led to defects which were apparent only at birth or within a short time after birth. Retinitis pigmentosa and the macular degenerations, however, may become apparent early in life or have a delayed onset into middle age, demonstrating that the genetic defect does not have to exert its effects until later life. Very recent studies in patients with retinitis pigmentosa show extensive alteration of the electroretinogram very early in life, prior to development of ophthalmoscopic evidence of the disease.

A number of conditions, now classified with senile degenerations, also may be due to a predetermined gene disturbance, for example, the occurrence of presenile and senile cataracts in many members of certain families, and the definite hereditary pattern of open angle glaucoma in other families.

Definitions. Some confusion exists about the exact meaning of words used to describe many congenital and developmental abnormalities. A definition may be helpful in understanding subsequent descriptions. *Developmental* abnormalities include those occurring between the time of fertilization of the ovum and the adult stage of development. Under this is included *congenital* abnormalities. An example would be a developmental cataract of the primary lens fibers (embryonal cataract), which also is congenital (present at birth). Another example is the discovery of glaucoma in a 5 month old child who has enlarged corneas and other signs of anomalous development of the anterior eye. An *anomaly* is any deviation from the usual form of any part or organ. A *variation* is a minor anomaly—a fairly common, mild deviation from the normal of a type, for example, the presence of a cilioretinal artery. Function may not be disturbed appreciably. An *abnormality* (abnormity) is a deviation in form, structure, or position of greater extent than a variation, e.g., congenital aniridia, congenital dislocation of the lens. An *arrest* indicates that normal development of a structure stopped at a stage short of completion of growth. A *simple arrest* of development means that no further growth occurred in the affected part, e.g., the anterior chamber angle in congenital glaucoma. An *arrest with aberration* indicates that there was abnormal development of the tissue after the arrest, e.g., microphthalmia with a cyst in the orbit. Arrested development in one part may cause a secondary anomalous condition of surrounding parts, e.g., the lack of development of the neural ectoderm in the absence of the lens, and failure of development of the choriocapillaris due to absence of the retinal pigment epithelium. An *aberration* is a variation or deviation from normal form, structure or course, resulting in an arrangement that is anatomically abnormal for the species, such as an inversion of the disk.

Anomalies Affecting the Eye as a Whole

Gross deformities of the eye most often have their onset early in embryonic life, and usually are diffuse and profound. They can be classified according to the stage of onset: prior to the formation of the optic vesicle, or following development of this structure.

Anophthalmos. Anophthalmos may arise in three ways:

1. There is failure of outgrowth of the optic vesicle from the forebrain. The failure must occur at a period after formation of the forebrain (2 mm. stage), because many of these infants exhibit no other nervous system defect.

2. The entire forebrain and its derivatives, the optic vesicles, fail to form.

3. Formation, followed by complete regression of the vesicle, so that no trace of an eye can be found in the orbit. This condition has been produced experimentally in various animals, especially in mice and rats, by the use of injurious agents. Some strains of rats and mice have anophthalmos but a hereditary type of transmission has not been found.

Anophthalmos most often is bilateral. Some reports describe anophthalmos on one side, and microphthalmos on the opposite. Heredity plays a part in the development of this condition in humans, although the mode of inheritance is uncertain.

The orbits are usually small but well formed. The eyelids are somewhat concave, but well developed. The conjunctival sac is reduced in size. An eye usually cannot be felt in the orbit on palpation. The muscles may be present and well developed. Autopsies of some infants with true bilateral anophthalmos show an absence of the chiasm, small geniculate bodies, and small optic foramina. Serial sections of the orbit show no eyeball. Other cases show some tissue in the orbit near its apex which is composed of a fibrous vascular pigmented tissue and necrotic retina. Hemicephalic infants may show a partial formation of the optic nerve.

Cyclopia. Cyclopia is a rather rare anomaly in which all the elements of the two eyes appear in the midline region of the forehead to form a single structure of varying composition. This condition appears to be due to some factors acting on the anterior end of the neural plate at a very early stage. The condition which leads to cyclopia appears to be a defect of the determinizer-inducer mechanism rather than a primary defect of the optic plate. Atypical differentiation of the mesoderm in the region of the future optic vesicles occurs, and as a result the areas of neural ectoderm which are predestined to form the eyes remain in contact with each other (particularly the medial portions) to a variable degree, producing this defect. Most experimental embryologists agree that the very great regularity of the pattern in those cyclopic eyes which remain as double structures mitigates against the theory that two eyes are first formed, then fuse to form the cyclopean eye.

This condition always is congenital, and since it is connected with other abnormalities which are incompatible with life, cannot be hereditary.

On examination of the cyclopean fetus the striking feature is the replacement of the two normal eyes by a single or double median eye (Fig. 61–1). Anomalous development of the nose is usual, this structure either being absent, or replaced by a proboscis-like structure located above the eye.

Usually the two eyes are fused along their medial aspects, and are enclosed in one orbit. Very rarely the two eyes are fused into a single eye which is placed in the midline in one orbit.

Microscopically there may be many major or minor defects in the various tissues of these eyes, especially in the retina and uveal tract. There may be persistence of the hyaloid system and tunica vasculosa lentis. Some of the inner choroid usually fails to develop in the areas of contact between the two eyes if the pigment epithelium fails to form and become pigmented. Folding and rosette-formation may occur at various sites in the retina, particularly near the ora serrata. The optic nerve or nerves may show various defects, such as colobomas, optic pits, or varying degrees of fusion. The extraocular muscles often are well developed, and vary in number.

Eyes which are fused usually have small corneas and are joined by a bridge of sclera. The anterior chamber angle structures usually are poorly developed, and there may be an absence of trabecular meshwork and the canal of Schlemm. The sclera commonly is missing between two fused eyes, the choroid, retina, and vitreous occupying a single large space.

Congenital cystic eyeball. Congenital cystic eyeball must be distinguished from microphthalmos with a cyst, in which there is a small eyeball with an attached orbital cyst

(Fig. 61–2). In congenital cystic eyeball there is failure of invagination of the optic vesicle, so that the orbit contains a cystic structure of varying size. Examination shows the lids and conjunctiva to be normal. The cyst has a bluish color, due to the contained fluid and the uveal pigment. Microscopic examination may show the anterior layers to contain some of the neuroectodermal elements, but these usually have disappeared by birth, due to stretching of the vesicle. Such cysts may be uniloculated or multiloculated, depending on the growth and position of adjacent tissues. Sometimes the ocular muscle insertions are seen in the wall of the cyst, which is composed principally of fibrous connective tissue. The remaining orbital structures usually are normal.

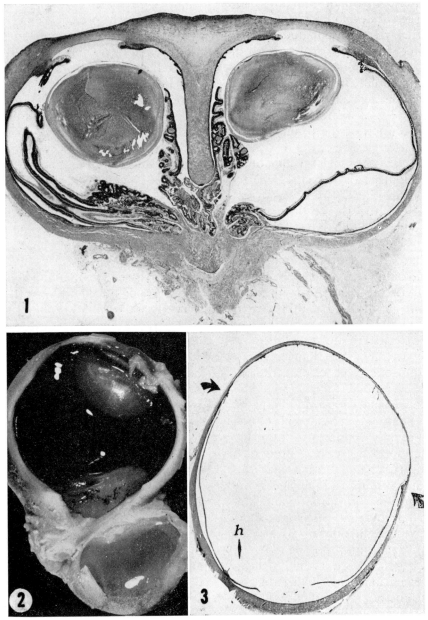

Figure 61.

1. Cyclopia. ×5. AFIP Acc. 51488.
2. Microphthalmos with orbital cyst. AFIP Acc. 505533.
3. Microphthalmos, congenital aphakia, and persistent hyaloid vessels (h). ×3. The limbal zone is indicated by arrows. AFIP Acc. 896509.

Arrest at the stage of partial invagination of the vesicle by the developing lens may lead to lesser degrees of cyst formation. In some instances the optic vesicle invaginates incompletely, leading to the condition known as congenital nonattachment of the retina.

Microphthalmos. Microphthalmos occurs after development of the primary optic vesicle. The term applies in those instances where an eye has formed, no matter how primitive. This condition arises in man between the 7 and 14 mm. stages of development, when the optic vesicle already has invaginated but the fetal cleft has not closed. A very rare form of this condition is exemplified by pure microphthalmos (nanophthalmos) in which a small but otherwise normal eye is found in the orbit. Most types of microphthalmos are the result of involution of the primary optic vesicle and failure of closure of the fetal cleft. Another group is associated with an abnormality in development of the surface ectoderm, in which case there may be failure of lens formation and an eye containing only retina surrounded by sclera is formed (Fig. 61–3).

Microphthalmos frequently accompanies other ocular anomalies (e.g., persistent hyperplastic primary vitreous), and it may be associated with more generalized malformations such as dyscranium, urogenital defects and polydactylia. Its causes are multiple but those which are most frequent are secondary to a genetic defect or some type of infection of the embryo.

MICROPHTHALMOS DUE TO FETAL INFECTION. Microphthalmos developing as a result of late fetal infections usually is due to intrauterine atrophy of a well-formed eye. Infections such as toxoplasmosis, rubella, and other virus diseases, may produce widespread damage to the intraocular structures, with atrophy and failure of further development. Such eyes show moderate to severe reduction in size, small corneas which may or may not be opaque, posterior synechias, cataract, retinal detachment, and degeneration of the uveal tract.

MICROPHTHALMOS DUE TO FAILURE OF CLOSURE OF THE FETAL FISSURE. Infection or other causes lead to a varying degree of microphthalmos with or without cyst formation (Fig. 62). Examination shows either an eye of reduced size without evidence of an adjacent orbital cyst, or one which is overshadowed by a cyst which bulges forward beneath the conjunctiva. The lid fissure usually is narrowed, and the orbit somewhat sunken. The small eye has a clear cornea, moderately deep anterior chamber, often has an iris coloboma, and may show a cataract. If there has been eversion of the retina through the unclosed fissure a large or small cyst may be observed. On sectioning, the eye often, but not always, appears quite deformed. Many of the ocular structures are present, especially the lens which is large in proportion to the size of the eye. A coloboma may be present in the iris, ciliary body, and choroid. The cyst usually lies in the lower orbit posteriorly and its outer lining most often is fibrous and varies greatly in thickness, being quite attenuated if the cyst reaches a fair size. The wall may be continuous with the sclera; by the time of removal, however, the continuity may be disturbed. The choroid most often is absent in the wall of the cyst, and the lining usually is composed of a mixture of neural and mesenchymal tissues. The cyst wall also may be lined by retinal pigment epithelium, and the cavity is filled with a clear fluid.

In most specimens there is true ectasia of the colobomatous defect, in which case retina is everted to form a lining of the cyst wall. In such case the cavity of the cyst is in direct continuity with the vitreous chamber. In true cysts, however, there is overgrowth of the outer portion of the optic cup and the cavity of the cyst opens into the space between the retina proper and its pigment epithelium.

Developmental enlargement of the eye. The eye may be enlarged at birth (megaloglobus), or become enlarged within the neonatal period. The latter types of enlargement occur in congenital glaucoma, von Recklinghausen's neurofibromatosis, myopia, and the Sturge-Weber syndrome. With respect to neurofibromatosis comparable enlargements of other body structures may occur. For example, neurofibromatous hemihypertrophy of the face, digits, or an entire extremity may be observed. There may be marked disfigurement of the globe, lids, or orbit (Figs. 63, 64). Ocular involvement often leads to increase in size of the globe due to secondary glaucoma. There is a deep anterior chamber with an ill-defined iris structure. Microscopic sections

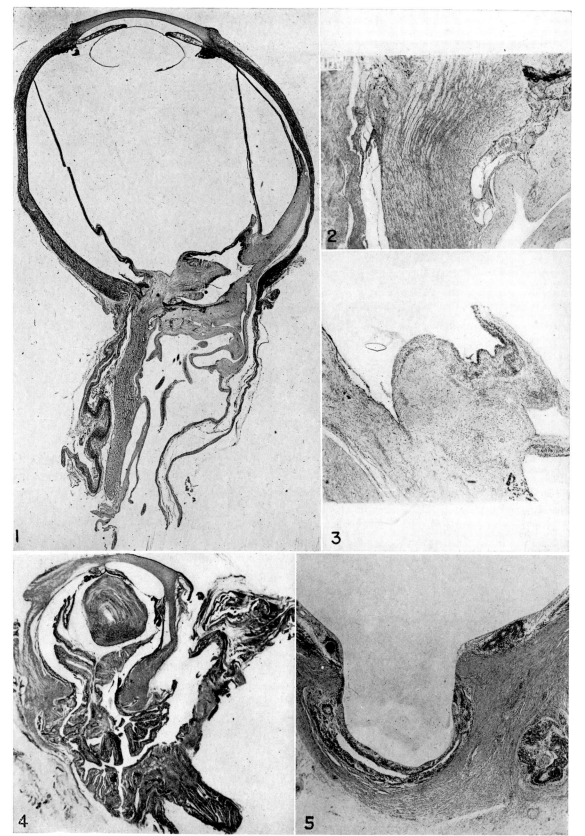

Figure 62. Congenital Cyst of Optic Nerve with Encephalocele. Congenital Abnormalities

1. Congenital cyst of optic nerve with encephalocele extending into globe. (Dvorak-Theobald, G., and Middleton, W. H.: Tr. Am. Acad. Ophth. *55:277–279*, 1951.)

2. Neural tissue entering globe (Dvorak-Theobald and Middleton, *loc. cit.*)

3. Blending of neural tissue with retina. (Dvorak-Theobald and Middleton, *loc. cit.*)

4. Microphthalmos with orbital cyst due to nonclosure of fetal cleft. Retinal tissue in cyst. Coloboma of iris. Coloboma of optic nerve. Persistent pupillary membrane. AFIP Acc. 22911.

5. Coloboma of choroid and retina with sclera ectasia. ×48. AFIP Acc. 40932.

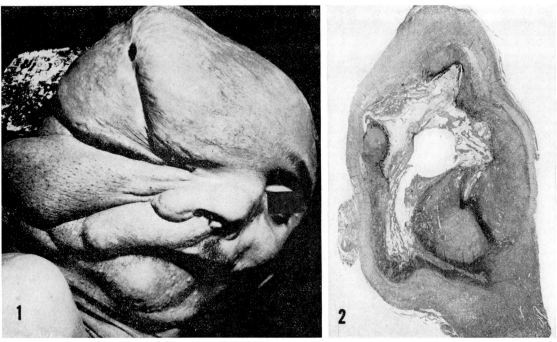

Figure 63. Neurofibromatosis with extreme disfigurement of one side of head and ipsilateral microphthalmos. AFIP Acc. 897676, contributed by Dr. J. M. B. Bloodworth.

show focal neurofibromas, nevi, and diffuse thickening of the uveal tract.

Albinism. Albinism is due to a genetically determined metabolic defect characterized by failure to convert precursors or intermediary products into melanin. The enzymes concerned with these biochemical reactions are under the control of specific genes, the mutation of which may lead to interference with formation of the final product. Increasing numbers of such inborn errors of metabolism are being discovered and studied. It is believed by some that a number of enzymes are concerned in the manufacture of melanin, but Lerner and Fitzpatrick have presented evidence that albinism specifically is the result of the absence of the enzyme tyrosinase.

Albinism may appear in a variety of forms, involving all pigmented structures (complete form), or only some structures of the body. Frequently patients who appear to be complete albinos do have a small amount of pigment in the retinal pigment epithelium and in the uvea. Carriers may exhibit minor forms of albinism.

Nystagmus, photophobia, defective vision, and a considerable refractive error are prominent symptoms. The iris appears pink and translucent, and the fundus shows an absence of retinal and choroidal pigment, clearly revealing the tangled network of choroidal vessels. The macular area usually is more pink. It has been demonstrated that heterozygous females may be carriers of albinism, and Falls observed a peculiar ophthalmoscopic picture in all female carriers in two American families in which male members exhibited ocular albinism. This finding has been verified by a number of subsequent observations. The fundus of such female carriers showed a coarse macular pigmentation. Peripherally an irregular, polymorphous pattern of granular pigmentation was seen.

The pink color of the iris and pupil produced by shining a light into the eye results from the lack of pigment in the iris stroma and epithelium and the reflection of light from the vessels in the posterior eye. Microscopic examination of the iris shows a fairly complete or partial absence of pigment not only in the iris melanocytes, but in the epithelial layers on the posterior surface (Fig. 65–1). The stroma and other cells appear normal. A similar partial or fairly complete absence of pigment is found in other parts of the eye, e.g. the retinal epithelium, ciliary body, and choroidal melanocytes (Fig. 65–2) Microscopic examination of human eyes rarely has been done in the *pure* form of albinism and most of the specimens examined have been of the imperfect or partial type. These usually have shown small amounts of pigment in the retinal epithelium even though the uveal melanocytes may have been amelanotic. Recently, partial albinism and its related ocular symptoms have been recognized as important features of the Chédiak-Higashi syndrome (Fig. 66) (Donohue & Bain, 1957).

Congenital abnormalities have been noted elsewhere in the eye as well as in other portions of the body in albinotic patients. Foveal aplasia, retinal aplasia, duplication of some portions of the posterior retina, partial aniridia, and congenital persistence of the pupillary membrane have been described.

Rawles and other biologists have furnished evidence that most melanocytes arise from the neural crest, and migrate peripherally at a very early stage in embryonic life. The factors responsible for the degree and direction

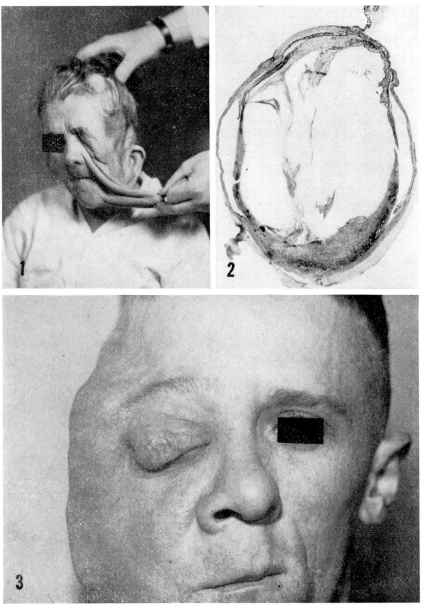

Figure 64. Facial, orbital, and ocular malformation in von Recklinghausen's disease.

1 and 2. AFIP Acc. 32609.

3. AFIP Neg. 55–17512, contributed by Dr. L. L. Calkins.

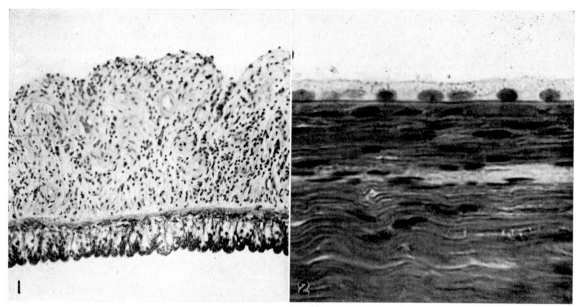

Figure 65.   Albinism

1. Iris in albinism. ×145. AFIP Acc. 88459.
2. Choroid and retinal pigment epithelium in albinism. ×860. AFIP Acc. 88459.

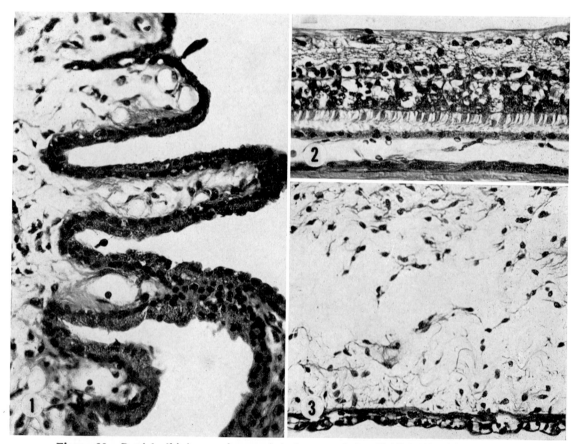

Figure 66.   Partial albinism, a characteristic feature of the Chédiak-Higashi syndrome.

1. Ciliary processes. ×300. AFIP Acc. 947298.
2. Retina and choroid. ×300. AFIP Acc. 947298.
3. Iris. ×300. AFIP Acc. 947298.

of spread of these cells from the neural crest are not known but it is certain that they follow certain patterns and usually do not cross the midline either dorsally or ventrally. Humoral agents such as thyroxine and the sex hormones, and enzymes such as tyrosinase play a part in determining the pigment pattern, but the degree to which they may modify pigmentary processes is as yet undetermined.

Genetic influences in the determination of pigmentation are important, as was indicated in the previous discussion. It is known that many strains of fruit fly (Drosophila melanogaster) possess, or are susceptible to, melanotic tumors, and that the susceptibility to such growth is transmitted by specific chromosomes. In certain instances even the genes responsible for these tumors have been determined positionally on a specific part of the affected chromosome.

Excessive melanin pigmentation. Excessive melanin pigmentation occurs physiologically (e.g., in pregnancy and after exposure to ultraviolet radiation) and in such pathologic conditions as Addison's disease, pernicious anemia and acanthosis nigricans.

Normally, in the newborn of white races, the pigment cells are present in the hair, skin and uveal tract but the pigment content is small. The amount of pigment gradually increases after birth, probably influenced by hormonal and other factors. In dark races considerable pigment is present in the hair, skin, and eyes at birth, but it also increases after birth.

Melanocytosis oculi. Congenital hyperpigmentation of the uveal tract of one eye, and a lesser hyperpigmentation of the sclera, episclera, and disk region is not uncommon. Clinically the affected eye is darker in color. Microscopically there is an increase in the number of melanocytes in the affected tissues. The melanocytes often appear larger and have more coarse fibers than normal. Melanomas rarely arise in such eyes. This condition is closely related to oculodermal melanocytosis.

Oculodermal melanocytosis. Fitzpatrick and co-workers reviewed this pigmentary disease which involves the skin about the eye, the conjunctiva, sclera and uveal tract. This unilateral condition may involve the entire eye or only a segment, and either may be apparent at birth, or is observed at or beyond puberty. There characteristically is hyperchromia of the affected iris. Clumps of dark pigment may be seen in the sclera and conjunctiva. In typical cases fundus examination may show a darker red reflex as compared to the fellow eye. Microscopic examination shows typical branching melanocytes in large numbers throughout the uveal tract, in the lamina cribrosa of the optic nerve, in the sclera and episclera (especially about the emissaria), and beneath the conjunctival epithelium (Fig. 67). The granules in these cells are dark brown or black. The entire uveal tract, especially the iris, may be thickened and more cellular than normal. Malignant melanomas may develop in such eyes, but the incidence is certainly much smaller than Doherty's often cited figure of twenty-five per cent. When there is such involvement of the eyeball, the eyelid, and adjacent face (extrasacral Mongolian spot), the condition is known as oculodermal melanocytosis or the nevus of Ota. This unilateral condition seems to be most common in Orientals, although a number of cases have been reported in Caucasians and Negroes. The pigmentation usually is present at birth, but may not be observed until puberty or early adult life. The pigmentation spreads progressively over the face and conjunctiva. The skin lesions may appear in various hues from black to slate blue, and dark brown to light brown. The upper and lower lids, frontal and temporal skin areas, buccal mucosa, gingiva, palate, cheek, conjunctiva, sclera, uveal tract, and even the orbit and cranial bones may be involved.

Biopsy of the affected skin or mucous membranes reveals no hyperpigmentation of the epithelial structures. The melanocytes are located deep in the dermis and in this respect resemble the changes seen in blue nevus. Malignant change is rare.

Myopia. *Stationary* (simple) myopia is of low degree, develops during youth, and ceases to progress significantly after completion of body growth.

In *progressive* myopia the changes commence during youth and increase steadily

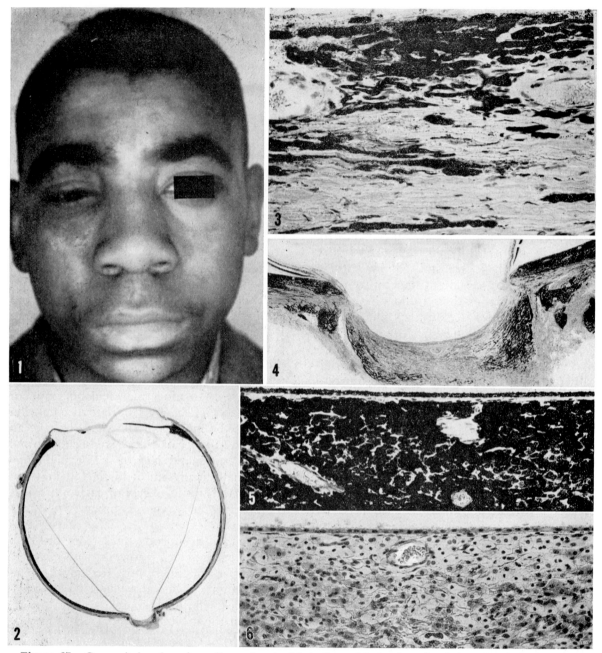

Figure 67. Congenital melanosis oculi associated with ipsilateral hyperchromia of the skin of the face (oculodermal melanocytosis or nevus of Ota), and mucous membranes of fauces. There is diffuse thickening of the uvea (2, 5, and 6), sclera and episclera (3), optic disk and ciliary vessels and nerves (4) by plump and branching melanocytes. 6 reveals a bleached section of choroid. AFIP Acc. 138761.

throughout life, often to very high amounts. This type of eye develops distinctive changes.

Myopia of modest degree is not associated with disease of the ocular tissues and simple myopic eyes vary little from emmetropic eyes. Abnormal myopic eyes exhibit a group of interesting changes, which vary with the stage and degree of myopia. Myopia has been attributed to many causes, and the hereditary aspects of this condition are important. Myopia is often associated with prematurity and retrolental fibroplasia.

Statistical analyses of the distribution of refractive errors in a given population and within given families show a significant correlation between the radius of corneal curvature, depth of the anterior chamber, refractive power of the lens, axial length of the eyeball, and the refractive error. If the necessary combination of factors is present the individual becomes highly myopic during the growth period. The myopia is due to enlargement and lengthening of the posterior segment of the eyeball (Fig. 68), and a good

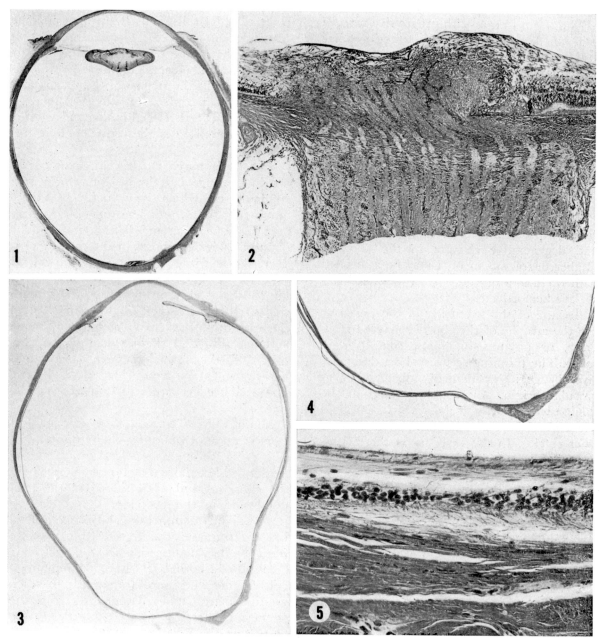

Figure 68. Axial Enlargement of Globe in Myopia

1 and 2. Five year old child who died with the Chédiak-Higashi syndrome. At 2½ years of age the patient had 6 diopters of myopia. AFIP Acc. 947298.

3, 4, and 5. Advanced myopia in a 69-year-old white person with secondary glaucoma. There is a large posterior polar staphyloma and the retina and choroid reveal marked degeneration. AFIP Acc. 693274.

In each picture the temporal side is toward the left. The malformation of the optic disk characteristic of myopia (see also Fig. 70) is shown in 2 but there is also an unrelated papilledema.

part of this lengthening occurs during the period of active growth. Anatomic studies of eyes with progressive myopia show extensive changes in the posterior segment. In eyes with myopia of up to three diopters there may be little anatomic change, except for the region of the optic nerve.

The *sclera* in eyes with progressive myopia is thinned, especially in the posterior polar region and on each side of the optic nerve. An equatorial staphyloma may form as a result of this thinning and stretching. The scleral collagen and elastic tissues show no particular abnormality to account for the thinning.

The *choroid* becomes atrophic as the myopia progresses, but the severity of the changes are not always correlated with the degree of myopia. It has been postulated that the general lengthening and thinning of the posterior eye produces secondary vascular lesions and degenerative changes in the choroid. Higher degrees of myopia may be associated with occlusions of choroidal vessels and secondary hemorrhage.

Because of the stretching of the posterior eye the atrophy of the choroid may be moderate, or progress to almost complete absence. The thinning seems to be a degenerative change rather than of inflammatory or vascular origin. Splits may develop in the lamina vitrea, forming clefts which appear to branch and have a reticular appearance (lacquer cracks). In the early stages there is reduction in choroidal thickness due to loss of the stroma and obliteration of some of the vessels. The melanocytes gradually degenerate, lose their pigment, and disappear. There may be widespread loss of the choriocapillaris (Fig. 68). The outer retina usually shows some degeneration as a result of these changes in the choroidal vessels.

In some highly myopic eyes (12 to 15 diopters) distortion or blurring of central vision may develop due to tears in Bruch's membrane and choriocapillaris, with subretinal hemorrhage at the macula. All this eventually leads to a pigmented scar (Fuchs's dark spot at the macula). With the ophthalmoscope this type of lesion appears dark, due to scarring and proliferation of the retinal pigment at the site of the hemorrhage.

In the *retina,* the receptors and pigment epithelium first show changes. They degenerate slowly and progressively, especially in the staphylomatous areas. If tears occur in the lamina vitrea proliferation of connective tissue occurs beneath the retina, fusing these structures. Pigment proliferation may occur from adjacent cells, and clumps may become embedded in the scar. Cystic degeneration and atrophy of the retinal tissues may occur at the macula. General attenuation and atrophy occur in the stroma of the retina, and the normal peripheral cystic degeneration may be intensified. This thinning and atrophy probably predisposes the retina to hole formation.

The *optic nerve* changes in myopic eyes are interesting, and the disk may present a configuration which is virtually pathognomonic (Fig. 69). Ophthalmoscopically, the myopic nerve head is somewhat flattened on the temporal side. Temporal to the disk there is a crescentic white area, known as a scleral crescent. A somewhat pigmented and vascular choroidal crescent lies to the temporal side of the latter (Fig. 70). Presumably, as the posterior eye enlarges and the sclera becomes thin and slightly ectatic, the choroid and the retinal pigment epithelium are drawn away from their normal position at the edge of the disk, producing the conus.

Microscopic examination reveals an extreme degree of obliquity of the optic nerve as it passes through the scleral canal, and remarkable deviations from normal on both the temporal and nasal sides. On the temporal side in the region of the conus, the retinal pigment epithelium and Bruch's membrane terminate at a considerable distance from the disk margin thus leaving a variable amount of choroid uncovered by pigment epithelium. The choroid also fails to reach the disk margin and adjacent to the disk the sclera and scleral canal are exposed. On the nasal side the reverse situation is observed. There the choroid, Bruch's membrane, and the pigment epithelium overlap the nerve head, not infrequently covering half of the scleral foramen. These histologic features of the myopic disk are contrasted with the normal in Fig. 70.

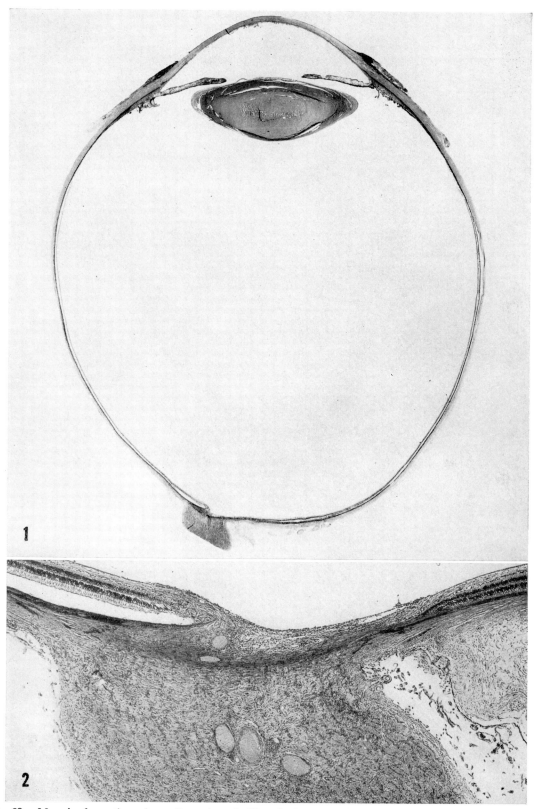

Figure 69.   Myopic elongation of eye, flattening of ciliary body, and deformity of optic nerve head (see Fig. 70)
Temporal side is to the right. AFIP Acc. 41014. 1. ×5. 2. ×40.

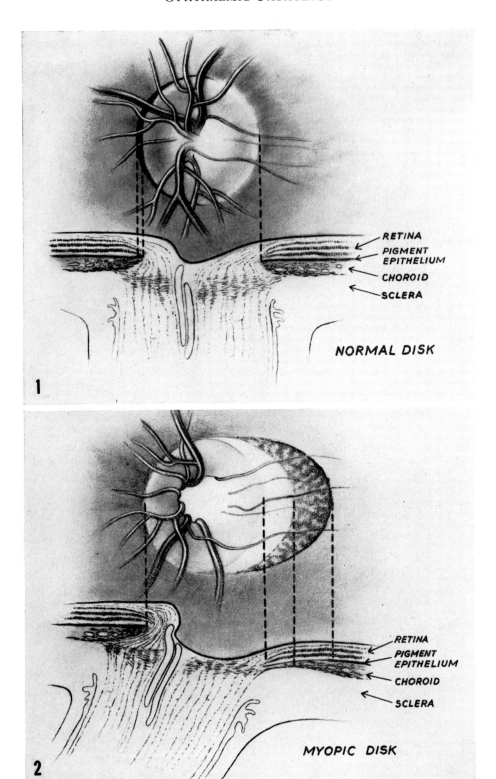

Figure 70. In the myopic eye the choroid, lamina vitrea, and pigment epithelium do not reach the edge of the nerve head on the temporal side (right side of illustrations); this accounts for the temporal crescents of exposed choroid and sclera. On the nasal side the pigment epithelium and lamina vitrea form a shelf-like projection into the nerve head around which the vessels must pass to enter the retina.

Very few changes have been found in the anterior part of the eye which could be said to be typical of myopia.

Vitreous opacities are extremely common in myopic eyes, possibly due to degenerative changes and liquefaction. These will be discussed in Chapter X.

Studies of the refractive error in patients with retinal detachment show that 50 to 60 per cent have myopia; however, only about 5 per cent of myopic patients develop retinal detachment. The probable cause of the detachment in highly myopic patients already has been discussed briefly and will be covered in more detail in Chapter VIII. Glaucoma, which occurs in at least 15 per cent of highly myopic patients, is of the open angle type and often is undetected unless applanation tonometry is used or scleral rigidity is considered. Cataract formation is common in highly myopic patients, being of the posterior subcapsular type and slowly progressive.

Capsular pseudoexfoliation. A peculiar disease of undetermined etiology and pathogenesis, often confused with true exfoliation of the lens capsule, is considered here because of the multiplicity of ocular structures involved and to emphasize the belief that it is not solely a lenticular disorder. The condition has been termed by Theobald "pseudo-exfoliation of the lens capsule." True exfoliation is described in Chapter XI.

The clinical manifestations of pseudoexfoliation of the lens capsule were first adequately described in 1925 by Vogt. He noted that 75 per cent of his cases had glaucoma and indicated that the glaucoma in these cases should be classified as glaucoma capsulare.

This condition has been studied intensively by a number of observers. During the 1920's the material was thought to result either from a rubbing of the iris on the lens capsule, deposition from the iris pigment epithelium on the lens, or a deposition of a substance from the aqueous humor.

Recent investigators have revived the idea that the material is a substance deposited from aqueous humor on the adjacent *tissues*. Gifford, however, believes it is derived from the lens capsule.

Pseudoexfoliation of the lens capsule seems to be more frequent in Norway and Sweden than in other countries, and the incidence of glaucoma in cases with pseudoexfoliation varies from 40 to 90 per cent of the reported series, depending on the geographic location. Similarly, open angle glaucoma cases have an incidence of pseudoexfoliation varying between 4 per cent and 86 per cent. According to Bellows, cataract is found in about 40 per cent of cases with pseudoexfoliation.

Examination of these cases shows deposits of gray fluffy "dandruff" on the lens, zonule, iris surface, pupillary margin, cornea and the trabecula. After dilatation of the pupil the central zone of the lens has a powdery or gray appearance. There is a zone of normal lens adjacent to this, appearing as a circular band. More peripheral to this is another powdery gray zone. With gonioscopy the trabecular meshwork usually shows heavy pigmentation in these cases, and the reason for this is uncertain.

Microscopically the lens capsule may or may not show thickening and stain intensely with eosin. Accretions were shown by Theobald to lie on the lens capsule in the pupil (Fig. 71), and as far back as the equator, but they were found to be separated from the lens capsule by a clear staining line (trichrome stain). The accretions in the pupillary area are short and stubby and are arranged in tufts and bundles standing side by side on the lens surface like shrubs in a hedge. Midway between the pupillary border and the equator the accretions are feathery and branched in appearance. On the zonule at the equator they are soft and fluffy. They are found on the ciliary epithelium, zonule, posterior iris, anterior iris surface, and in the trabecular meshwork (Fig. 71). Pigment also is present in macrophages and the trabecular endothelial cells.

Histochemical stains have been made in these cases by Theobald, Gifford and Ashton. They have demonstrated that the material stains positively with PAS and colloidal iron and that it has the staining characteristics of the normal zonule. This would appear to suggest that it is derived from the zonular lamella of the lens and the zonule, rather than from the lens capsule or aqueous.

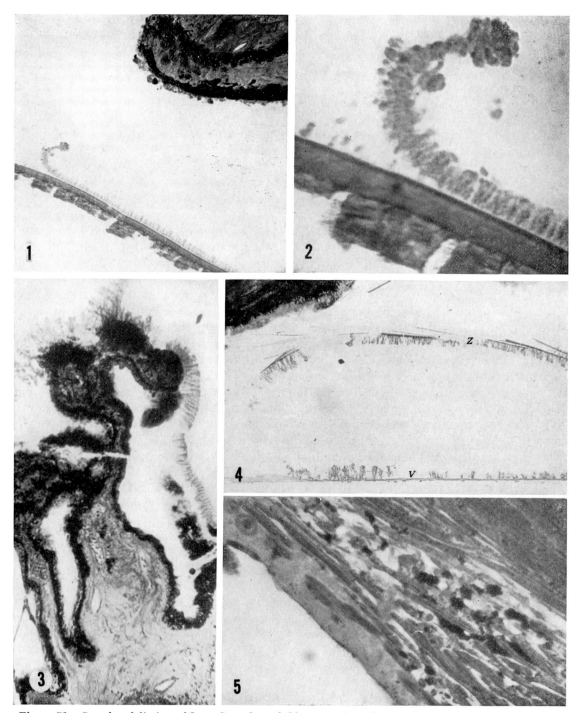

Figure 71. Pseudoexfoliation of Lens Capsule and Glaucoma Capsulocuticulare. From Theobald (1954).

1. Accretions on anterior lens surface, peeling off in form of a curl; similar deposits on posterior surface of iris.
2. Anterior lens surface at higher magnification.
3. Accretions on ciliary processes.
4. Accretions on zonular fibers (z)and on face of vitreous body (v).
5. Similar material fills the intertrabecular spaces.

OCULAR INFLAMMATION

The terms used to define the types of widespread intraocular inflammation have changed over a period of years. Some have persisted and are satisfactory, while others have become obsolete. The changes in the concepts of infections and inflammations will be discussed in Chapter V. As a result of improved health and new therapeutic measures, ocular infections now are less common and severe. Each advance, however, creates new problems, and organisms with altered resistance have changed the character of infections and their pathologic counterparts.

An attempt will be made to discuss diffuse ocular inflammation both from a clinical as well as a histopathologic aspect. The classification which is used corresponds to present concepts of inflammatory and infectious processes. It should be understood, however, that an ideal classification is difficult because in the early stage the inflammatory process may present the features of a suppurative process, and at a later date it may become predominantly nonsuppurative. Some organisms may elicit an early suppurative reaction, followed within a short period by conversion of the exudate to that seen in a chronic inflammation. At other times the process may be suppurative in the region of the most active disease and be nonsuppurative away from this area. These facts should be borne in mind in the interpretation of any slides which are being studied.

Classification:

I. Suppurative
   A. Panophthalmitis
   B. Endophthalmitis
      1. Diffuse
      2. Localized
II. Nonsuppurative
   A. Panophthalmitis
      1. Nongranulomatous
      2. Granulomatous
   B. Endophthalmitis
      1. Nongranulomatous
      2. Granulomatous
   C. Uveitis
      1. Nongranulomatous
      2. Granulomatous

Intraocular inflammations also may be classified according to source:

I. Exogenous
   A. Penetrating wounds
   B. Foreign bodies
   C. Corneal ulcers
   D. Spread from adjacent tissue (orbit, sinuses, etc.)
II. Endogenous
   A. Metastasis of bacteria, fungi, etc. from a focus elsewhere in the body
   B. Necrosis of tissue (tumors, etc.)
   C. Spread from adjacent tissue (optic nerve)

More localized ocular inflammations, such as uveitis, will be covered in Chapter VII.

Suppurative Ocular Inflammations

Panophthalmitis. Inasmuch as intraocular inflammations may involve many tissues or be restricted in extent, it would seem logical to apply the term panophthalmitis to those which are widespread in the eye, and also involve the outer coat and Tenon's capsule; endophthalmitis designates those inflammations which involve only the ocular cavities and their adjacent structures.

Panophthalmitis varies somewhat in its gross and microscopic appearance, depending on the cause. It varies from: (1) the typical type in which there is a fulminating suppurative process with varying degrees of destruction of the retina and uveal tract, abscess formation in the vitreous and anterior chamber, necrosis of the cornea and limbus, extension through the scleral emissaria to produce a tenonitis and orbital cellulitis and rupture of the eye; (2) a less fulminating form in which the inflammatory process, though diffuse and severe, is characterized by lymphocytic and plasma cell infiltration. It should be pointed out, however, that in suppurative panophthalmitis, even though the principal cell in the exudate is the polymorphonuclear leukocyte, quite often the inflammatory process in the choroid is characterized by lymphocytic infiltration.

The clinical manifestations of *panophthalmitis* include pain, congestion and edema of the lids and conjunctiva, exophthalmos, haziness of the cornea, and purulent exudate in the anterior chamber. Edema and congestion of the lids and other external ocular structures as well as exophthalmos are produced by extension of the intraocular inflammation into Tenon's capsule and orbital tissues. Microscopic examination shows that this extension of the inflammatory process to the tissues outside of the eye occurs through the scleral emissaria.

This acute type of panophthalmitis most often is attributed to lacerated wounds, intraocular foreign bodies, and extension of corneal infections, and may follow various surgical procedures. Other cases, rare in recent years, result from septicemia or bacterial metastasis to the choroid or retina from a remote infection (e.g., meningococcemia, pneumonia, endocarditis, or puerperal sepsis). Glaucomatous eyes with bullous keratopathy may develop a bacterial infection of the cornea with perforation, followed by panophthalmitis. Other patients with lagophthalmos due to scars, pemphigus, and lid cancer may develop corneal ulcers which perforate and cause panophthalmitis. The necrosis of intraocular tissues often results in severe ocular inflammation resembling panophthalmitis. This occurs in melanomas of the choroid and ciliary body and is not rare in retinoblastomas. Extension to the eye of infections from neighboring structures, e.g., the sinuses and orbit, is rather uncommon.

Many organisms may cause suppurative panophthalmitis. The most common are: Staphylococcus aureus, Pseudomonas aeruginosa, Streptococcus pyogenes, Diplococcus pneumoniae, and the coliform organisms. Less commonly, Proteus vulgaris, Cl. perfringens, and fungi are encountered. Staphylococcus aureus infections seem to be the most common, although Pseudomonas aeruginosa infections have become frequent, largely due to contamination of surgical solutions.

Following establishment of the inflammation the tough and relatively impenetrable corneoscleral coat tends to confine inflammatory reactions within its boundaries. The flow of the intraocular fluids, causing diffusion of toxic or chemotactic substances liberated from a localized lesion within the eye, usually leads to the involvement of the eyeball as a whole. The reactions of the eye to inflammatory agents tend, therefore, to a certain uniformity with relatively little regard to the particular site at which the damaging agent makes its first appearance or produces its most intensely destructive lesion. With progressive spread of the infecting agent the suppurative process soon involves all the contents of the eye, and extends into the surrounding tissues.

The pathologic picture which develops in the eye in these acute infections is of considerable interest (Fig. 72). The peculiar structure of the eye with its large avascular cavity accounts for the frequent separation of the cellular part of the inflammatory reaction from the vascular part. The spaces about the perforating vessels become choked with polymorphonuclear leukocytes; most often there is a diffuse purulent infiltration in the choroid, and usually a marked infiltration in the retina (Fig. 72). The retina becomes edematous; often a serous or seropurulent exudate forms beneath it and separates it from the choroid. Following this it usually becomes necrotic. The retinal perivascular infiltration extends down along the central vessels into the optic nerve (Fig. 73), and frequently some of the inflammatory exudate accumulates in the meningeal sheaths of the nerve. Leukocytes migrate into the vitreous in great numbers, clinging to the vitreous sheets in much the same way that the cells in tissue cultures cling to the fibers of the clot in which the culture is implanted. Over the surface of the ciliary body, where the infiltration of the vitreous usually is most intense, this forms an arresting picture, for the leukocytes are seen strung out along the sheets which radiate fan-wise from the surface. The circulation of the intraocular fluids carries infectious material and cells into the anterior chamber, where the cells settle down as a *hypopyon* under the influence of gravity (Fig. 73). The iris is found to be swollen and densely infiltrated with cells which enter its stroma from the iris vessels and also from the anterior chamber.

In severe infections a peripheral annular infiltrate (ring abscess of the cornea) of increasing density forms in the deep cornea but later tends to involve the more superficial layers, finally ulcerating and giving rise to a trough (Fig. 74).

As the process advances the intraocular

contents become disorganized beyond recognition, and if the infection is sufficiently severe, perforation of the globe and evacuation of the purulent material eventually result. There is a potential danger of meningitis in these cases, due either to the extension of the process along the sheath of the optic nerve or to the development of orbital cellulitis and cavernous sinus thrombophlebitis.

Not in all instances is the infection so severe that it converts the whole contents of the globe into one large abscess and causes

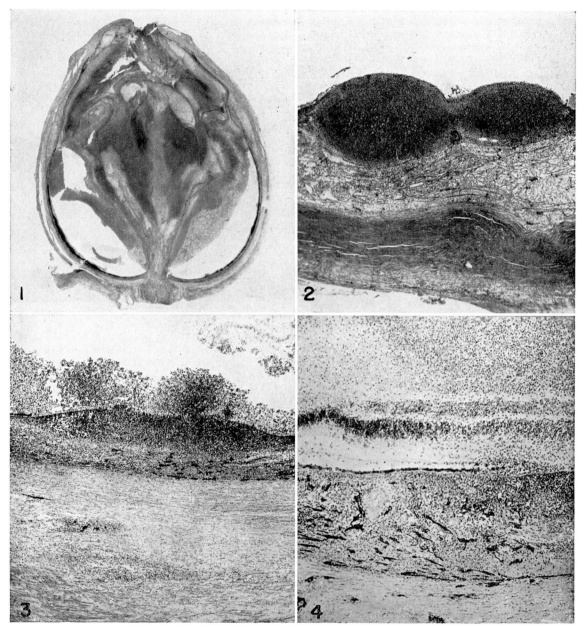

Figure 72. Panophthalmitis

1. Acute purulent panophthalmitis with perforated corneal ulcer, prolapse of iris and extrusion of lens. Vitreous abscess. Detachment and destruction of retina. AFIP Acc. 28817.

2. Abscesses in choriocapillaris. ×100. AFIP Acc. 183550.

3. Abscess in choriocapillaris breaking through Bruch's membrane into subretinal space. ×48. AFIP Acc. 170851.

4. Purulent exudate in choroid. Localized destruction of Bruch's membrane. Partial destruction of retina. Purulent exudate in vitreous. ×100. AFIP Acc. 170851.

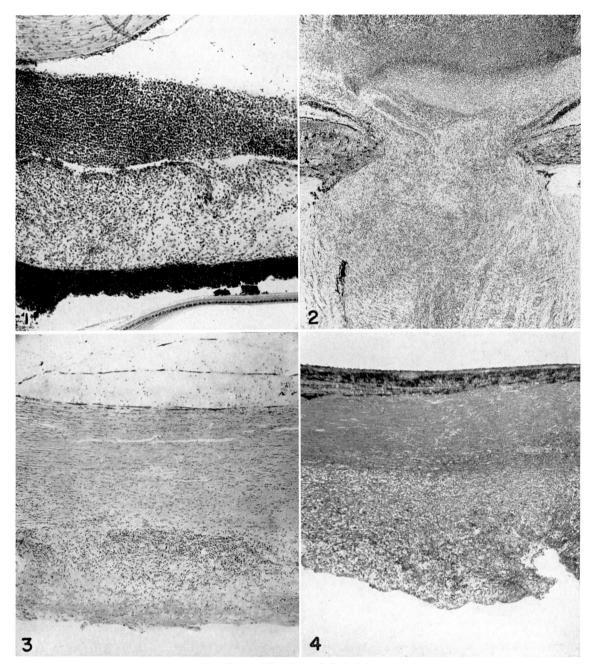

Figure 73. Panophthalmitis

1. Acute iritis. Purulent exudate in anterior chamber forming hypopyon. ×100. AFIP Acc. 24075.

2. Polymorphonuclear leukocytes infiltrating optic nerve. ×48. AFIP Acc. 170851.

3. Acute scleritis and episcleritis. Polymorphonuclear leukocytes infiltrating sclera and episclera. ×100. AFIP Acc. 170851.

4. Acute purulent episcleritis with orbital cellulitis. ×75. AFIP Acc. 159519.

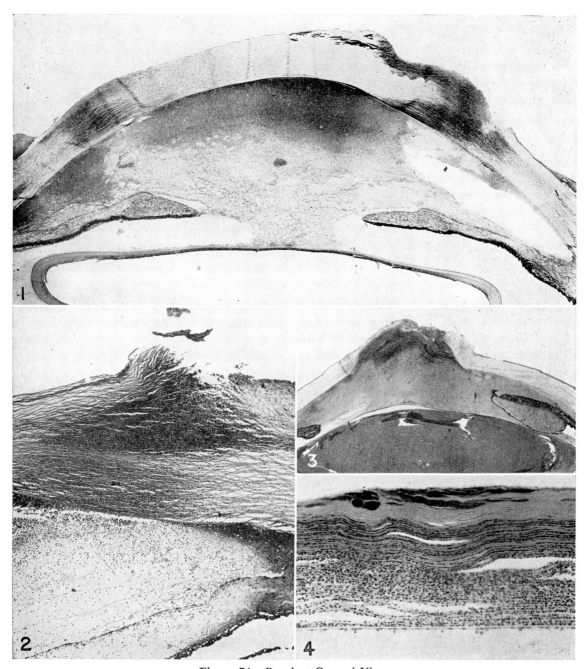

Figure 74. Purulent Corneal Ulcer

1. Ring abscess with ulceration, right. Hypopyon (purulent exudate in anterior chamber). AFIP Acc. 46889.
2. Ring abscess with ulceration and necrosis of peripheral lamellas. ×70. AFIP Acc. 28176.
3. Central perforating ulcer. Hypopyon. ×18. AFIP Acc. 55783.
4. Acute purulent corneal ulcer. Deeply staining bacterial colonies in outer lamellas. Polymorphonuclear leuko-cytes infiltrate deep lamellas and cling to posterior surface. ×125. AFIP Acc. 201278.

rupture. Quite often the infection more or less becomes walled off, the site of the abscess depending on the point of original infection, but even then there is infiltration of neutrophils in the rest of the globe. These parts of the picture are dependent upon the anatomy of the eye and the currents of its fluids, and upon the diffusion throughout the eye of the toxic products of the bacteria and of the injured tissues.

Macrophages reach the eye through the blood vessels and also develop by local proliferation of histiocytes. These cells rapidly migrate toward the focus of infection. Not all reach that focus, for many are caught in the fluid currents of the eye and are washed either into the anterior chamber and toward the canal of Schlemm, or into the perivascular spaces of the retina and toward the optic nerve. No doubt they are joined by many cells that have come closer to the focus and have gorged themselves with the chemotactic substances.

Extension of the intraocular inflammation or the active infection into the emissaria leads to more or less inflammation of Tenon's capsule and the adjacent soft tissues of the orbit. The capsule over the sclera shows edema, vascular dilatation, and diffuse and perivascular lymphocytic and polymorphonuclear leukocytic infiltration. The nearby orbital tissues show similar subacute inflammatory changes (Figs. 73–3, 73–4).

When the infection is walled off or the eye ruptures, granulation tissue begins to form and the usual picture of a subsiding abscess develops. The polymorphonuclear cells die, and lymphocytes and plasma cells predominate. Eventually a dense scar is formed, chiefly through organization of the exudate by fibrous tissue. The subsequent course depends upon whether the infection was diffuse or was located in the anterior or posterior segment of the eye. In any case the less involved portion tends to regain a more or less normal appearance, though there will always remain some adhesions between the iris and lens, and some disorganization and loss of function of the retina. Most often the disorganized eye gradually shrinks and becomes phthisical. The characteristic findings in this type of atrophy with disorganization are described subsequently in this chapter.

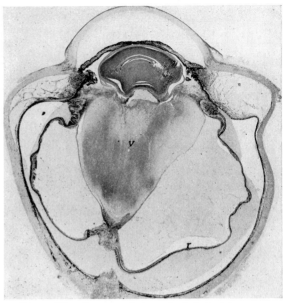

Figure 75. Suppurative endophthalmitis, a complication of meningococcic meningitis. Purulent exudate infiltrates the vitreous body (v) which has become detached from the retina (r). Proteinaceous exudate fills the preretinal and subretinal spaces. The serous detachment of the ciliary body reflects the hypotonic state of this eye. ×5. AFIP Acc. 35073.

Suppurative endophthalmitis. In suppurative endophthalmitis the inflammation involves the ocular cavities and their immediate adjacent structures (Fig. 75). The inflammatory changes are quite similar to those seen in suppurative panophthalmitis, the only difference being that in endophthalmitis there is an absence of extension of the inflammation to Tenon's capsule or the adjacent soft tissues of the orbit. Clinically, the eye with suppurative endophthalmitis shows much less edema and chemosis, and there is less lid edema and no protrusion of the eye. Minor variations in this clinical picture are dependent on the specific cause and pathogenesis of the endophthalmitis. For example, *metastatic ophthalmia* is characterized by the appearance of a white, purulent exudate in the vitreous cavity of an eye which is less inflamed anteriorly. The infectious agent metastasizes to one of the intraocular tissues, produces a suppurative inflammation, and the exudate gathers in the vitreous cavity (Fig. 75).

Most postoperative infections may involve the anterior segment or spread to produce a diffuse endophthalmitis. Following surgical procedures for glaucoma, infections are especially likely to localize anteriorly because the lens-zonule area acts as a protective barrier. Suppurative infections in aphakic eyes most often spread widely through the eye.

Fungus infections may occur in the eye following injuries and operations (Fig. 76) or during the course of other fungal infections such as actinomycosis of the lungs, sporotrichosis, mucormycosis of the sinuses (Fig. 77), or aspergillosis. Similar mycotic infections have also been reported in the eyes of patients who showed no other evidence of systemic disease and in whom the portal of entry remained obscure (Fig. 78). The endophthalmitis which follows such infections is characterized by an insidious onset, clouding of vision by vitreous opacities, pain, redness,

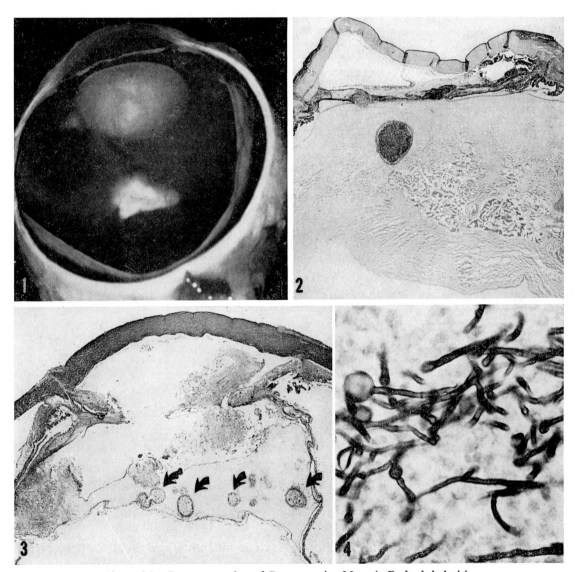

Figure 76. Post-traumatic and Postoperative Mycotic Endophthalmitis

1. Localized vitreous abscess 6 weeks after penetrating wound. AFIP Acc. 741873.

2. Discrete fungal abscess in anterior vitreous approximately 3½ months after uneventful cataract extraction. AFIP Acc. 704186.

3. Many small discrete mycotic abscesses in the vitreous (arrows) and a large lesion on inner surface of the ciliary body (left side of photograph) about five months after intracapsular lens extraction. AFIP Acc. 868441.

4. The saprophytic fungi responsible for intraocular infections following accidental or surgical trauma are easily demonstrated by special staining techniques but they can be identified specifically only by mycologic methods. Gomori's methenamine silver stain, ×630. AFIP Acc. 743097. (From Fine and Zimmerman, 1959.)

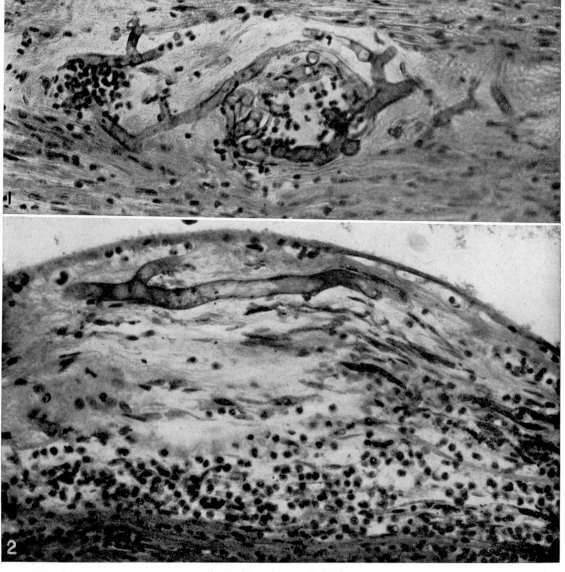

Figure 77. Fungus Infection

1. Mucor mycelia surrounding circulus arteriosus major in ciliary body. Slight chronic inflammatory reaction. ×375. AFIP Acc. 87679.

2. Mucor mycelium in choroid. Mild lymphocytic and histiocytic reaction. ×300. AFIP Acc. 87679.

chemosis, and a certain amount of systemic reaction.

The noninfectious type of suppurative endophthalmitis accompanying necrosis of tumors appears to be due to hemorrhage and necrosis of the tumor tissue. The inflammation is characterized by polymorphonuclear leukocytic and lymphocytic infiltration into the retina, choroid, and vitreous, and a re-

active inflammation in other ocular tissues. Glaucoma may develop, further obscuring the presence of a tumor in the inflamed eye. In some retinoblastomas a massive shedding of tumor cells with migration into the aqueous may cause a pseudohypopyon.

Intraocular foreign bodies may lead to a mixture of suppurative endophthalmitis and granulomatous inflammation within the eye.

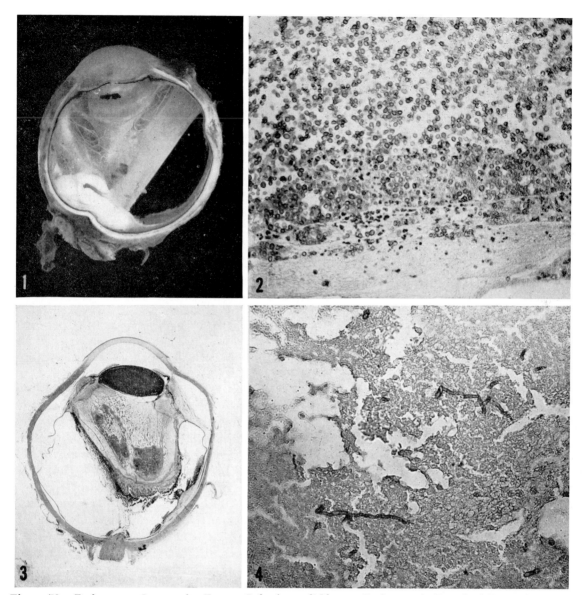

Figure 78. Endogenous Intraocular Fungus Infections of Obscure Pathogenesis (Portal of Entry Unknown)

1 and 2. Cryptococcal infections (from de Buen, Foerster, and Zimmerman, 1954). 1. AFIP Acc. 599915. 2. Mucicarmine stain, ×290. AFIP Acc. 161194.

3 and 4. Probable Aspergillus infection (from Harley & Mishler, 1959). AFIP Acc. 785857. 4. Gridley fungus stain, ×250.

The outcome of these various examples of focal and diffuse suppurative endophthalmitis varies with the cause, severity, duration and complications. It is possible, with therapy, for fairly complete resolution to take place in eyes with early endophthalmitis due to corneal ulcers, wounds, foreign bodies, and operations. Most often, however, the tissue damage, followed by repair, leads to extensive alteration in the function of the eye.

Glaucoma, cataract, cyclitic membrane, occlusion and seclusion of the pupil, and retinal and uveal detachment all may be sequelae of endophthalmitis.

Nonsuppurative Inflammation

Nongranulomatous panophthalmitis. Nonsuppurative inflammations often become

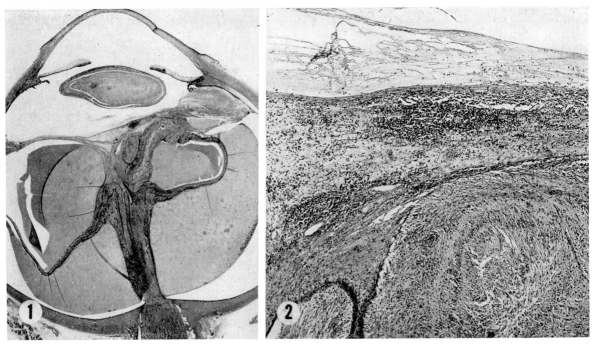

Figure 79. Chronic nongranulomatous endophthalmitis. There is a preretinal inflammatory membrane that is infiltrated by lymphocytes and plasma cells. 1. ×4. 2. ×45. AFIP Acc. 759207.

diffuse and extend through the emissaria to Tenon's capsule and adjacent orbit. This very common type of inflammation warrants discussion as a form of panophthalmitis. Surgical and other trauma which produce hemorrhage in the eye, and endogenous infections most often produce nonsuppurative panophthalmitis.

Ocular wounds and foreign bodies most often cause extensive destruction of tissue with hemorrhage. Even if infection does not result a violent diffuse nongranulomatous inflammation ensues which is characterized by a predominant lymphocytic and plasma cell infiltration. Granulation tissue forms in many areas, and healing by connective tissue replacement leads to scarring of the tissues and atrophy of the eye.

Nongranulomatous endophthalmitis. Nongranulomatous endophthalmitis has most of the features of panophthalmitis except for extraocular extension. Mechanical trauma and surgical procedures are common causes. Persistent endophthalmitis may follow lens extraction, especially of the extracapsular type, and may be caused by a low-grade infection, a fungus infection, or result from phacoanaphylaxis.

Maternal infections such as rubella may produce widespread endophthalmitis, leading to microphthalmos. The most common type of endophthalmitis is that which occurs in patients with *endogenous diffuse uveitis.* This will be discussed in Chapter VII, but at this point it seems appropriate to review the reactions of the eye as a whole to a focus of subacute or chronic inflammation.

The histologic picture is characterized by much less destruction of tissue than in the purulent cases and the invading cells are fewer in number (Fig. 79). Mononuclear wandering cells are seen surrounding the perforating vessels of the sclera, the infiltration being most dense about the vessels that are closest to the lesion. Diffuse or focal infiltration of the choroid is the rule. The infiltration is intense around the retinal blood vessels, especially the veins, and these vessels often are capped by a clump of wandering cells on the inner limiting membrane. All types of mononuclear wandering cells are seen, but very large ones appear to be more common in such inflammations of the eye than in nonspecific inflammatory lesions elsewhere in the body, except, perhaps, in the respiratory mucosa. It may be that the loose structure of the eye facilitates the recognition of the large cells which exhibit a strong tendency to agglutinate, forming clumps of sufficient size to be seen with the naked eye. These clumps of cells are prominent in the sheaths of the retinal vessels.

Over the surface of the ciliary body and in the vitreous and zonule, the wandering cells are seen in considerable number, either isolated or in clumps. These cells are carried forward by the flow of intraocular currents, and they are to be found on the back of the iris, at the pupillary margin, and on the anterior surface of the iris, where they often can be recognized clinically as gray translucent nodules. The aqueous becomes turbid with protein and floating cells, and the latter are deposited in clumps on the back of the cornea, usually in a triangle with its base down, in the lower quadrant (keratic precipitates).

In sections, the deposits of cells on the anterior surface of the iris are conspicuous, and smaller numbers of cells penetrate the iris stroma, the perivascular spaces of the iris, and the anterior part of the ciliary body. Even when inflammations are located primarily far back in the globe, relatively large numbers of cells accumulate at the bottom of the anterior chamber, in and about the canal of Schlemm and in the sheaths of the vessels with which the canal is connected. At this stage transitory elevations of intraocular pressure are frequent, due perhaps to trabecular inflammation and the blocking of the outflow channels with wandering cells and detritus.

Inflammations of this type often heal completely, leaving nothing more than a scar at the site of the focal lesion which was responsible for the dissemination of the inflammatory process. In more severe cases and those in which there have been frequently recurring attacks, organization of the inflammatory exudate takes place in various parts of the eye, most conspicuously over the surface of the retina or ciliary body, where active proliferation of epithelial cells and fibroblasts is often noted. The subsequent course of these severe cases of subacute and chronic endophthalmitis is the same as that of the milder cases of purulent infection. When the lesion is limited essentially to the anterior segment of the eyeball, adhesions develop which may produce secondary glaucoma. When the posterior segment is severely involved, an exudate from the ciliary body forms a scar behind the lens (cyclitic membrane) (Fig. 80). The retina detaches and the eyeball becomes soft and eventually shrinks (Fig. 81). Recurrent focal attacks of a subacute character, in many instances accompanied by hemorrhage into the disorganized tissues, as in phthisis bulbi, may lead to enucleation because of the severe pain.

Granulomatous panophthalmitis. The granulomatous form of panophthalmitis may follow injury with introduction of foreign bodies. It also may be due to post-traumatic fungus infection, and perforation of the lens leading to subsequent autosensitization to lens protein. The tissues react by producing phagocytic cells—at first polymorphonuclears, and later macrophages. These surround the foreign substance and attempt to destroy and phagocytize it. Characteristically some of the large mononuclears become transformed into epithelioid and giant cells. A massive lymphocytic and plasma cell response also occurs, and soon the eye is involved in widespread diffuse and perivascular inflammation.

Rarely, this type of panophthalmitis is the result of an endogenous granulomatous disease such as blastomycosis or tuberculosis, especially in those patients with active pulmonary disease (Fig. 23). It also may occur in patients receiving corticosteroid therapy who are not suspected of being tuberculous. In such eyes the disease pursues a rapid course, involving all tissues, and frequently causes perforation of the cornea or limbus. It can be seen that such infection, predominantly granulomatous in nature, can lead to explosive inflammations in which the necrosis overshadows the granulomatous process. Other diseases usually produce more localized lesions and will be discussed in Chapter VII. Syphilis rarely has been established as a cause of such inflammations.

Granulomatous endophthalmitis. Granulomatous endophthalmitis most often is diffuse with a tendency to be more severe in one portion of the eye. The etiology of such lesions is much the same as that given for panophthalmitis. Fungi may enter the eye via the optic nerve or blood stream and produce an endophthalmitis of a granulomatous type.

A type of granulomatous inflammation occasionally is produced in the eye by the microfilarias and the larvas of various helminths (Fig. 27). This is discussed in Chapter X.

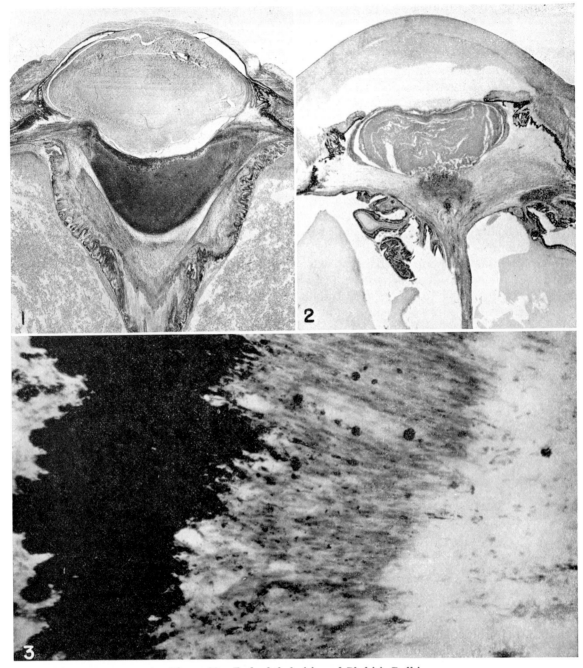

Figure 80. Endophthalmitis and Phthisis Bulbi

1. Abscess in vitreous. Beginning organization of a pyogenic cyclitic membrane, detaching retina. AFIP Acc. 24594.

2. Almost complete replacement of abscess by cyclitic membrane. AFIP Acc. 17990.

3. Proliferation of ciliary epithelium into cyclitic membrane. ×205. AFIP Acc. 17945.

Another important parasitic cause of granulomatous endophthalmitis is cysticercus. As long as the cysticercus remains viable there is no significant inflammatory reaction. When the parasite dies or is inadvertently ruptured during surgical removal, a violent inflammatory reaction ensues which may be decidedly granulomatous in character (Fig. 26).

The type of granulomatous endophthalmitis which follows injury to the lens or lens surgery will be discussed in Chapter III.

The organisms or noninfectious agents

which cause a granulomatous type of endophthalmitis result in a reaction characterized by epithelioid and giant cells, diffuse lymphocytic and plasma cell infiltration, and relatively less fibrosis than one encounters after pyogenic inflammations. Pyogenic organisms cause a predominantly polymorphonuclear leukocytic response with severe tissue damage, and massive reparative fibrosis. These two types of reactions in well developed lesions tend to be mutually exclusive, but it must be remembered that combina-

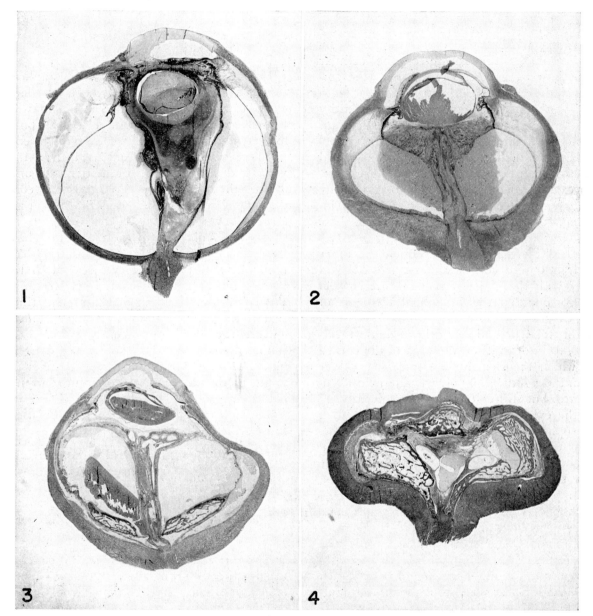

Figure 81. Endophthalmitis, Atrophia Bulbi, and Phthisis Bulbi

1. Acute endophthalmitis with vitreous abscess. Detachment of retina, ciliary body and peripheral choroid. Beginning atrophy of globe. ×3. AFIP Acc. 56281.

2. Cyclitic membrane replacing vitreous abscess. Detachment and gliosis of retina. Subretinal serous exudate. Detachment of ciliary body and peripheral choroid. Moderate atrophy of globe. Thickening of sclera. ×4. AFIP Acc. 54885.

3. Old cyclitic membrane and retinal detachment. Ossification of choroid. Atrophy of globe. ×3. AFIP Acc. 189580.

4. Advanced atrophy of globe. Ossification of choroid and cyclitic membrane. Thickening of sclera. ×3. AFIP Acc. 112917.

tions are not unknown. Also in any lesion where considerable tissue is destroyed, the irritating material so derived, be it from a nongranulomatous or granulomatous infection, will cause a polymorphonuclear and lymphocytic cell and plasma cell response at the periphery of the lesion.

The type of cellular response in the anterior segment of the eye usually can be determined without difficulty on clinical examination by the nature of the cellular deposits on the posterior surface of the cornea and in the iris. It is often possible to make a shrewd clinical guess as to the identity of the cells precipitated upon the back of the cornea merely from observations *in vivo,* either with the naked eye or with the corneal microscope. Polymorphonuclear leukocytes, for example, show no tendency to agglutinate when suspended in the aqueous and, in inflammatory lesions of the eye in which these cells predominate, the corneal precipitates are extremely fine. On inspection the inner surface of the cornea appears frosted, and only with the higher powers of the corneal microscope can the individual elements of the deposit be resolved. Lymphocytes show a slight tendency to agglutinate and, therefore, form deposits on the back of the cornea in which the elements are somewhat larger than those formed of polymorphonuclear leukocytes but still below the limits of visibility to the eye, though they are easily seen with the ophthalmoscope or slit lamp microscope. It is only rarely, however, that a pure lymphocytic inflammatory reaction occurs in the eye. Usually plasma cells and larger mononuclear phagocytes are present in considerable numbers. A strong tendency to agglutinate with each other and with the corneal endothelium is characteristic of these cells and the resulting deposits often are visible without magnification. They are of a yellowish color and appear waxy, thus resembling mutton fat. Cells of this type are especially abundant in tuberculosis, sympathetic ophthalmia, and sarcoidosis, and the presence of "mutton fat" deposits on the inner surface of the cornea should lead the clinician to classify the lesion as granulomatous and to consider all those conditions which might cause a granulomatous reaction. The precipitates on the posterior surface of the cornea always are accompanied by similar deposits in or on the surface of the iris. Granulomatous inflammations frequently include epithelioid and lymphocytic nodular lesions in the iris stroma and epithelioid cell accumulations in the pigment ruff at the pupillary margin of the iris (Koeppe nodules).

Sequelae of Panophthalmitis and Endophthalmitis

Inasmuch as a number of the complications of these inflammations such as glaucoma, cataract, and retinal detachment will be covered in subsequent chapters, only atrophy and phthisis bulbi will be discussed.

These terms have been used over the years, and there have been arguments for and against their use under certain clinical conditions. Originally it was thought that atrophic eyes following injury were apt to show bouts of inflammation and therefore were likely to develop sympathetic ophthalmia, but that phthisical eyes tended to remain quiet and were very unlikely to cause this condition. It is felt at the present time that if the atrophy follows an open wound, and if the eye is recurrently inflamed it should be considered as potentially dangerous. The terms atrophy and phthisis refer to stages in the degeneration of injured or inflamed eyes.

The following classification may be used to describe such eyes:

1. Atrophy of the eyeball without shrinkage (e.g., postglaucomatous atrophy).
2. Atrophy of the eyeball with shrinkage (usual type of atrophy).
3. Atrophy of the eyeball with disorganization (phthisis bulbi).

Atrophy without shrinkage. These eyes usually are of normal size but may be enlarged or slightly smaller than normal. The ocular tissues in this type of atrophy usually have been affected by long-standing glaucoma. Vision usually is absent. The fundus may or may not be seen, and the lens may be cataractous. Microscopic examination shows a relatively well-preserved internal architecture, but there is diffuse atrophy of the various ocular tissues. There may be a moderate serous separation of the retina and choroid, a cyclitic membrane, varying cataractous changes, and anterior and posterior synechias.

Atrophy with shrinkage. The eye definitely is reduced in size, is soft, and there may be marked squaring (Fig. 81–1, 2). The cornea may be scarred, and frequently is small and flattened. The anterior chamber may be absent, and anterior or posterior synechias are present. The lens is cataractous. Again, the internal architecture is relatively well preserved, the uveal tract is more or less intact, and the retina and vitreous frequently are detached. A cyclitic membrane may be present. The sclera does not show the great thickening which is seen in phthisical eyes.

Atrophy with disorganization (phthisis bulbi). Phthisis bulbi, on the other hand,

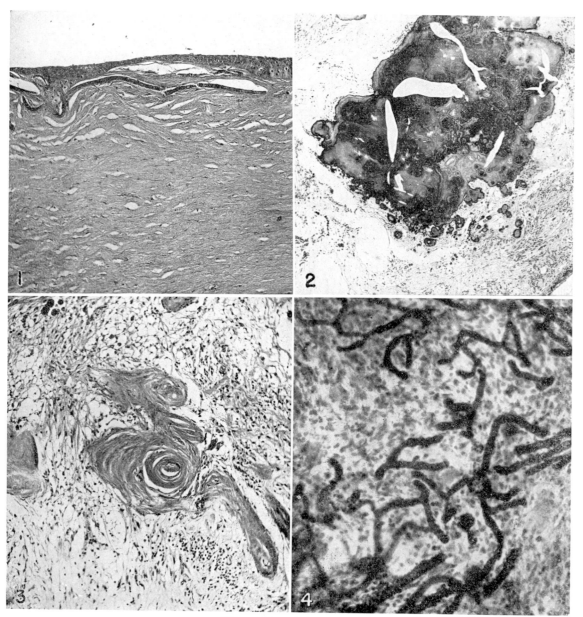

Figure 82.   Phthisis Bulbi

1. Vascularization of corneal substantia. Degenerated superficial corneal scar. Fragmented and calcified Bowman's membrane. Irregularities in corneal epithelium. ×145. AFIP Acc. 484175.

2. Drusen in detached retina. ×125. AFIP Acc. 339661.

3. Obliterated blood vessels in detached and gliosed retina. ×100. AFIP Acc. 176195.

4. Siderocalcific degeneration of capillaries in detached retina. ×160. AFIP Acc. 29400.

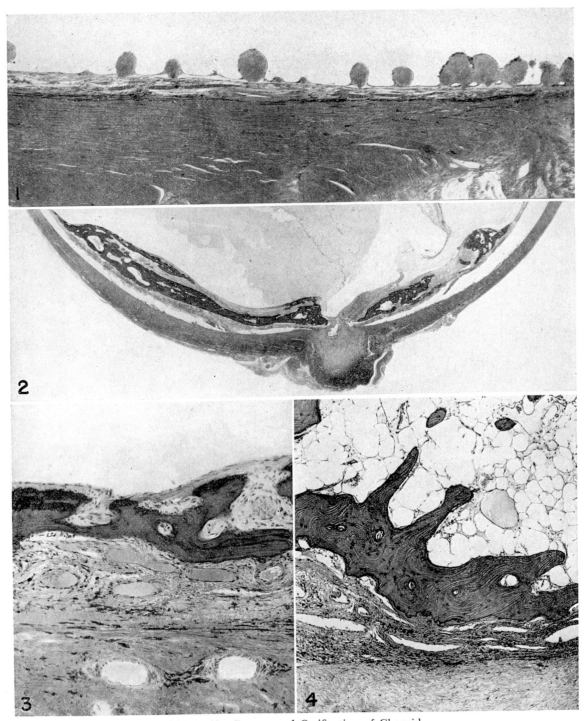

Figure 83. Drusen and Ossification of Choroid

1. Drusen on Bruch's membrane in retinal detachment. Atrophy of choroid. ×5. AFIP Acc. 96423.
2. Ossification of choroid. ×6. AFIP Acc. 98600.
3. Ossification of choroid showing characteristic involvement of choriocapillaris and inner surface. ×125. AFIP Acc. 208848.
4. Ossification of choroid. Fat in marrow spaces. ×75. AFIP Acc. 315182.

occurs in eyes which have been severely injured with loss of tissue or in those which have become disorganized as a result of panophthalmitis. The entire eye is reduced to a dense white structure 16 to 18 mm. in diameter. The cornea is shrunken, flat, and opaque, and the sclera is tremendously thickened and very white. The contents of the eye are replaced by scar tissue which involves the choroid and the totally detached retina, and forms a dense cyclitic membrane. Characteristic is the bone formation which often lines the entire choroid (Figs. 81–3, 81–4).

Microscopically, in contrast to atrophic eyes, the phthisical eye shows extreme disorganization, replacement fibrosis, and reduction in size. The cornea is narrowed in diameter, markedly thickened, scarred and irregular (Fig. 82–1). The scarred area is usually vascularized. If there has been a wound, layers of connective tissue extend into the eye from its deeper aspect to become continuous with other damaged tissue, especially a cyclitic membrane. The sclera is extremely thickened and irregular. The choroid is thickened and its vessels dilated, and the retina is totally disorganized and often partially calcified (Fig. 82) as a result of contraction of vitreous membranes.

Beneath the detached retina the pigment epithelium proliferates and secretes globular masses of hyaline material, which are called "warts" or "drusen," on the lamina vitrea (Fig. 83–1). Hyaline degeneration also occurs in the thick layers of connective tissue lining and infiltrating the choroid. The drusen and connective tissue scar later may become hyalinized, then calcified, and finally, the calcified deposits may become organized into cancellous bone (Fig. 83). If sufficient time is allowed to elapse, bone formation may be extensive, involving the whole choroid, extending into the anterior eye to the mass of scar tissue behind the lens. These changes often are seen also in atrophic eyes which are reduced in size. It is not known why such eyes often show bony degeneration. They may develop recurrent attacks of inflammation, most often because of spontaneous hemorrhages from the degenerating scar tissue. Some pain and congestion often accompany these attacks. Such symptoms, and the unsightliness of the eye usually provide a reason for enucleation.

Very often the destructive effects of the reparative process in such eyes are more severe than those of the original infection. Much of the repair consists in fibroblastic organization of the inflammatory exudates, forming opaque sheets of scar tissue in the ocular cavity and producing detachment of the retina.

REFERENCES

Ashton, N. [Discussion on: Gifford, H.: A Clinical and Pathological Study of Exfoliation of the Lens Capsule.] Trans. Am. Ophth. Soc. 55:215, 1957.

Bellows, J. G.: Cataract and Anomalies of the Lens; Growth, Structure, Composition, Metabolism, Disorders, and Treatment of the Crystalline Lens. St. Louis, C. V. Mosby, 1944, p. 494.

Boell, E. J.: Biochemical and Physiological Analysis of Organizer Action. Growth 6 (Supplement): 37–53. 1942.

de Buen, S., Zimmerman, L. E., and Foerster, H. C.: Patologia ocular en la criptococosis. Rev. Inst. Salub. y. Enferm. Trop. 14:163–172, 1954.

Danielli, J. F., and Brown, R., eds.: Symposia of the Society of Experimental Biology. No. II. Growth in Relation to Differentiation and Morphogenesis. New York, Cambridge University Press and Academic Press, 1948.

Doherty, W. B.: Cases of Melanosis Oculi with Microscopic Findings. Amer. J. Ophthal. 10:1–8, (Jan.) 1927.

Donohue, W. L., and Bain, H. W.: Chédiak-Higashi Syndrome: A Lethal Familial Disease with Anomalous Inclusions in the Leukocytes and Constitutional Stigmata. Report of a Case with Necropsy. Pediatrics 20:416–430, 1957.

Druault, A., and Druault, S.: Eye of the Newborn. Ann. Oculist. 179:375–388, (July) 1946.

Falls, Harold F.: Sex-linked Ocular Albinism Displaying Typical Fundus Changes in the Female Heterozygote. Amer. J. Ophthal. 34:41–50 (May) 1951.

Fine, B., and Zimmerman, L. E.: Exogenous Intraocular Fungus Infections: with Particular Reference to Complications of Intraocular Surgery. Amer. J. Ophthal. 48:151–165, (Aug.) 1959.

Fitzpatrick, T. B., Zeller, R., Kukita, A., and Kitamura, H.: Ocular and Dermal Melanocytosis. A.M.A. Arch. Ophthal. 56:830–832, (Dec.) 1956.

Gifford, H.: A Clinical and Pathological Study of Exfoliation of the Lens Capsule. Amer. J. Ophthal. 46:508–524, (Oct.) 1958.

Hamilton, W. J., Boyd, J. D., and Mossman, H. W.: Human Embryology (Prenatal Development of Form and Function). Baltimore, Williams and Wilkins Co., 1945, pp. 102–111.

Harley, R. D., and Mishler, J. E.: Endogenous Intraocular Fungus Infection. Trans. Amer. Acad. Ophthal. *63*:264–271, 1959.

Lerner, A. B., and Fitzpatrick, T. B.: Biochemistry of Melanin Formation. Physiol. Rev. *30*:91–126, (Jan.) 1950.

Needham, J.: Biochemistry and Morphogenesis. London, Cambridge University Press, 1942.

Rawles, Mary E.: Origin of the Mammalian Pigment Cell and Its Role in the Pigmentation of Hair. In: Conference on the Biology of Normal and Atypical Pigment Cell Growth. 3rd. edition, New York, 1951. Pigment Cell Growth; Proceeding edited by Myron Gordon. New York, Academic Press, 1953, pp. 1–15.

Spemann, H.:Über den Anteil von Implantat und Wirkskeim au der Orientierung und Beschaffenheit der induzierten Embryonalanlage. Arch. f. Entwcklngsmechn. d. Organ. *123*:389–517, (Feb.) 1931.

Theobald, G. D.: Pseudoexfoliation of the Lens Capsule; Relation to "True" Exfoliation of the Lens Capsule as Reported in the Literature and Role in Production of Glaucoma Capsulocuticulare. Amer. J. Ophthal. *37*:1–12, (Jan.) 1954.

Vogt, A.: Ein neues Spaltlampenbild des Pupillengebietes: Hellblauer Pupillensaumfilz mit Häutchenbildung auf der Linsenvorderkapsel. Klin. Monstsbl. f. Augen. *75*:1–12, 1925.

Chapter **III**

Injury to the Eye

(Accidental and Surgical)

This chapter deals primarily with injury to the eyeball as a whole; the subsequent chapters will cover in more detail injuries to individual structures. Mechanical injury in its many forms probably is the most common cause of eye disease. Injuries most often result from accidents of various types, and may be due to surgery. The nature and location of the injury frequently determines the final outcome, as do such secondary factors as the introduction of infectious and noninfectious foreign material and the availability of immediate treatment. The type of treatment also is important and includes proper wound closure, repositioning or excision of tissue, control of hemorrhage, anti-infectious therapy, and anti-inflammatory measures. The initial damage either may be moderate or so destructive that enucleation is required within a few hours. Removal may be delayed for weeks or years, often becoming necessary because of recurrent hemorrhage and inflammation. The injury may be localized and simple or widespread and extremely complicated.

Mechanical injuries of the eye may result from contusions, penetrating or perforating wounds. The effects of these injuries differ greatly, not only in the mechanism of the injury and character of the lesions, but also in the complications, course, and sequelae. Nonpenetrating wounds outnumber those which are penetrating, but they usually are less severe. Penetrating injuries may cause no permanent loss of vision, but most often they result in loss of vision, or of the eye.

A penetrating wound of an individual tissue indicates that the wound enters into but not through the tissue, whereas a perforating wound of that tissue signifies complete severance of the layers of the tissue. Therefore, it is proper to speak of a penetrating wound of the *eyeball*, indicating that the laceration extends into the eye, but not completely through it. A penetrating wound of the *cornea* might involve only the epithelium, or extend down to Descemet's membrane, but would not extend into the anterior chamber, in contrast to a perforating wound of the cornea, which would extend completely through the cornea into the anterior chamber. Perforating and penetrating wounds may be produced in several ways: lacerations,

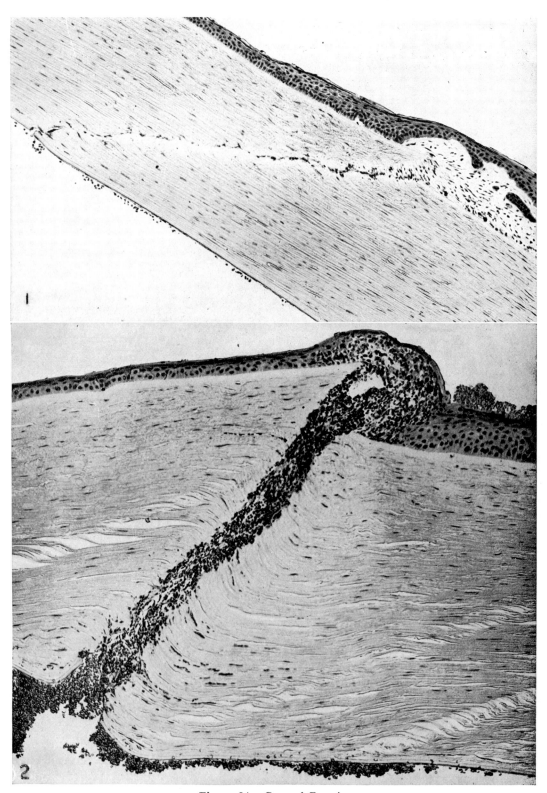

Figure 84.   Corneal Repair

1. Paracentesis. Breaks in Bowman's and Descemet's membranes. Superficial healing. ×125. AFIP Acc. 176476.

2. Paracentesis two weeks before enucleation. Repair of epithelium over wound. Escape of hemorrhage from anterior chamber through wound. ×150. AFIP Acc. 38925.

punctures, missiles, surgical incisions, or contusion with rupture. Their effects depend upon the site of the wound as well as on its extent. The perforation may vary tremendously in degree as to linear extent as well as in depth. Generally if the wound involves the anterior segment, the cornea, iris, and lens are damaged; if the posterior segment is penetrated, the sclera, choroid, retina, and vitreous are affected.

SURGICAL VS. ACCIDENTAL TRAUMA

Surgical incisions. Surgical trauma differs from accidental trauma in many respects. The incision is made at a site selected so as to accomplish the desired purpose with the least accompanying damage. Accidental perforation, however, may occur almost at any position. For example, although cataract incisions vary somewhat in location and angu-

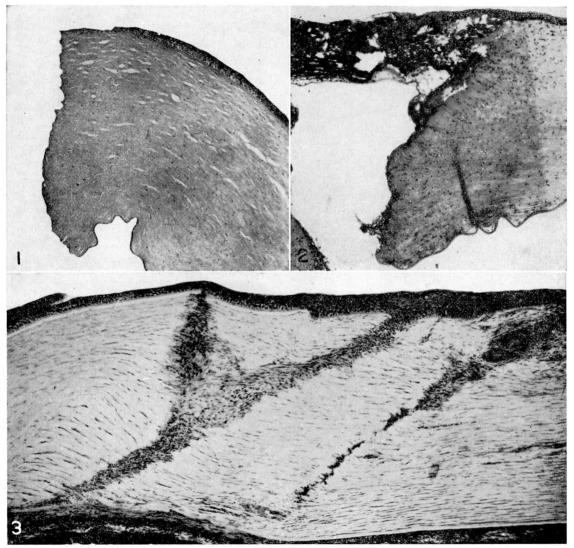

Figure 85. Corneal Repair

1. Perforating wound of cornea one hour before enucleation. Edema of epithelium and stroma. No inflammatory cell infiltration. ×40. AFIP Acc. 70703.

2. Recent corneal perforation. Fibrinous mass in wound. Edema and polymorphonuclear leukocytic infiltration, wound margin. ×70. AFIP Acc. 68691.

3. Old and recent wounds of cornea with anterior synechia. ×91. AFIP Acc. 28646.

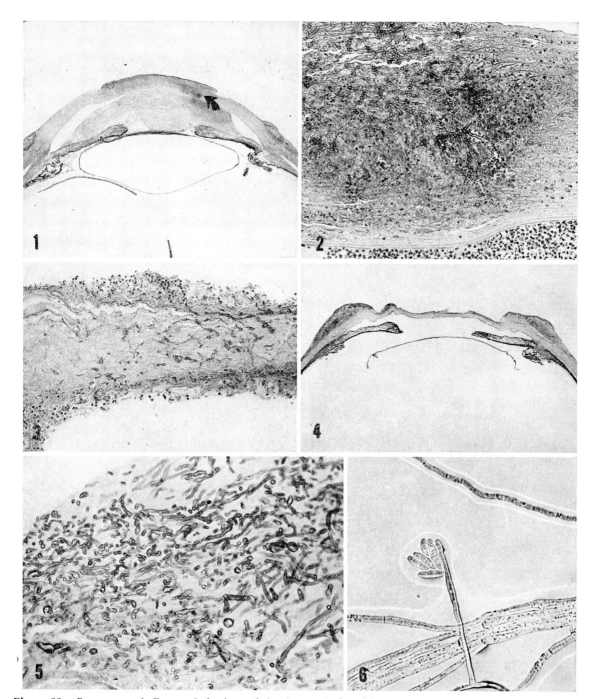

Figure 88. Post-traumatic Fungus Infections of the Cornea Induced by Antibiotic and Corticosteroid Therapy

1. Ring ulcer, deep mycotic abscess of cornea (arrow), and hypopyon. ×6. AFIP Neg. 57–342.

2. Mycelial forms of a fungus, probably a species of Aspergillus, in abscess shown by arrow in 1. ×165. AFIP Neg. 57–340.

3. Mycelial forms of a fungus invade the anterior chamber from the corneal stroma; this field is from center of lesion shown in 4. ×115. AFIP Neg. 57–355.

4. Diffuse necrotizing keratitis with perforation of cornea and hypotony. ×5. AFIP Neg. 57–354.

5. Diffuse growth of Cephalosporium in corneal stroma. Gridley fungus stain, ×305. AFIP Acc. 791062.

6. Fusarium sp. cultured from corneal ulcer, ×395. AFIP Acc. 793806.

lation according to the techniques employed, they all are essentially limbal, avoiding uveal tissue and the visual area of cornea. Certain glaucoma operations are designed to promote drainage of aqueous, but the routes of leakage are contrived to avoid damage to important structures and to provide controlled filtration to physiologic tissue spaces. Poor location of incisions in these and other operations may result in complications or loss of the eye.

Surgical wounds usually are neat and clean, with minimal crushing of adjacent tissues (Fig. 84). Accidental wounds more often are ragged and irregular, with more or less devitalized edges (Fig. 85). Surgical wounds are placed for accurate closure and their edges usually are exactly reapproximated. Wounds of chance may fit together poorly, if at all, and their surgical repair often represents the best that can be made of an unfavorable situation. Surgical incisions are made under aseptic and mechanically clean conditions, with a minimum of opportunity for introduction of infectious organisms or foreign material. Operations, whenever possible, are performed on relatively soft globes to reduce the risk of accidental extrusion of ocular contents. Accidental trauma is the result of force applied to the eye so that contents of the globe may be forced into or out through the wound (Figs. 86, 87).

All of the factors mentioned above combine to affect the outcome of the trauma. Wounds made without proper preparation, asepsis, and antisepsis are prone to infection. The condition and location of the wound edges seriously affect healing. Foreign matter in the wound may prevent healing and foreign bodies deeper in the globe may set up various types of reactions depending on the nature of the alien substance. Some of these factors may be influenced by treatment. Antimicrobial therapy may control infectious processes, and anti-inflammatory measures may reduce the tissue reaction to trauma, to foreign material, and to infection. This last form of treatment, in some instances may seriously depress the normal defenses and favor growth of infectious agents (Figs. 76, 88).

CONTUSIONS AND CONCUSSIONS

Contusion of the eyeball may be direct or indirect. *Indirect* contusion or concussion may result from blast injuries, plane crashes, falls, and gunshot head injuries. These may lead to intraocular hemorrhage, and to retinal detachment.

Direct injuries which are not so severe as to cause rupture of the globe may nevertheless produce a variety of changes. Displacement and rupture of the parts of the uveal tract, lens, retina, and optic nerve may result.

Iris. Contusion of the iris may produce a variety of effects, such as rupture, injury to the sphincter with mydriasis, stromal atrophy, or injury to the pigment layer. Ruptures of the iris, either at the pupillary margin or at the root (iridodialysis) (Figs. 89, 90) are particularly serious as they may cause hemorrhage into the anterior chamber and glaucoma. Tears in the iris stroma resulting from blows may be radial or localized at the iris root. Such traumatic colobomas can be bridged by the scar of an organizing hemorrhage, but often remain unhealed.

Cyclodialysis or a tear through the scleral spur with separation of the ciliary body (Fig. 90) is less common but may produce similar hemorrhages by rupturing the anterior ciliary vessels. The most serious effect of contusion in this area is to the anterior ciliary body. A tear most often commences in the anterior portion external to the iris root and extends backward toward the major circle, severing some of its branches. It is this type of injury which most often produces severe anterior chamber hemorrhage, especially that which is recurrent and leads to severe glaucoma. After subsidence of the effects of this type of injury, microscopic examination shows the angle on the injured side to be much deeper and rounded, because of the ciliary body tear (Fig. 91). Associated with this is damage to the aqueous outflow passages which leads to a type of chronic secondary glaucoma (Fig. 91). This type of glaucoma may develop in-

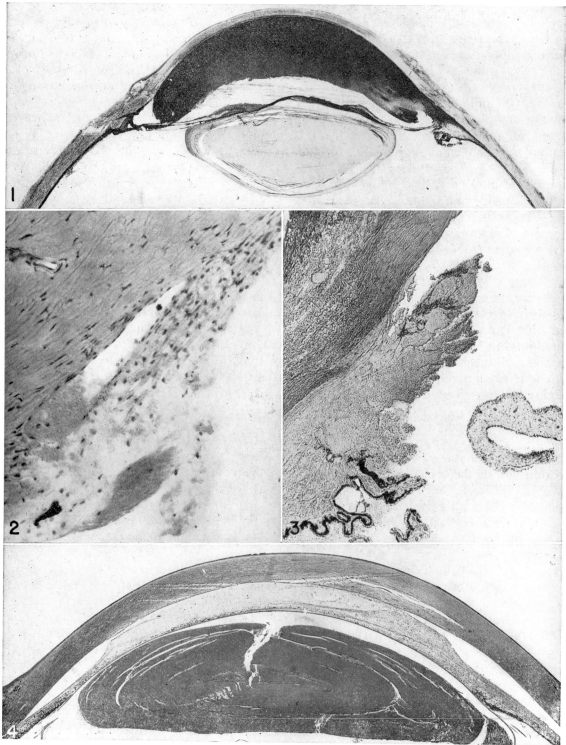

Figure 89. Contusion

1. Hemorrhage in anterior chamber from rupture of filtration angle and pupillary zone of iris. ×6. AFIP Acc. 24062.

2. Rupture of filtration angle. ×240. AFIP Acc. 91571.

3. Iridodialysis. ×35. AFIP Acc. 101534.

4. Organized hemorrhage in anterior chamber. ×15. AFIP Acc. 104773.

sidiously long after the immediate effects of the contusion have subsided and the injury has been forgotten. In such cases the glaucoma is often mistakenly interpreted as a unilateral chronic simple glaucoma until the excessively deep recess of the anterior chamber angle is recognized and its significance realized (d'Ombrain, 1949; Wolff and Zimmerman).

Hyphema, or hemorrhage in the anterior chamber, is one of the most important consequences of contusion. The amount of blood varies widely. Small hemorrhages do not clot, the red cells being suspended in the aqueous humor, whereas in larger hemorrhages the anterior chamber is filled with blood and clotting is common.

The hemorrhage may disappear both by degeneration of the cells and by their diffusion through the trabecular outflow channels and iris. Persistent or recurrent hemorrhage may lead to formation of iris membranes and adhesions between the iris, cornea and lens. Seclusion and occlusion of

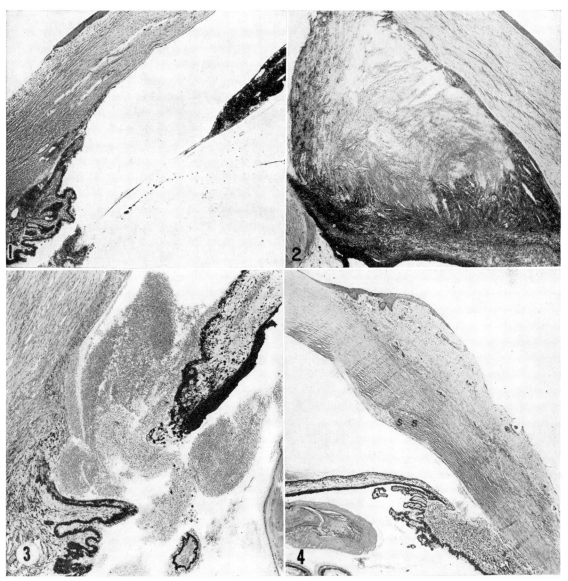

Figure 90. Contusion

1. Iridodialysis. Adhesion of ciliary process to corneoscleral trabeculas. ×30. AFIP Acc. 116864.
2. Cholesterol slits in organized hemorrhage in anterior chamber. ×35. AFIP Acc. 29626.
3. Iridodialysis. Hemorrhage in anterior chamber. ×38. AFIP Acc. 513807.
4. Cyclodialysis. The ciliary body is torn away from the scleral spur (ss). ×16. AFIP Acc. 800407.

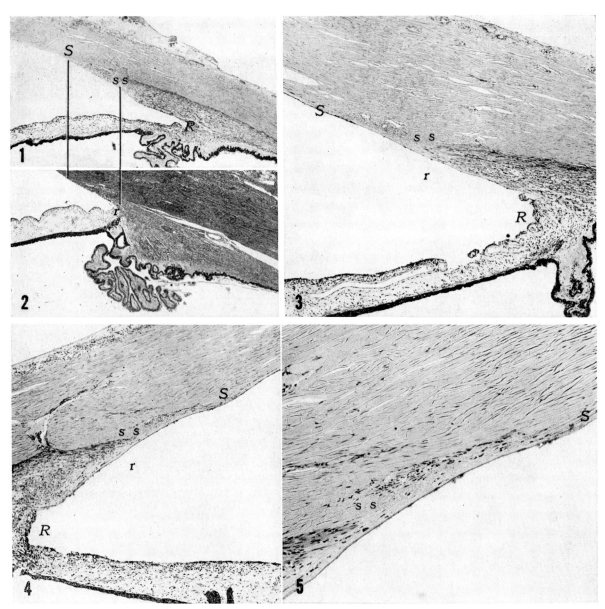

Figure 91. Post-contusion Deformity of Chamber Angle

Deepening of anterior chamber angle produced by contusion of eye, often associated with ipsilateral chronic glaucoma of insidious onset long after the injury. In 1 the abnormally deep recess (R) of the anterior chamber angle is compared with the normal chamber angle position (r) and other normal relationships shown in 2: normally the chamber angle is at the level of the scleral spur (s s); the position of Schwalbe's line (S) is in normal relationship to the trabecula but appears farther forward than normal in 1, 3, and 4 because of the retro-displacement of the iris root. Degeneration of the trabecula and hyaline membrane covering its inner surface are shown in 5. 1. ×21. AFIP Acc. 61457. 2. ×21. AFIP Acc. 814227. 3 and 4. ×50. AFIP Acc. 849004. 5. ×125. AFIP Acc. 849004.

the pupil may occur. Rarely, the anterior chamber may become filled with fibrous tissue. Recurrent hemorrhages later occur as a sequela of such scar formation.

Secondary glaucoma is one of the most important results of severe contusion and often is the cause of eventual loss of the eye.

It usually is associated with recurrent large anterior chamber hemorrhages in which the blood clots become dark-colored, the so-called "eight-ball" type. The flow of aqueous may be blocked directly by the clot, which becomes organized and firmly adherent to iris and cornea around the angle.

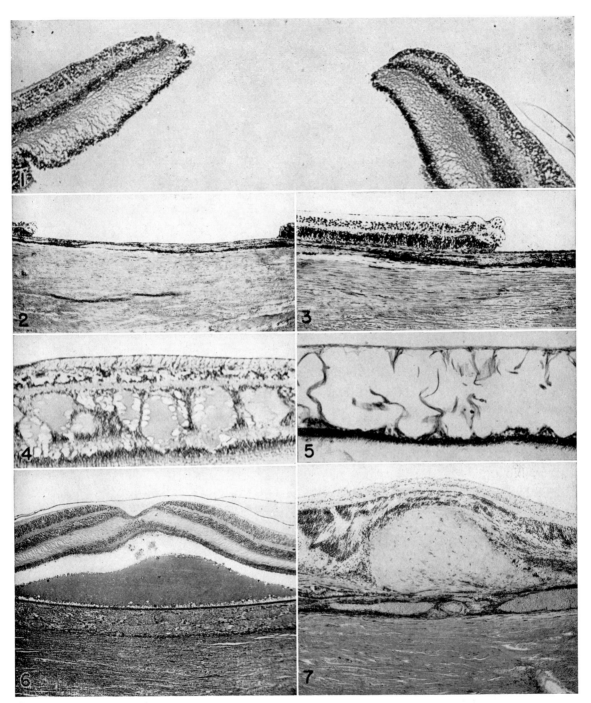

Figure 92. Contusion

1. Hole in macula, recent. ×75. AFIP Acc. 158930.
2. Hole in macula, old. ×45. AFIP Acc. 212454.
3. Margin of macular hole. ×75. AFIP Acc. 212454.
4. Serous exudates in retina. ×48. AFIP Acc. 232679.
5. Cystoid degeneration of retina in area of serous exudation. ×120. AFIP Acc. 107046.
6. Submacular serous exudation. ×48. AFIP Acc. 232679.
7. Organized submacular hemorrhage. ×75. AFIP Acc. 191956.

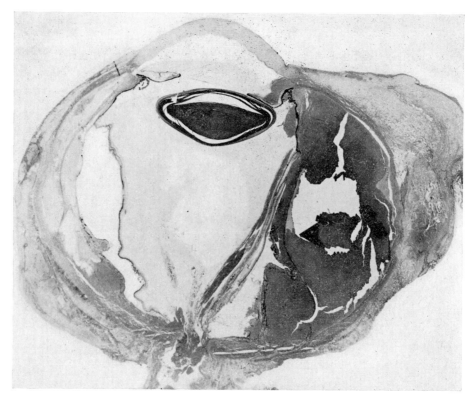

Figure 93. Contusion. Avulsion of optic nerve. Rupture of filtration angle. Massive suprachoroidal hemorrhage. AFIP Acc. 104621.

When increased intraocular pressure is associated with hemorrhage in the anterior chamber, blood staining of the cornea may occur by passage of hemoglobin through the corneal endothelium into the stroma. For this to occur, damage to the corneal endothelium usually is necessary, and, if this damage is sufficiently severe, the cornea may be stained with blood pigment even without increased intraocular pressure (see Chapter VI).

Rupture of the ciliary processes is rather uncommon and if bleeding occurs the blood usually finds its way into the anterior chamber, particularly when the zonular fibers have been damaged. Blunt injuries often produce choroidal tears and hemorrhage. These injuries may lead to extensive choroidal and subchoroidal fibrosis and finally to ossification. Subretinal hemorrhages or serous exudates may cause retinal detachment. Superficial retinal hemorrhages between the nerve fiber layer and the internal limiting membrane may rupture into the vitreous. As in the anterior chamber, the blood may be absorbed or become organized by the proliferation of fibrovascular tissue arising from the retina (retinitis proliferans). Farther anteriorly a similar process may lead to formation of a retrolental mass of organized hemorrhage anchored on each side at the ora serrata (cyclitic membrane). Large vitreous hemorrhages tend to settle inferiorly where they eventually form diffuse fibrous masses of tissue.

Always associated with hemorrhage is a certain amount of inflammatory reaction represented (1) by phagocytic cells which are active in "absorption," (2) by formation of granulation tissue, and (3) by a persistent mild inflammatory reaction to damaged tissue. Infections are rare in injured eyes which do not have penetrating wounds. Secondary intraocular pyogenic reactions occasionally are seen when infection of the orbit has followed injury to the lids, the conjunctiva, or the orbital tissues.

Edema of the retina may follow contusion and usually is most intense in the macular region. The edema may lead to cystoid degeneration of the macula followed by development of a retinal hole at the fovea (Fig. 92). A retinal tear at the ora serrata (retinal dialysis or disinsertion) may occur and be followed by retinal detachment. Tears in the retina near the disk generally are a consequence of avulsion of the optic nerve rather than of simple contusion (Fig. 93).

A more interesting feature resulting from blunt injuries to the eye is concussion of the retina (commotio retinae). As in concussion of the brain, the pathogenesis of this lesion is not understood. It is characterized by widespread edema of the retina, often associated with retinal hemorrhages of various sizes. The ophthalmoscopic picture of a snow-white retina, most dense at the posterior pole, flecked with hemorrhages is most striking but is not necessarily associated with great loss of vision, for the edema and hemorrhages commonly are absorbed without much residual damage.

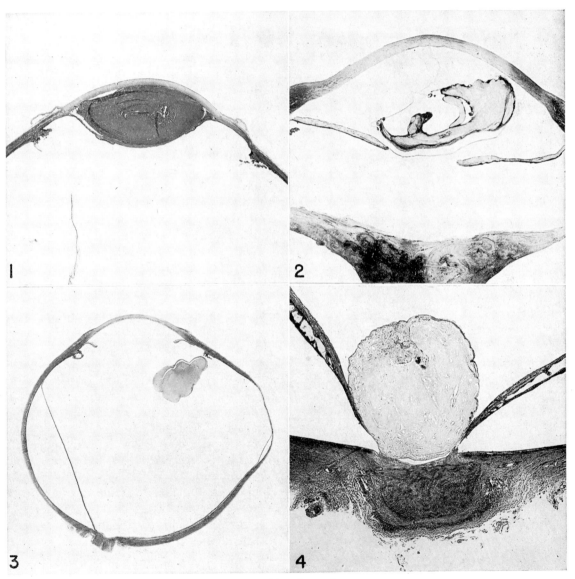

Figure 94. Contusion

1. Dislocation of lens into anterior chamber. AFIP Acc. 133591.
2. Dislocation of lens into anterior chamber. Calcareous cataract. AFIP Acc. 175620.
3. Subluxation and degeneration of lens resulting in irregular contour. AFIP Acc. 159084.
4. Dislocation of lens to optic disk. Advanced degeneration of lens substance. AFIP Acc. 264250.

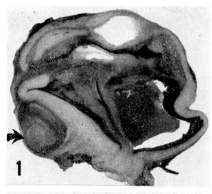

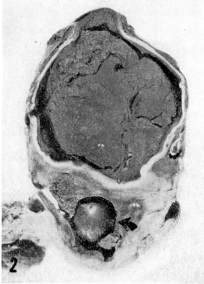

Figure 95. Contusion of eye with rupture of sclera. In both instances the lens (arrows) has been dislocated into the retrobulbar orbital tissues. 1. AFIP Acc. 646985. 2. AFIP Acc. 646933.

Retinal hemorrhages either may be absorbed without residue or are followed by cystoid degeneration or massive gliosis. The latter condition following retinal hemorrhages in children may be mistaken for retinoblastoma. The degree of glial proliferation may be so great that the posterior segment is largely filled with bizarre hypertrophic glia and prominent blood vessels.

Contusion of the globe also may produce dislocation of the lens. If part of the zonular fibers are ruptured, subluxation may result, but the lens, even though freely movable, remains in the hyaloid fossa. If the zonule is completely ruptured, dislocation can occur either into the anterior chamber or posteriorly into the vitreous. Anterior chamber

dislocations lead to block of the pupil and filtration angle, producing glaucoma. If the lens remains in this location, an inflammatory reaction results, with formation of adhesions between the iris, lens, and cornea. If dislocation is incomplete or posterior, glaucoma may be produced, but the mechanism is unknown (Fig. 94).

Contusion cataract usually occurs without rupture of the lens capsule. As a result the opacity is in the posterior cortex, is of the rosette type, and is probably due to separation of the lens fibers from the suture lines. Rupture of the lens capsule, particularly at the equator, occasionally is caused by severe contusions. Cataract may develop in lenses dislocated at the time of injury. Clinically, following contusion, a ring of pigment (Vossius' ring) is often seen on the anterior surface of the lens capsule. This has been interpreted either as melanin from the pigment epithelium of the iris, or as hemosiderin limited in its distribution by the anterior insertion of the zonular fibers.

Blunt trauma may involve sufficient force to cause rupture of the globe (Fig. 95). The rupture may occur at the site of the application of force but often is located elsewhere. The internal pressure caused by the blow may cause a rupture at an anatomically weak area, such as the thin equatorial sclera or limbus over Schlemm's canal, or one which is weakened by disease, such as a deep corneal ulcer or a staphyloma. The majority of these ruptures are so explosive that extensive loss of the ocular contents and massive hemorrhage ensue. This results in collapse and disorganization of the eye, followed by inflammation and phthisis.

Those concussive effects which are produced by indirect force, for example, a bomb blast, or underwater explosion, lead to tissue changes in the more vascular ocular tissues, such as the uveal tract and retina. The concussion wave leads to a rise in intravascular pressure and spasm, and a later paralysis. Slowing of the blood stream and leakage of fluid and blood from the walls result. Damage occurs in the retinal cells with subsequent degeneration. The retina usually shows edema and some hemorrhage, especially posteriorly.

PENETRATING AND PERFORATING WOUNDS

Anterior Wounds

Penetrating and perforating wounds of the anterior segment are common. Those which are complicated usually are more extensive and involve a number of tissues, and quite often are followed by serious sequelae such as glaucoma, endophthalmitis, and atrophy of the eyeball. Uncomplicated wounds often are small, are not accompanied by such severe involvement of internal structures, and are less likely to have serious sequelae.

Uncomplicated. Perforating wounds of the conjunctiva usually heal rapidly by proliferation of fibroblasts from the stromal cells and of epithelium from the wound edges. Corneal wounds heal by activity of the corneal stromal cells, histiocytes, the epithelium, and the endothelium, without formation of granulation tissue (Fig. 96). The resulting scar may be so uniform that it is difficult to detect clinically as well as in microscopic sections. Wounds of the limbus and sclera rarely are uncomplicated because of the proximity of vessels, the filtration area and anterior chamber, the lens, and the vitreous. Small puncture wounds or lacerations may lead to relatively slight intraocular damage, and heal without sequelae. If the wound produces a defect in the iris it is interesting that if no inflammation occurs, the gap fails to close. Apparently a stimulus to healing is lacking. Similar small wounds in the lens capsule may gape very little, and be sealed by proliferation of epithelium or by adhesion of the adjacent iris.

Complicated. Complicated wounds most often are characterized by their large size, irregular shape, more extensive involvement of the intraocular tissues, frequent loss or incarceration of portions of the intraocular tissues, and prolonged inflammation during healing (Figs. 97 to 99). Complicated corneal and limbal wounds often are jagged and are associated with tears and prolapse of the iris. Laceration of the lens capsule is frequent, with incarceration or prolapse of capsule and cortex. The vitreous may be prolapsed into the anterior chamber, or between the lips of the wound, and ciliary body injuries may cause extensive hemorrhage into the posterior and anterior chambers and the vitreous.

Surgical correction of such injuries usually involves excision of iris, removal of incarcerated lens tissue and prevention of adherence of vitreous to the wound. Even though there is accurate closure of the wound edges, adhesions most often form between the deep wound surface and the intraocular tissues. The hemorrhage and inflammatory exudate in the anterior chamber organize into dense fibrous bands. A corneal leukoma often results, and sequelae include glaucoma, recurrent iridocyclitis, and atrophy of the eyeball with disorganization of its contents.

According to Dunnington (1951), the wounds of cataract operations usually are not completely approximated throughout their depth and tend to gape internally. The defect gradually is bridged by fibrous tissue which slowly contracts and pulls the edges together. Incarceration of lens capsule or iris in such a wound may result in localized areas of nonunion. This occurs unintentionally in the course of cataract operations but is done deliberately in iris inclusion operations to control glaucoma.

A number of important complications may arise as a relatively *early* effect of the anterior ocular injury. These include infection, cataract, glaucoma, endophthalmitis due to trauma and lens hypersensitivity, and hemorrhage, which may be either moderate or of the expulsive type.

Later complications include glaucoma, endophthalmitis due to recurrent hemorrhage, epithelial ingrowth into the anterior chamber, and retinal detachment. Many of these complications will be discussed in detail in subsequent chapters, but others are of such importance they should be considered here.

Early Complications

Cataract usually results from interruption of the lens capsule. Small wounds often seal and the damage to the cortex remains localized. Most commonly, however, the injury leads to a complete cataract.

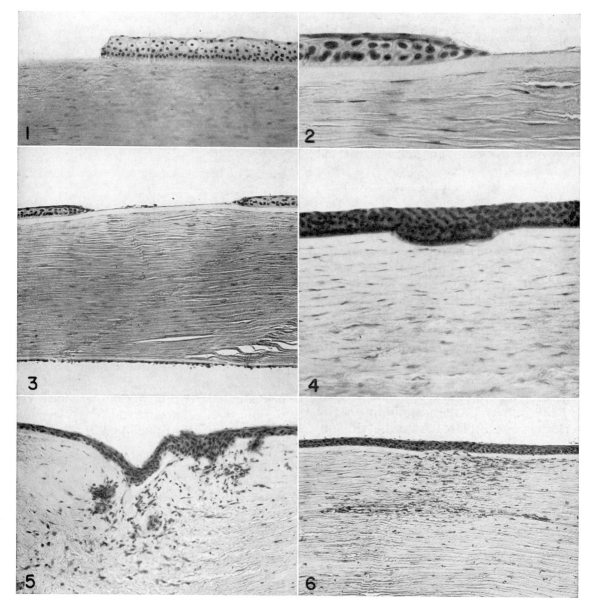

Figure 96. Superficial Corneal Injuries

1. Abrasion of corneal epithelium after enucleation. Sharp epithelial margin. No evidence of repair. ×125. AFIP Acc. 136747.

2. Abrasion of corneal epithelium before enucleation. Smooth epithelial margin. Beginning extension of cells of basal layer into defect. ×400. AFIP Acc. 201565.

3. Corneal abrasion. Beginning repair. ×125. AFIP Acc. 201565.

4. Epithelial facet at site of foreign body which caused small break in Bowman's membrane. ×300. AFIP Acc. 28249.

5. Fibroblastic proliferation and few chronic inflammatory cells in recent superficial corneal wound. New-formed epithelium covers wound. ×125. AFIP Acc. 480850.

6. Healing scar of superficial corneal wound. Fibroblastic proliferation in superficial stroma. Break in Bowman's membrane. Complete repair of epithelium. ×75. AFIP Acc. 148893.

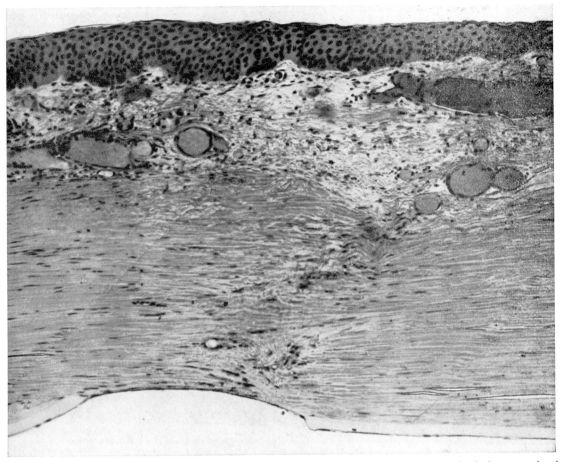

Figure 97. Corneal repair. Somewhat vascular scar of iridectomy performed two months before enucleation. Wide break in Descemet's membrane. ×200. AFIP Acc. 56280.

Glaucoma results from hemorrhage, peripheral anterior synechias, and organization of fibrous tissue in the angle and pupillary region.

Endophthalmitis and *panophthalmitis* of varying severity almost always follow penetrating and perforating injuries. These may be the result of infection or hemorrhage, necrosis of tissue, and, at times, phacoanaphylaxis. The ocular changes in endophthalmitis and panophthalmitis have been given in the previous chapter. Sympathetic ophthalmia will be discussed in Chapter VII. It seems appropriate to discuss phacoanaphylactic endophthalmitis here because of its special nature and the wide effects it produces in the eye.

Endophthalmitis phaco-anaphylactica is the appropriate term introduced by Verhoeff and Lemoine for the lens-induced endophthalmitis which previously was described by Straub.

The concept of bilaterality in this disease later was emphasized by Courtney who reported seven cases of bilateral inflammation following extracapsular operation for senile cataract. Autosensitization to lens protein is believed to be responsible for the disease, although the histopathologic lesion characteristic of phaco-anaphylaxis of humans has not been reproduced in experimental animals. As Woods has recently emphasized, there is no good evidence to support the concept of phacotoxic uveitis or endophthalmitis. It has never been shown in man or animals that normal or cataractous lenses contain toxic substances capable of producing an endophthalmitis. A possible exception is observed in phacolytic glaucoma which is discussed in Chapter XII.

Clinically the phaco-anaphylaxis usually follows injury to the lens of one eye, and it ordinarily affects only the injured eye. In rare cases the inflammation also involves the

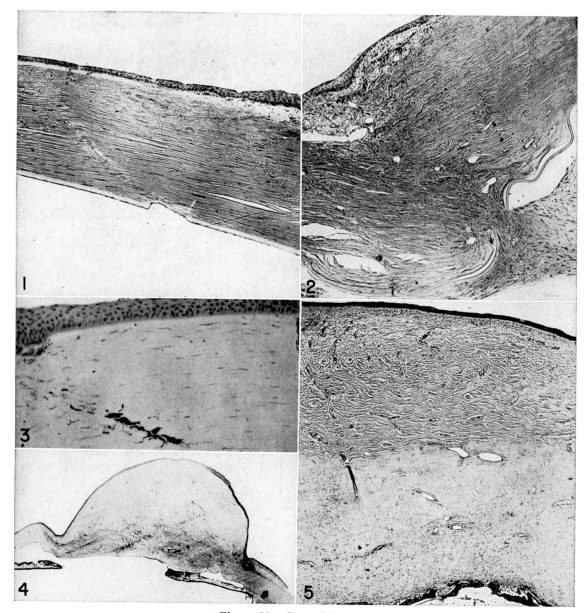

Figure 98. Corneal Repair

1. Healed linear scar of perforating wound of cornea. Narrow break in Bowman's membrane. Wide break in Descemet's membrane. Surface epithelium completely replaced. ×75. AFIP Acc. 271517.

2. Broad scar of cataract extraction extending through Descemet's membrane near limbus. ×75. AFIP Acc. 114455.

3. Pigment from iris in scar of operative wound. ×120. AFIP Acc. 54296.

4. Hypertrophic scar of foreign body injury followed by ulcer. ×20. AFIP Acc. 115850.

5. Keloidal kerato-iridic scar following corneal perforation. ×48. AFIP Acc. 292418.

fellow (uninjured) eye, producing a syndrome that resembles sympathetic ophthalmia. It has been the observation of several ophthalmic pathologists (most recently by Blodi) that phaco-anaphylaxis and sympathetic ophthalmia occur simultaneously more often than would be expected by chance alone, but statistical proof is lacking. The inflammation may develop insidiously or acutely with congestion, a hazy cornea, white keratic precipitates, and an intense cellular exudation into the anterior chamber. The exudate in the region of the lens may be serofibrinous or, rarely, purulent.

Microscopically the inflammatory reaction in phaco-anaphylaxis is centered around the damaged lens which is extensively infiltrated by polymorphonuclear leukocytes (Fig. 100). Surrounding the lens, especially where its capsule is broken, is a zone of large mononuclear cells some of which are transformed into epithelioid and giant cells. The adjacent iris and ciliary body are intensely inflamed and are infiltrated with lymphocytes and plasma cells. Typically the iris is firmly bound to the lens by an inflammatory membrane. The choroid and retina have a variable mononuclear infiltration, mainly around the vessels and on the inner limiting membrane of the retina over the vessels.

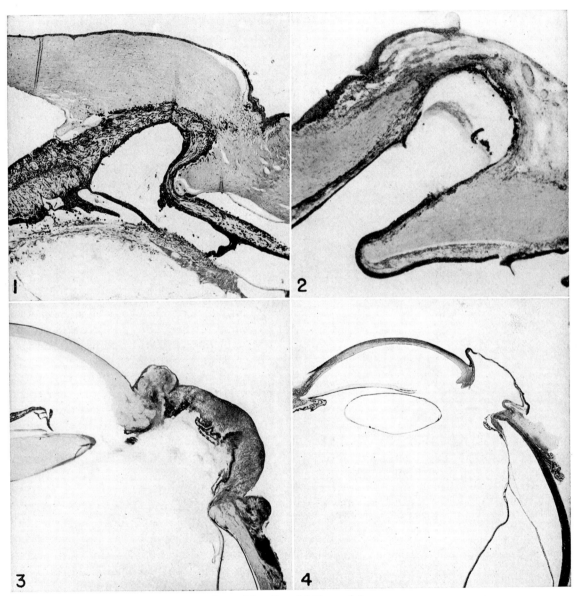

Figure 99. Cystoid Corneal Scar

1. Iris loop in scar of operative wound preventing approximation of deep corneal lamellas. ×48. AFIP Acc. 212598.

2. Iris loop preventing closure of wound margins. Cystoid kerato-iridic scar covered by conjunctiva and lined by iris pigment epithelium. ×85. AFIP Acc. 31974.

3. Cystoid kerato-iridic scar lined by iris pigment epithelium, following perforating wound of limbus with prolapse of iris and ciliary body. AFIP Acc. 21478.

4. Cystoid scar of perforating wound at limbus. AFIP Acc. 161046.

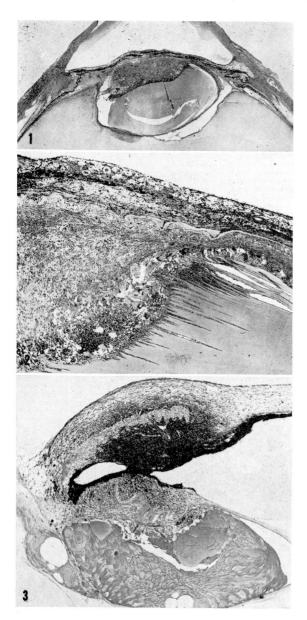

Figure 100. Lens-induced endophthalmitis following traumatic rupture of lens capsule (phaco-anaphylaxis).

1. Exuberant proliferation of chronic inflammatory cells and connective tissue with replacement of absorbed lens cortex and nucleus at site of injury. ×10. AFIP Acc. 339621.

2. The inflammatory reaction has a distinctly granulomatous component with many multinucleated giant cells. ×53. AFIP Acc. 339621.

3. Nongranulomatous chronic iritis, presumed to be phacogenic. ×50. AFIP Acc. 749639.

It is not known how the injury or operation on the first eye produces a subsequent inflammation in the fellow eye, but it is assumed that the second eye develops a hyper-sensitivity reaction to lens protein escaping from the intact but usually cataractous lens in the uninjured eye. Phacolytic glaucoma, an entirely different process which is apparently independent of autosensitization, will be described in Chapter XII.

Expulsive hemorrhage. Another serious immediate complication of penetrating anterior eye injuries is expulsive hemorrhage which is characterized by an immediate massive choroidal hemorrhage following an operative procedure or injury (Fig. 101–1). Occasionally the hemorrhage appears after 6 to 24 hours. The blood fills the choroid, detaching it from the sclera, forcing the retina and vitreous toward the wound, and eventually resulting in loss of iris, lens, vitreous and retina. At times the choroid and ciliary body are completely detached and are everted through the wound edges. Less severe hemorrhage also may occur after surgery and injuries, and its frequency is greater than is generally appreciated (Fig. 101). In such instances the hemorrhage occurs as a more or less broad zone at the equator.

Late Complications

The later complications of anterior ocular wounds will be discussed in detail in subsequent chapters. Glaucoma most often results either from pupillary block by occlusion or seclusion of the pupil with formation of peripheral anterior synechias, or from trabecular fibrosis. Endophthalmitis is due to recurrent inflammation produced by degeneration and hemorrhage into scar tissue.

Epithelial ingrowth. Epithelial ingrowth into the anterior chamber is a relatively common complication of injuries as well as of surgical procedures. It is produced by delayed or faulty coaptation of the corneal or limbal wound edges.

Where surface epithelium has access to such a wound, it may proliferate through the tract and enter the eye to line the cornea and angle; this epithelial downgrowth eventually produces glaucoma (Fig. 102). Surface epithelium also has a tendency to line suture tracts. Epithelialization of the anterior chamber should be distinguished from pearl-like implantation cysts of the iris, which result

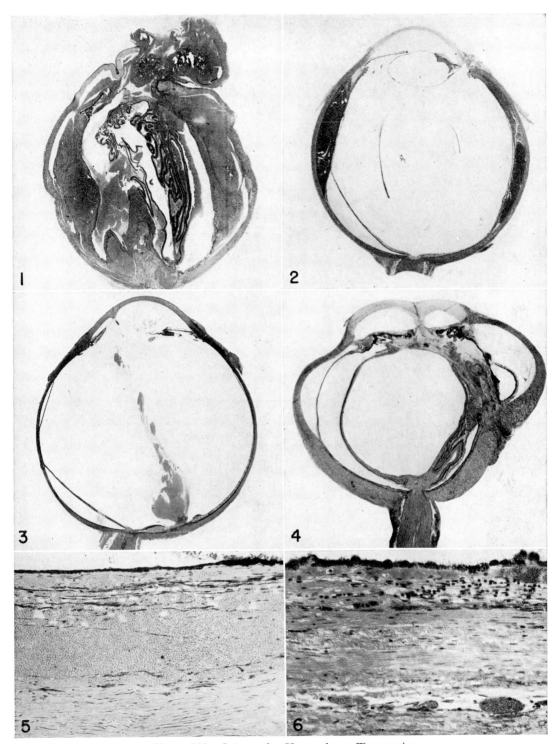

Figure 101. Intraocular Hemorrhage, Traumatic

1. Expulsive hemorrhage following penetrating wound at limbus. AFIP Acc. 98147.
2. Suprachoroidal hemorrhage following penetrating wound at limbus. AFIP Acc. 199434.
3. Hemorrhage in track of foreign body which perforated cornea and lodged in macula. AFIP Acc. 87408.
4. Organized hemorrhage forming traction band between corneal scar of entrance and scleral scar of exit. AFIP Acc. 23545.
5. Suprachoroidal hemorrhage, recent. ×125. AFIP Acc. 214528.
6. Organized suprachoroidal hemorrhage. ×185. AFIP Acc. 184424.

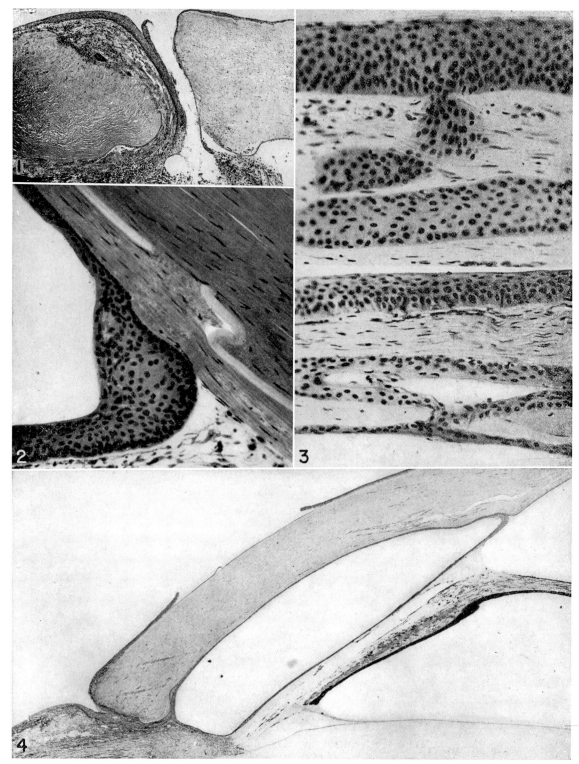

Figure 102. Epithelialization of Cornea and Anterior Chamber

1. Epithelialization of recent corneal wound. ×40. AFIP Acc. 187218.

2. Epithelialization of anterior chamber following cataract extraction. Break in Descemet's membrane indicates site of operation. ×240. AFIP Acc. 55491.

3. Solid and cystoid epithelial implants in different fields of one cornea, following injury. AFIP Acc. 218092.

4. Cystoid epithelialization of anterior chamber following cataract extraction. Continuity between surface and intraocular epithelium is evident in wound. ×30. AFIP Acc. 114455.

from introduction of eyelashes into the iris with subsequent growth. Such cysts, however, usually remain small and confined to the iris. The cysts which result from ordinary epithelial downgrowth may become very large and fill the anterior chamber. The downgrowth following cataract extraction is associated with delayed reformation of the anterior chamber, which results from a leaking wound.

Posterior Wounds

Perforating wounds of the posterior sclera are not common. Most often they follow blows and automobile accidents. This type of injury is most frequent in the temporal sclera posterior to the ora serrata. Puncture wounds usually produce no severe damage even though they perforate the choroid and retina. A small amount of vitreous often is incarcerated in the wound, and healing is accompanied by formation of a light connective tissue scar which may contain blood vessels and extend a short distance into the adjacent vitreous. Detachment of the retina usually does not occur. Larger wounds almost always are complicated by loss of vitreous, bleeding, and severe damage to the choroid and retina. The complications and sequelae are much the same as those which follow anterior scleral wounds, except that vitreous loss usually is more extensive, and vital structures may be affected. Some of the complications of all these types of injury have been mentioned. Retinal detachment may develop, especially if vitreous loss is followed by formation of vitreous bands in the reparative stage. Atrophy with disorganization of the eyeball is common.

FOREIGN BODIES

The effects of foreign bodies which are introduced into the eye depend on the size, location, and number of particles introduced, the material of which they are composed, their initial damage, and the length of time they are retained. Gold, silver, platinum, glass, and many plastic materials are relatively well tolerated (Fig. 103). Lead and zinc are less well tolerated, while iron, particularly soft iron, and copper are oxidized and absorbed more rapidly, sometimes leading to generalized siderosis and chalcosis. Limestone elicits a marked reaction.

In eyes removed from soldiers during World War II, Wilder found that the reaction to primary missiles in the eye often was complicated by accompanying nonmagnetic materials, such as paint, vegetable matter, shale, clay, skin, bone and cilia. It is clear that even in the absence of such obvious particulate material, the cleanliness of the primary missile has much to do with the outcome. Clean metallic foreign bodies incite a minimal inflammatory reaction, whereas animal and vegetable fibers characteristically provoke a foreign body reaction with numerous giant cells. Vegetable matter is often accompanied by pyogenic bacteria and fungi, but sterile organic materials (e.g., cotton fibers introduced during surgical operations) can provoke a similar though usually milder reaction (Fig. 30).

The degree of siderosis resulting from retained ferrous foreign bodies and the rapidity with which it develops depend largely on the size, hardness, and number of the ferrous particles, on the position in the eye, and on their encapsulation by organizing hemorrhage. If the foreign body is promptly encapsulated, the siderosis is localized to the surrounding tissues. These tissues and the exudates surrounding them become discolored and often exhibit marked affinity for hematoxylin. When the iron is absorbed, it is distributed throughout the eye in an ionized form which histochemically cannot be distinguished from hemosiderin. Within the cells of the affected tissues it combines with the proteins to form insoluble salts, thus interfering with metabolic activity in the cells. The effect of the iron-protein complex is pronounced on the retinal cells, which have a high metabolic activity. Extreme damage occurs to the neuronal and supporting cells. The experiments of Cibis, in dogs which were given saccharated iron parenterally over

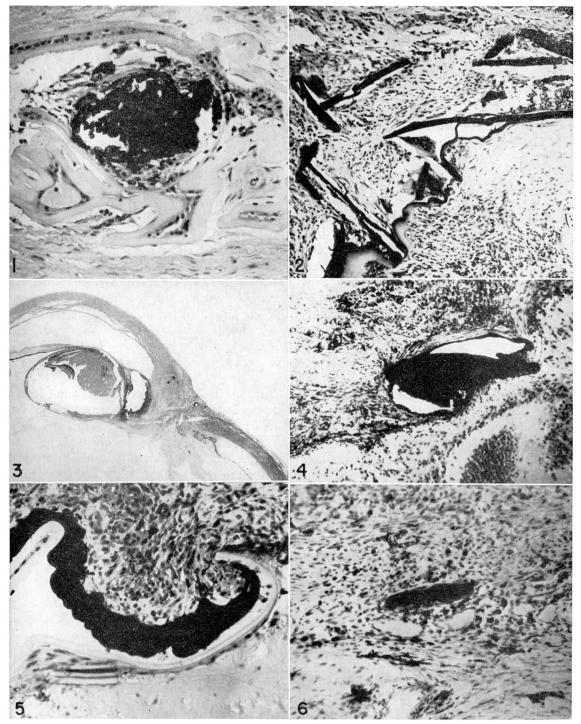

Figure 103. Intraocular Foreign Bodies

1. Ferrous foreign body in lens capsule incarcerated in an inflammatory cyclitic membrane. AFIP Acc. 95810.

2. Multiple ferrous foreign bodies in an inflammatory cyclitic membrane. AFIP Acc. 83318.

3. Pigmentation of scar tissue around site of ferrous foreign body in posterior chamber. AFIP Acc. 117881.

4. Lead particles in inflammatory tissue in vitreous chamber. AFIP Acc. 110885.

5. Copper wire in lens. Early anterior subcapsular cataract. Lens capsule recoiled outward at site of entrance. AFIP Acc. 107401.

6. Paint fragment in choroid. Steel foreign body to which paint had been attached had been removed by magnet extraction. AFIP Acc. 112894.

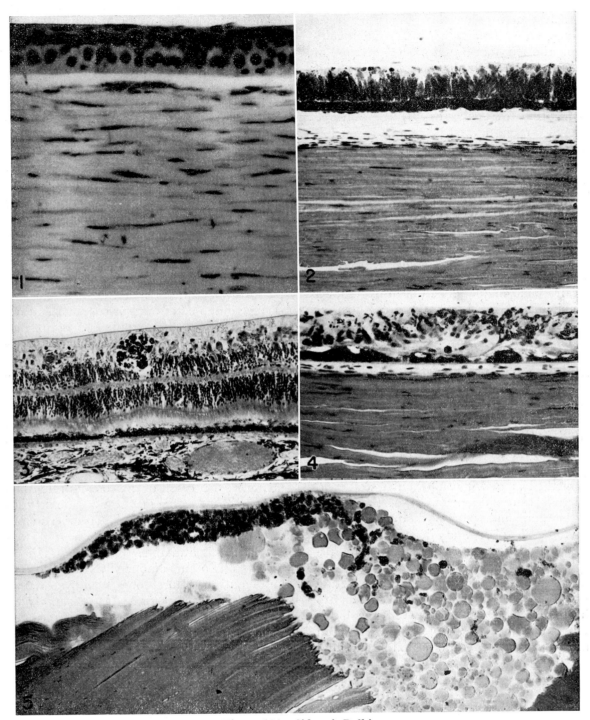

Figure 104. Siderosis Bulbi

1. Iron pigment phagocytized by corneal corpuscles. ×375. **AFIP Acc.** 54227.
2. Iron pigment in normally nonpigmented ciliary epithelium. ×185. **AFIP Acc.** 182503.
3. Iron pigment around retinal vessel. ×100. **AFIP Acc.** 105307.
4. Pigmentation and atrophy of retina. ×185. **AFIP Acc.** 182503.
5. Iron pigment in subcapsular epithelium of lens. Degenerated lens fibers forming morgagnian globules. ×170. **AFIP Acc.** 54227.

a period of years, demonstrate dramatically the effect of iron on the retina and other tissues. Other studies by this same investigator showed that intravitreal injection of saccharated iron could produce severe effects on the retinal vessels and cells. It is known that severe intraocular hemorrhage may lead to hemosiderosis, with exactly the same effects as those produced by retained iron foreign bodies.

Histologic signs of siderosis appear in varying interludes following injury (Fig. 104). The iris epithelium and dilator muscle, the ciliary epithelium, the retina, the retinal pigment epithelium and the epithelium of the lens reveal the greatest affinity for iron, but the endothelium and stromal cells of the cornea, the corneoscleral trabecula and the uveal stroma may also become involved. In nonpigmented structures the iron deposits may give the tissues a rusty macroscopic appearance and the brown pigment often can be seen microscopically without special stains. When present in small quantities or when taken up by pigmented cells it is necessary to use histochemical methods (e.g., Prussian blue reaction) in order to demonstrate the iron.

Iron in the lens epithelium may stimulate epithelial proliferation to produce a heavily pigmented anterior subcapsular cataract. Siderosis causes degeneration of the ciliary epithelium, and patchy disappearance of melanin. The pigmentary degeneration of the retina usually is more intense at the periphery. It appears within phagocytes around the blood vessels and also produces a diffuse retinal discoloration. Eventually, owing to the toxic effects of the dissolved metal, the retina undergoes widespread degeneration until it is converted into a glial strand, and its blood vessels undergo obliterative changes. Glaucoma is a frequent complication. Whether this is due to toxic effects on the ciliary body or to alterations in the outflow channels is uncertain, though the latter seems more likely.

The increasing industrial use of steel alloys containing little or no iron has added new complications to industrial accidents. Some of these alloys have little or no ferromagnetism and hence cannot be removed with a magnet. On the other hand, vanadium, tungsten, chromium, and nickel are less readily oxidized by the tissue fluids and hence are a less dangerous source of toxic ions than is iron itself.

Copper is oxidized almost as readily as iron and the cupric ion is at least as toxic as the ferric. Consequently, intraocular foreign bodies composed of brass or copper are nearly as damaging as those composed of iron or steel. Attempts at surgical removal of these nonmagnetic metals rarely are successful.

Vogt described lenticular chalcosis due to a copper foreign body lodged in the cornea which also produced deposits in the epithelium and in Bowman's membrane. Loddoni and Duc demonstrated this metal in the corneal epithelium and Descemet's membrane by introducing copper into the eye experimentally. In cases of prolonged retention, atrophy of the retina may result. The deposits in the cornea and lens may be observed clinically, but no satisfactory histochemical test for copper is available.

Argyrosis occurs among silversmiths or follows continued local or systemic medicinal use of silver compounds. It particularly affects Bowman's membrane of the cornea and Bruch's membrane of the choroid, causing deep pigmentation of these structures.

SURGICAL FOREIGN BODIES

Foreign bodies may be introduced surgically either by accident or by intention. Accidentally introduced foreign bodies include glass, cotton fibers, cilia, bits of rubber from irrigating bulbs, as well as bacteria, fungi, and viruses (Figs. 8, 76, 105). All of these have been considered under accidental trauma. Surgeons take advantage of the tolerance of ocular tissues to certain material by intentionally introducing such useful foreign bodies as buried sutures, setons (silk, plastic, or nonirritating metals), acrylic lenses, and various space-occupying plastics in detachment operations. However, all of these cause

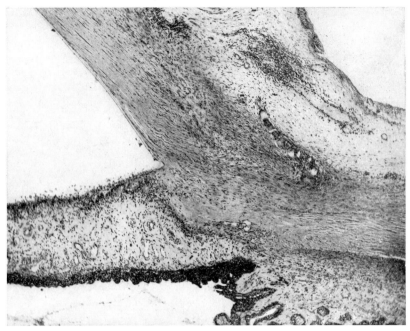

Figure 105. Intraocular foreign bodies. Foreign body reaction to cotton fibers in scar of cataract extraction. ×75. AFIP Acc. 300453.

some reaction in adjacent tissues. Occasionally the reaction is excessive and has disastrous consequences. More often, particularly when the tissue response is suppressed by anti-inflammatory therapy, the reaction is minimal and the material well tolerated. Nevertheless, the combination of a foreign body, however inert, and bacterial contamination usually is more than the eye can tolerate.

BURNS

Chemical and thermal burns of the surface of the eyeball and lids are common accidents. They produce necrosis of the tissues to a depth determined by the nature and concentration of the agent and the extent and duration of contact. The necrotic tissue is sloughed off, and healing is accompanied by very dense scar formation. Burns of the skin of the lids may produce a scar leading to ectropion of the lids. Conjunctival burns quite often are followed by shrinkage and extensive adhesions between the eyeball and the lids (symblepharon). Burns of the cornea result in a variable amount of inflammation and necrosis and often cause extensive scarring. Chemical burns due to lime are especially apt to produce severe destruction of the conjunctiva and cornea. Lye, ammonia, various acids, sulfur dioxide, phenol, and innumerable other industrial chemicals have caused corneal burns (Fig. 106). Thermal burns usually are less severe than those due to chemicals because the contact with the heat is of shorter duration.

Acid burns were studied experimentally by Friedenwald, Hughes and Herrmann and were found to be essentially nonprogressive and were less likely to have a late relapse of the inflammation. The penetration of the acid is limited by the buffering reaction of the tissues and the lesions tend to be sharply demarcated. Healing following such burns generally is rapid.

Hughes found that the severity of alkali burns depended less on the character of the cation than on alkali concentration. Alkali burns more often produce severe damage than do acid burns. The impression is universal that alkali burns are progressive,

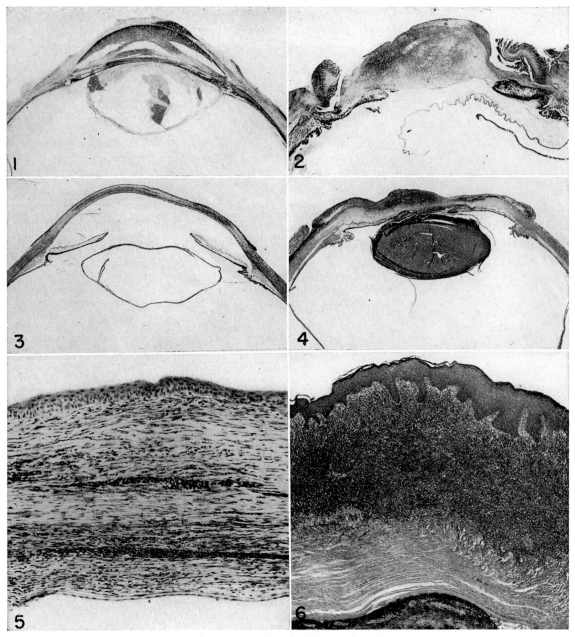

Figure 106. Chemical Burns, Cornea

1. Sulfuric acid burn. Hypopyon ulcer. AFIP Acc. 279070.
2. Lime burn. Destruction of cornea. Hypopyon ulcer. AFIP Acc. 56653.
3. Mustard gas burn. Interstitial keratitis. AFIP Acc. 191010.
4. Ammonia burn. Recurrent keratitis. AFIP Acc. 38830.
5. Mustard gas burn. Interstitial keratitis. ×125. AFIP Acc. 191010.
6. Ammonia burn. Recurrent chronic ulceration. Epidermidalization of epithelium. ×48. AFIP Acc. 38830.

mainly because tissues so damaged initially have a normal appearance, but gradually become more opaque. This is borne out experimentally by the observation that the buffering capacity of tissue against alkali is weaker than against acids, and the fact that the agent continues to act for an hour or more, even though irrigation is efficient.

Tear gas vapor causes pain, lacrimation, and epithelial exfoliation, but the lesions often heal without damage. Direct exposure, however, may lead to severe necrosis. Mild burns from mustard gas vapor clear up within a few weeks, but those which are more severe produce a necrotizing lesion of the cornea. Vascularization with permanent opacities and a tendency to recurrent inflammation with further corneal damage is a sequela of such an injury. Mustard gas burns of the eye have been studied extensively by a number of investigators. Exposure to threshold doses of mustard gas causes inhibition of mitosis in the corneal epithelium. With larger doses the epithelium becomes stippled and the eye irritated. The cohesion between epithelium and stroma is reduced, and nuclear fragmentation or karyorrhexis is noted in the epithelial cells. Complete recovery is still possible at this dosage level. With still more severe exposure the stromal cells are killed and an inflammatory reaction with vascularization and scarring ensues. Lewisite produces instantaneous irritation and blepharospasm, with histologic changes in the anterior segment as early as ten minutes after exposure to either the liquid or the vapor.

Deliberate burns of the choroid are created surgically to form chorioretinal adhesions and cure retinal detachment. These burns are produced by electric currents, chemicals, concentrated light rays, or direct heat. The edges of a sclerotomy wound may be cauterized in glaucoma surgery to help form a lasting fistula. Inadvertent fistulas may result from cauterization of bleeding vessels in other incisions and interfere with sound wound healing.

RADIANT ENERGY

In addition to the mechanical, chemical, and thermal trauma previously described, the eye may be subjected to injury from radiant energy. The resulting ocular damage depends on the wave length of the radiation, the amount absorbed by the tissues, and the tissue affected. Ocular lesions can be produced by radiant energy of almost any wave length. The tissue reactions to these radiations are very complex and, in spite of extensive study, still are incompletely understood. The details of local damage will be considered in the other chapters and only a general survey is given here.

Ordinary visible light radiations in moderate amounts may be unpleasant to the eye but cause no permanent damage. Photophobia and discomfort are particularly noticeable in fatigued or inflamed eyes. The unpleasant sensations of glare and flicker are extremely difficult to interpret. Painful photophobia probably is due to a strong miosis and accommodative spasms. Injury may result from more prolonged exposure, such as eclipse blindness, and severe retinal damage may occur. The burn is due to the concentration of the radiant energy in a very small area, producing local heating and consequent necrosis. Advantage is taken of this effect in therapeutic photocoagulation. The heating effect occurs in the pigment epithelium, which absorbs light and converts it to heat. Necrosis occurs in the pigment cells and secondary effects develop in the adjacent rods and cones. Wave lengths shorter than those which are visible are absorbed by the lens and do not reach the retina. Therefore, unless the eye is aphakic, the retina is not injured by ultraviolet light. Lesions of the retina in experimental animals after exposure to intense radiation from an arc lamp, therefore, are due to the visible and the infrared heat effects, but are not due to the ultraviolet irradiation.

Infrared radiant waves (800–1600 mu) are very strongly absorbed by the lens. If sufficient energy is delivered, definite injury can be produced. Cataracts due to this type of heat may occur in glass blowers, iron puddlers, and other workers whose occupations expose them to intense heat for long periods. True exfoliation of the lens capsule also may occur in such workers.

The cornea absorbs ultraviolet wave lengths shorter than 295 mu. Consequently, such radiation may burn this tissue while those beneath it are protected.

Radiation from x-rays, radium, neutrons, or atomic blasts may be absorbed in various parts of the eye and produce damage. Lens injury is quite common, and the effects of radiation on the lens are fairly well understood. Corneal and conjunctival burns also may occur. The late effects of radiation damage include glaucoma, massive intraocular hemorrhage, generalized necrosis, and inflammation. Flick observed retinal lesions, chiefly exudates and hemorrhages, in 50 per cent of patients with radiation sickness. Similar fundus changes were observed in the Japanese population following the atom bomb explosions. Round, snow-white, and slightly elevated exudates appear at the level of the retinal vessels but apparently have no relation to them. These fundus lesions probably contain cytoid bodies. The retinal lesions clear without permanent damage in patients who recover.

The effects of electric shock on the eye are not well known. Direct electrical stimulation of the optic nerve produces visual sensations. Exposure of the eye to a nearby flash of lightning or a powerful electric spark produces conjunctivitis, but this is an ultraviolet and not an electric effect. After a person has been struck by lightning or after he has been shocked by a powerful current, cataracts may develop. They may appear with amazing rapidity and become mature. The injury probably produces necrosis of the lens epithelium followed by secondary changes in the lens fibers.

ENDOGENOUS POISONS

Injury to the eyes may be produced by circulating substances in the blood. Four classes are recognized: (1) toxins of certain bacteria (Corynebacterium diphtheriae and Clostridium botulinum) which produce paralysis of the ocular muscles, a condition which will not be discussed here, since it belongs rather in the domain of neurology; (2) poisons, such as naphthalene and ergot, which cause cataract and are discussed in Chapter XI; (3) organic compounds, mainly alkaloids and other drugs, which bring about aberrations of visual perception. The delimitation of this group is exceedingly difficult, for nearly any drug, when given in excess, may cause an alteration of visual perception. There is an almost continuous gradation, ranging from the visual hallucination of a truly psychogenic delirium and the bizarre sights described by acute alcoholics and narcotic addicts, through the peculiar visual disturbances which are sometimes produced by salicylates and by digitalis. Simple disturbances of color perception, such as xanthopsia (all colors appearing yellow) are caused by drugs such as santonin. Little is known concerning the mechanism by which these visual disturbances are produced. Except for the last mentioned, they are believed to result from action on the brain rather than on the eye. Their effect is transitory and there are no permanent clinical or histologic residua. Atabrine (quinacrine) taken internally in the prophylaxis or treatment of malaria has produced transitory edema of the corneal epithelium in patients, some of whom later developed hepatitis; (4) a group of drugs that cause optic atrophy. Among these are tobacco and alcohol, especially wood alcohol; the arsenicals, especially Atoxyl and tryparsamide; lead and other metallic poisons; and finally, certain alkaloids, notably quinine and the closely allied Optochin. The action of tobacco after long continued use by an extremely small number of susceptible persons is peculiar. Atrophy of the papillomacular bundle of fibers in the optic nerve is produced and, correspondingly, a small central or paracentral scotoma. It is not known whether the primary site of this injury is in the optic nerve or the retina. A similar lesion is at times seen in chronic alcoholics and has been attributed to a lack of vitamin B. Wood alcohol, on the other hand, attacks all the nerve fibers, often causing complete loss of vision. It has been stated that the initial injury in this intoxication is in the retinal ganglion cells. Potts and Johnson have postulated that methanol produces further inhibition of retinal glycolysis by the formation of formaldehyde. The mechanism by which the arsenicals produce optic atrophy has not been ascertained. In regard to quinine, much emphasis has been laid upon the great narrowing of the retinal arteries which generally occurs at the onset of the visual impairment, and it has been thought that the blindness and optic atrophy are the result of retinal ischemia. Direct action on the ganglion cells of the retina, however, cannot be ruled out. Anoxemia in carbon monoxide poisoning or, rarely, in exsanguination from massive hemorrhage may occasionally cause optic atrophy.

REFERENCES

Blodi, F. C.: Sympathetic Uveitis as an Allergic Phenomenon. With a Study of its Association with Phacoanaphylactic Uveitis and a Report on the Pathological Findings in Sympathizing Eyes. Trans. Amer. Acad. Ophthal. Otolaryng. 63:642–649, 1959.

Buschke, W., Friedenwald, J. S., and Moses, S. G.: Effects of Ultraviolet Irradiation on Corneal Epithelium: Mitosis, Nuclear Fragmentation, Posttraumatic Cell Movements, Loss of Tissue Cohesion. J. Cell. Comp. Physiol. 26:147–164, 1945.

Chamberlain, W. P., Jr., and Boles, D. J.: Edema of Cornea Precipitated by Quinacrine (Atabrine). A.M.A. Arch. Ophthal. 35:120–134, 1946.

Cibis, P. A., Brown, E. B., and Hong, S.: Ocular Effects of Systemic Siderosis. Amer. J. Ophthal. 44:158–172 (Oct.) 1957.

Courtney, R. H.: Endophthalmitis with Secondary Glaucoma Accompanying Absorption of the Crystalline Lens. Trans. Amer. Ophthal. Soc. 40:355–369, 1942.

Cross, A. G.: The Ocular Sequelae of Head Injury. Ann. Roy. Coll. Surg. Engl. 2:233–240, 1948.

d'Ombrain, A.: Traumatic or "Concussion" Chronic Glaucoma. Brit. J. Ophthal. 33:495, 1949.

Dunnington, J. H.: Healing of Incisions for Cataract Extractions. Amer. J. Ophthal. 34:36–45, 1951.

Dunnington, J. H.: Ocular Wound Healing with Particular Reference to Cataract Incision. A.M.A. Arch. Ophthal. 56:639–659 (Nov.) 1956.

Dunnington, J. H.: Tissue Responses in Ocular Wounds. Amer. J. Ophthal. 43:667–678, 1957.

Flick, J. J.: Ocular Lesions following the Atomic Bombing of Hiroshima and Nagasaki. Amer. J. Ophthal. 31:137–154, 1948.

Friedenwald, J. S., Hughes, W. F., Jr., and Herrmann, H.: Acid-base Tolerance of Cornea. A.M.A. Arch. Ophthal. 31:279–283, 1944.

Gundersen, T.: Observations on the Vossius Ring. Trans. Amer. Ophthal. Soc. 43:149–162, 1945.

Gundersen, T.: Surgery of Intraocular Foreign Bodies. Trans. Amer. Acad. Ophthal. Otolaryng. 52:604–613, 1947.

Hughes, W. F., Jr.: Alkali Burns of the Eye. I. Review of Literature and Summary of Present Knowledge. A.M.A. Arch. Ophthal. 35:423–449, 1946.

Hughes, W. F., Jr.: Alkali Burns of the Eye. II. Clinical and Pathologic Course. A.M.A., Arch. Ophthal. 36:189–214, 1946.

Loddoni, G., and Duc, C.: La Senescenza dell' Occhio Umano. Boll. D'Oculi. 27:139–192, 1948.

Lorenz, E., and Dunn, T. B.: Ocular Lesions Induced by Acute Exposure of the Whole Body of Newborn Mice to Roentgen Radiation. A.M.A. Arch. Ophthal. 43:742–749, 1950.

Oaks, L. W., Dorman, J. E., and Petty, R. W.: Tear Gas Burns of the Eye. Trans. Pac. Coast Otoophth. Soc. 39:237–256, 1958.

Potts, A. M., and Johnson, L. V.: Studies on the Visual Toxicity of Methanol. I. The Effect of Methanol and Its Degradation Products on Retinal Metabolism Amer. J. Ophthal. 35:107–113, 1952.

Rones, B., and Wilder, H. C.: Nonperforating Ocular Injuries in Soldiers. Amer. J. Ophthal. 30:1143–1160, 1947.

Schlaegel, T. F., Jr.: Ocular Histopathology of Some Nagasaki Atomic-bomb Casualties. Amer. J. Ophthal. 30:127–135, 1947.

Straub, M.: Inflammation of the Eye Caused by Lenticular Material Dissolved in Eye Lymph. Amsterdam, J. H. deBussy, 1919. Cited in Woods, A. C.: Adventure in Ophthalmology. Amer. J. Ophthal. 48:463–472, 1959.

Struble, G. C., and Kreft, A. J.: War Injuries of the Eyes and Visual Pathways. War Med. 8:290–304, 1945.

Verhoeff, F. H., Bell, L., and Walker, C. B.: The Pathological Effects of Radiant Energy in the Eye. Proc. Amer. Acad. Arts and Sciences 51: No. 13, 1916.

Verhoeff, F. H., and Lemoine, A. N.: Endophthalmitis Phacoanaphylactica. Trans. Intern. Cong. Ophth. 1:234–284, (April) 1922.

Vogt, A.: Kupfercataract. Schweiz. Med. Wschr. Basel 52:205, 1922.

Wilder, H. C.: Intraocular Foreign Bodies in Soldiers. Amer. J. Ophthal. 31:57–64, 1948.

Wilder, H. C., and Maynard, R. M.: Ocular Changes Produced by Total Body Irradiation. Amer. J. Path. 27:1–19, 1951.

Wolff, S. M., and Zimmerman, L. E.: Chronic Secondary Glaucoma Associated with Retrodisplacement of Iris Root and Deepening of the Anterior Chamber Angle Secondary to Contusion. To be published.

Woods, A. C.: Adventure in Ophthalmology. Amer. J. Ophthal. 48:463–472 (Oct.) 1959.

Yamashita, T., and Cibis, P. A.: Staining of the Retina with Saccharated Iron Oxide. A.M.A. Arch. Ophthal. 61:698–708, 1959.

Chapter IV

Lids and Lacrimal

Drainage Apparatus

The pathogenesis of eyelid lesions depends on the type, character, and localization of the causative agent and, to a great extent, on the anatomic arrangement of the lid tissues (Fig. 107).

ANATOMY AND HISTOLOGY

Each lid is composed of four layers and, in spite of some anatomic differences between the upper and lower lids, their pathologic reactions are quite similar. The palpebral conjunctiva forms the innermost layer, and the skin the most external layer. Between these two is a more superficial muscular layer (orbicularis oculi) and a deeper tarsal layer. In the upper lid, the insertions of the levator palpebrae superioris and of Müller's muscle help form the muscle layer. The junction between skin and conjunctiva is located near the posterior edge of the lid margin just posterior to the openings of the Meibomian gland ducts (Figs. 107, 108). Anterior to the latter and posterior to the lashes, a pigmented sulcus (gray line) extends over most of the length of the lid. The lid can be split surgically along this line dividing it into two layers, an anterior one formed of skin and obicularis muscle, and a posterior one composed of tarsus and conjunctiva.

The skin of the eyelids is elastic in younger persons and is quite thin. The subcutaneous tissue is loose and delicate.

The basal cell layer of the epidermis (Figs. 37, 107) consists of a single row of cells resting on a basement membrane which is firmly adherent to the corium. The cells are columnar with their long axes at right angles to the skin surface. Intercellular bridges connect these cells with each other and with the overlying cells. They contain variable quantities of melanin pigment. Several layers of prickle cells, which are polygonal and have well-developed intercellular bridges, lie superficial to the basal layer. They are derived from the basal cells and form the stratum malpighii.

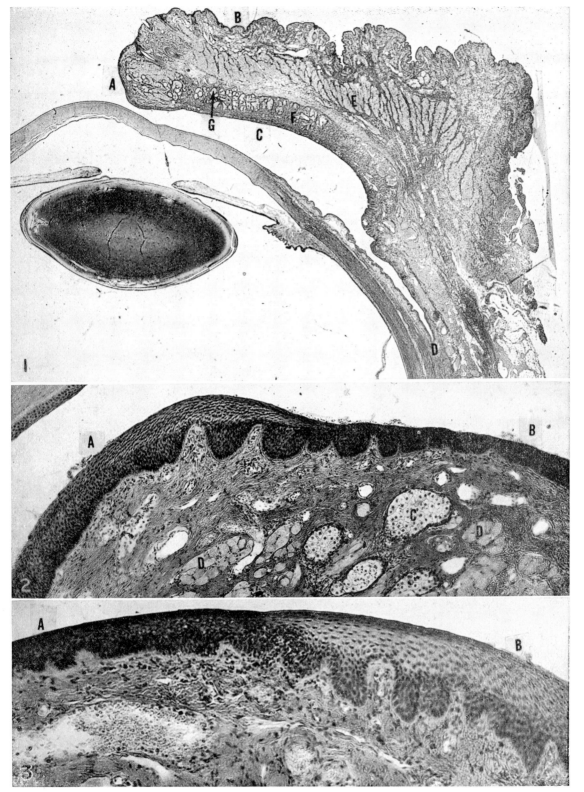

Figure 107. Normal Eyelid

1. Upper lid. A, lid margin. B, dermal surface. C, conjunctival surface. D, fornix. E, orbicularis muscle (sphincter palpebrae). F, tarsal plate. G, meibomian glands. ×8. AFIP Neg. 103947.

2. Lid margin. A, conjunctival epithelium. B, epidermal epithelium. C, sebaceous glands. D, pars marginalis of orbicularis muscle. ×75. AFIP Neg. 103950.

3. Lid margin. A, epidermal epithelium. B, conjunctival epithelium. ×50. AFIP Neg. 103945.

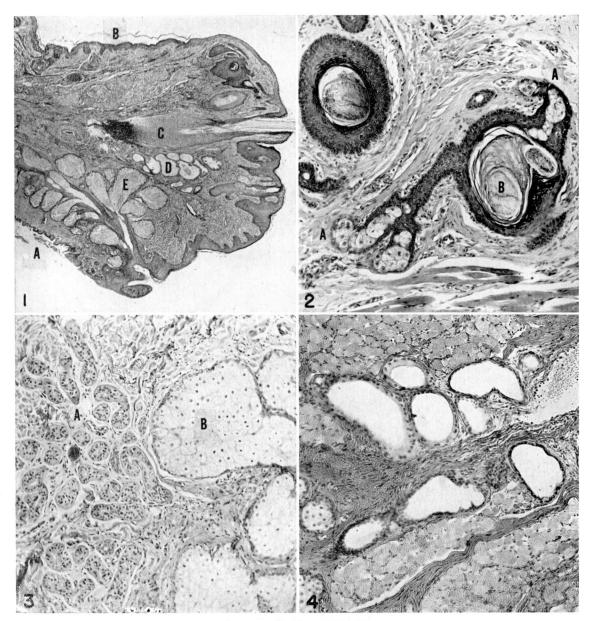

Figure 108. Normal Eyelid

1. Lid margin. A, conjunctival surface. B, dermal surface. C, hair follicle containing hair shaft. D, gland of Moll. E, meibomian gland. ×24. AFIP Acc. 171463.

2. A, glands of Zeis (sebaceous glands). B, hair follicle containing hair shaft. ×125. AFIP Acc. 325133.

3. A, glands of Wolfring (accessory lacrimal glands). B, meibomian glands (modified sebaceous glands). ×125 AFIP Acc. 482185.

4. Glands of Moll (modified sweat glands) dilated. ×90. AFIP Neg. 103949.

Outside these is the granular layer, a row of elongated, flat cells which contain coarse keratohyaline granules. This layer often is inconspicuous in the lid. The most external layer of the skin is the horny layer which consists of flattened keratinized cells without nuclei.

A variety of epidermal appendages are present in the lids. The sebaceous glands of the skin are holocrine glands. They have no lumen and their secretion is formed by decomposition of the cells. They empty through a duct into a hair follicle. The sebaceous glands of the lashes (Zeis) empty into the follicles of the cilia (Figs. 107, 108). Their cells have a foamy cytoplasm and empty into a sac and duct which is lined by a stratified squamous epithelium. The duct epithelium is continuous with that of the epidermis and the external root sheath of the hair.

The sweat glands are tubular and more deeply placed. The secretory portion is lined by two layers of cells, an inner one composed of large cuboidal secretory cells, and an outer one of small, cylindrical cells, the myo-epithelial elements. The ducts are lined by two layers of small cuboidal cells and empty onto the skin surface. Related glands, probably apocrine in type, lie near the palpebral margin and empty into the follicles of the lashes (glands of Moll) (Fig. 108).

The hair of the skin of the lid is scanty and fine, and differs but little from that in other areas. The two or three rows of lashes are unusually strong and long, and do not have arrectores muscles.

The corium (or dermis) in the skin of the lids is loose and delicate. In conformity with skin elsewhere the dividing line between epidermis and corium is irregular. Prolongations of the epidermis dip into the corium (rete pegs or ridges; epidermal papillas) and between them the corium extends upward (dermal papillas).

Collagenous, elastic and reticular fibers and ground substance form the structure of this layer; nerve fibers and blood vessels also are found.

The subcutis of the lids is very loose and contains but little fat. It is very loosely adherent to the underlying muscle, and because of this a rapid and intense swelling of the lids is common following hemorrhage, edema and acute inflammation.

The *orbicularis* muscle forms an elliptical sheet of concentrically arranged striated fibers within the eyelids. In the upper lid the tendon of the levator palpebrae superioris passes through it to insert into the skin and tarsus. Deep to it lies the smooth muscle layer of Müller. Alterations in these muscular structures may lead to ptosis, ectropion or entropion. The *orbital septum* is a thin fibrous fascia which helps to form the anterior aspect of the bony orbital cavity. All pathologic processes posterior to this diaphragm are considered to be intraorbital.

The *tarsi* are flat, semilunar plates which contribute to the rigidity to the lids. They are made up of dense collagenous tissue and elastic fibers. They contain the sebaceous tarsal (meibomian) glands, the ducts of which open into the lid margin (Figs. 107, 108). The epithelium of the tarsal conjunctiva is stratified columnar, but islands of squamous epithelium are usually found. The conjunctival stroma is thin and very closely adherent to the tarsus.

GROWTH AND AGING

Senile atrophy. The wrinkling of the skin in aged persons is caused by thickening and loss of elasticity of the tissues of the corium. The collagen fibers show a basophilic degeneration (Fig. 109) and may form large masses of degenerating fibers which take elastic stains (elastosis).

Blepharochalasis is characterized by atrophy of the skin which becomes so lax that it hangs down in a large fold over the lid margin (Fig. 109). The epithelium becomes thin and the rete ridges are diminished or absent. The corium is thin and loses its elastic fibers. Characteristic is the great proliferation of capillary endothelium, especially in the vascular tuft at the base of

the hair follicles and in the net normally surrounding the sweat glands. In both these regions globular masses of convoluted capillaries can be seen. Orbital fat may prolapse into the lid, aggravating the ptosis.

The relaxation of the tarsal ligaments and tarsi, which occurs in older patients as a result of loss of elastic tissue, often leads to poor apposition between the lids and eyeball. In such patients the lids can be everted with great ease.

Defects in the orbital septum. Dehiscences in the orbital septum may occur in old age. Orbital fat can prolapse through the openings. These prolapses have, at times, been misinterpreted as orbital lipomas.

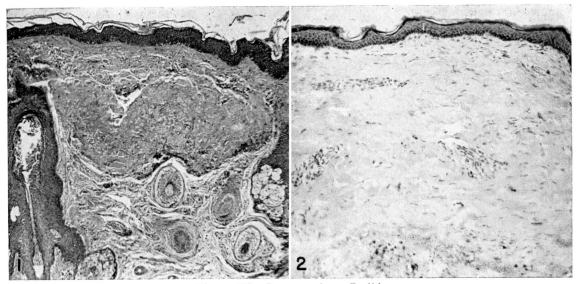

Figure 109. Degenerations, Eyelid

1. Senile degeneration, eyelid. ×75. AFIP Acc. 484011.
2. Blepharochalasis, long standing. Fibrosis of lid. Atrophy of surface epithelium. ×125. AFIP Acc. 484772.

CONGENITAL AND DEVELOPMENTAL ANOMALIES

Epidermoid cyst. These cysts may lie in the superficial or deep tissues of the lid and orbit and are found in almost any position (Fig. 110). They are lined by a squamous surface epithelium, the innermost layer of which is composed of hornified cells. Desquamated keratinized cells fill the cyst cav-

ity. Epidermoid cysts differ from the dermoid type by the lack of dermal appendages in their wall and by the absence of sebaceous contents. Sebaceous cysts are similar to the epidermoid variety except that they are filled with sebaceous material.

Milium. A milium is a small pinhead-

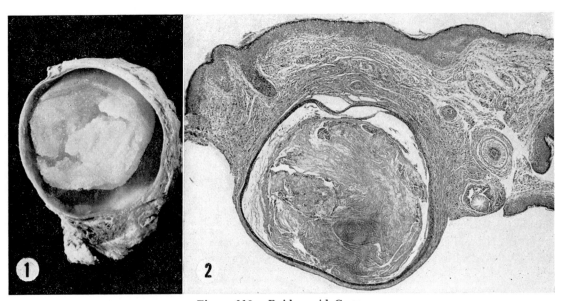

Figure 110. Epidermoid Cysts

1. AFIP Acc. 281885.
2. ×48, AFIP Acc. 486713.

sized elevation in the skin of the lids. Numerous milia may be present and they appear as a white, round, slightly elevated lesion. They are often congenital, but may be derived from dilated, scarred hair follicles or from sebaceous glands. The cyst lies in the superficial dermis, is lined by several layers of flat epithelium, and contains keratin. Sebaceous material is absent.

Dermoid cyst. This cyst usually occurs between brow and nose, at the temporal brow line, and near the inner canthus. It often is attached to the periosteum and may have extensions into the orbit. Its contents may be clear, oily, or nearly solid.

The fibrous wall of the cyst is lined by several layers of flat epithelium, the innermost of which may be keratinized. Characteristically, dermal appendages are present (Fig. 111). The contents include epithelial cells, hair, fat and cholesterol. When these elements escape through breaks in the epithelial lining of the cyst a granulomatous foreign body reaction may develop in the adjacent tissues (Fig. 112). Ossification and calcification of these cysts have been described.

Distichiasis. This anomaly is characterized by the presence of an accessory row of lashes. The primary defect is in the Meibomian glands which are smaller than normal, may be absent, or are replaced by abnormal sebaceous glands. These glands open into the row of abnormal lash follicles. The glands of Moll usually are hypertrophic. The tarsus

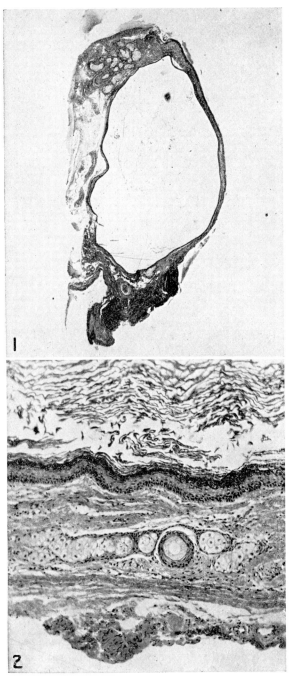

Figure 111

1. Dermoid cyst, orbit. ×24. AFIP Acc. 200051.
2. Dermoid cyst. Squamous epithelium lining. Keratic debris in lumen. Sebaceous glands and hair follicles in wall. ×125. AFIP Acc. 72852.

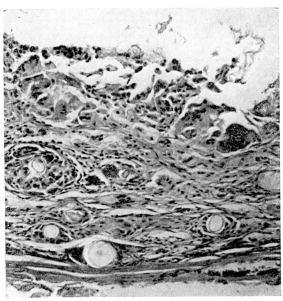

Figure 112. Dermoid Cyst

Foreign body giant cell reaction to degenerated sebaceous debris, replacing epithelial lining. ×180. AFIP Acc. 307524.

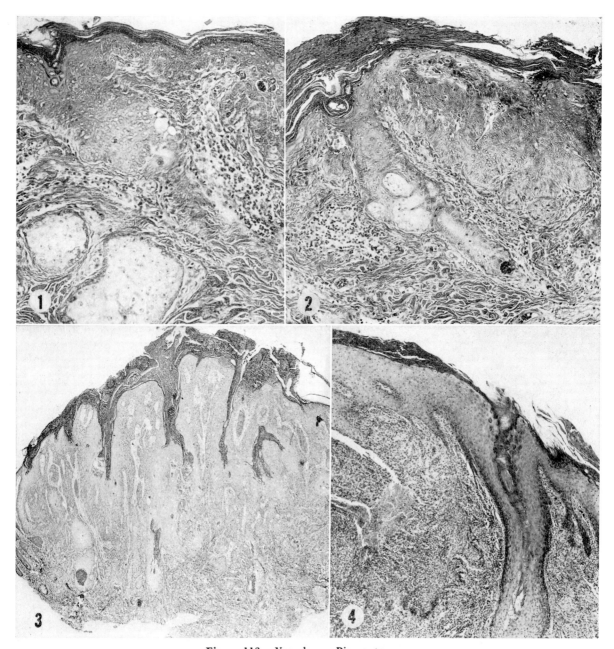

Figure 113. Xeroderma Pigmentosum

1 and 2. Irregular acanthosis, hyperkeratosis, parakeratosis, and dyskeratosis with nonspecific chronic inflammation in the corium. ×150 and 115, respectively.

3. Early squamous cell carcinoma, ×19.

4. Edge of basal cell carcinoma, ×50.

All from same case, AFIP Acc. 596894.

may be rudimentary or absent. This abnormality often is associated with other malformations, such as congenital ectropion and shortening of the palpebral fissure.

Ankyloblepharon. A dense adhesion of the lids at the inner canthus occurs in this condition. It is complete in cryptophthalmos and the eye itself often is malformed. In *ankyloblepharon filiforme adnatum* bridges of skin connect the upper with the lower lid. These bridges consist of epidermis and corium and are covered posteriorly with conjunctiva.

Congenital ptosis. Congenital ptosis usually is a hereditary condition and may be associated with other malformations, such as

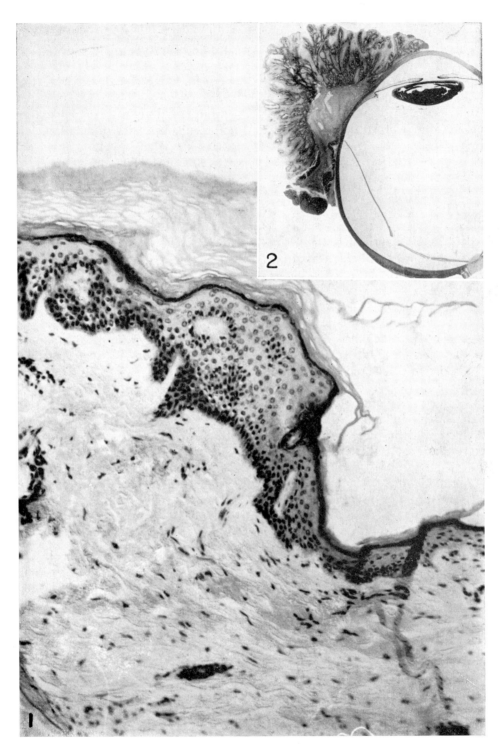

Figure 114. Xeroderma Pigmentosum

1. Patchy atrophy of prickle cell layer with acanthosis and hyperkeratosis in other areas. Pigment in basal layer. ×200. AFIP Acc. 56481.

2. Squamous cell carcinoma of bulbar conjunctiva in patient with xeroderma pigmentosum. AFIP Acc. 129202.

epicanthus. In congenital ptosis the levator muscle may be poorly formed or is absent. The superior rectus muscle, which is embryologically closely related to the levator, also may be affected. In a large series in which the anterior part of the muscle was examined histologically by Berke and Wadsworth the more marked cases showed no striated muscle. The smooth muscle of Müller was normal in all these cases.

Xeroderma pigmentosum. A congenital hypersensitivity to light seems to be responsible for the skin changes in this disease. The portions of skin which usually are exposed to light are affected first and the lids therefore are involved early. The earliest changes consist of areas of pigmentation which alternate with patches of atrophic skin. In the affected areas there is papillary overgrowth, followed by ulceration.

The histologic picture of the early stage is nonspecific. The basal cell layer becomes pigmented and the prickle cell layer somewhat irregular. Hyperkeratosis develops and the upper dermis shows edema and perivascular inflammatory infiltration. Later there is atrophy of the skin, increasing hyperpigmentation, acanthosis, and dyskeratosis (Figs. 113, 114). Atypical multinucleated cells are found in the epidermis. Finally squamous and basal cell epitheliomas and melanomas may develop (Fig. 113). The conjunctiva and cornea also may be involved (Fig. 114).

INFLAMMATIONS

The character of the inflammatory reaction varies with the cause and site of the pathologic process. The multilayered structure of the lid often modifies the process and limits its extension to certain planes.

Dermatitis. Mild inflammations of the skin are characterized by hyperemia, edema, and serous exudation. If the exudation increases, fluid accumulates among the epithelial cells, producing vesicles. The epithelial cells may degenerate and develop parakeratosis. Tissue necrosis, ulceration, and intense leukocytic infiltration may be seen in more severe infections. Under certain conditions, the inflammation commences in the dermis and affects the epidermis secondarily.

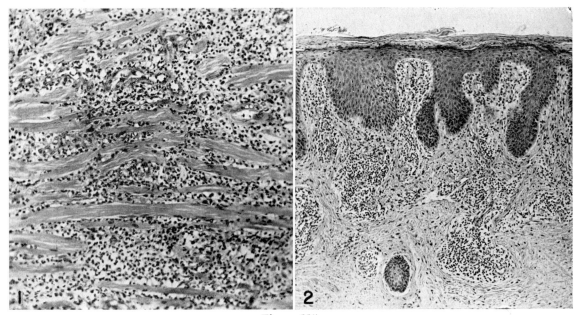

Figure 115

1. Acute purulent infiltration of palpebral muscle. ×125. AFIP Acc. 45355.

2. Chronic blepharitis. Lymphocytic infiltration and fibrosis of dermis. Hyperplasia and parakeratosis of epithelium. ×75. AFIP Acc. 59233.

Cellulitis. Acute cellulitis may involve the subcutis and tarsus and be characterized by a diffuse polymorphonuclear leukocytic infiltration, a massive edema, and hyperemia. An abscess may form which often breaks through the skin. Extension of the inflammation to the deeper structures results in an orbital cellulitis.

Erysipelas occurs in the face and especially in the lids. This streptococcal infection of the skin may lead to necrosis and a secondary keratoconjunctivitis. An intense polymorphonuclear and lymphocytic infiltration is found in the corium. The blood and lymph vessels are widely dilated.

Blepharitis. Two principal types of blepharitis are known: the seborrheic form and the infectious. Frequently these are

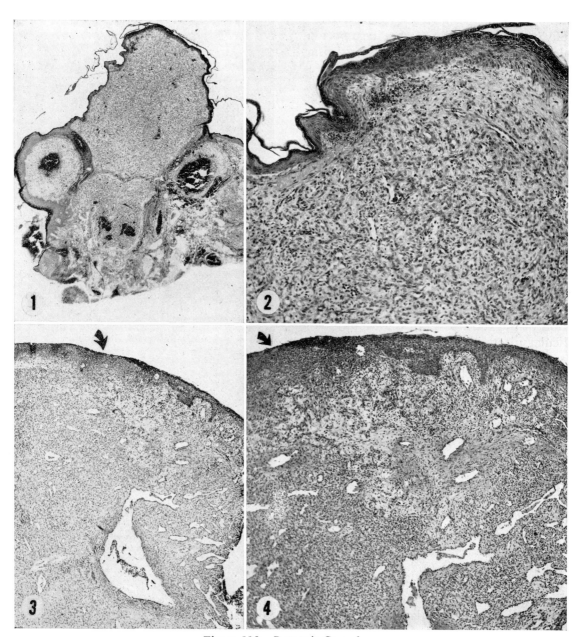

Figure 116. Pyogenic Granuloma

1 and 2. Epidermis is intact over this pedunculated mass of exuberant granulation tissue. ×20 and ×115, respectively. AFIP Acc. 635222.

3 and 4. The epidermis covering this lesion is partially ulcerated (arrows). ×25 and ×50, respectively. AFIP Acc. 712539.

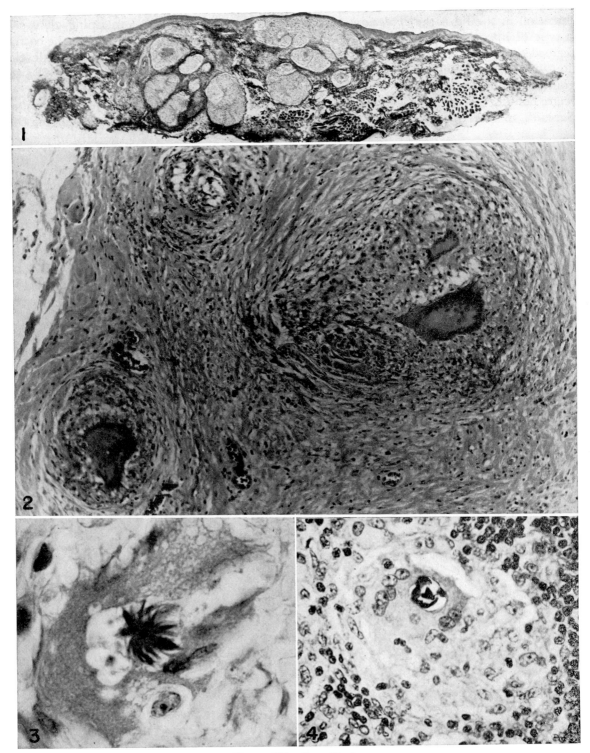

Figure 119. Sarcoidosis

1. Granulomatous lesion, eyelid. ×45. AFIP Acc. 54803.

2. Discrete noncaseating aggregations of epithelioid cells, surrounded by fibrous tissue. Centrally placed giant cells. Minimal chronic inflammatory cell infiltration. ×240. AFIP Acc. 84537.

3. Asteroid in giant cell. ×1360. AFIP Acc. 62800.

4. Schaumann body in giant cell. ×500. AFIP Acc. 108499.

and connective tissue. Several distinctive, but not pathognomonic, inclusions may be found in the giant cells: asteroid bodies, Schaumann bodies, and birefringent calcium oxalate crystals (Fig. 119). In *lupus pernio* there is a marked dilation of the capillaries in the upper corium together with sarcoid tubercles in the subcutis.

Syphilis. Syphilis may affect the lids in the primary, secondary, and tertiary stages. The primary lesion appears as a skin ulcer with indurated margins and with the healing of this ulcer, a dense scar may follow. The regional lymph nodes are enlarged. The syphilitic exanthema may be macular, papular, or pustular. The gumma may affect the skin or the tarsus (syphilitic tarsitis).

Tuberculosis. The most important lesion among the tuberculous affections involving the lid is *lupus vulgaris*. It is secondary to lesions elsewhere on the face. The lupus nodules consist of an accumulation of small tubercles, usually containing tubercle bacilli, at the actively spreading edge of the lesion. Ulceration and scar formation occur in the center of the affected area. Extensive destruction of the lids and cicatricial ectropion follow.

Leprosy. According to Holmes, the neural form of leprosy frequently affects the lids (Fig. 120). The lesions result from a chronic interstitial neuritis with destruction of the nerve fibers and proliferation of fibrous tissue. They appear as erythematous, well-circumscribed, depigmented patches. Lagophthalmos, loss of eyebrows and lashes, and entropion or ectropion of the lids occur. The tuberculoid lesions, however, rarely are seen in the lids.

Histologically the lesions of tuberculoid leprosy consist of tubercle-like structures composed of epithelioid cells (Fig. 120). Invasion or destruction of the nerves is characteristic. In tuberculoid leprosy acid-fast bacilli are extremely difficult to demonstrate and there is no necrosis.

Lepromatous leprosy may affect the brows or the upper lid (Fig. 120). Red, elevated granulomas (lepromas) are characteristic; these may produce marked enlargement of the lids and brow. Nodules of various sizes can be seen and palpated in and around the lids.

Granulomatous infiltration occurs in the dermis with many histiocytes (lepra cells) which have an abundant, foamy cytoplasm containing large clumps of Mycobacterium leprae.

Fungus disease. Numerous fungus diseases may affect the lids, often being secondary to infection elsewhere on the face (Fig. 121). In the cutaneous form of North American *blastomycosis* (Gilchrist's disease) the skin of the face and lids often is involved. Large fungating verrucous plaques and ulcerating granulomas appear and the active borders show numerous minute abscesses. Histologically there characteristically is pronounced pseudoepitheliomatous hyperplasia of the epidermis (Fig. 40). Tuberculoid granulomas containing giant cells of the Langhans' type and microabscesses composed of polymorphonuclear leukocytes are found. The typical budding double-contoured cells of Blastomyces dermatitidis are seen in the microabscesses and granulomas. The lesions heal with a great deal of scarring and cicatricial ectropion. Littman and Zimmerman have described similar facial lesions in *cryptococcosis*.

Sporotrichosis may be localized to the lids as a primary infection or be secondary to involvement of the face. Granulation tissue containing microabscesses and foci of granulomatous inflammation are characteristic. The organisms rarely are demonstrable histologically, even with the aid of special stains. The diagnosis must be established by culture or animal inoculation.

The lids may be infected by *Actinomyces*. Granulation tissue and large abscesses form. Colonies of the fungus may be large enough to be visible macroscopically as sulfur granules. The gram-positive branching filaments, typically surrounded by eosinophilic deposits, are usually found with the foci of suppuration.

Protozoal infections. Among the *protozoal infections*, cutaneous leishmaniasis most often is seen in the lids. The corium is infiltrated diffusely with lymphocytes, plasma cells and epithelioid cells. Leishman-Donovan bodies can be found on sections stained with the Giemsa stain. Granulomatous lesions may also be stimulated by nematode larvae (Fig. 121).

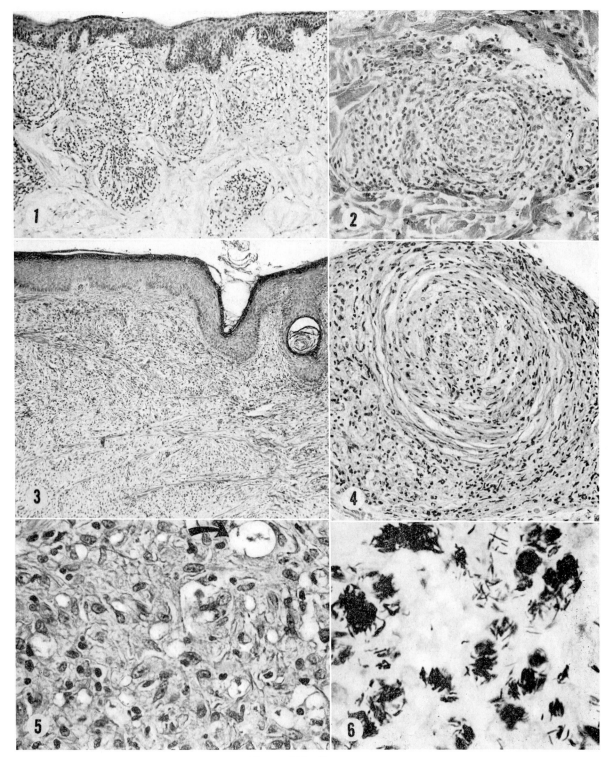

Figure 120. Leprosy

1. Tuberculoid leprosy, skin. ×80. AFIP Neg. No. 56–19556.
2. Tuberculoid leprosy, dermal nerve. ×200. AFIP Acc. 658941.
3. Lepromatous leprosy, skin. ×80. AFIP Acc. 922173.
4. Lepromatous leprosy, dermal nerve. ×200. AFIP Acc. 922173.
5. Lepromatous leprosy, skin. Epithelioid cells, foamy macrophages, and globi (arrow). ×440. AFIP Acc. 922173
6. Lepra bacilli demonstrated by Fite-Faraco acid-fast stain. ×1020. AFIP Acc. 644253.
(Courtesy of Dr. C. H. Binford.)

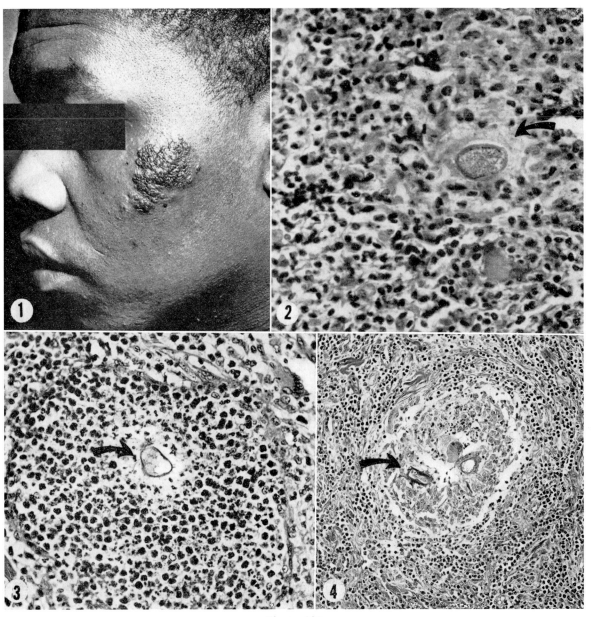

Figure 121

1 and 2. Pseudoepitheliomatous hyperplasia and granulomatous inflammation due to coccidioidomycosis. Arrow indicates spherule of *C. immitis* in a giant cell. AFIP Acc. 802823.

3 and 4. Suppurative and granulomatous lesions with marked eosinophilia, probably due to nematodiasis. The foreign bodies contained within the abscess in 3 and within the epithelioid tubercle in 4 are believed to represent degenerating nematode larvae. ×220 and ×125, respectively. AFIP Acc. 930290.

Viral Infections

Vaccinia. Vaccinia of the lids often is due to self-inoculation by a child with an active smallpox vaccination. At times nonimmunized adults accidentally are infected by a child who is being actively immunized. Vesicles and pustules form between the horny and prickle cell layers. The cells of the prickle cell layer become detached, and lie as round spheres within the vesicles. There is a marked proliferation of epithelial cells around the lesions. The papillas of the corium participate in this inflammation. Eosinophilic cytoplasmic inclusions (Guarnieri bodies) can be demonstrated in the epithelial cells under appropriate conditions.

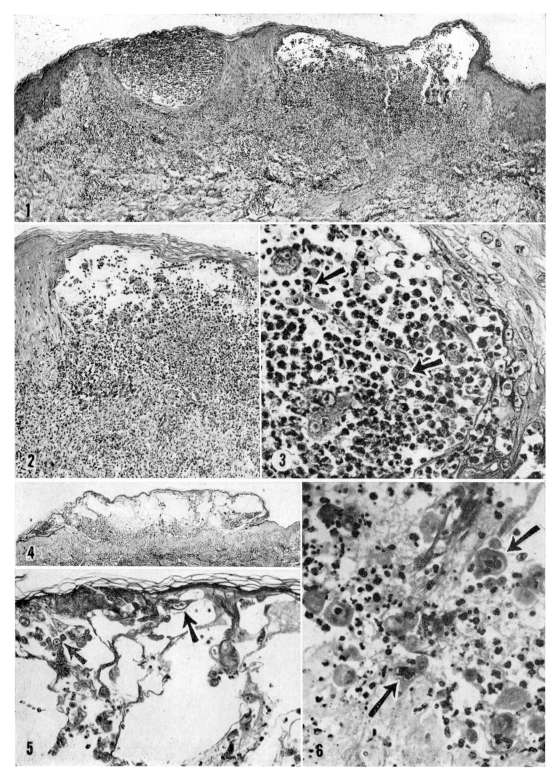

Figure 122. Herpetic Lesions of Skin

1, 2 and 3. Advanced stages with intraepidermal pustules and subacute inflammatory reaction in dermis. Arrows indicate intranuclear inclusion bodies in epidermal cells. AFIP Acc. 660418.   1. ×55.   2. ×115.   3. ×380.

4, 5 and 6. Early stages with intraepidermal vesicles resulting from "ballooning" and disintegration of infected epidermal cells. Arrows indicate intranuclear inclusion bodies in epidermal cells. AFIP Acc. 566812.   4. ×26. 5. ×215.   6. ×400.

Herpes simplex and zoster. Herpes simplex and herpes zoster produce a pathologic picture practically identical with that of vaccinia. The intra-epidermal vesicles are associated with a marked degeneration of epithelial cells (ballooning and reticular degeneration) (Fig. 122). Intranuclear inclusion bodies are found in both conditions (Fig. 122).

Molluscum contagiosum. Molluscum contagiosum is a virus infection which produces a hyperplastic papular lesion on the lid surface or margin. A small, round, moderately

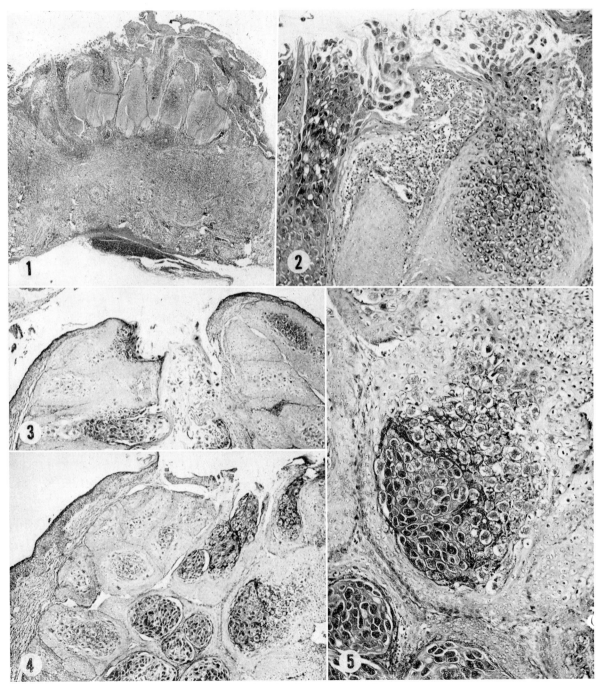

Figure 123. Molluscum Contagiosum

1 and 2. ×17 and ×80, respectively. AFIP Acc. 733646.
3, 4 and 5. ×42, ×50 and ×125, respectively. AFIP Acc. 213759.

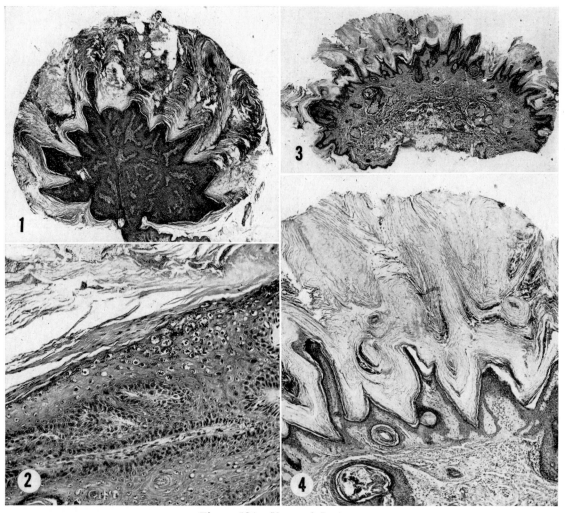

Figure 124. Verrucal Lesions

1 and 2. Verruca vulgaris. ×19 and ×115, respectively. AFIP Acc. 327919.
3 and 4. Nevus verrucosus. ×12 and ×50, respectively. AFIP Acc. 598101.

elevated nodule forms. Its center often is umbilicated and a yellowish, cheesy material can be expressed.

Histologically these nodules are character-ized by a peculiar type of acanthosis, with convoluted infoldings of the epithelium which account for the umbilicated center (Fig. 123). The epithelial cells at the surface become markedly degenerated, slough off, and fill the central cavity. The molluscum cells (bodies) are enlarged cells of the stratum granulosum and spinosum, which contain the cytoplasmic inclusions. These inclusions are homogeneous and eosinophilic (Fig. 123). When the nodule is on the lid margin, the virus particles are liberated into the con-junctival sac and often produce a follicular conjunctivitis and superficial keratitis.

Verruca. Verruca vulgaris and verruca plana which are caused by identical or closely related strains of virus occur fairly frequently on the lids. Verruca vulgaris is characterized by a solid, elevated growth with a papillomatous surface. Verruca plana is a smoother, flatter lesion and may be pig-mented.

Histologically in verruca vulgaris there is papillary proliferation with hyperkeratosis, acanthosis and parakeratosis (Fig. 124). Char-acteristic are large, vacuolated cells in the granular layer and shadow cells in the horny layer (Fig. 124). In verruca plana the same vacuolated, large cells occur in the superficial layers of the epidermis. Conjunctivitis and keratitis also may occur from lid margin ver-rucas.

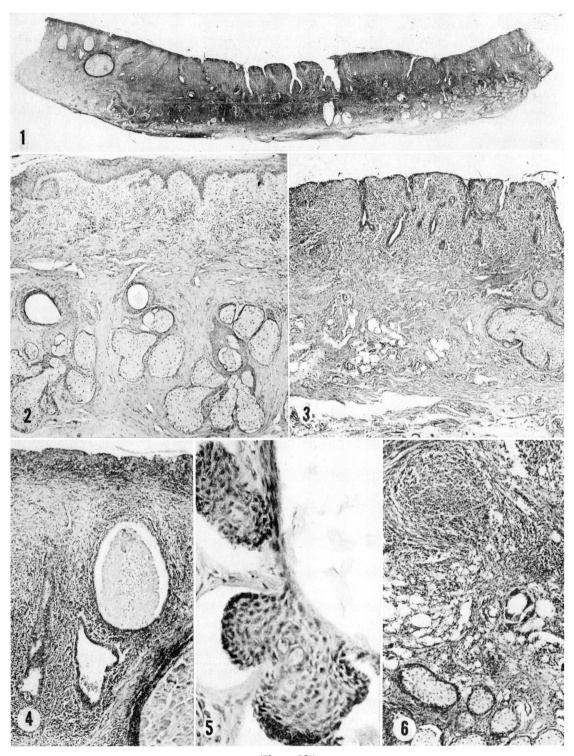

Figure 125

1, 2 and 3. Trachomatous blepharitis and tarsitis.   1. ×6.   2. ×50.   3. ×40.

4, 5 and 6. Secondary changes include: cystic dilatation and squamous metaplasia of meibomian glands and their ducts and formation of chalazions.   4. ×50.   5. ×265.   6. ×80.

AFIP Acc. 942688.

Trachoma. Trachoma primarily affects the conjunctiva and therefore is discussed in Chapter V. In most cases the tarsus is involved and in severe cases all the layers of the lid are affected. Signs of such involvement are ptosis, palpebral edema and thickening of the tarsus. The tarsus appears grey-red, thickened and edematous. Microscopically, the inflammation is diffuse with perivascular accumulations of lymphocytes and plasma cells. The tarsal glands also may be directly invaded and destroyed by the inflammatory process (Fig. 125). Softening of the tarsus occurs as a result of necrosis of its connective tissue.

In all cases in which the trachomatous process has reached a certain severity, a myositis of the orbicularis muscle is present. The inflammation presents itself as an interstitial, lymphocytic infiltration with edema. Later this is followed by the formation and overgrowth of connective tissue, leading to a pressure atrophy of muscle fibers. Müller's muscle of the upper lid frequently is involved in a similar manner.

Healing occurs by transformation and absorption of the exudate, and by proliferation of connective tissue. The newly formed connective tissue occludes the ducts of the palpebral glands. The young connective tissue later is replaced by scar tissue which becomes hyalinized and contributes to the deformity. In the cicatricial stage the tarsus shrinks and assumes a curved, dome shape with an anterior convexity. This distortion produces the most aggravating complications of entropion and trichiasis. At times, the tarsus becomes quite atrophic and is transformed into a thin layer of connective tissue.

Dermatologic Conditions

This group comprises first of all a large class of purely dermatologic lesions which also may affect the lids. Among them are psoriasis, lichen planus, solar dermatitis and acne rosacea. These lesions are relatively rare in the lids and of minor importance to the ophthalmologist. They are too numerous to be discussed here. Their histologic features can be found in textbooks of dermatology or works on pathology of the skin. The group

of vesicular and bullous diseases will be discussed in Chapter V.

Contact dermatitis. Contact dermatitis probably is the most common cutaneous disease of the lids. The thin epidermis with its small, underdeveloped glands makes the skin of the lids susceptible to drying and external irritants, e.g., cosmetics. In the acute forms the skin is edematous and there is a diffuse erythema with oozing and crusting. Vesicles may be present. In the chronic forms scaling and lichenification predominate.

Histologically there is at first an edema of the corium with diffuse lymphocytic infiltration. The infiltration increases as the disease progresses. Hyperplastic changes soon appear in the epidermis (acanthosis, parakeratosis, and cornification).

Lupus erythematosus. The discoid type of lupus erythematosus often is seen on the lids, either as an isolated patch or as part of a more generalized affection of the face. The affected areas show well-circumscribed patches of erythema and infiltration which show a characteristic pale-blue color. There is some scaling and atrophy of the skin. Scar formation may ensue. The histologic picture is characterized by irregular atrophy, acanthosis, hyperkeratosis, thickening of the granular layer, liquefaction degeneration of the basal cell layer, atrophy of the stratum malpighii, keratotic plugging and degeneration of hair follicles, lymphocytic perivasculitis, and a basophilic degeneration of the collagen (Fig. 126).

The erythema of acute disseminated lupus erythematosus also may involve the lids. The edema is quite pronounced, and the skin changes are more diffuse, ill-defined and purplish. Fibrinoid degeneration of collagen and edema of the upper dermis are present.

Scleroderma. The lids may be affected in systemic scleroderma along with the face, neck, and hands. Edema and erythema of the skin initially are present, followed by a marked induration and hypertrophy. This is followed by atrophy resulting in a thin, smooth, white shining skin. The lid folds are flattened and finally disappear. The entire facial musculature becomes atrophic. The esophagus, heart, and lungs may be involved.

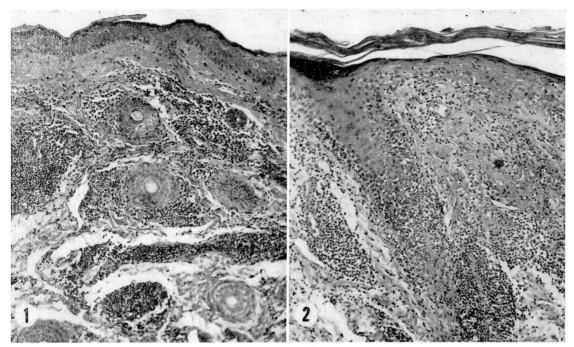

Figure 126. Lupus Erythematosus

Irregular atrophy, acanthosis, and hyperkeratosis; thickened granular layer, liquefaction degeneration of basal cell layer, lymphocytic infiltration about blood vessels and skin appendages, degeneration of connective tissues of dermis and of hair follicles.
1. ×125. AFIP Acc. 180887.
2. ×125. AFIP Acc. 136646.

In circumscribed scleroderma (morphea) isolated areas of the skin are involved. At first the affected patches are brown or violet. Later they become white because of sclerosis. The lids may become involved when a lesion of the frontal skin area extends below the brow. The resulting scar has the appearance of an old injury (coup de sabre). This variety is benign and the internal organs are not involved.

Inflammatory cells and edema are seen around the vessels of the corium only in the early phase of the disease. The collagen fibers become thick and irregular and undergo a severe degeneration. Atrophy occurs in the end stage.

Dermatomyositis. The lids may be the primary site of involvement in dermatomyositis. The skin lesions consist of well-circumscribed areas of edema and erythema. The face, chest and arms are the main sites of involvement. The myositis causes pain, weakness and finally atrophy of the muscles.

The histologic picture of the active phase is usually that of a nonspecific dermatitis. The collagen fibers later become thickened and homogeneous and the muscle fibers show various degrees of inflammation and degeneration.

Inflammations of the Lid Glands

External hordeolum. An external hordeolum (stye) results from a purulent inflammation of the accessory glands and the follicle of a cilium. It frequently is a complication of staphylococcic blepharitis. The inflammation, which begins as a painful swelling and edema of the lid, soon becomes localized. The purulent exudate often breaks through the skin near the lash line. Healing often is prompt, but adjacent follicles may become infected.

The basic histologic feature is a purulent folliculitis, followed by a perifolliculitis. The adjacent glands of Zeis and Moll are involved and at times there develops a cellulitis in the nearby tissues. Finally an abscess is formed followed by necrosis of the skin

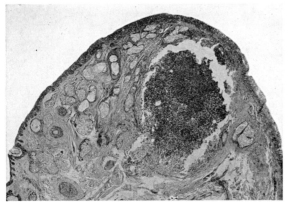

Figure 127.   Focal Inflammation, Eyelid

Hordeolum, eyelid of monkey. ×48. AFIP Acc. 142890.

and spontaneous evacuation occurs at the lid margin (Fig. 127).

Internal hordeolum. An internal hordeolum is a purulent inflammation of a meibomian gland. Obstruction of the duct of a meibomian gland followed by a secondary staphylococcic infection produces such a lesion. Swelling, redness, and pain occur and a localized area of inflammation soon appears. If the lid is everted, a circumscribed elevation is seen in the tarsus and purulent exudate may be observed to come from a break in the abscess wall. The inflammation may

spread and a cellulitis of the soft tissue develops.

Microscopically the tarsus shows a localized abscess which quite often involves the orbicularis and conjunctiva and may break through the conjunctiva (Fig. 128). A considerable amount of scar tissue may follow such an infection.

Chalazion. Chronic inflammation of a meibomian or a Zeis gland produces a chalazion. The evolution of this condition is slow and painless, beginning with a localized thickening of the tarsus which soon is visible through the skin surface. There is little inflammation of the lid or conjunctiva. The lesion may rupture through the conjunctiva and appear as a polypoid mass containing chiefly granulation tissue (internal chalazion). Rarely will it perforate the tarsus and lie as a soft tumor under the skin. It also may develop from a duct of one of these glands and then be localized at the margin of the lids (marginal chalazion).

Microscopic examination shows a granulomatous reaction due to the liberated fat (Fig. 129). A connective tissue capsule often forms around the lesion. The essential feature is the formation of the focal granulomas and abscesses around fat which is discharged from

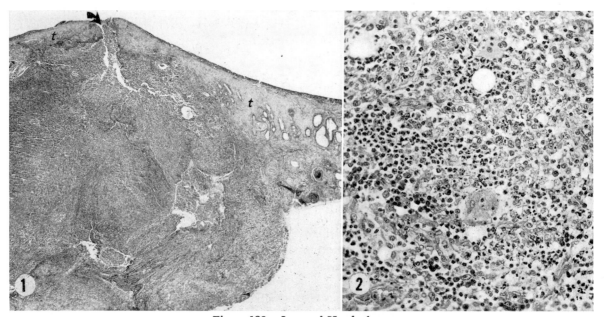

Figure 128.   Internal Hordeolum

1. A chronic abscess has thickened the lid, destroyed much of the tarsus (t), and erupted through the conjunctival surface (arrow). ×17. AFIP Acc. 98605.

2. The tissue reaction is both suppurative and granulomatous. ×165. AFIP Acc. 98605.

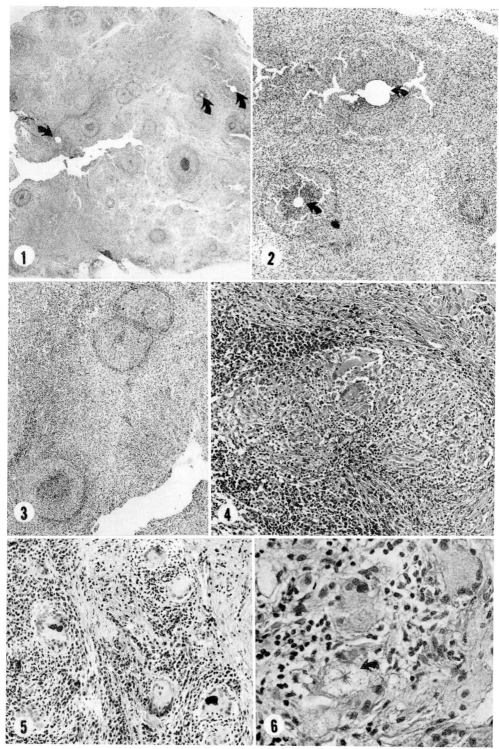

Figure 129.   Chalazion

1, 2 and 3. Multiple discrete lipogranulomas at varying stages of development. Vacuoles in center of some of the lesions (arrows) mark sites of pools of fat liberated from meibomian gland and dissolved away during preparation of sections. ×15, ×63, and ×50, respectively. AFIP Acc. 769807.

4. Late sclerosing stage after absorption of fat and disappearance of polymorphonuclear leukocytes. ×130. AFIP Acc. 732397.

5. Schaumann bodies in giant cells. ×145. AFIP Acc. 780091.

6. Asteroid body (arrow). ×395. AFIP Acc. 692858.

the sebaceous glands. Giant cells and epithelioid cells, lymphocytes and plasma cells are seen. These lipogranulomas may resemble the lesions of tuberculosis or sarcoidosis and the inexperienced examiner may easily misinterpret an innocuous chalazion. Even crystalloids, asteroids, and Schaumann bodies may be found (Fig. 129).

METABOLIC DISEASES

Xanthelasma. Yellow plaques may occur in the skin of the lids in patients with hypercholesteremia. They are more common, however, in female patients with normal serum cholesterol levels at around the fifth decade. The lesions appear as yellowish, flat, irregularly outlined patches. They usually begin at the inner canthus and spread laterally. They are benign but may cause difficulty because of their appearance.

Microscopic sections show large, pale-staining, fat-laden histiocytes throughout the corium and in the subcutis (Fig. 130). They are distributed mainly around the blood vessels and skin appendages. In paraffin sections their cytoplasm appears foamy, but frozen sections stained with Sudan show them to be filled with fat. Touton giant cells usually are absent. Ordinarily there is no tissue necrosis and no inflammatory reaction. Fibrotic changes may occur.

In view of the histologic identity of the xanthelasma with hypercholesteremic xanthomas, the suspicion is warranted that even these localized lesions are associated with some disturbance of lipid metabolism and transport. A true tuberous xanthoma also may occur in the lids.

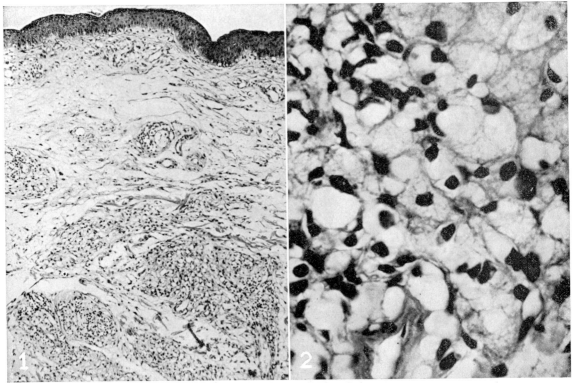

Figure 130. Xanthelasma

1. Accumulations of lipoidal histiocytes around blood vessels. Moderate atrophy of surface epithelium. ×175. AFIP 26555.

2. Large foamy cells with small eccentric pyknotic nuclei (lipoidal histiocytes). ×810. AFIP Acc. 26555.

Juvenile xanthogranuloma. Another type of cutaneous xanthoma has been seen in infants and children. It has been called nevoxanthoendothelioma, but the term juvenile xanthogranuloma (Fig. 131) seems more appropriate (Helwig and Hackney, 1954). These yellowish cutaneous lesions which range from a few millimeters to 1.5 cm. in diameter tend to involve the head and neck most often. While the eyelid, conjunctiva, and orbit may be affected, the most important ocular manifestations are the result of involvement of the iris. (See p. 449.) Microscopically the lesions in the corium are comprised of spindle and polygonal cells containing fat. A variable number of Touton giant cells are present and in some cases eosinophils are numerous. Except for the intraocular complications, these juvenile xanthogranulomas are characteristically benign lesions which regress spontaneously and are not associated with the visceral manifestation and progressive curse of Letterer-Siwe and Hand-Schüller-Christian diseases.

Amyloid. Amyloidosis refers to a group of disorders of diverse etiology and pathogenesis which are characterized pathologically by a special type of hyaline degeneration (Fig. 132). An abnormal glycoprotein which reacts with iodine in the same manner as starch to produce a mahogany-red color is deposited in the affected tissues. The most common cause of this condition is chronic infection (secondary amyloidosis) in which case excessive proliferation of plasma cells is believed to be responsible for the production of the amyloid deposits.

Lid depositions of amyloid usually are associated with similar deposits in the conjunctiva. Chronic infections such as trachoma and syphilis may lead to a tumor-like thickening of the lid with formation of a grey-red, rubbery granulation tissue when viewed through the conjunctiva. Similar lesions may develop spontaneously without an antecedent chronic blepharoconjunctivitis.

Histologic sections show the amyloid to be deposited in all layers of the lid, sometimes replacing the tarsus. The deposits may stimulate a foreign body reaction.

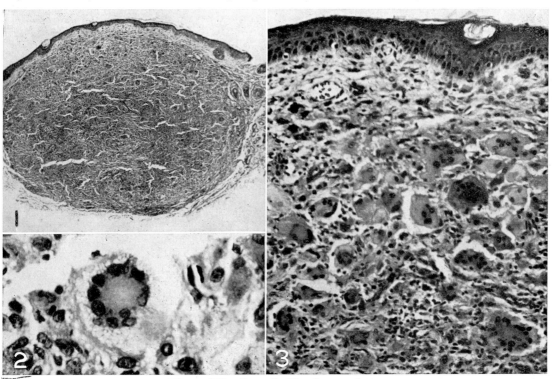

Figure 131. Juvenile Xanthogranuloma

1. Lesion from eyelid. ×30. AFIP Acc. 136738.
2. Touton giant cells in same lesion. × 185. AFIP Acc. 136738.
3. Touton giant cell in same lesion. × 500. AFIP Acc. 136738.

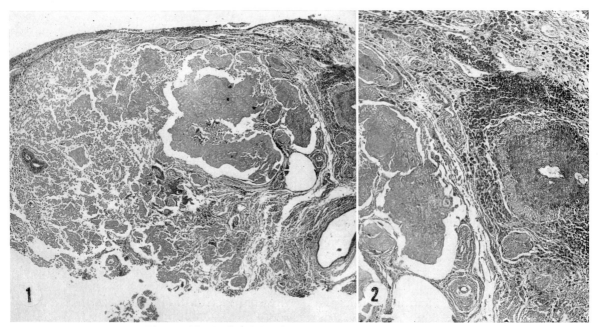

Figure 132. Isolated Amyloid Tumor Mass, Inner Canthus

1. ×50. AFIP Acc. 868840.   2. ×115, AFIP Acc. 868840.

Hyaline degeneration greatly resembling but not staining like amyloid occurs at times in the lids (Fig. 109). It most often is secondary to other diseases, especially trachoma and vernal conjunctivitis.

Calcium. Dystrophic calcification may occur in the tarsus secondary to chronic inflammation, trauma, foreign bodies, injection of irritants, etc.

Comedo. Comedones (blackheads) may occur in the skin of the lid and appear as black areas at the site of pilosebaceous fol-

licles. Caused by an occlusion of the follicular orifice, they contain keratotic debris and inspissated secretion (Fig. 133).

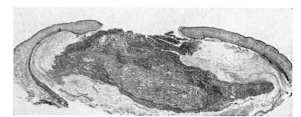

Figure 133. Comedo, Eyelid
×7. AFIP Acc. 236456.

NEOPLASMS AND RELATED CONDITIONS

Sudoriferous cysts. Sudoriferous cysts usually occur at the lid margin, and are rare on the skin of the lids. They are filled with a clear fluid and may reach a considerable size. They usually arise from a blocked excretory duct of a Moll's gland, are lined by two or more layers of flat or cuboidal epithelium, and are surrounded by a thin connective tissue capsule (Fig. 134–1). They may become large enough to compress and replace adjacent sebaceous glands and hair follicles.

Sebaceous cysts. Cysts of the Zeis or the

meibomian glands are rare. Meibomian gland cysts most often are true retention cysts. They are secondary to a variety of obstructive lesions in the lids and are lined with squamous epithelium and filled with sebaceous material and keratin (Fig. 134–2).

Sebaceous cysts of the skin occur in areas where there are large and numerous hair follicles. Therefore, they are more frequent in the brows. They are solid white or yellowish and appear as small or large tumor-like elevations beneath a normal skin. Their

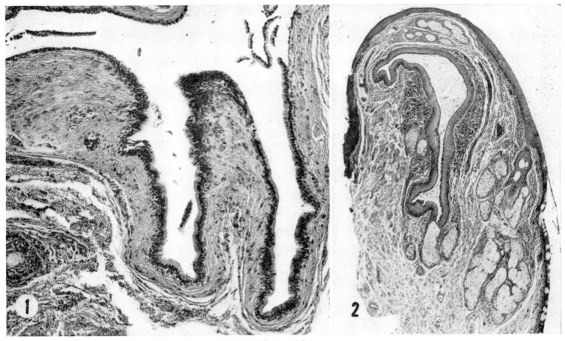

Figure 134.

1. Sudoriferous cyst of eyelid. ×110. AFIP Acc. 750918.   2. Sebaceous cyst of eyelid. ×48. AFIP Acc. 501320.

consistency is soft to rubbery, depending on the nature of the contents. They lie in the subcutis but are attached to the skin in the region of the orifice of the sebaceous duct.

The capsule of the cysts consists of a dense connective tissue lined by several layers of partly vacuolated glandular cells which do not show keratinization. The cavity usually is filled with a fatty or oily mass. Calcification may occur.

Benign Epithelial Neoplasms and Non-neoplastic Tumors

Seborrheic keratosis. Seborrheic keratosis (basal cell papilloma, seborrheic wart, senile verruca) is one of the most frequently observed skin lesions occurring on the lids. It appears as a superficial brown to brown-black excrescence which is well circumscribed and slightly elevated. This lesion is characterized by outward acanthosis and there are no extensions into the dermis (Fig. 135). This causes it to appear like a button stuck on

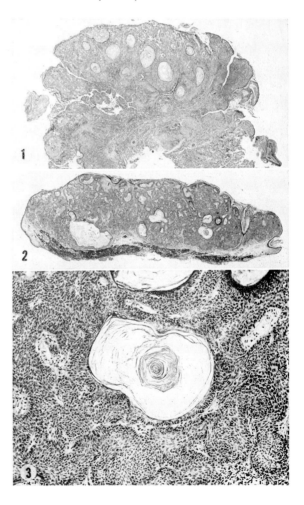

Figure 135. Seborrheic Keratosis
1. ×14. AFIP Acc. 866115.
2. ×15. AFIP Acc. 688965.
3. ×115. AFIP Acc. 688965.

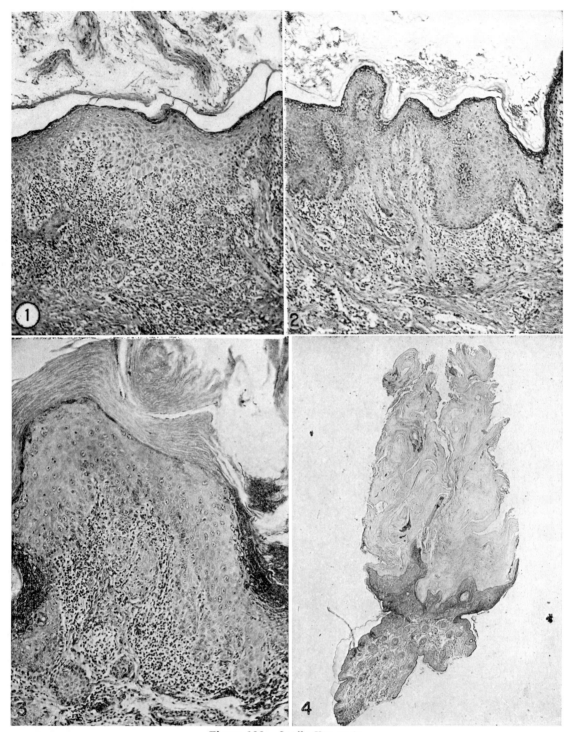

Figure 136. Senile Keratosis

1. ×75. AFIP Acc. 186215.
2. ×48. AFIP Acc. 106215.
3. ×125. AFIP Acc. 314073.
4. Cutaneous horn. ×13. AFIP Acc. 138845.

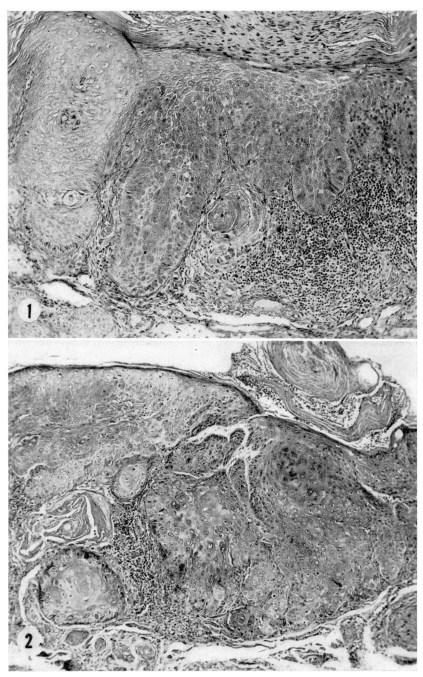

Figure 137. Senile Keratosis with Early Carcinomatous Change

1. ×115. AFIP Acc. 933270.
2. ×80. AFIP Acc. 933270.

the skin surface. Usually there is no surrounding inflammation. It may become inflamed, leading to much confusion in the differential diagnosis, being mistaken for basal or squamous cell epithelioma.

The proliferating cells mostly are of the basal cell type and may contain much pigment. Thus they may be confused with pigmented basal cell epitheliomas or even with melanomas. Trapped among these proliferating cells are concentric layers of horny material (keratin cysts) which should not be confused with the epithelial pearls of a squamous cell carcinoma.

Senile keratosis. Senile keratosis is a benign lesion which is especially important because of its tendency to develop into a squamous cell carcinoma (Figs. 136, 137). It appears as a slightly pigmented, well-circumscribed, somewhat elevated lesion in the epidermis. Sometimes it appears as a cutaneous horn. It is composed of hyperkeratotic, acanthotic, and dyskeratotic epithelium. Bizarre epithelial cells and many mitoses usually are present. The dermal papillas and underlying tissues are infiltrated by large numbers of chronic inflammatory cells.

Papillomas. Papillomas are common benign tumors of the lids (Fig. 138). They may occur as a sessile tumor at the lid margin or as a pedunculated lesion on the skin and often recur if incompletely excised.

The tumor consists of finger-like processes (papillas) of a vascularized connective tissue which is covered with a hyperplastic squamous epithelium. There is normal palisading of the basal cell layer but the basement membrane remains intact. The epithelium is usually acanthotic, parakeratotic and hyperkeratotic.

Benign calcifying epithelioma, hair matrixoma. The benign calcifying epithelioma of Malherbe usually occurs in young adults and is more common in females. According to Helwig, this benign tumor arises from hair matrix cells. The tumor is comprised of variable proportions of necrotic and viable epithelial cells (Fig. 139). The latter may appear pleomorphic, contain many mitotic figures, and simulate an invasive carcinoma. In the necrotic areas pale cells without nuclei are found (shadow cells), and there may be extensive calcification. Ossification is uncommon. The tumor is surrounded by connective tissue which contains numerous foreign body giant cells (Fig. 139-3). The lesion may appear to be malignant histologically but it does not metastasize.

Keratoacanthoma. The keratoacanthoma (molluscum sebaceum, molluscum pseudocarcinomatosum) is a benign lesion which often is mistaken for a low grade squamous cell epithelioma (Fig. 140). It is characterized by a rapid growth but after six to eight weeks the maximal size of 1 to 2 cm. is reached. Spontaneous regression may follow. The general configuration of this lesion resembles that of a molluscum contagiosum, and a crater filled with keratin is formed (Figs. 141, 142). The acanthotic and dyskeratotic epidermal cells grow toward the corium simulating an early invasive squamous cell carcinoma.

Inverted follicular keratosis. Another morphologically specific type of keratosis which has a distinct predilection for the face, and which is often confused with carcinoma by both the clinician and the pathologist, is inverted follicular keratosis. The lesion usu-

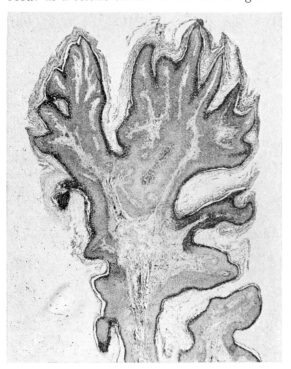

Figure 138. Papilloma of Eyelid
There are numerous papillary projections with the corium extending into the papillas. The acanthotic epidermis is also hyperkeratotic.

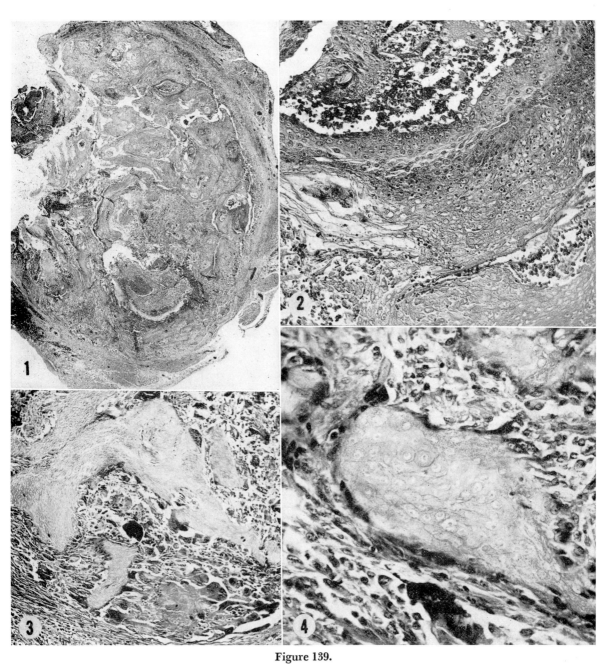

Figure 139.

Benign calcifying epithelioma of Malherbe, eyelid. AFIP Acc. 645171. 1. ×15. 2. ×180. 3. ×80. 4. ×305.

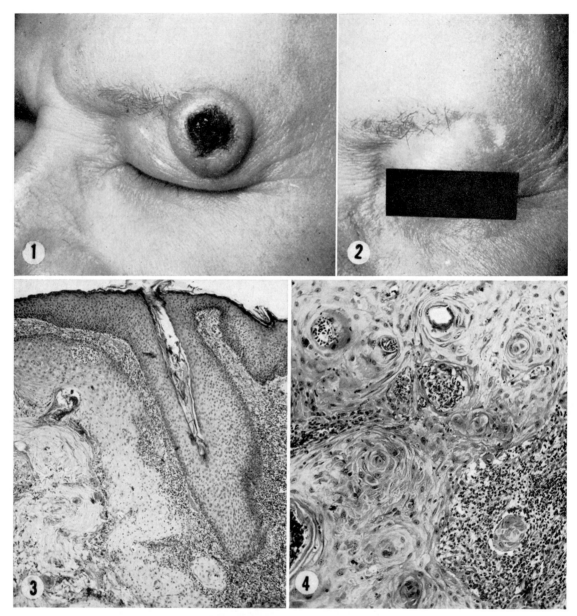

Figure 140. Keratoacanthoma

1. About 8 weeks after onset.
2. Complete involution after 12 weeks' treatment with podophyllum.
3 and 4. Biopsy of lesion. ×50 and ×115, respectively.
Case reported by Kallos (1958). AFIP Acc. 960693.

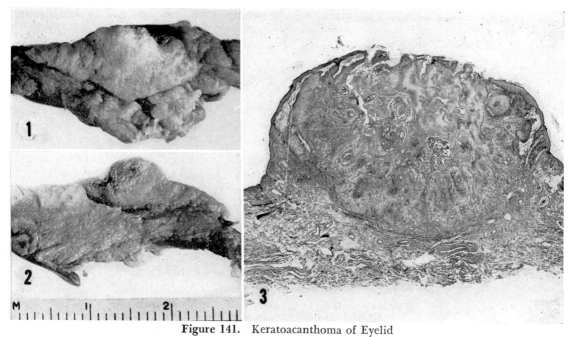

Figure 141. Keratoacanthoma of Eyelid

The lesion was originally thought to be a squamous cell carcinoma. AFIP Acc. 784356.

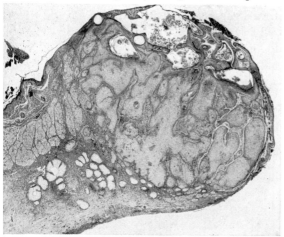

Figure 142.

Keratoacanthoma of eyelid originally considered to be a basal cell carcinoma (clinically). × 15. AFIP Acc. 819080.

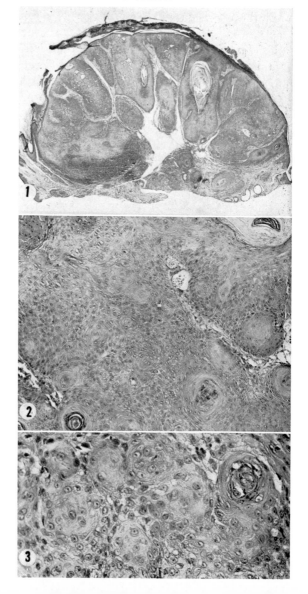

Figure 143. Inverted Follicular Keratosis

1. This lesion was originally thought to be a basal cell carcinoma. ×16. AFIP Acc. 844610.

2. Typical squamous eddies from a recurrent lesion first interpreted as a squamous cell carcinoma. ×115. AFIP Acc. 784873.

3. Same case as 2. ×305.

ally presents as a single papillary or nodular projection from the surface. Its name is derived from its outstanding histopathologic characteristics—an inverted configuration resembling that of molluscum contagiosum and keratoacanthoma and the presence of innumerable "squamous eddies" (Helwig, 1954). These are flattened, concentrically oriented epidermal cells which are seen throughout the broad areas of acanthosis (Fig. 143). There is no evidence that this lesion gives rise to malignant tumors.

Other keratotic lesions. A variety of pseudoepitheliomatous lesions of diverse etiology occur on the eyelids. Often the cause is entirely obscure and the best the pathologist can do is to label the lesion "pseudoepitheliomatous hyperplasia, etiology undetermined" (Fig. 145) or "benign keratosis, type uncertain" (Fig. 144).

Adnexal Neoplasms

Trichoepithelioma. The trichoepithelioma is a benign neoplasm which differentiates toward the hair follicle. Characteristic are the horn cysts. These consist of a keratin core which is demarcated by a layer of basal cells (Fig. 146). Solid strands of basal cells frequently accompany these cysts. The tumor may arise from the cilia and appear at the lid margin.

Sweat gland adenoma. Benign tumors of the sweat glands in the skin of the lids are quite frequent (Fig. 147). They occur commonly in the lower lid. They appear as small plaques or dimples. Essentially, all these lesions are adenomas, but according to the degree of differentiation the name varies.

Sebaceous adenomas. Benign tumors of the meibomian glands arise in the tarsus and lie close to or continuous with a meibomian gland. They include simple hyperplasias, true adenomas and hamartomas (Figs. 148, 149). The hyperplasia is an overgrowth and multiplication of sebaceous gland cells which produce a lesion resembling a neoplasm. Hamartomas and true adenomas show a loss of the normal glandular pattern. The former is the result of a congenital malformation while the latter is an acquired neoplasm. Acinar organization is still present in both, but the central duct arrangement is absent. These are sharply localized tumors which compress the adjacent tissues but do not invade them.

Benign tumors of the glands of Zeis are uncommon. In their structure they imitate a sebaceous gland but contain cilia. They lie anterior to the mucocutaneous junction.

Benign tumors of the sebaceous glands of the skin of the lids are rare. True adenomas may occur. The lids may be involved in the hamartomatous enlargement of these glands (adenoma sebaceum) which occurs in tuberous sclerosis (Fig. 150).

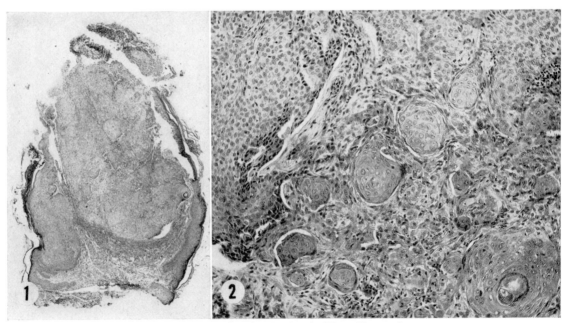

Figure 144.   Benign Keratosis, Type Uncertain
1. ×23. 2. ×115. AFIP Acc. 738582.

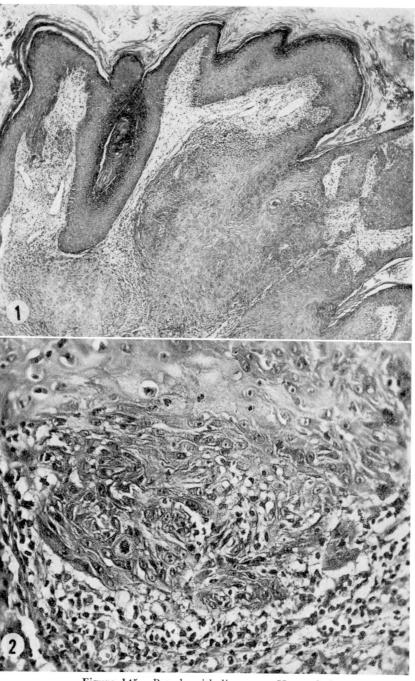

Figure 145. Pseudoepitheliomatous Hyperplasia

1. ×50. AFIP Acc. 853800.
2. ×305. AFIP Acc. 853800.

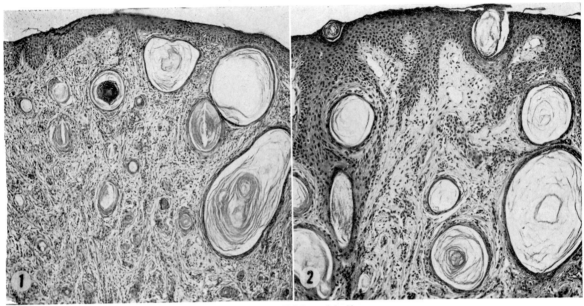

Figure 146.   Trichoepithelioma

1. ×80. AFIP Acc. 811519.
2. ×115. AFIP Acc. 811519.

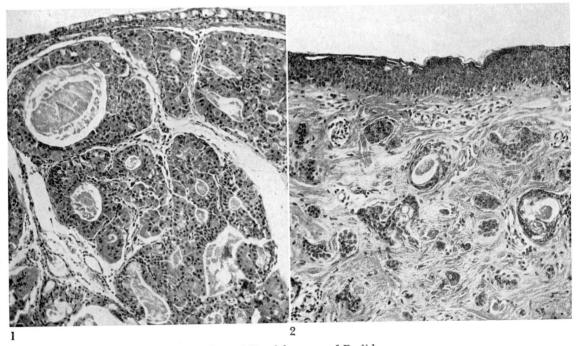

Figure 147.   Adenomas of Eyelid

1. Adenoma of uncertain histogenesis. ×125. AFIP Acc. 283871.
2. Syringoma (adenoma of sweat gland ducts). ×125. AFIP Acc. 282867.

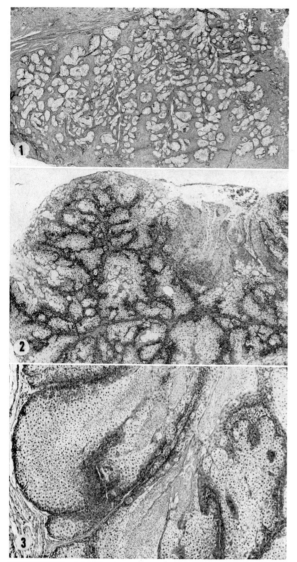

Figure 148.

1. Adenomatoid hyperplasia, meibomian gland.
×22. AFIP Acc. 514703.

2. Adenoma, meibomian gland. ×56. AFIP Acc.
209672.

3. Adenoma, meibomian gland. ×80. AFIP Acc.
942326.

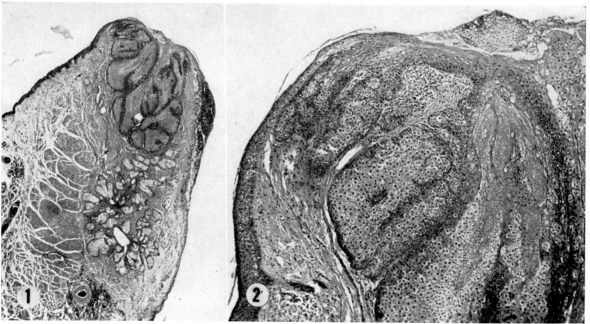

Figure 149. Adenoma, Meibomian Gland

1. ×14. AFIP Acc. 942326.   2. ×80. AFIP Acc. 942326.

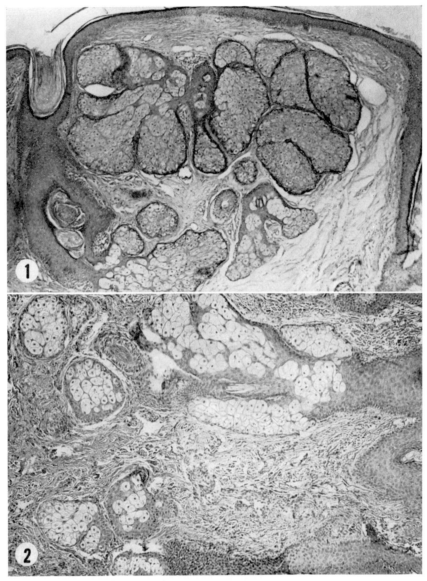

Figure 150.   Sebaceous Gland Lesions

1. Senile hyperplasia of sebaceous glands. ×75. University of California Acc. 59–43.

2. Hamartomatous lesions of sebaceous glands (adenoma sebaceum) and of other dermal tissues in tuberous sclerosis. ×80. AFIP Acc. 219474–108. (Courtesy of Dr. H. Z. Lund from Tumors of the Skin, Atlas of Tumor Pathology, Fascicle 2, Fig. 100, 1957.)

Pigmented Lesions

Ephelis and lentigo. Ephelis (freckle) is characterized merely by increased amounts of melanin in the epidermis. Lentigo contains, in addition to hyperpigmentation, an increased number of melanocytic clear cells associated with elongation of rete ridges. Distinct nests of nevus cells are absent (Fig. 153).

Nevi. Benign nevi occur frequently on the surface of the lid or on the lid margin. There is a definite hormonal influence on melanogenesis and the increased pigmentation of congenital nevi during puberty or pregnancy may be a physiologic event and not a sign of tumor growth.

Nevus cells form nests, sometimes strands and sheets. The cells are larger than basal cells and somewhat polygonal, with definite cell outlines. The nuclei are irregular, and often are wedge-shaped. Nucleoli generally are absent or poorly developed. Nevus giant cells are common. The degree of pigmentation varies and may be absent.

Dermal nevus. In the lids, as elsewhere in the skin, nevi can be classified according to their location. The dermal type is the most common, its cell being located entirely in the dermis (Fig. 151). It represents the common mole so frequently found in the skin. The surface may be smooth but usually is elevated and may be distinctly papillomatous (Fig. 152). If a nevus contains hair, the evidence is strong that it is intradermal. This is an important point since these dermal nevi do not become malignant. A thin layer of connective tissue lies between the tumor and the epidermis. The nevus cells may extend into the subcutis and even the lid muscles may be infiltrated. This type rarely is apparent before puberty.

Junctional nevus. The junctional type of nevus arises in the deep layers of the surface epithelium and does not involve the adjacent dermis (Fig. 153). It appears as a flat, smooth lesion. There is a loss of cohesion of the basal cells and, frequently, of other cells of the epidermis. Pigmentation of the basal cells is variable. This type of nevus is potentially malignant. The development of frank malignancy is preceded by cellular pleomorphism, anaplasia, hyperchromatism, mitotic figures and an inflammatory reaction in the adjacent dermis.

Compound nevus. The compound nevus contains both junctional and dermal elements (Fig. 153). It is more common than the pure junctional nevus, but like it may undergo malignant changes.

Juvenile nevus. A particularly disturbing lesion is known as "juvenile nevus." It appears prior to puberty and, though histologically it resembles malignant melanoma in the adult, the clinical course is entirely benign.

Blue nevus. A blue nevus may occur on the face. It is a slightly elevated lesion of blue-to-gray-to-black color. The color depends upon the depth of the lesion and upon the quantity of melanin deposited. The lesions are present at birth or appear shortly thereafter. They do not change in size (Fig. 151).

Histologically the blue nevus consists of an accumulation of melanocytes in the deeper part of the dermis. The cells are ovoid or spindle-shaped and often have long branching processes (Fig. 67). Usually they are heavily laden with melanin. A more cellular type of blue nevus exists which may undergo malignant change on rare occasions.

These extrasacral Mongolian spots are seen more frequently in the Oriental races and in Negroes, and may be associated with ipsilateral hyperpigmentation of the uvea.

Hamartomas and Other Benign Tumors

Neurofibromatosis. The lids may be involved in generalized neurofibromatosis (von Recklinghausen's disease). Isolated lid neurofibromas without other signs of this syndrome are common. In other cases the lids may become enormously enlarged and large masses of racemose cords (plexiform neuroma) (Fig. 154) and tumors (neuromatoid elephantiasis) may develop. Neurofibromatosis of the lid may be associated with orbital and intraocular neurofibromatosis and with glaucoma (Figs. 63, 64).

These tumors are formed by a proliferation of Schwann cells and connective tissue elements, but special stains may also demonstrate the presence of neural fibers.

Isolated tumors of the nerve sheaths also may occur in the lids (schwannoma, neurilemoma). They are well circumscribed, often encapsulated tumors in the dermis or the subcutaneous tissue. Their consistency

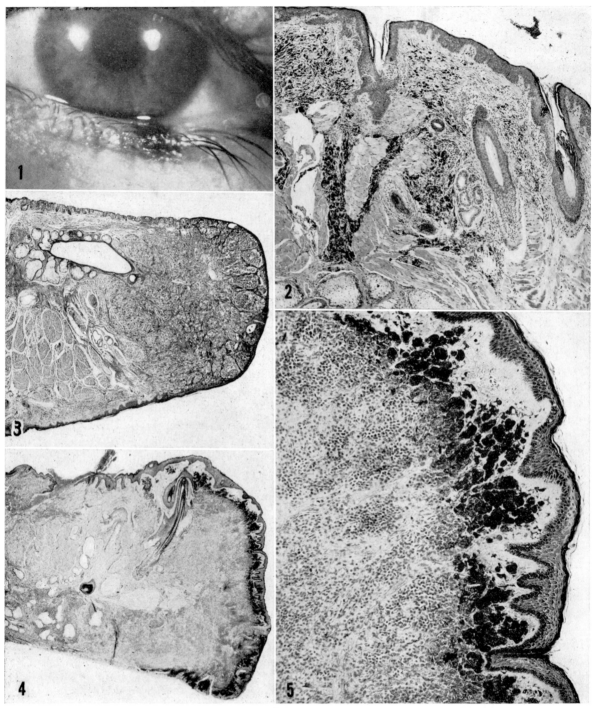

Figure 151.

1 and 2. Blue nevus. Courtesy of Dr. A. B. Reese. The heavily pigmented dermal melanocytes are situated deep in the lid amongst the skin appendages and within the orbicularis muscle. ×50. AFIP Acc. 334467.

3. Lightly pigmented dermal nevus of lid margin with obstruction and dilatation of duct of meibomian gland. ×16. AFIP Acc. 933242.

4 and 5. Heavily pigmented dermal nevus of lid margin. ×16 and ×115, respectively. AFIP Acc. 686089.

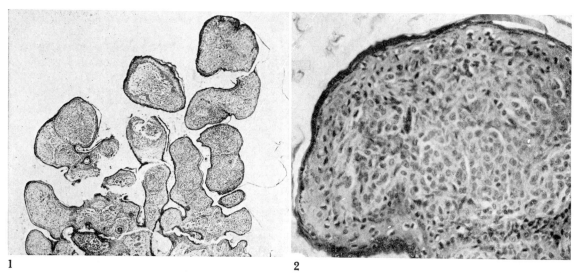

Figure 152. Papillary Dermal Nevus, Eyelid

1. ×45. AFIP Acc. 119510.   2. ×275. AFIP Acc. 119510.

may vary from firm to soft when cystic degeneration occurs.

Characteristic of this tumor is the parallel arrangement of nuclei in rows (palisading) (Fig. 155). A herringbone pattern of alternating rows of nuclei and fibers is often visible. The nuclei are usually long and slender. There is a fibrillar matrix in this solid (Antoni A) type; sometimes hyalinized foci (Verocay bodies) may appear. A mucoid degeneration of the connective tissue with the appearance of microcysts is characteristic of the soft type (Antoni B).

Fibroma, lipoma, chondroma, and osteoma all are very rare in the lids. A benign rhabdomyoma or a granular cell myoblastoma may arise in the orbicularis muscle fibers.

Hemangioma. Angiomatous tumors usually are congenital and are classified as hamartomas. The port-wine stain (nevus flammeus) is a telangiectatic type of hemangioma. It appears as a dark-red or blue discoloration of the skin of the lids. It consists of dilated and newly formed capillaries and veins in the dermis. These lesions remain stationary and usually do not change in size or appearance. The lid involvement usually is part of an extensive lesion that covers one-half of the face, following the distribution of a branch of the trigeminal nerve. Such a lesion may be accompanied by ipsilateral

glaucoma, with or without choroidal hemangioma, and by a meningeal hemangioma (Sturge-Weber syndrome).

Capillary hemangiomas (strawberry marks) are elevated, soft, red tumors. They consist of endothelial cells which may form solid cords (angioblastic hemangioma) or numerous capillaries (Fig. 156). Most often both types occur together. In the natural history of these tumors, there often occurs an early replacement of vascular tissue by dense connective tissue. The vessels become obliterated and the tumor shrinks. This histologic phenomenon of sclerosis accounts for the usual spontaneous disappearance of the clinical lesions.

Cavernous hemangiomas are large, soft, subcutaneous tumors. Large, thin-walled cavities are formed and filled with blood. The cavities are lined with a single layer of endothelium (Fig. 157). Sclerosis also may occur. Frequently a hemangioma is of the mixed type and contains capillary as well as cavernous elements.

Hemangiosarcomas, including Kaposi's hemorrhagic sarcoma, have been observed in the lids, but these are exceedingly rare tumors.

Lymphangiomas of the face or of the orbit may involve the lids. Hemorrhage into these lymph vessels may lead to an erroneous diagnosis of hemangioma.

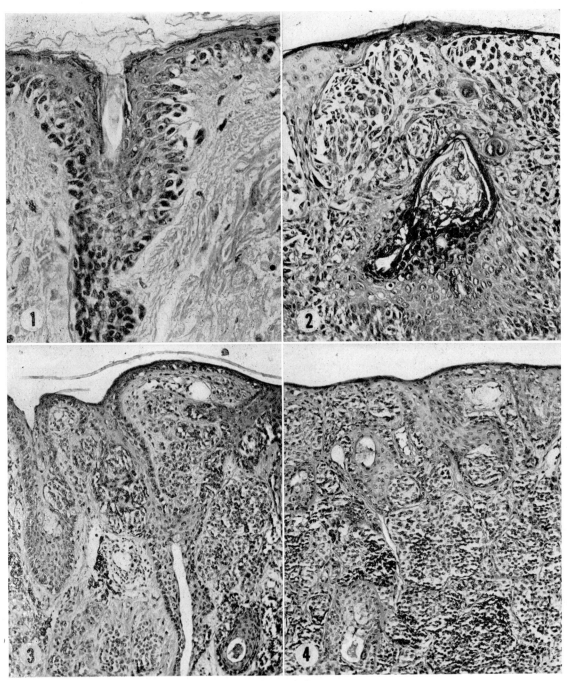

Figure 153.

1. Lentigo. ×265. AFIP Acc. 838056.

2. Elevated junctional nevus with marked activity but no definite evidence of malignant change. ×170. AFIP Acc. 909836.

3 and 4. Compound nevus. ×115. AFIP Acc. 928640.

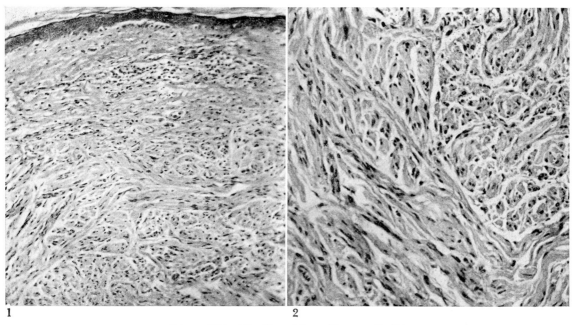

Figure 154. Plexiform Neurofibroma, Eyelid

1. ×125. AFIP Acc. 260641.
2. ×180. AFIP Acc. 260641.

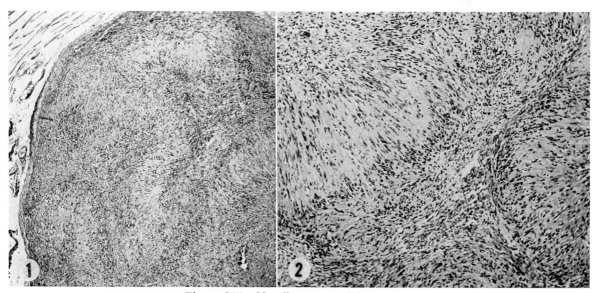

Figure 155. Neurilemoma or Schwannoma

A discrete encapsulated subcutaneous nodule with conspicuous palisading of the Schwann cell nuclei.   1. ×42.
2. ×90. AFIP Acc. 648520.

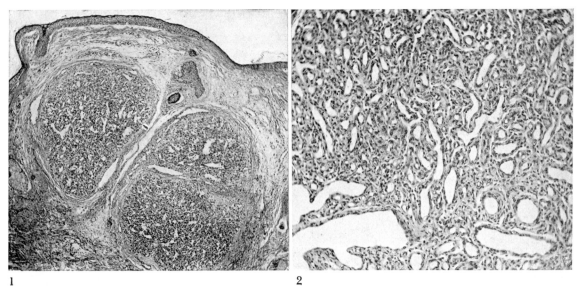

1   2

Figure 156

1. Hemangioma, capillary, in adult. ×48. AFIP Acc. 212330.
2. Hemangioma, capillary. ×135. AFIP Acc. 91274.

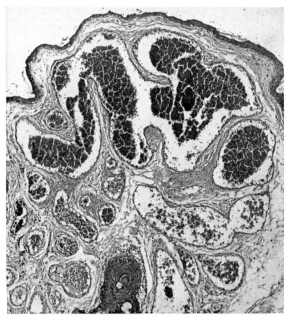

Figure 157

Hemangioma, cavernous, eyelid. ×48. AFIP Acc. 499506.

Malignant Tumors

Basal cell epithelioma. The basal cell carcinoma is the most common malignant tumor of the lids, and the skin about the eye is a most frequent site of occurrence of basal cell carcinoma. Well over 90 per cent of all epitheliomas of the lids are of the basal cell type. They occur most frequently in the lower lid, are next most common at the inner canthus, then at the outer canthus, and least common in the upper lid. They often appear as small nodular tumors, containing characteristic dilated vessels in their surface. The nodule grows slowly and finally ulcerates. The fully developed tumor then appears as a slowly enlarging ulcer surrounded by an elevated, pearly margin (rodent ulcer) (Fig. 158). They often contain large deposits of melanin. The tumor also may remain superficial in the skin and be slightly elevated, red, and scaly, with a pearly border. The clinical and histologic appearance of these tumors varies markedly from case to case. In the early stages they usually are well circumscribed. Some become highly invasive, but do not metastasize. In spite of repeated excisions they may invade deep into the orbit. In the more advanced stages, the tumor may proliferate into a large, cauliflower-like mass and destroy the entire lid and adjacent tissues.

The tumor cells resemble those of the basal cell layer of the epithelium. They have a rather scanty cytoplasm so that the deeply staining, non-nucleolated nuclei appear densely packed. The rather uniform appearance and deep basophilia are quite characteristic and help differentiate the basal cell

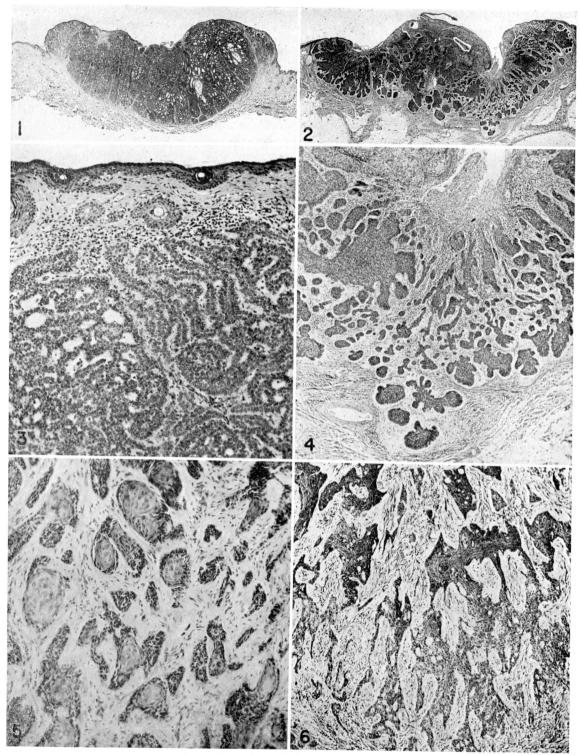

Figure 158. Basal Cell Carcinoma, Eyelid

1. Circumscribed basal cell carcinoma. ×10. AFIP Acc. 288649.
2. Ulcerated basal cell carcinoma. ×8. AFIP Acc. 113123.
3. Adnexal type basal cell carcinoma. ×125. AFIP Acc. 230088.
4. Ulcerated basal cell carcinoma. ×48. AFIP Acc. 113123.
5. Keratinizing basal cell carcinoma. ×125. AFIP Acc. 293651.
6. Infiltrative and cicatrizing basal cell carcinoma invading orbit. ×75. AFIP Acc. 37436.

carcinoma from the squamous cell carcinoma. The arrangement of the tumor cells varies a great deal. Most frequent is the solid or primordial type (Fig. 158–1). Here the cells grow in solid cords or sheets showing polarization (palisading of nuclei) at the periphery. The cells arrange themselves with the oval nuclei pointing toward the center of the mass. Varying degrees of inflammation and connective tissue proliferation surround the tumor. Superficial ulceration is often present. Melanin pigment may be found in the cells of certain tumors. Rarely, the connective tissue proliferation is exaggerated (scirrhous form), and long, thin strands of tumor cells are seen to be embedded in a dense stroma (Fig. 158–6). Occasionally the tumor is very superficial and multiple small epitheliomas are attached to the epidermis. Cysts may appear in the center of the tumor mass. They are caused by a central degeneration and necrosis of the tumor cells (Fig. 159–1). Squamous metaplasia and keratinization may be found in certain basal cell epitheliomas (Fig. 158–5). Such tumors should not be called basosquamous cell carcinomas because their prognosis is no worse than that of other basal cell carcinomas.

If the neoplasm shows signs of greater differentiation, tubular and gland-like structures may be formed (Figs. 158–3, 159–2). These tumors often resemble epitheliomas of skin appendages (Fig. 146). They may grow within the tarsus or at the lid margin and for a long time the skin and conjunctiva remain freely movable over them. Large polypoid areas, with little or no evidence of ulceration, may be observed (Fig. 159). They may resemble a chalazion, and in the beginning it is impossible to make an exact diagnosis except by examination of a biopsy specimen. Any chalazion, therefore, which does not respond to the usual treatment should be studied microscopically.

Meibomian gland carcinoma. Meibomian gland carcinomas are slowly growing, yellow-white tumors in the tarsal portion of the lids. In the early stage the clinical picture may be that of a chalazion. Eventually the tumor erodes the lid margin or the conjunctiva to produce a nodular or lobulated mass. Metastasis to the regional lymph nodes may

occur. The arrangement of the tumor cells varies. Most frequently it is acinar, resembling and imitating the normal structure of the gland (Fig. 160), but the cells also may be arranged in sheets, solid cords or small clusters. Considerable cytologic variation may be encountered, but at least certain portions of the tumor contain large cells with abundant vacuolated cytoplasm. Frozen sections stained for fat reveal a large amount of lipid in the vacuolated cells and in the necrotic central areas of certain lobules (Fig. 160–2). Mitotic figures are often conspicuous. In the poorly differentiated areas these sebaceous gland tumors may imitate a squamous carcinoma. Pagetoid invasion of the epidermis of the lid margin may be seen (Fig. 161).

Other adenocarcinomas. Malignant tumors of the glands of Zeis are rare. They arise at the lid margin. Clinically they first resemble marginal chalazions. Their clinical behavior is similar to that of meibomian gland carcinomas, and like them they are microscopically typical sebaceous gland carcinomas.

Malignant tumors of the glands of Moll are quite rare. The principal lesion is an epithelioma stemming from this special apocrine sweat gland. The mucin which is present in the cells is strongly PAS-positive. The tumors usually are isolated from the surface epithelium and acini develop which resemble the original gland.

Squamous cell epithelioma. The squamous cell carcinoma (epidermoid carcinoma) is comparatively rare in the lids and less than five per cent of all malignant epithelial tumors in this location are of the squamous cell type. A variety of benign tumors and non-neoplastic lesions have been misinterpreted as squamous cell carcinoma. Among such lesions are the previously described keratocanthoma, inverted follicular keratosis, inflamed seborrheic keratosis, and pseudo-epitheliomatous hyperplasia (see pp. 195 thru 199 and Figs. 135, and 140 to 145). Keratoses are much more common on the lids than are squamous cell epitheliomas, but these are rarely of the type from which squamous cell carcinomas develop. The true precancerous dermatoses (e.g., senile keratosis, xeroderma pigmentosa, radiation keratosis) all occur on the lids (Figs. 113, 114, 136, 137), but they

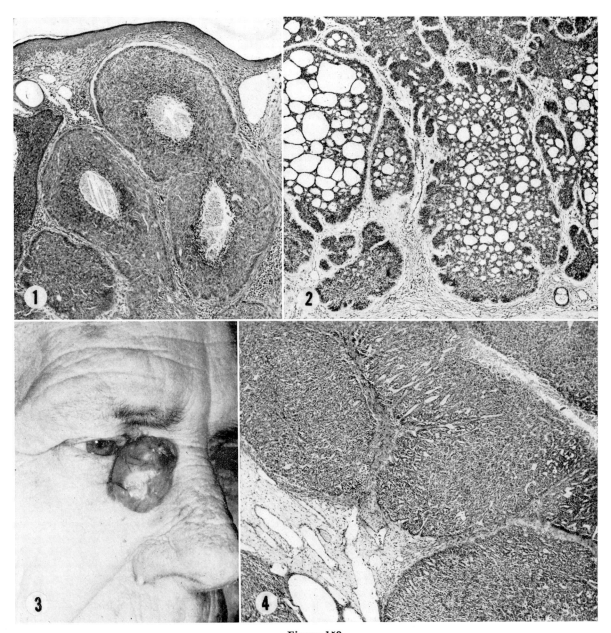

Figure 159.

1. Basal cell carcinoma with central necrosis and pseudocyst formation. ×50. AFIP Acc. 49500.
2. Adenoid cystic carcinoma pattern in basal cell carcinoma. ×50. AFIP Acc. 73666.
3 and 4. Polypoid basal cell carcinoma, adnexal type. AFIP Acc. 962128. (Courtesy J. M. Dixon, M.D.)
4. ×50.

are observed much less often than other keratotic lesions.

Grossly the squamous cell carcinoma may resemble basal cell epitheliomas, except that its richness in keratin may produce a pearly shagreen. The lesions ulcerate early but their progress is usually slower than that of keratoacanthoma. They may metastasize to the regional lymph nodes. If the tumor is in the upper lid, the preauricular nodes are involved whereas if the tumor is in the lower lid, spread is to the submaxillary nodes. The tumor usually appears as a shallow ulcer with a granular, red base which frequently is covered by a crust. There is an elevated, hard border.

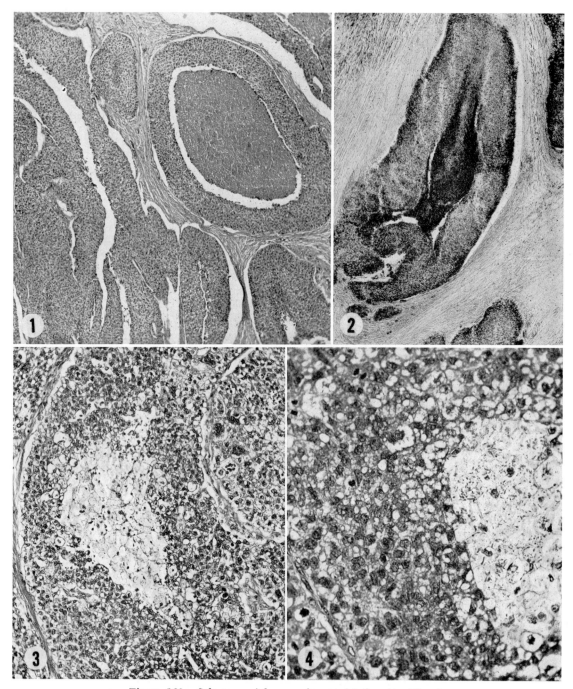

Figure 160. Sebaceous Adenocarcinoma, Meibomian Gland

Tumor cells rich in sebaceous material become necrotic in center of lobules.
1. H and E. ×48. AFIP Acc. 541358.
2. Oil red O stain for fat. ×60. AFIP Acc. 541358.
3. H and E. ×130. AFIP Acc. 804889.
4. H and E. ×305. AFIP Acc. 804889.

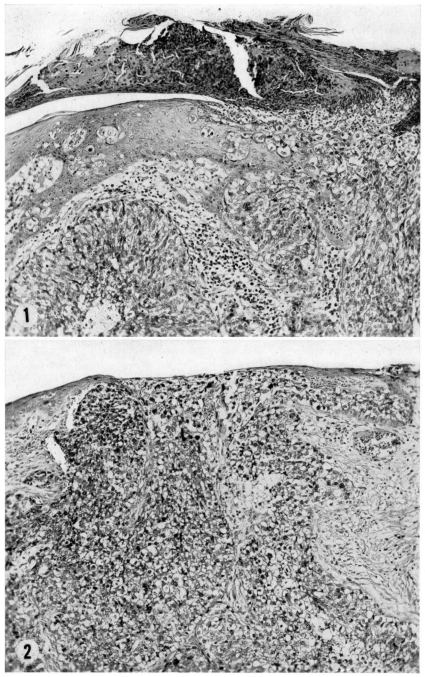

Figure 161.

Pagetoid invasion of epidermal surface of eyelid by carcinoma cells from an underlying meibomian gland tumor ×115. AFIP Acc. 804889.

Histologically the neoplasm consists of atypical, pleomorphic prickle cells which proliferate in a haphazard fashion (Fig. 137). The tumor cells along the periphery fail to exhibit the regularity and palisaded nuclei observed in basal cell carcinoma. There is much variation in cytology and degree of differentiation in these neoplasms (Fig. 162). Epithelial pearls, consisting of concentric layers of keratinized tumor cells with a central core of acellular keratin, are present in the better differentiated tumors. Individual tumor cells often show intracellular keratinization, and dyskeratosis is a prominent feature. If the tumor grows rapidly, keratinization may not occur, pearls are absent, and the cells remain undifferentiated.

Malignant melanoma. Malignant melanomas may arise either from a junctional or a compound nevus (Figs. 153, 163) but rarely, if ever, from a dermal nevus. Often, however, microscopic examination fails to disclose evidence of a pre-existing benign tumor, possibly because the malignant melanoma has so completely overgrown the original lesion. The degree of pigmentation varies as it does in benign nevi and some of these tumors contain relatively little pigment. Usually the tumor appears as a pigmented, enlarging nodule on the lid surface or margin. It grows until it becomes a fungating mass surrounded by smaller, pigmented lesions. The first metastases may occur in the regional lymph nodes or in distant organs. Local recurrence is frequent following simple excision. The prognosis of malignant melanomas of the eyelid is very much worse than in the case of conjunctival melanomas.

Microscopically, malignant melanomas differ from benign nevi mainly in their cytologic characteristics. In compound nevi the cells appear to mature, become smaller, and are surrounded by connective tissue fibrils as they progress from the epidermal to the deep dermal component. In malignant melanomas this tendency for the cells to mature is not observed. The tumor cells are large and pleomorphic; they contain large nuclei and prominent nucleoli (Fig. 163). Formation of discrete organoid clusters is inconspicuous and when such aggregations are observed their constituent cells appear to have lost their cohesiveness. Mitoses may or may not be numerous. Ulceration is common and secondary inflammation is observed in most cases.

Malignant melanoma of the lid is rare in children and, even though the histologic picture may suggest malignancy, the clinical course most often is that of a benign nevus.

Lymphoma. The lids may be the site of an isolated lymphoid infiltration. Both eyes often are affected symmetrically. These "lymphomas" of the lids often are associated with similar lesions of the conjunctiva, orbit or salivary glands. Even such extensive lymphomas may be quite benign and may remain confined to the head and neck. The tumor usually is predominantly lymphocytic, but reticulum cells and plasma cells may be present in significant numbers. These tumors usually are quite benign and it is probable that many instances of so-called "malignant" lymphoma in the lids, orbit, and conjunctiva are really benign reactive lymphatic hyperplasias. In these cases the formation of reactive germinal centers has been mistakenly called giant follicular lymphoma. It is, however, probable that the lids, together with many organs, are affected in a systemic malignant lymphoma.

Most lymphoid lid tumors are accompanied by a normal blood picture. In some patients, however, a leukemia may be present or may follow. This is especially true in small children in whom a mass in the lid may represent the first manifestation of acute leukemia. In these cases the cytologic picture differs from the reactive lymphoid hyperplasias in that the tumor cells are immature and obviously malignant.

The lids may be involved in mycosis fungoides, which begins as an erythematous eruption resembling eczema, psoriasis, or generalized exfoliative dermatitis. Subsequently, well defined elevated plaques develop and eventually tumor masses are formed. A great variety of inflammatory cells including eosinophils and immature reticulum cells are seen in the early stages, while in the tumor stage the process may be indistinguishable microscopically from Hodgkins disease or reticulum cell sarcoma.

Rhabdomyosarcoma. This tumor, especially the undifferentiated or embryonal type, may occur in the subcutis of the lids. It is practically confined to children in the first decade of life.

Metastatic tumors. These occur rarely in the lids. The gastrointestinal tract, the breast, and the kidney have been described as primary sites.

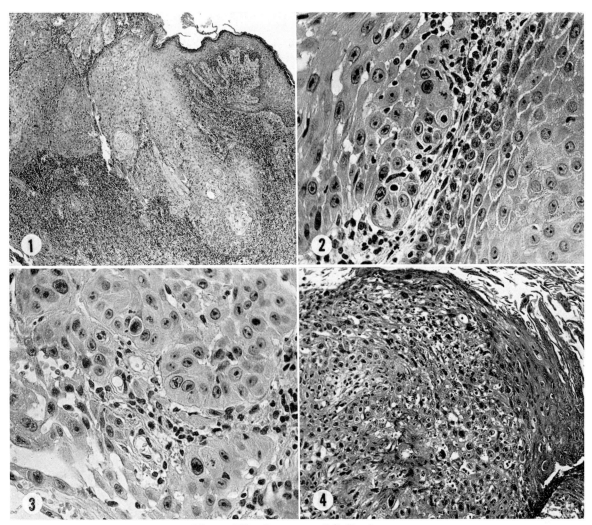

Figure 162.   Squamous Cell Carcinoma

1. ×36. AFIP Acc. 700309.
2. ×120. AFIP Acc. 700309.
In 1 and 2 the anaplastic squamous cells of the carcinoma on the left may be contrasted with the hypertrophic squamous cells of the adjacent acanthotic but non-neoplastic epidermis on the right.
3. ×120. AFIP Acc. 700309.
4. A more highly anaplastic undifferentiated squamous cell carcinoma. ×145. AFIP Acc. 650064.

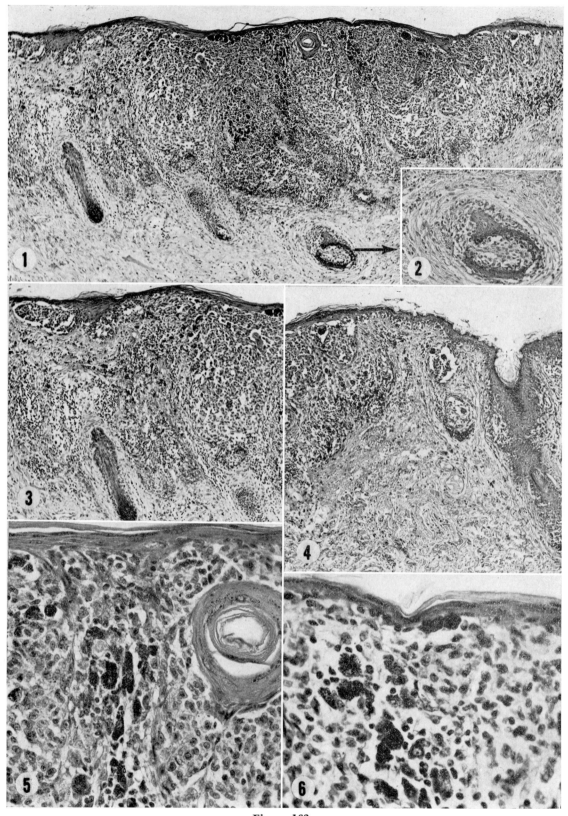

Figure 163.

Malignant melanoma arising in a compound nevus of outer canthal region. AFIP Acc. 838056.
1. ×65.   2. ×115.   3 and 4. ×75.   5. ×265.   6. ×380.

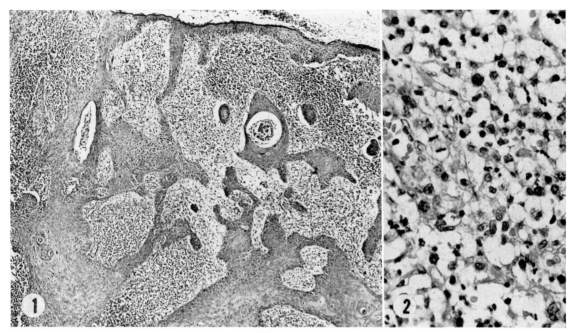

Figure 164.

Reticulum cell sarcoma and pseudoepitheliomatous hyperplasia of eyelid. This was the initial clinical manifesta
tion of the malignant lymphoma which proved fatal. AFIP Acc. 928317.   1. ×50.   2. ×380.

EXCRETORY LACRIMAL APPARATUS

Anatomy

The lacrimal passages consist of the lacrimal canaliculi with their external openings (puncta), the lacrimal sac, and the nasolacrimal duct. The punctum is seen as a small papilla on the lid margin surrounded by a sphincter derived from the orbicularis. The canaliculi are small tubes lined with stratified squamous epithelium. They run vertically for a short distance from the puncta, then turn horizontally in the lacrimal part of the lid margin to the lacrimal sac.

The lacrimal sac lies in the lacrimal fossa in the inferior nasal quadrant of the orbit, entirely surrounded by periosteum. Histologically, it is lined by two layers of columnar ciliated epithelium containing scattered goblet cells. The epithelium rests on a highly refractile basal membrane. The stroma consists of a loose, reticular connective tissue which contains numerous elastic fibers and many lymphocytes. In some areas true lymph follicles are formed. The submucosal tissue consists of a dense, fibrous tissue with many elastic fibers. Folds (duplicatures) of the mucosal lining may occur in the sac but are especially frequent at both ends of the duct.

The nasolacrimal duct is a continuation of the sac inferiorly through the bony canal into the nose, opening into the inferior meatus. Histologically, it resembles the sac and actually they are a single structure, the sac merely being the intraorbital portion.

Congenital Anomalies

Fistulas. A fistula may lead from the sac into the subcutaneous tissues of the lower lid, and to the conjunctival sac. The tract is lined by several layers of cuboidal epithelium which is not keratinized, and resembles that of the canaliculi.

Atresia of the duct. During the eighth fetal month the duct opens into the nasal cavity. It is sometimes still closed by a mucosal fold in newborn infants. This fold may open spontaneously with growth.

Atresia of the punctum. This may occur with or without atresia of the canaliculus.

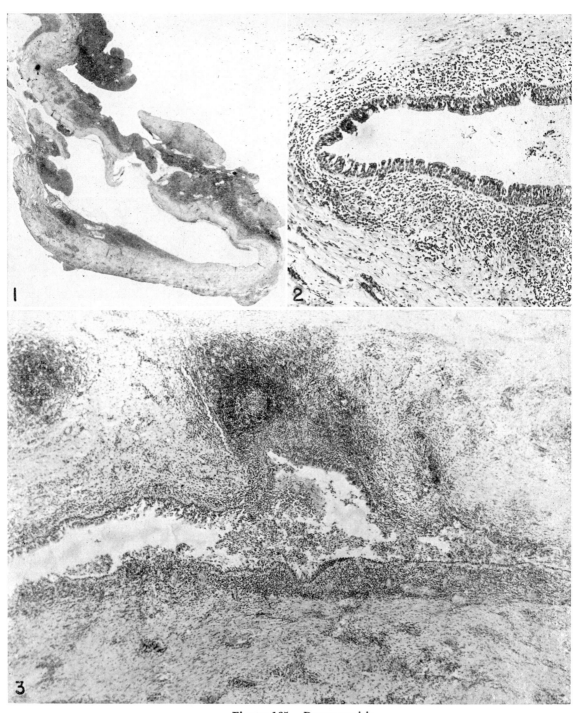

Figure 165. Dacryocystitis

1. Acute dacryocystitis. Destruction of epithelial lining and rupture of wall of sac. AFIP Acc. 28276.
2. Chronic dacryocystitis. Lymphocytic infiltration in wall of sac. ×125. AFIP Acc. 491021.
3. Recurrent dacryocystitis. Lymph follicle in wall, purulent exudate in lumen. ×91. AFIP Acc. 21464.

An acquired obliteration of the punctum may occur after a senile eversion or a long-standing blepharitis.

Cysts. Cystic outpouchings from the canaliculi or from the sac may extend out into the adjacent orbit and lid.

Inflammations

Dacryocystitis. Inflammations of the lacrimal sac usually are caused by a permanent or temporary obstruction of the flow of the tears into the nose. A temporary closure may occur due to swelling of the mucosal lining in infections of the nose. A permanent stenosis usually is the result of a congenital defect plus a chronic infection of the nose or a paranasal sinus. The stagnating tears become infected and cause an inflammatory irritation of the mucous membrane with proliferation of the epithelium, hyperemia, and a purulent exudation into the sac. The

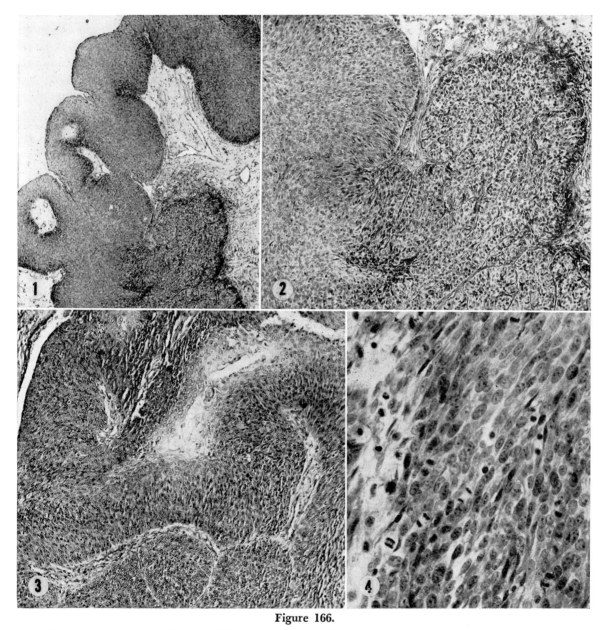

Figure 166.

1 and 2. Early squamous carcinoma arising in a papilloma of lacrimal sac. ×50 and ×115, respectively. AFIP Acc. 912043.

3 and 4. Transitional cell carcinoma of lacrimal sac. ×110 and ×380, respectively. AFIP Acc. 697113.

sac may become dilated, forming a pyocele with thin walls.

Histologically, the walls usually are thickened and the lumen is enlarged (Fig. 165). The mucosa is markedly folded. The epithelium may become hyperplastic and inflamed and there are numerous goblet cells. The deeper layers show a diffuse round cell infiltration. Necrosis of the epithelium and ulceration toward the lumen may occur (Fig. 165). In the acute cases a true abscess may develop which may rupture and drain through the skin resulting in a permanent external fistula. Postinflammatory stones (dacryoliths) may develop. If a mucocele develops, the mucosa and submucosa are markedly atrophic.

A tuberculous infection of the sac usually is secondary to one affecting adjacent structures (conjunctiva, nose, skin, bone). Fistula formation is common. The lacrimal sac may be involved in a gummatous process which completely blocks the drainage. A leprotic process of the overlying skin also may affect the sac.

Trachoma of the sac may occur during a severe conjunctival infection. Coalescing follicles often are found in the wall. The epithelium is destroyed and a marked fibroblastic proliferation may follow shrinkage of the scar tissue, leading to stenosis of the sac.

Mycotic infections of the sac are common after partial atresia of the duct. Actinomycosis, rhinosporidiosis and other fungus infections also may cause dacryocystitis. Some fungi, especially Streptothrix, may proliferate in the sac and form large casts which can be expressed through the nasal opening by pressure at the internal canthus. Recurrences are common. The cast can be fixed in formalin and sectioned, or smears prepared and stained with Giemsa. Quite often the material observed is amorphous, in which case it may be derived from inspissated mucus. At other times the hyphas of the fungus can be observed.

Inflammations of the canaliculi. Inflammation and concretions in the canaliculi usually are due to infection with one of the Actinomyces (Streptothrix) or other fungi. The canaliculi may become scarred after a severe conjunctival infection, e.g., trachoma, or after application of such miotics as furmethide.

Tumors

Tumors of the lacrimal sac are relatively rare. In the early stages of development, epiphora is the only clinical symptom. Later a round, hard mass may be visible and palpable in the area of the sac. Finally, if the tumor is malignant, it may invade the lids and the orbit.

Epithelial tumors. Ashton reported that epithelial tumors constitute about 50 per cent of all the reported neoplasms of the lacrimal sac. Their histologic appearance and natural history are quite similar to those of the papillomas and transitional carcinomas of the nose and paranasal sinuses (Fig. 166). These tumors typically are associated with severe chronic inflammation, but it is not established whether they cause obstruction and infection or whether the neoplasms are sequelae of a chronic inflammatory process.

Connective tissue tumors. Most of the nonepithelial tumors in this location represent inflammatory pseudotumors, but lymphomas and a variety of other tumors have been reported.

REFERENCES

Allen, A. C. Reorientation on Histogenesis and Clinical Significance of Cutaneous Nevi and Melanomas. Cancer 2:28–56, (Jan.), 1949.

Allen, A. C.: The Skin—A Clinicopathologic Treatise. St. Louis, C. V. Mosby Company, 1954.

Ashton, N., Choyce, D. P., Fison, L. G.: Carcinoma of Lacrimal Sac. Brit. J. Ophthal. 35:366–376, (June), 1951.

Ashton, N., and Rey, A.: Hyaline Infiltration of Eyelid. Brit. J. Ophthal. 35:125–133, (March), 1951.

Berke, R. N., and Wadsworth, J. A. C.: Histology of Levator Muscle in Congenital and Acquired Ptosis. A.M.A. Arch. Ophthal. 53:413–428, 1955.

Foot, N. C.: Adnexal Carcinoma of Skin. Amer. J. Path. 23:1–27, (Jan.), 1947.

Helwig, E. B.: Seminar on the Skin: Neoplasms and Dermatoses. Proc. Twentieth Seminar, American Society Clinical Pathologists, Sept. 11, 1954, Wash., D. C.

Helwig, E. B., and Hackney, V. C.: Juvenile Xanthogranuloma (Nevo-xanthoendothelioma). Amer. J. Path. 30:625, 1954.

Holmes, W. J.: Leprosy of the Eye. Trans. Amer. Ophthal. Soc. 55:145–187, 1957.

Jones, I. S.: Tumors of the Lacrimal Sac. Amer. J. Ophthal. 42:561–566, 1956.

Kallos, A.: Giant Keratoacanthoma. A.M.A. Arch. Derm. 78:207–209, 1958.

Lever, W. F.: Histopathology of the Skin. Second edition, Philadelphia, J. B. Lippincott Company, 1954.

Lund, Herbert Z.: Tumors of the Skin, Atlas of Tumor Pathology, Section I, Fascicle 2, Washington, D.C., Armed Forces Institute of Pathology, 1957.

Reese, A. B.: Tumors of the Eye. New York, Paul B. Hoeber, 1951.

Reese, A. B.: Tumors of the Eye and Adnexa, Atlas of Tumor Pathology, Section X, Fascicle 38, Washington, D. C., Armed Forces Institute of Pathology, 1956.

Scuderi, G.: Istopatologia del Tracoma. Torino, Edizione Minerva Medica, 1957.

Stout, A.: Tumors of the Peripheral Nervous System, Atlas of Tumor Pathology, Section II, Fascicle 6, Washington, D.C., Armed Forces Institute of Pathology, 1956.

Straatsma, B. R.: Meibomian Gland Tumors. A.M.A. Arch. Ophthal. 56:71–93, 1956.

Chapter **V**

Conjunctiva

ANATOMY AND HISTOLOGY

The conjunctiva is a mucous membrane which, as part of the external tegument, covers the posterior surface of the lids and the anterior surface of the globe with the exception of the cornea. Even though it is a continuous membrane it is convenient for practical and clinical purposes to subdivide it into several regions.

The *palpebral* conjunctiva is firmly adherent to the tarsus, and is thin and transparent. On the lid margin it unites with the skin, forming the mucocutaneous junction (page 168). The conjunctiva of the upper and lower fornices unites the lid and bulbar conjunctiva. In the fornix the conjunctiva lies in a number of folds which are loosely attached to the orbital septum. These folds ensure the mobility of the globe and enlarge the secretory surface. The *bulbar* conjunctiva is loosely adherent to the sclera. The *semilunar fold* is a soft, movable fold of the bulbar conjunctiva which lies near the inner canthus between the caruncle and the globe. It corresponds to the third lid of certain mammals and can be moved actively in some animals (nictitating membrane).

The caruncle is formed by another fold near the inner canthus. It also is a transition zone, combining mucous membrane and cutaneous elements which are intermixed. It is composed of a head, which lies in the lacrimal lake, and a tail, blending with the skin at the canthus.

Histology. Two or more layers of cylindrical cells of a stratified columnar type cover most of the conjunctiva. Stratified squamous epithelium is present only at the palpebral margin and over the sclera near the limbus. The basal cells always are cylindrical and more deep staining, and may contain pigment near the limbus. The cylindrical epithelium over the tarsal conjunctiva is much less constant in form than in the bulbar conjunctiva. Often it is interrupted by islands of squamous epithelium, and in some conjunctivas the entire tarsus may be covered with this type of epithelium.

Round or oval goblet cells normally are present in the superficial layers of the epithelium (Fig. 167). They are much larger than the epithelial cells and their mucous content pushes the nucleus to one side.

The stroma consists of connective tissue which is dense and thin over the tarsus and loose and wide in the fornix and over the globe (Fig. 167). At the limbus the connective tissue forms papillas, comparable to those of the dermis. Lymphoid tissue is present in the superficial stroma commencing at the subtarsal sulcus and extends around the fornices

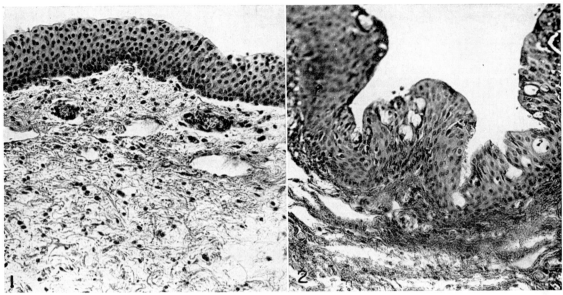

Figure 167. Normal Conjunctiva
1. Nonkeratinizing conjunctival epithelium. ×185. AFIP Acc. 482595.
2. Mucous cells in conjunctival epithelium from fornix. ×185. AFIP Acc. 218650.

toward the limbus. In some areas this tissue forms follicle-like structures which do not have germinal centers. This layer of subepithelial adenoid tissue develops only after the age of three to four months. Branched melanocytes may be found in the bulbar conjunctiva just under the epithelial layers.

Commencing at the superior margin of the upper tarsus the stromal connective tissue becomes more abundant and forms the crests and furrows which develop into folds in both fornices. Between these folds the epithelium may sink down into the stroma to form crypts (pseudoglands of Henle).

Accessory lacrimal glands, with a structure identical to the lacrimal gland, often are found in the substantia propria. There are approximately forty such glands in the upper and six in the lower fornix (glands of Krause). Three or more additional glands lie at the superior margin of the upper tarsus (glands of Wolfring) (Fig. 108).

The epithelium of the semilunar fold is similar to that of the surrounding conjunctiva and contains numerous goblet cells. Cartilage may be present in the substantia propria in this region.

The epithelium of the caruncle is thick and of the stratified squamous type. A number of lanugo hairs with numerous large sebaceous glands are found in its head. The substantia propria of the caruncle contains elastic fibers and striated muscle fibers from the lacrimal part of the orbicularis oculi muscle (Horner's muscle). Accessory lacrimal and sweat glands also may be found here.

CONGENITAL ANOMALIES

Dermoid. Dermoids, either solid or cystic (Fig. 111), are congenital misplacements and represent inclusions of epidermal and associated connective tissues during the closure of fetal clefts. The solid dermoid is the usual type found at the limbus (Fig. 168). It is composed of dense, collagenous connective tissue covered by stratified squamous epithelium which sometimes has a granular layer and produces keratin, but usually is thin and does not show rete pegs. Extending into the underlying tissue are hair follicles with shafts and sebaceous glands. Occasionally nerve bundles, fat (dermolipoma), and aberrant lacrimal and sweat glands may be present (Fig. 168). Dermoids may occur on the cornea as fibrofatty masses with projecting hairs.

Dermolipomas. A type of solid dermoid,

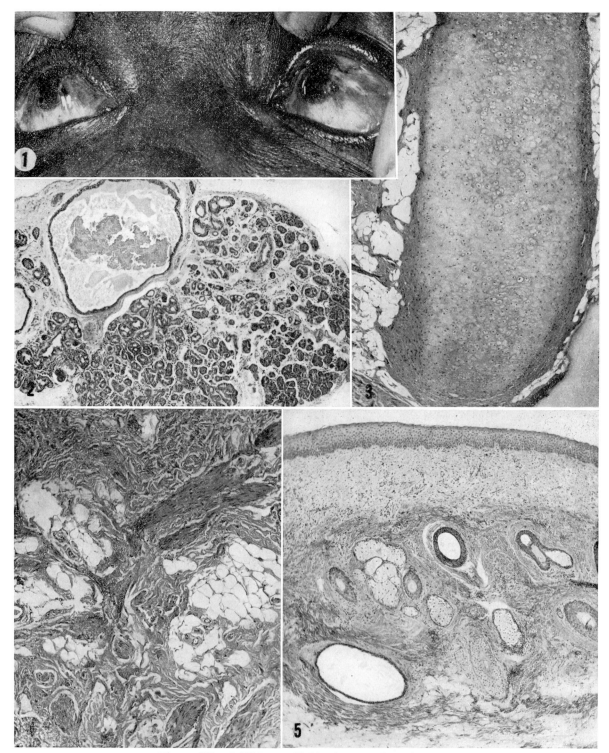

Figure 168. Solid Dermoid Choristomas of Conjunctiva

1 to 4. Unusual example with bilateral involvement of nasal and temporal conjunctiva and cornea. AFIP Acc 934481.

2. Lacrimal gland tissue. ×50. AFIP Acc. 934481.

3. Cartilage. ×50. AFIP Acc. 934481.

4. Fibroadipose connective tissue and smooth muscle bundles. ×80. AFIP Acc. 934481.

5. Ordinary type of limbal dermoid containing hair follicles, sweat and sebaceous glands, and fibroadipose tissue. ×75. AFIP Acc. 203027.

containing few or no epithelial structures and a disproportionate amount of fat, is called a dermolipoma. Dermolipomas are yellowish, soft, lobulated tumors which usually are situated near the outer canthus. These tumors extend upward and outward, between the lateral and superior rectus muscles. They either have a smooth surface or are covered by a somewhat leathery epithelium and may grow to a considerable size, extending forward toward the cornea and backward into the orbit.

Intrascleral nerve loops. The long ciliary nerves, as they pass forward in the suprachoroidea of the ciliary body sometimes send U-shaped loops into the sclera and at times appear subconjunctivally 4 to 7 mm. from the limbus. They are smooth, elevated, tender, and sometimes are pigmented (Fig. 59).

INFLAMMATIONS

General considerations. The various parts of the conjunctiva react to injury in a varying manner. The epithelial cells may be damaged either by the noxious agent itself or secondarily by inflammatory changes in the stroma. The cells may become edematous or they may degenerate with nuclear pyknosis and cell death. Occasional leukocytes normally are found among the epithelial cells, but as a result of inflammation they become much more numerous (Fig. 169). Neutrophils, eosinophils, basophils, plasma cells and lymphocytes are seen, depending on the type of inflammation. They arise from the stroma and migrate or diffuse through the surface. The goblet cells proliferate markedly in chronic conjunctivitis (Fig. 169–3). The epithelium may also proliferate in chronic inflammations, forming cords and channels which may result in retention cysts or concrements. Such retention cysts also may result from papillary hypertrophy when epithelium between enlarged papillas becomes trapped and secretion accumulates. In chronic conjunctivitis the epithelium becomes hyperplastic and, under certain conditions may keratinize (Fig. 169–5, 6). This is seen in exposure keratitis, tear deficiences, neoplasms, and in vitamin A deficiency.

The most conspicuous clinical sign of acute inflammation is hyperemia, which, because it is due to dilatation of the posterior conjunctival vessels, is most marked in the fornix and diminishes toward the limbus (Fig. 170–1, 2). If the anterior ciliary vessels also are involved, the pericorneal area is congested, suggesting that the inflammation has involved the deeper structures of the eye or the cornea.

The inflammatory edema (chemosis) is caused by exudation of fluid and cells into the loose tissue (Fig. 170–1, 2). In the acute stage, polymorphonuclear leukocytes predominate and are replaced later by lymphocytes and plasma cells. At times necrosis followed by ulceration occurs over an intense focus of inflammation.

The conjunctival secretion normally contains mucus and a few degenerating epithelial cells. Cytologic evaluation of pathologic secretions may be of great diagnostic help. A polymorphonuclear leukocytic reaction (Fig. 171) is characteristic of bacterial conjunctivitis, the exceptions being those due to Neisseria catarrhalis and the diplobacillus of Morax-Axenfeld (Moraxella lacunata). Eosinophilic leukocytes may be found in allergic forms of conjunctivitis, especially vernal conjunctivitis (Fig. 172–1, 2). Basophilic leukocytes also may be found in the secretion of an allergic conjunctivitis (Fig. 172–3). Mononuclear cells (especially lymphocytes) usually are found in the exudate produced in viral conjunctivitis (Fig. 173). The exceptions are those due to the atypical viruses of the psittacosis-lymphogranuloma venereum group which, in the acute phase, produce a purulent discharge. If follicles have ruptured, plasma cells (Fig. 173) and large macrophages (Leber cells) are observed in the exudate of trachomatous conjunctivitis (Fig. 174).

In order to examine the cells found in such an exudate, scrapings should be taken from the conjunctival surface with a platinum spatula. Such a spatula has the advantage that it can be sterilized easily by heat and quickly cools in air. The scraping then should be stained according to the Gram method to find the microorganisms present in the con-

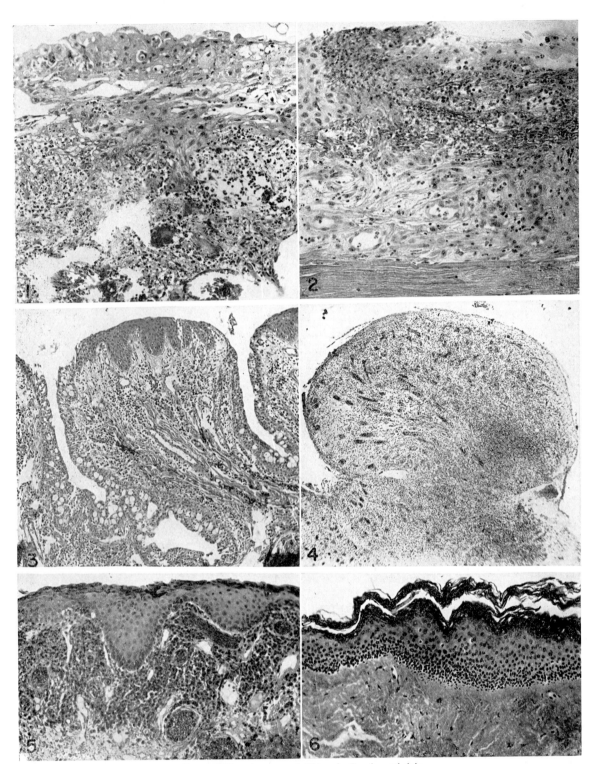

Figure 169. Acute and Chronic Conjunctivitis

1. Acute bacterial conjunctivitis. Polymorphonuclear leukocytic response to colonies of cocci, and tissue destruction. Edema and hyperplasia of epithelium. ×160. AFIP Acc. 65138.

2. Acute conjunctivitis. Purulent infiltration of epithelium, with ulceration. Inflammatory granulation tissue replacing stroma. ×275. AFIP Acc. 77220.

3. Chronic conjunctivitis. Formation of vascular papillae infiltrated by lymphocytes and plasma cells. Hyperplasia of epithelium at surface. Increase in mucous cells in crypts. Epithelial adhesions in crypts forming cystic inclusions. ×75. AFIP Acc. 194376.

4. Granuloma pyogenicum. ×45. AFIP Acc. 71434.

5. Chronic conjunctivitis. Subepithelial chronic inflammatory cell infiltration. Epithelial hyperplasia. ×125. AFIP Acc. 38830.

6. Chronic conjunctivitis, old. Epidermidalization with keratinization of epithelium. Hyalinization of stroma. ×125. AFIP Acc. 338247.

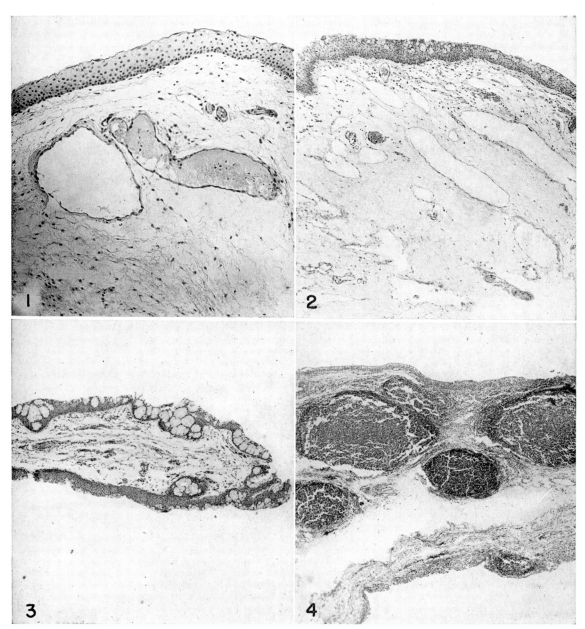

Figure 170. Reaction to Irritation, Conjunctiva

1. Chemosis, consistent with angioneurotic edema. Dilatation of blood vessels. ×125. AFIP Acc. 131909.

2. Chemosis. Dilatation of lymph spaces simulating lymphangioma. Marked edema. Mild chronic inflammatory cell infiltration. ×62. AFIP Acc. 96541.

3. Increase in mucous cells. ×48. AFIP Acc. 136737.

4. Lymph follicle formation in chronic conjunctivitis. ×45. AFIP Acc. 49329.

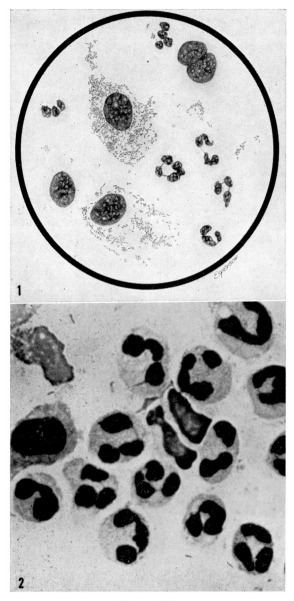

Figure 171.

1. Polymorphonuclear leukocytic exudate in Koch-Weeks bacillus conjunctivitis (artist's drawing).

2. Polymorphonuclear leukocytic exudate in pneumococcal conjunctivitis. Giemsa stained smear. ×2280. (Courtesy of Dr. Phillips Thygeson.)

junctival sac. Giemsa stains should be made to evaluate the cytologic characteristics of the exudate.

Certain infectious and toxic agents either produce a coagulative necrosis of mucous membranes or provoke an outpouring of fibrinous and serous exudate from the underlying capillaries with the formation of "false

membranes." These consist of coagulated exudate firmly adherent to the degenerating epithelium. Frequently when these membranes are stripped off they lead to bleeding from the underlying capillary bed. Such "membranous" or "pseudomembranous" inflammations are observed in epidemic keratoconjunctivitis, streptococcal conjunctivitis, diphtheria, the Stevens-Johnson syndrome, and after chemical burns, especially those produced by alkalis. Pseudomembranes should not be confused with true membranes, composed of necrotic tissue and granulation tissue (Fig. 175–1, 2).

The formation and hypertrophy of lymph follicles is a common occurrence in many types of conjunctival disease (Fig. 176). These follicles usually are found between the margin of the tarsus and the fornix. Follicular hypertrophy is a common reaction to viral infections of the conjunctiva. Most chemical agents do not produce follicular hyperplasia; however, a few drugs such as eserine and other miotics, also may produce a follicular reaction in the conjunctiva. Clinically, follicles appear as grayish or whitish elevations of round or oval shape. They are practically avascular and on slit lamp examination small conjunctival vessels can be seen to encircle the follicle without reaching its center.

Papillary hypertrophy (Fig. 177) is a nonspecific reaction occurring in the chronic and acute forms of conjunctivitis. Papillaformation depends on the attachment of fine fibrils between the epithelium and the tarsus. The accumulation of an inflammatory exudate between these irregularly placed fibrils produces the papillas. This exudation may be transformed into granulation and connective tissue (Fig. 169–3, 4).

Papillas may be relatively small and give the surface a velvety appearance. In other instances the proliferations are of the giant, pavement type. On slit lamp examination a small vessel can be seen to enter the center of the papilla and branch beneath the surface.

Some infectious conjunctival inflammations are endogenous and primarily affect the stroma. Epithelial scrapings rarely reveal the cause in such infections, and a biopsy may be necessary to establish the correct diagnosis.

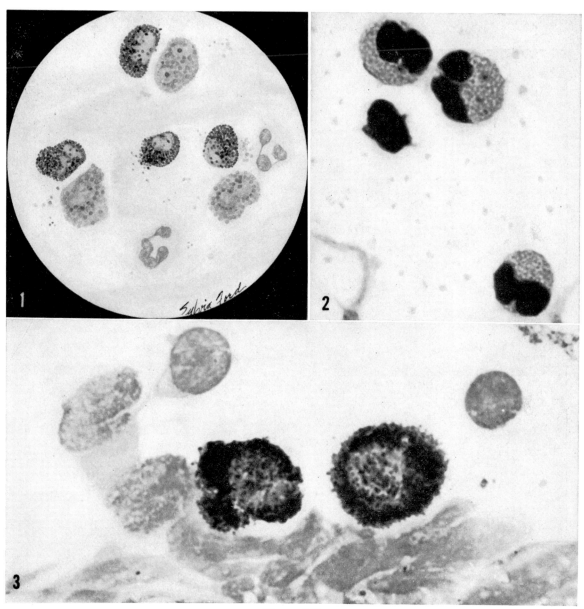

Figure 172.

1. Eosinophilic leukocytes in exudate of vernal conjunctivitis. Artist's drawing.
2. Eosinophils in Giemsa-stained smear of conjunctival scrapings in vernal conjunctivitis. ×2280.
3. Basophils in Giemsa-stained smear of conjunctival scraping in chronic conjunctivitis of unknown etiology ×2280. (Courtesy of Dr. Phillips Thygeson.)

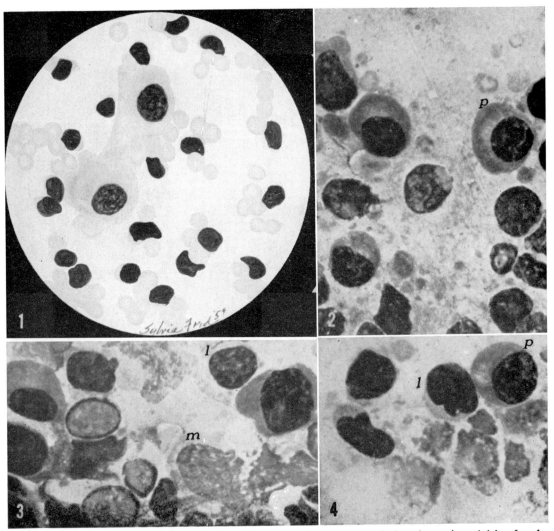

Figure 173.   Mononuclear exudate in conjunctival scraping from a case of chronic conjunctivitis of **unknown** etiology.

1. Artist's drawing reveals two macrophages, many lymphocytes and erythrocytes.

2 to 4. Giemsa-stained smears contain an admixture of plasma cells (p), lymphocytes (l), and macrophages **(m)**. ×1600.

(Courtesy of Dr. Phillips Thygeson.)

Into this group belong the Leptothrix conjunctivitis, tuberculous conjunctivitis which has not led to ulceration, and other granulomatous inflammations.

Bacterial conjunctivitis. The majority of conjunctival inflammations are of exogenous bacterial origin. The susceptibility of the conjunctiva to various infectious agents differs from that of the mucous membrane of the nose. Any bacteria which are capable of producing an inflammation of mucous membranes may involve the conjunctiva. The most frequent offenders are the pneumococcus, diplobacillus of Morax-Axenfeld, influenza bacillus, the Koch-Weeks bacillus, the streptococcus, the gonococcus, and the pathogenic forms of staphylococcus. In order to prove that a microorganism may be the cause of conjunctival infections, it has to be shown that it *grows* on normal epithelial cells and is not a saprophyte. The most frequent saprophytes in the conjunctiva are the xerosis bacillus and Staphylococcus albus. The exception is the pathogenic staphylococcus which may grow in the mucous films on the conjunctival surface, yet can produce a toxin

which results in a conjunctivitis. Occasionally, streptococci, diplobacilli and coliform organisms may grow on the surface of cells and on debris. The predominant organism in an acute epidemic of conjunctivitis varies greatly with time and geographical location; for example, pneumococcal infections are more common in northern countries in winter, and Koch-Weeks infections are more common in southern countries in the spring and fall.

The toxins of the gonococcus damage the epithelial cells and cause a severe inflammatory reaction with marked hyperemia and purulent exudation. The damaged cells are shed, and the new-formed cells which replace them are more resistant and phagocytize the cocci.

The diplobacillus of Morax-Axenfeld first causes an inflammation of the skin at the outer canthus. This is followed by inflammation of the conjunctiva. The skin at and near the palpebral margin becomes thin and its epithelium shows marked edema and parakeratosis. The bacilli are found in the superficial layers of the skin epithelium.

Other organisms may cause histopathologic

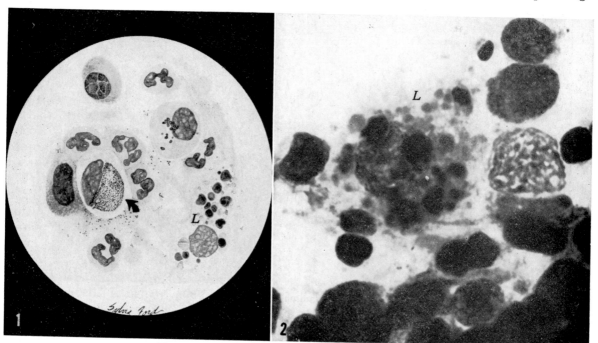

Figure 174. Exudate in Trachomatous Conjunctivitis

1. Artist's drawing showing a cytoplasmic inclusion body (arrow) and a large Leber cell (L) containing ingested cellular debris.

2. Leber cell (L) containing many particles of cellular debris in Giemsa-stained smear of conjunctival scraping in trachoma. ×2280. (Courtesy of Dr. Phillips Thygeson.)

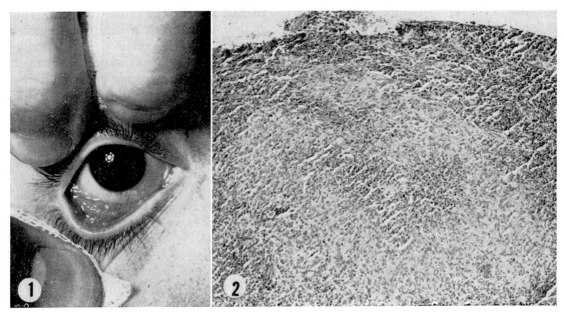

Figure 180. Oculoglandular conjunctivitis due to cat-scratch disease (from the cases reported by Margileth, 1957).

1. Clinical appearance of granulomatous lesions of palpebral conjunctiva and outer fornix. AFIP Neg. 57–7988–1.

2. Conjunctival granuloma. A broad zone of epithelioid cells surrounds a central necrotic focus containing polymorphonuclear leukocytes. Plasma cells and lymphocytes infiltrate the surrounding tissues. ×115. AFIP Acc. 801923.

Viral Conjunctivitis

Trachoma. Trachoma, according to Scuderi, still is the most important and widespread eye disease in the world. This disease has become less common in North America and Europe during the past twenty years.

The virus of trachoma belongs to the group of large atypical viruses (Chlamydozoaceae) to which also belong the viruses of lymphogranuloma venereum and psittacosis. The trachoma virus appears as minute elementary bodies and as large basophilic initial bodies which form the cytoplasmic inclusion bodies of Halberstaedter and Prowazek (Fig. 181). The isolation and cultivation of this virus recently was achieved. It can grow in the yolksac of an embryonated chicken egg. T'ang et al. have made successful serial passages and a human volunteer has been infected after the eighth passage.

Trachoma often begins as a mild infection, but occasionally it is acute and severe. It usually is bilateral, although one eye may be more severely affected. It affects the conjunctiva and lids in a variable manner depending on the climate, age of the patient, and presence or absence of secondary infection. Generally the infection follows a pattern first classified by MacCallan. According to this classification there are four stages of the disease:

Stage 1. There are minute conjunctival follicles and subepithelial infiltrates which give the conjunctiva a velvety appearance.

Stage 2. The conjunctiva becomes thickened and roughened. Two substages may be seen:

    2A. A follicular reaction predominates.

    2B. A papillary reaction predominates.

Stage 3. Widespread cicatrization and contraction occur. Sequelae appear.

Stage 4. Complete arrest of the disease.

Histopathology. During stage 1 a marked hyperplasia of the epithelium occurs. The epithelial cells, which contain inclusions, show signs of cloudy swelling and degeneration. Many lymphocytes infiltrate between the epithelial cells, and the stroma is edematous and hyperemic and is infiltrated with numerous inflammatory cells, mostly lymphocytes. Follicles appear at this time in the stroma, and there is edema, hyperemia and diffuse infiltration with lymphocytes and plasma cells (Fig. 182).

After a period of activity the conjunctiva

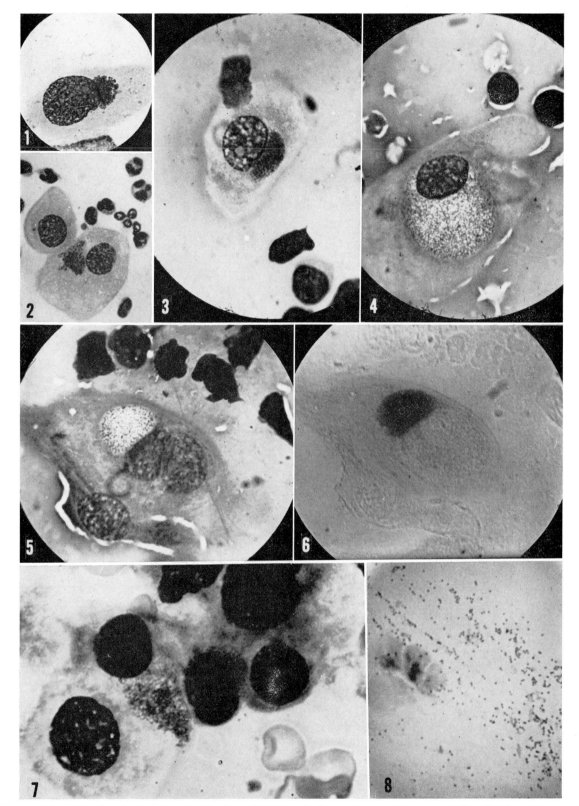

Figure 181. Cytoplasmic inclusion bodies in epithelial cells in trachoma. (Courtesy of Dr. Phillips Thygeson.)

1. Young inclusion body composed of swollen forms, the so-called initial bodies. Giemsa stain.

2 and 3. Slightly more mature inclusion bodies. Giemsa stains.

4 and 5. Larger mature inclusion bodies composed of elementary bodies. Giemsa stains.

6. Same cell shown in 5 but stained with Lugol's solution to demonstrate the carbohydrate matrix in which the elementary bodies are suspended.

7 and 8. Free elementary bodies in cells and exudate.

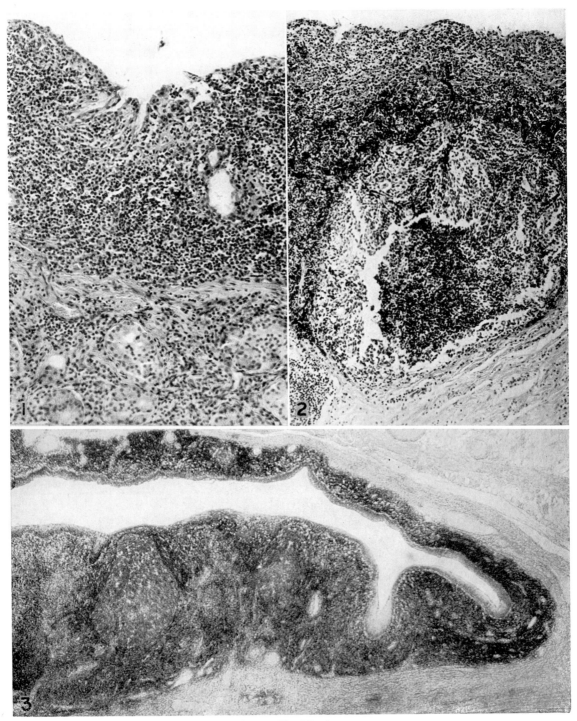

Figure 182. Trachoma

1. Trachoma, eyelid. ×160. AFIP Acc. 33894.
2. Follicle formation and dense chronic inflammatory cell infiltration, conjunctiva. ×160. AFIP Acc. 33894.
3. Trachoma. Involvement of conjunctiva of eye, fornix and lid. ×39. AFIP Acc. 36980.

adenoviruses may produce conjunctival and pharyngeal inflammations (pharyngoconjunctival fever). An acute follicular conjunctivitis is characteristic, the acute follicular conjunctivitis of Béal being the most typical. During the acute phase there is conjunctivitis with regional adenopathy. The follicles occur mainly in the palpebral conjunctiva and fornix of the lower lid. The bulbar conjunctiva is edematous and hyperemic. The cornea may show small gray epithelial opacities of a transient type.

Vaccinia. Involvement of the conjunctiva may occur in vaccinia. An ulcerated pustule containing polymorphonuclear cells and lymphocytes may develop on the conjunctiva.

Measles. An acute catarrhal conjunctivitis appears most regularly in the course of measles and the typical Koplik's spots are found on the caruncle and conjunctiva. The most characteristic and frequent lesion is, however, an epithelial keratitis.

Conjunctivitis Due to Fungi, Parasites and Animal Irritants

Fungi. Actinomyces (Streptothrix) has been described in Chapter IV.

Leptotrichia buccalis already has been mentioned as a possible cause for the clinical picture of Parinaud's oculoglandular syndrome. In this condition small, yellow conjunctival nodules form, consisting of lymphocytes, epithelioid cells, polymorphonuclear leukocytes and giant cells. These cells surround areas of necrosis containing the organisms. Pityrosporum ovale is the fungus most frequently found in the conjunctiva. It usually occurs in seborrheic blepharitis and often is associated with pathogenic staphylococci. It is not known to produce tissue alteration by itself.

Other fungus diseases are rare. Among the more important are those due to Rhinosporidium seeberi which produces polypoid or flat lesions in the conjunctiva (Fig. 184). Microscopically the nodules contain numerous subepithelial cysts which are filled with Rhinosporidium. Sporotrichosis is associated with ulcerated, yellow nodules in the conjunctiva, and enlargement of the preauricular nodes.

Parasites. Parasitic infections of the conjunctiva are rare. Schistosoma hematobium, the blood fluke (flat worm) which is a common cause of bladder and colonic infections in Egypt, may give rise to ectopic lesions, including conjunctival granulomas containing eggs (Fig. 185). Filariasis (Fig. 185–4), paragonimiasis, sparganosis and trichinosis are other parasitic diseases in which the conjunctiva and eyelids may be involved. External ocular myiasis may be produced by the deposition of larvas or eggs from flies into the conjunctival sac.

Ophthalmia nodosa is caused by the hairs of caterpillars. The hairs produce a severe foreign body reaction and numerous granulomas develop, which contain foreign body giant cells and macrophages surrounding the caterpillar hair (Fig. 186). Ultimately a thick fibrous capsule may enclose the nodule. In many cases the hair is absorbed and the lesion subsides. Occasionally hairs penetrate into the sclera and anterior chamber to produce an endophthalmitis.

Allergic Conjunctivitis

Vernal conjunctivitis. Vernal conjunctivitis usually occurs in adolescents and is more common in boys. It often is worse at some seasons, usually the spring, and is active for seven to ten years. According to Beigelman, in the palpebral form the most severe changes occur in the upper tarsal conjunctiva. At first the palpebral conjunctiva is hyperemic and is covered by a thin milky-white pseudomembrane. Eventually the subepithelial layers are affected, and a papillary hypertrophy dominates the picture (Fig. 187–1, 2, 3). Individual papillas may become so large that they are flattened by the cornea (Fig. 177).

At the onset of the disease, hypertrophy of the epithelial cells seems to be the rule, but regressive changes soon appear as the result of a poor blood supply to the infiltrated stroma, and they atrophy and finally are desquamated. Over the height of large papillas only a single layer of epithelial cells may be present. In the crevices and folds between papillas these cells undergo mucoid degeneration to form retention cysts. In areas with flatter papillas the epithelium may show some hyperplasia (Fig. 187–1, 2, 3).

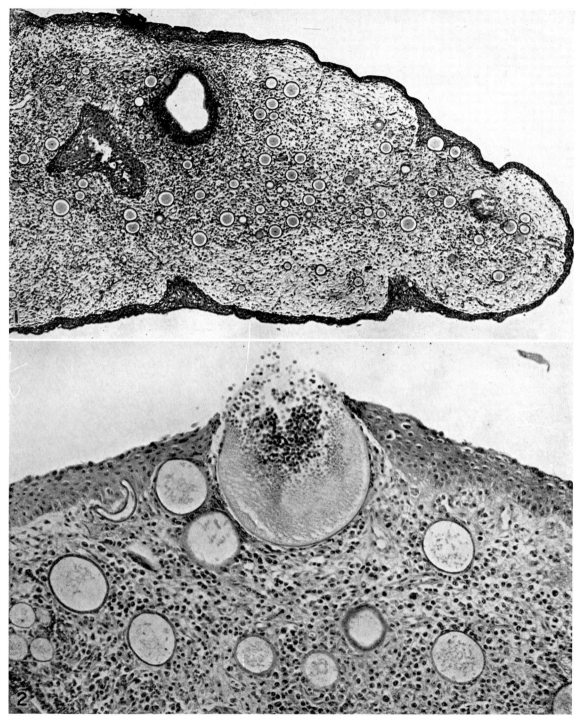

Figure 184. Rhinosporidiosis

1. *Rhinosporidium seeberi* in conjunctival stroma. ×70. AFIP Acc. 61934.
2. Rupture of sporangium with escape of spores. ×230. AFIP Acc. 105982.

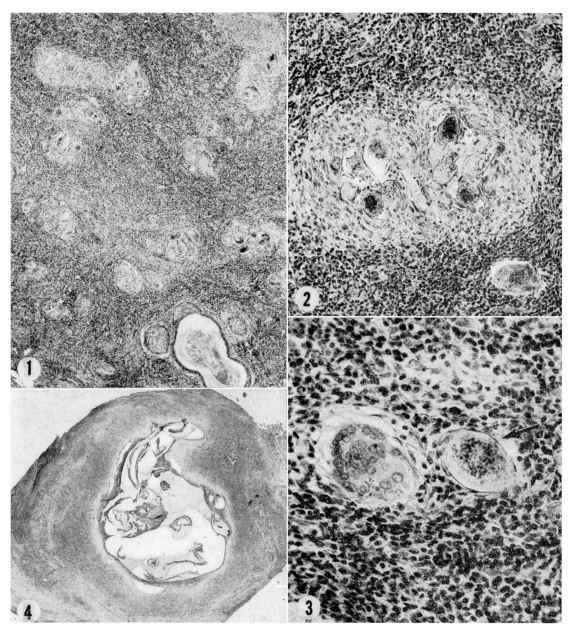

Figure 185.

1. Granulomatous inflammation of conjunctiva due to schistosomiasis. Case reported by Mohamed (1956). **AFIP** Acc. 930098. ×45.

2. Epithelioid cells surround a group of schistosome eggs from same case. ×165.

3. Embryonated egg (arrow) and a multinucleated giant cell in same lesion. ×305.

4. Filariasis of conjunctiva. The parasite, Filaria bancrofti, occupies the cystoid space within the inflammatory mass. Courtesy of Dr. A. F. Mohamed, Giza, Cairo, AFIP Acc. 930098. ×10.

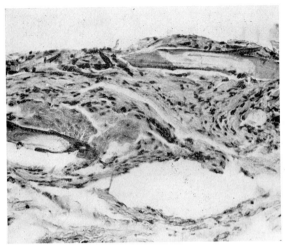

Figure 186.   Ophthalmia Nodosa

Caterpillar hairs imbedded in bulbar conjunctiva and episclera have provoked a foreign body granulomatous reaction. ×192. University of California Acc. 59–829A.

The most conspicuous and severe changes occur in the stroma. In the early stages the perivascular and diffuse infiltration of lymphocytes and plasma cells predominate. Less frequent are polymorphonuclear leukocytes, macrophages and fibroblasts. Characteristic are the numerous eosinophilic leukocytes which appear in the stroma and migrate through the epithelium to appear in the secretion. Soon the collagen develops interesting changes. It proliferates so markedly that the inflammatory exudate of the papillas is largely replaced (Fig. 187–2). The tissue soon becomes avascular and hyalinized, especially in the superficial layers of the stroma near the epithelium. The vessel walls also show similar changes. The epithelial layer does not show such alterations.

Limbal vernal catarrh. The clinical picture of limbal vernal catarrh is different from

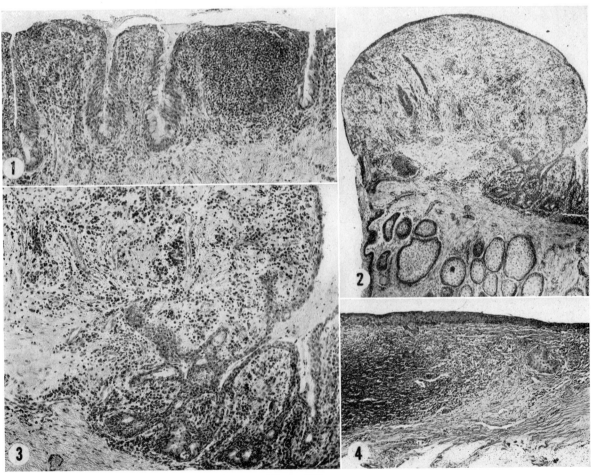

Figure 187.

1 to 3. Palpebral involvement in vernal conjunctivitis. ×115, ×50, and ×115 respectively. AFIP Acc. 28901.
4. Limbal form of vernal conjunctivitis. ×50. AFIP Acc. 927318.

that of the palpebral form; however, the underlying pathologic changes are quite similar. The exudation and proliferation in the conjunctiva lead to grayish, waxy papillas at the limbus, especially in the interpalpebral fissure. The excrescences may reach a height of several millimeters and often extend onto the cornea. Histologically (Fig. 187–4) there is a similar excessive proliferation of connective tissue which may reach tumor-like dimensions. The same type of hyaline degeneration of the collagen fibers occurs and the infiltration of inflammatory cells gradually is replaced. The epithelium also may undergo a balloon type of degeneration, leading to formation of localized pockets containing degenerated cellular debris and eosinophils (Trantas' dots).

Phlyctenular conjunctivitis. Phlyctenular conjunctivitis is a condition which is caused mainly by a hypersensitivity to bacterial proteins. Tuberculosis, otitis median, and staphylococcal blepharitis are especially common causes. Small, whitish nodules 2 to 3 mm. in size, surrounded by a zone of hyperemia appear in the bulbar conjunctiva, most frequently at the limbus or in the cornea. These nodules are formed by localized subepithelial accumulations of lymphocytes. The epithelium degenerates over the nodule and an ulcer forms with liberation of the degenerating contents into the conjunctival sac (Fig. 188).

Contact allergies. An acute allergic reaction may be produced by vegetable (pollen) or animal proteins or by relatively simple chemical compounds such as atropine, and topical anesthetics. Dermatitis of the lids with itching is a characteristic accompanying feature. This allergic reaction to drugs must be differentiated from a toxic reaction to drugs which is to be described.

In allergic reactions there is proliferation of the conjunctival epithelium, particularly of the goblet cells, and a stromal hyperemia, with edema, and a cellular infiltration which is rich in eosinophils. Eosinophils migrate into the epithelial layer and conjunctival sac.

Chemical conjunctivitis. The follicular reaction to some topical agents probably is not due to hypersensitivity but more likely is a toxic reaction. It most often is produced by the prolonged instillation of eserine or pilocarpine, and characteristic are the small follicles which appear in the lower fornix and tarsal conjunctiva. Histologically these follicles cannot be differentiated from those which occur in trachoma, except for the later development of necrosis in trachoma.

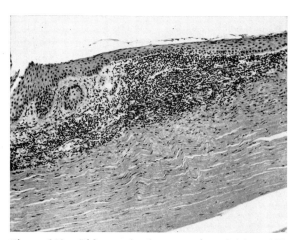

Figure 188. Phlyctenular keratoconjunctivitis. ×115. U. of Cal. Acc. 47–230. AFIP Neg. 60–5282.

THE CONJUNCTIVA IN SYSTEMIC DISEASES

Metabolic Disorders

Cystinosis. Cystinosis is an inborn metabolic error of amino acid metabolism which is based on a hereditary defect. The renal tubules are defective, and as a result, cystine is deposited in crystalline form in the various tissues. The cystine crystals may be deposited in the subepithelial tissue of the conjunctiva and in the cornea (Fig. 189). According to Braendstrup, biopsy of conjunctival tissue may be of great diagnostic value. The biopsy specimen should be fixed in absolute alcohol, since other fixatives dissolve and remove the cystine crystals.

Ochronosis. Ochronosis is a congenital and familial disturbance of protein metabolism, particularly of tyrosine and phenylala-

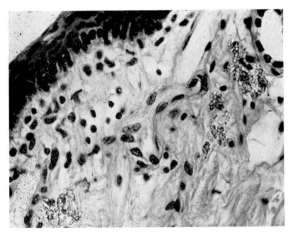

Figure 189. Clusters of cystine crystals in the substantia propria of the conjunctiva. From the case reported by Garron (1959). ×1120. AFIP Acc. 220211.

nine, with deposition of polymers of homogentisic acid in cartilage and fibrous tissues, causing them to become dark. According to Seitz, pigmentation occurs bilaterally in the sclera, conjunctiva, and cornea in the interpalpebral fissure. Large clumps of pigment are deposited in the collagen and elastic fibers (Fig. 190). These clumps of pigment produce little inflammatory reaction. The urine of such patients turns dark on standing, due to the excreted homogentisic acid (alkaptonuria).

Hypercalcemia. According to Walsh and Howard, the calcium deposits found in the hypercalcemia of parathyroid disease, vitamin D overdosage, and sarcoidosis lie immediately beneath the epithelium in the most superficial layers of the connective tissue. They are most intense near the limbus.

Dermatologic Diseases

Pemphigus. According to Lever, the conjunctiva may be involved in true pemphigus vulgaris. In some patients the conjunctival pemphigus has a benign course and even can precede onset of changes in other mucous membranes and skin. In rare cases the pathologic process may remain confined to the conjunctiva.

Subepidermal bullas are characteristic, the entire epithelium being detached from the underlying stroma. However, the bulla formation is not the most important part of the disease. A dense inflammatory reaction occurs in the dermis and in the substantia propria of the conjunctiva with edema, hyperemia and lymphocytic infiltration (Fig. 191). Scarring and shrinkage result from the destruction produced by the inflammatory reaction.

The affected conjunctiva becomes atrophic,

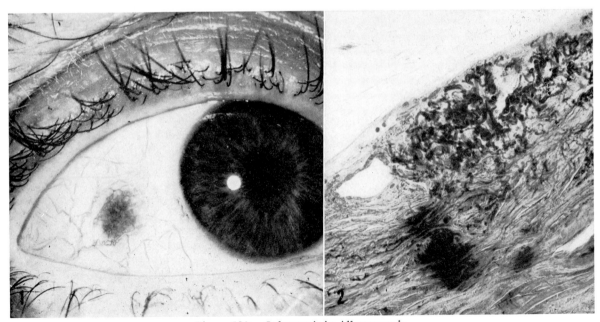

Figure 190.   Ochronosis in Alkaptonuria

The degenerative changes in the connective tissue fibers and the melanotic pigmentation are principally in the cornea and sclera (see also Fig. 289. Chapter VI). Case reported by Rones (1960). AFIP Acc. 871509.

the submucosal tissues being transformed into a vascular, hypertrophic, dense connective tissue. The epithelium is thickened, keratinized, and irregular. The process may advance upon the cornea in the form of a pannus and the puncta may become obliterated. The result is extensive symblepharon, dryness of the eye (xerophthalmia) and opacification of the cornea.

Essential shrinkage. Custodis has described essential shrinkage of the conjunctiva or benign mucous membrane pemphigoid as occurring mostly in women over fifty and characterized by a progressive scarring of the conjunctiva, drying of the eye and formation of a symblepharon. An inflammatory reaction occurs in the subepithelial layers and results in hypertrophy of the stromal connective tissue. Occasionally this condition has been accompanied by other skin diseases such as epidermolysis bullosa, dermatitis herpetiformis, and poikiloderma.

Stevens-Johnson syndrome. The Stevens-Johnson syndrome (mucocutaneous syndrome, erythema multiforme, ectodermosis erosiva pluriorificialis) may be associated with vesicular or ulcerative lesions in the mouth and the genitalia (Patz, 1950; François, 1954). A chronic, severe, nonspecific inflammatory reaction of the conjunctiva may be observed (Fig. 192). The conjunctivitis may be catarrhal, purulent or pseudomembranous. Frequently it is necrotizing and the necrosis of the epithelium leads to extensive cicatrization with formation of symblepharon, entropion, corneal ulcers and anterior uveitis.

Topical application of drugs, such as furmethide, DFP and other miotics can produce changes resembling essential shrinkage of the conjunctiva. Presumably this is a toxic effect of the drug on the mucous membrane. Chronic inflammation induced by the drug

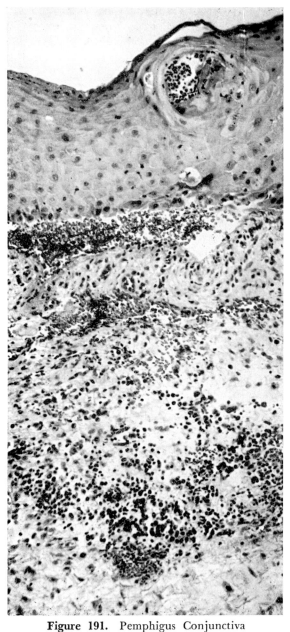

Figure 191. Pemphigus Conjunctiva

Bullous separation of epithelium. ×175. AFIP Neg. 47490.

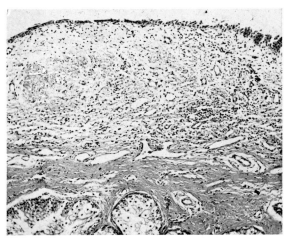

Figure 192. Nonspecific subacute inflammation of tarsal conjunctiva in the case of a 26 year old soldier who had "essential conjunctival shrinkage resembling trachoma" associated with erythema multiforme. ×115. AFIP Acc. 90352.

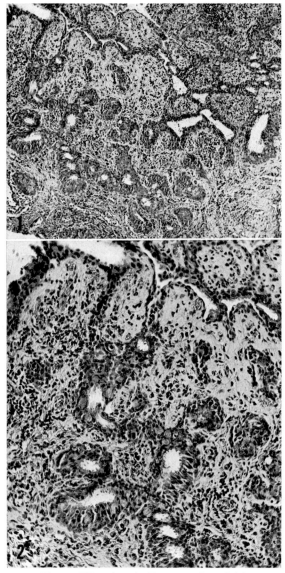

Figure 193.   Atopic Keratoconjunctivitis

Nonspecific chronic inflammation with marked stromal and epithelial proliferation.
  1. ×80. U. of Cal. Acc. 50–2. AFIP Neg. 60–5283.
  2. ×145. U. of Cal. Acc. 50–2. AFIP Neg. 60–5284.

leads to proliferation of stromal connective tissue, epithelial hyperplasia, and inflammation. Conjunctival shrinkage occurs with formation of symblepharon and shortening of the fornices.

Atopic dermatitis. In this condition the inflammatory reaction involves the lid surfaces, conjunctiva of the lids and eye, and the cornea. Secondary infection is common, especially by pathogenic staphylococci. The skin involvement is characterized by hyperemia, edema, epithelial hyperplasia, and acanthosis. Scaling is severe, and the skin soon becomes permanently thickened and slightly scarred. The conjunctiva shows hyperemia, edema, lymphocytic and plasma cell infiltration, and eosinophilia. The epithelium is hyperplastic, edematous, and there is an increase in the number of goblet cells (Fig. 193). The cornea shows stromal infiltration near the limbus, followed by vascularization (Hogan, 1953). Ulceration is rare, except following secondary infection

Atopic dermatitis is thought to be due to a hypersensitivity to inhalants or food, and a strong hereditary tendency has been observed. Most patients have a history of infantile eczema, followed by atopic dermatitis in adult life. The upper body and extremities characteristically are affected.

Involvement of the conjunctiva in other skin diseases is not rare. A chronic blepharoconjunctivitis with formation of limbal nodules may be associated with *acne rosacea* and extension to the cornea may occur. In xeroderma pigmentosum the conjunctiva may show changes similar to those described in Chapter IV, and exposure of the conjunctiva resulting from lid deformity produces keratinization of the epithelium.

DEGENERATIONS

Pinguecula. Pinguecula is a localized, yellowish-gray, elevated area close to the limbus in the interpalpebral fissure. It derives its name from the yellowish color which is produced by hypertrophic and degenerated connective tissue fibers, and not from fat as formerly was believed. Its pathogenesis is far from clear, but it appears to be determined genetically, and to assume tumorous proportions only in middle life or later (Cogan, Kuwabara, and Howard, 1959).

The epithelium over the surface is thin and flat, often being reduced to two layers. In the folds of the pinguecula several layers of cylindrical cells with goblet cells are found. The subepithelial layer is thin. The stroma shows marked degeneration of the collagen fibers which are transformed into masses of amorphous hyalin or accumulations of coiled and fragmented fibers. These fibers, because of their general appearances and stain characteristics, appear to be elastic tissue (senile elastosis) (Fig. 194). It is interesting, however, that the enzyme, elastase, does not affect these fibers (Cogan, Kuwabara, and Howard, 1959).

Calcium later may appear in the superficial layers.

Pterygium. Pterygium is characterized by elevated mass of thickened conjunctiva at the limbus in the interpalpebral fissure on one or the other side, more often nasally. The lesion extends onto the cornea and slowly

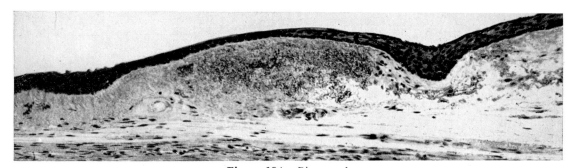

Figure 194. Pinguecula

Elastosis of conjunctival stroma; atrophy of overlying epithelium. ×120. AFIP Acc. 61823.

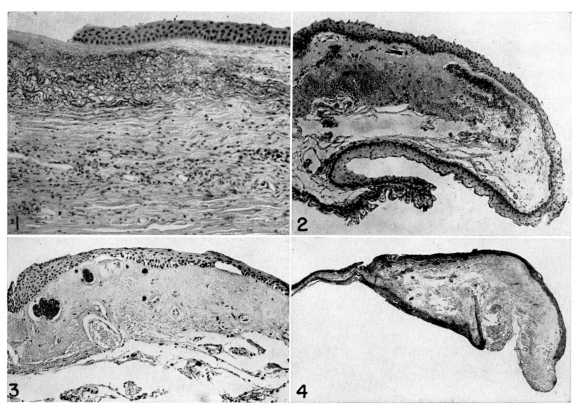

Figure 195. Pterygium

1. Elastosis of conjunctiva and peripheral corneal lamellas. Chronic inflammatory cell infiltration of substantia. ×130. AFIP Acc. 119276.

2. Pterygium. Degenerated elastica and hyalinization, conjunctival stroma. ×150. AFIP Acc. 36522.

3. Pterygium. Hyalinization of conjunctival stroma extending over cornea. Amorphous deposits are probably derived from degenerated elastic tissue. ×125. AFIP Acc. 315301.

4. Pterygium. Hyalinization of conjunctival stroma which extended over cornea. Atrophy of conjunctival epithelium. AFIP Neg. 47484.

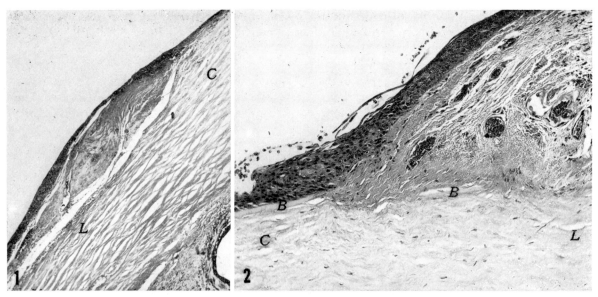

Figure 196. Pterygium Situated at Limbus (L) and Invading Cornea. (C).

1. Incidental observation in an eye enucleated for other reasons. ×47. AFIP Acc. 687301.
2. Excised pterygium. Observe breaks in Bowman's membrane (B). ×115, AFIP Acc. 959641.

progresses toward or across the pupillary area. The pathogenesis of pterygium is not known; however, the occurrence in the interpalpebral zone, and at an epithelial zone of change suggests an external irritant as a cause. Wind, sunlight, dust, etc., have been suggested as causal agents.

The stroma reveals connective tissue alterations similar to those observed in pingueculas. There is "senile elastosis" and the collagen fibers are hypertrophic, dense, and hyalinized, and may degenerate to form a granular basophilic material (Fig. 195). Many new vessels are seen in the stroma, often associated with accumulations of large mononuclear connective tissue cells.

Microscopically, the epithelium is more like that of the conjunctiva but is quite irregular, being thin in some areas and thickened in others. It often is converted to a stratified squamous type. At the head of the pterygium the corneal epithelium is elevated and attenuated by the invasion of the conjunctival connective tissue. In this area Bowman's membrane is absent while beyond this it is usually defective. Similar islands of connective tissue may form and elevate the corneal epithelium over dehiscences in Bowman's membrane central to the head of the pterygium (Fig. 196).

The epithelium overlying pingueculas and

pterygiums may exhibit a wide variety of degenerative and proliferative changes. At times the acanthosis and dyskeratosis are sufficiently disturbing that carcinoma-in-situ must be considered in differential diagnosis (Fig. 197). Rarely, however, does an invasive squamous cell carcinoma arise from these lesions.

Hyaline degeneration and amyloidosis. In localized, elevated lesions hyalin may be deposited extracellularly. According to Ashton and Rey, in some cases the deposited material may show staining reactions which are similar to or identical with those of amyloid and which have been described in Chapter IV (Fig. 198). A cellular infiltration usually precedes the degeneration and the deposits first appear around the vessels. Amyloidosis of the conjunctiva is rarely associated with systemic infections but may be secondary to local chronic inflammatory processes such as trachoma. Recently Pico has described two cases in which conjunctival amyloidosis occurred in patients who exhibited clinical and laboratory evidence of hypothyroidism (Fig. 199). He postulated that amyloidosis might be related to myxedema.

Xerosis. Drying of the conjunctiva may occur spontaneously, without known cause, in isolated areas, usually near the limbus or it may involve the entire surface. It may be due to a congenital defect of lacrimation (familial dysautonomia), to a vitamin A deficiency (Bitot's spot and keratomalacia), prolonged exposure of the eye (lagophthalmos, marked exophthalmos), acquired atrophy of the conjunctival glands (trachoma, pemphigus, etc.), x-radiation, and other causes.

Xerosis is characterized by epidermidalization of the conjunctival epithelium. Acanthosis, dyskeratosis and intercellular bridges may be prominent. At times there occurs a granular layer with keratinization, which may give the lesion the pearly surface which is so characteristic of Bitot's spot. The process of epidermidalization may be diffuse or appear as a localized, slightly elevated lesion in the interpalpebral fissure (tyloma).

Keratoconjunctivitis sicca. Patients with Sjögren's syndrome and keratoconjunctivitis sicca not only have dryness of the conjunctiva but also may have a dry mouth, nose and vagina, achlorhydria and chronic polyarthritis. This disease affects females past the menopause, is bilateral, and is thought to be of endocrine origin.

The conjunctival epithelium may be thickened or thinned. Thickening is due to

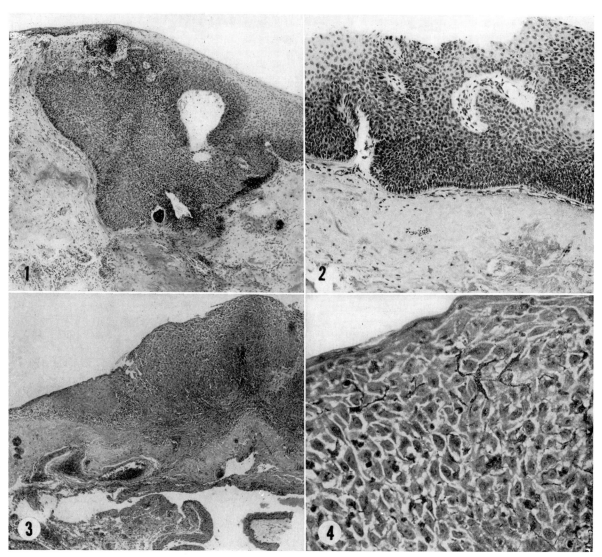

Figure 197.

1 and 2. Acanthosis and dyskeratosis associated with pterygium. ×50 and ×100, respectively. AFIP Acc. 819464.
3 and 4. Acanthosis and proliferation of dendritic melanocytes associated with pterygium. ×50 and 400, respectively. AFIP Acc. 709615.

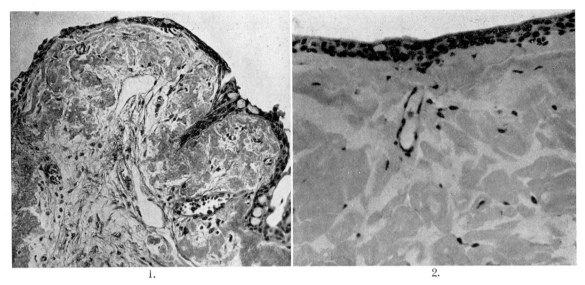

Figure 198.   Amyloidosis

1. Amyloidosis of conjunctival stroma. Subepithelial amyloid deposits which gave positive reaction with cresyl violet. ×275. AFIP Acc. 337450.

2. Amyloidosis. Amyloid deposits in conjunctival stroma. Atrophy of epithelium. ×260. AFIP Acc. 71546.

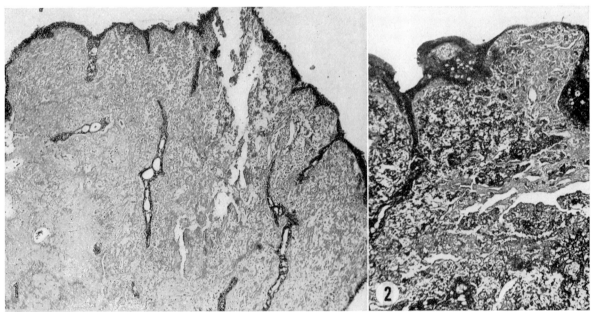

Figure 199.   Amyloidosis of conjunctiva associated with hypothyroidism and myxedema. Case reported by Pico, 1960. AFIP Acc. 953167.

1. H and E, ×50.
2. Cresyl violet, ×80.

marked intercellular and intracellular edema. The intercellular bridges become stretched and spongiosis results. Cystoid spaces soon appear in the epithelium and the cells may show a vacuolar degeneration. Portions of the superficial layers may be sloughed off, producing filaments, and accounting for an uneven surface. Keratin granules may be found in these cells, but no true cornification occurs. In the thinned areas there is an absence of edema and the epithelial cells are flattened giving the epithelium a lamellated appearance. The superficial cells may be shredded off.

Concrements. Longstanding chronic conjunctivitis may lead to formation of yellowish or gray, hard concretions in the superficial layers of the conjunctiva, especially in the lower fornix. They may be pigmented or calcified.

Histologically this amorphous, sometimes calcareous, material lies in a gland-like invagination of the epithelium. The cavities are lined by a thin conjunctival epithelium. There are two layers, a deep cuboidal and a superficial cylindrical one.

ABNORMAL PIGMENTATION

Racial variations. The basal cells of the limbal conjunctiva frequently contain melanin granules in their cytoplasm. This is a constant finding in the darker races but it is not infrequent in the white race (Fig. 200–1). The pigmentation is not congenital but develops after the sixth month of life. Hyperpigmentation may develop in areas that have been traumatized (Fig. 200–2) and in acanthotic plaques over pingueculas and pterygiums (Fig. 197–3, 4).

Melanosis. Congenital melanosis may occur in conjunctiva alone or be associated with ocular and facial melanocytosis. In either case the pigmented melanocytes lie in groups in the deeper submucosal layers, and aggregate especially around the emissaria of the vessels and nerves of the eyeball. In ocular melanocytosis there is an increase in the number of

melanocytes in the uveal tract, sclera, and conjunctiva. This condition may be combined with increased pigmentation in the skin of the lids and temporal areas (nevus of Ota) (see Chapter II and Fig. 67).

Systemic diseases. *Ochronosis* has been mentioned previously (p. 249). Conjunctival pigmentation occurs also in *icterus,* where bile pigments are deposited subepithelially, and in *Addison's disease* where melanin is found in the conjunctiva.

Exogenous. *Argyrosis* of the conjunctiva usually is due to a prolonged ingestion or topical administration of silver-containing drugs. It also is an occupational disease occurring in hatters and felt workers. Most of the metal lies immediately beneath the epithelium as fine grayish granules, but some silver deposits also can be found in the deeper

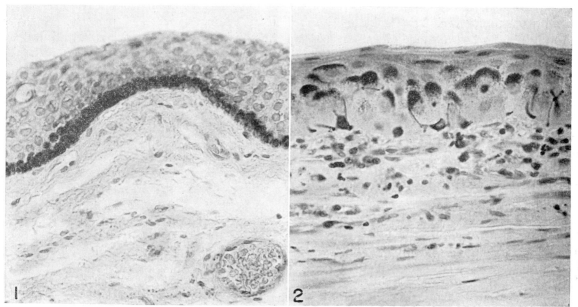

Figure 200. Pigmentation, Cornea and Conjunctiva

1. Hyperpigmentation of basal layer of conjunctival epithelium. ×400. AFIP Acc. 488522.
2. Melanocytes and melanin-containing epithelial cells, derived from conjunctiva but overlying cornea in epithelialization following trauma. The patient was a Negro. ×450. AFIP Acc. 62131.

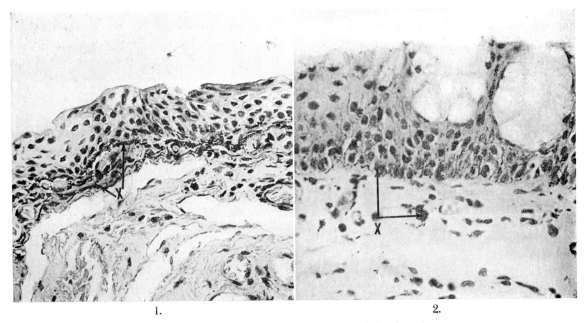

1.   2.

Figure 201. Pigmentation of Cornea and Conjunctiva

1. Argyrosis (X), conjunctiva. ×400. AFIP Acc. 88692.
2. Atabrine pigmentation (X), cornea. ×400. AFIP Acc. 136737.

epithelial layers (Fig. 201–1). The silver lies mostly around elastic fibers for which it has a great affinity. It also occurs in the vessel walls.

Atabrine may produce a discoloration of the conjunctiva in patients who are receiving the drug for malaria or who are exposed to it during its manufacture. This is believed to be the result of a brown metabolic intermediate of the drug which is deposited in and beneath the conjunctival epithelium (Fig. 201–2). The pigmentation is reversible when exposure to atabrine is discontinued.

Gold deposits can be found in the conjunctiva in cases of chrysiasis that occur after prolonged parenteral gold treatment. According to Roberts and Wolter, the gold is found subepithelially as well as among the epithelial cells.

Pigmentation of the conjunctiva may occur after repeated local applications of ointments containing *mercury.* According to Long and Danielson, this usually is accompanied by a discoloration of the skin of the lids.

Workers exposed to *aniline dyes,* especially quinone and hydroquinone, may acquire pigmentation of the conjunctiva and cornea in the interpalpebral fissure. According to Anderson and Oglesby, the pigment lies in the

basal cells of the epithelium and in the subepithelial tissue (see Chapter IV).

Pigmented foreign bodies may give rise to granulomatous nodules which occasionally are mistaken for melanotic tumors (Fig. 202).

Hematogenous. A hematogenous pigmentation may appear after extensive subconjunctival hemorrhages. The pigment usually is hemosiderin, which is deposited around the blood vessels and basal epithelium, and between the stromal fibers.

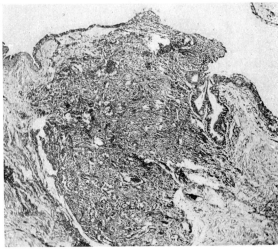

Figure 202. Pigmented foreign body granuloma of conjunctiva which clinically was considered a probable malignant melanoma. ×50. AFIP Acc. 958759.

NEOPLASMS AND RELATED CONDITIONS

Cysts

Epithelial. Epithelial cysts of the conjunctiva may occur after inflammation or trauma or they may be of obscure etiology. In some cases, surface epithelium is implanted in the substantia propria. The trapped epithelium first proliferates as a solid sheet; then the central part of the island of tissue disintegrates, leaving one or more cysts (Fig. 203). Retention cysts usually form in the upper or lower fornix. The excretory duct of a gland may be blocked by inspissated secretion, scar tissue, or inflammation. The glands of Krause frequently are the source of such cysts. They lie deep in the stroma and often are a sequel of a chronic inflammation. The cysts are lined by one or two layers of flat epithelial cells. Rarely, large multiloculated cysts lined by typical conjunctival epithelium are encountered (Fig. 204).

Lymphatic. Lymphatic cysts are superficial circumscribed ectasias of pre-existing lymph vessels. They are more frequent than epithelial cysts in the conjunctiva. It is doubtful that a clearcut distinction can be made between lymphangiectasias and lymphangiomas (Landing and Farber, 1956). They are extremely thin-walled and lined by endothelial cells. The epithelium over them may be normal or thinned. Hemorrhage may occur into the cysts either spontaneously or after trauma, but usually these cysts are filled with a clear fluid (Fig. 205).

Cystic nevi. Nevi on the bulbar conjunctiva are frequently cystic. These are considered on page 270.

Tumors

Papilloma. Papillomas are not rare in the conjunctiva. They occur more frequently at the limbus, on the caruncle, and at the lid margin. Those at the caruncle and lid margin usually are of the soft, pedunculated or sessile

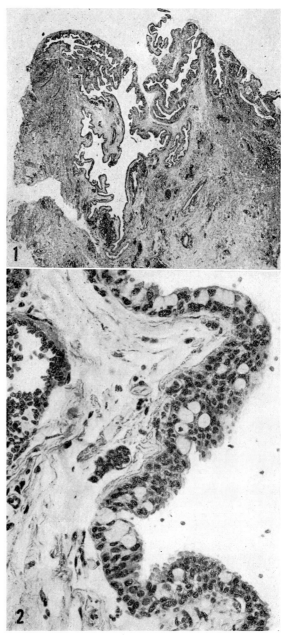

Figure 204.

1. Conjunctival cyst of upper inner canthal region ×11.

2. The cyst is lined by typical conjunctival epithelium. ×305. AFIP Acc. 962244.

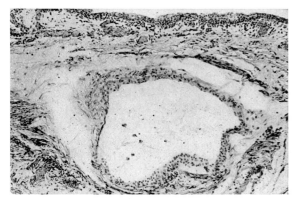

Figure 203. Epithelial inclusion cyst of conjunctiva. ×75. U. of Cal. Acc. 56–609.

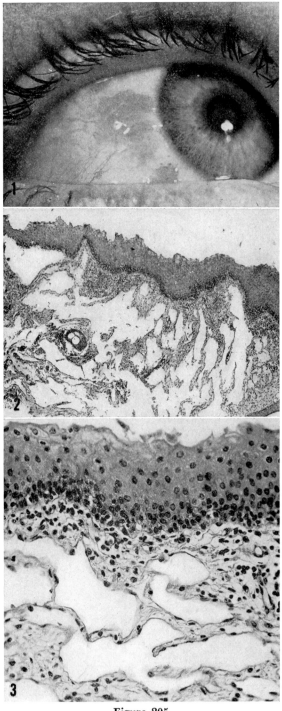

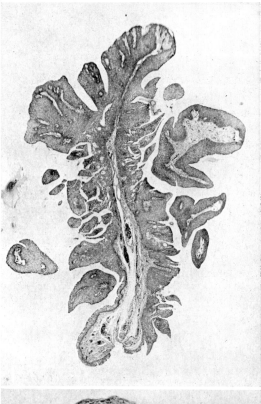

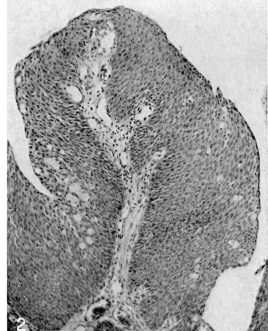

Figure 205.

1. Lymphangiectasia of bulbar conjunctiva. **The lesion** appeared cystic and there had been recurrent hemorrhages into the cysts. AFIP Acc. 824111. (Courtesy of Dr. L. C. Moss.)

2. ×50.

3. ×305.

Figure 206. Papilloma

1. Papilloma, bulbar conjunctiva. Nonkeratinizing epithelium. ×24. AFIP Acc. 215412.

2. Papilloma, conjunctiva. Mucous cells in non keratinizing epithelium. ×125. AFIP Acc. 230075.

type and appear as a grayish-red, fleshy elevation with an irregular surface which sometimes may be cauliflower-like. They often recur after removal because they are infectious. Papillomas at the limbus arise from a broad base, remain flat, and spread laterally onto the conjunctiva and cornea. There is less tendency for papilla-formation because of pressure from the lids.

These tumors have a core of connective tissue and are covered with a proliferating epithelium (Fig. 206). The goblet cells usually are retained in those at the lid margin but not in those of the limbus. The epithelium exhibits a tendency toward epidermidalization, although keratinization is usually

moderate. The basal membrane is always intact. The epithelium may, however, show some irregularities and eventually a malignant tumor may develop.

Dyskeratosis and carcinoma-in-situ. The limbus is a frequent site for the development of slow-growing opaque plaques of thickened epithelium exhibiting varying degrees of epidermidalization, acanthosis and dyskeratosis (Figs. 38–1, 39, 40–2). The clinical term, leukoplakia, is appropriate for these lesions (Fig. 207) and preferable to the designation of "epithelioma" which is often used. Microscopically these lesions rarely present unequivocal evidence of malignancy and they almost always follow a benign course. Many show changes that are very similar to those observed in the skin in senile keratosis (see Chapter IV) and these have often been labelled by the term "leukoplakic type of dyskeratosis" (Fig. 208) (Ash and Wilder, 1942). Less frequently the microscopic picture resembles that of Bowen's disease of the skin and that of the erythroplasia of Queyrat (a placoid lesion occurring on the glans penis). In these cases there is less acanthosis, more diffuse dyskeratosis, greater pleomorphism, more bizarre multinucleated giant cells and mitotic figures at all levels of the involved epithelium, and vacuolated cells containing pyknotic nuclei surrounded by a clear halo (Fig. 209). In still other cases the

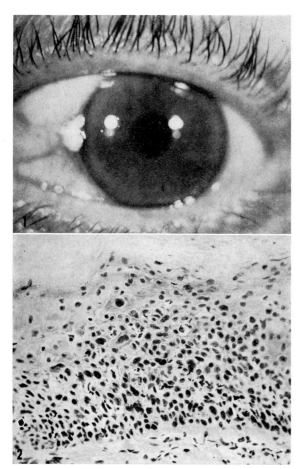

Figure 207.

1. Leukoplakic plaque on bulbar conjunctiva at nasal limbus. This was removed by simple excision.

2. Microscopically the affected epithelium reveals marked acanthosis, cellular pleomorphism, hyperchromatism, and loss of polarity. ×305. AFIP Acc. 824113. (Courtesy of Dr. G. V. Simpson.)

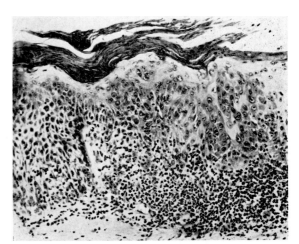

Figure 208. Leukoplakic type of dyskeratosis of bulbar conjunctiva with changes similar to those observed in senile keratosis; irregular acanthosis, marked parakeratosis, pleomorphism of prickle cells with loss of polarity, and heavy lymphocytic infiltration of subepithelial tissues. ×355. AFIP Acc. 70308.

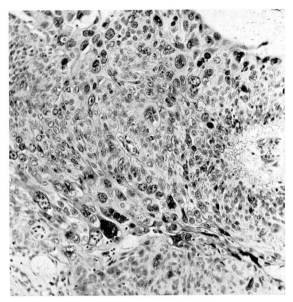

Figure 209. Bowenoid type of dyskeratosis of conjunctiva with many large bizarre multinucleated cells at all levels of the epithelium. ×145. AFIP Acc. 196541.

histopathologic picture (Figs. 210, 211) is not unlike that of carcinoma-in-situ of the cervix.

Squamous cell carcinoma. While invasive carcinoma may develop from any of these dyskeratotic, acanthotic plaques, there is a much greater tendency for the lesions to become papillomatous (Figs. 212, 213–3) and to spread along the epithelial surface into the cornea (Fig. 213–1, 2). Lateral extension along the bulbar conjunctiva into the fornices is uncommon. When invasion is observed it is usually restricted to minute foci in the substantia propria (Fig. 212) but only rarely do penetration of the sclera, intraocular extension (Figs. 213–4, 214), and metastasis occur.

Basal cell carcinoma rarely, if ever, arises in the conjunctiva. Some of the epithelial lesions which are associated with pterygiums and pingueculas exhibit basal cell proliferation, simulating basal cell carcinoma (Fig. 197).

Angiomas. All of the types of hemangiomas described in Chapter IV may occur in the conjunctiva (Figs. 156, 157). A common conjunctival hemangioma develops early in life, or is congenital. It is a small elevated dark-red tumor which moves freely with the conjunctiva. It occurs most frequently near the inner canthus, and is of the cavernous variety. Histologically there are large, thin-walled blood spaces. The conjunctiva also may be involved in hereditary hemorrhagic telangiectasia (Rendu-Osler). Congenital varicosities of the conjunctiva may be associated with more extensive malformations of the orbital and intracranial vasculature (Fig. 216).

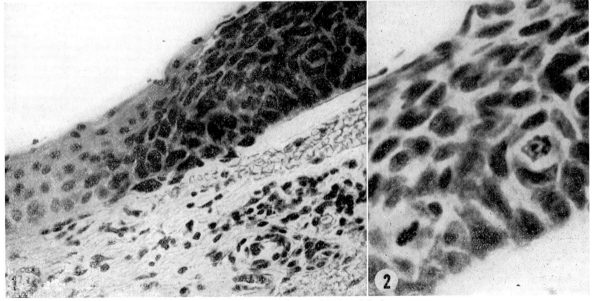

Figure 210.   Carcinoma-in-situ, Limbus

1. There is an abrupt transition from essentially normal epithelium on the left to the intraepithelial neoplasm. The affected cells are pleomorphic, hyperchromatic, and much larger than the normal. ×570. AFIP Acc. 272972
2. ×980. AFIP Acc. 272972.

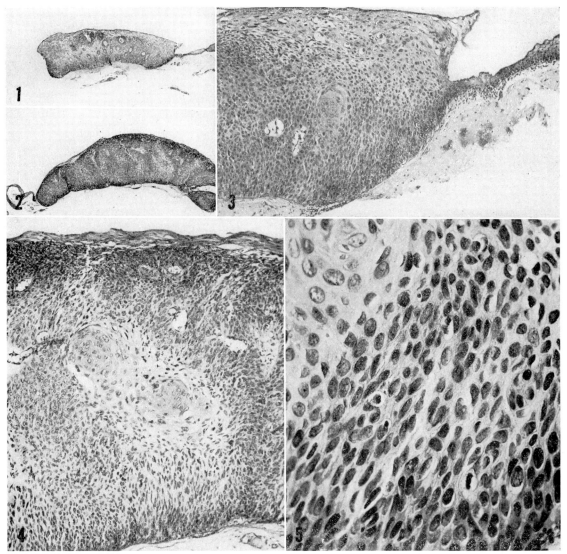

Figure 211. Placoid lesion excised from bulbar conjunctiva reveals changes consistent with carcinoma-in-situ. 1 and 2. ×13. 3. ×80. 4. ×90. 5. ×305. AFIP Acc. 873376.

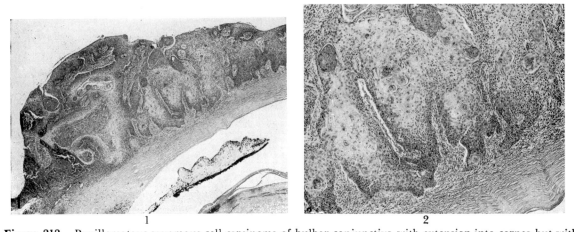

Figure 212. Papillomatous squamous cell carcinoma of bulbar conjunctiva with extension into cornea but with little invasion of stroma. 1. ×18. 2. ×50. AFIP Acc. 785865.

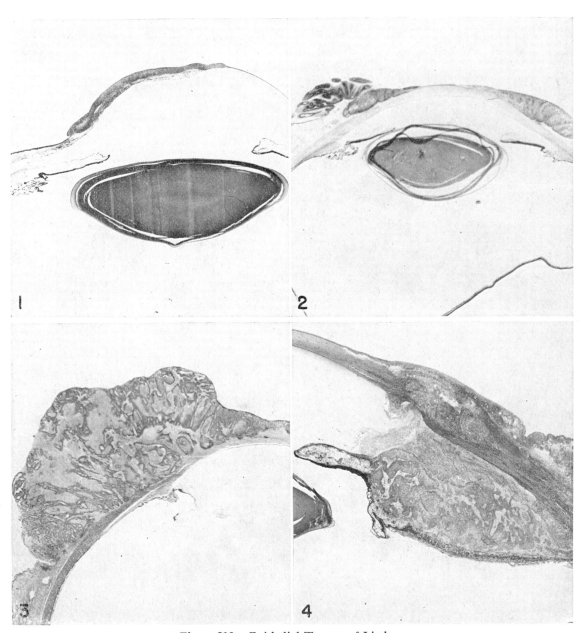

Figure 213. Epithelial Tumors of Limbus

1. Epidermidalization and dyskeratosis of conjunctival and corneal epithelium. ×7. AFIP Acc. 73701.
2. Papillary squamous cell carcinoma of the limbus, early, with involvement of the corneal epithelium. ×7. AFIP Acc. 61746.
3. Squamous cell carcinoma of limbus. ×5. AFIP Acc. 44334.
4. Squamous cell carcinoma of limbus extending through sclera into ciliary body and iris. ×7. AFIP Acc. 56348.

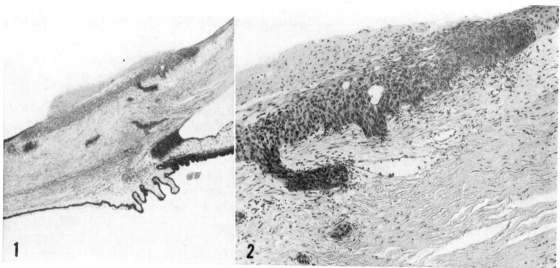

Figure 214.

1. Carcinoma of the bulbar conjunctiva with infiltration of stroma at corneoscleral junction and invasion of anterior chamber angle. ×29.

2. Much of the lesion at the surface retains the features of carcinoma-in-situ. ×85. AFIP Acc. 690246.

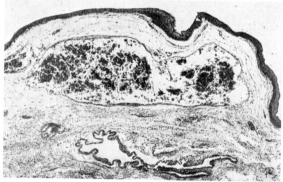

Figure 215. Cavernous hemangioma of conjunctiva. ×50. AFIP Acc. 524777.

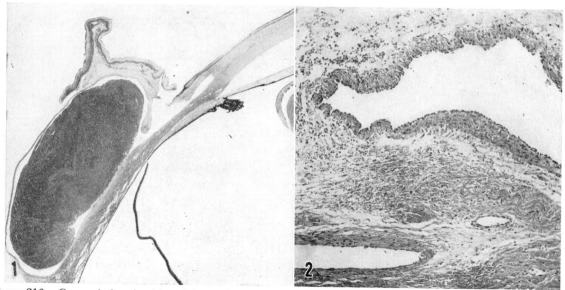

Figure 216. Congenital varicosities of the conjunctiva and episclera. There were associated orbital and intracranial vascular anomalies.

1. ×10.   2. ×110. AFIP Acc. 155685.

Cavernous lymphangiomas are rare and usually congenital (Fig. 217). They consist of lymph spaces of various sizes and of a cellular connective tissue. These can not be sharply separated from lymphangiectasias (Fig. 205).

Nevus. Nevi probably are the most common tumors of the conjunctiva and usually are of the junctional or compound type (Figs. 218, 219). Nevi that are entirely subepithelial (comparable to dermal nevi of the skin) are rarely encountered on the conjunctiva (Fig. 220). The structure of conjunctival nevi is quite similar to that of nevi in the skin (see Chapter IV). Peculiar to the conjunctival type, however, are the large number of epithelial inclusions. These may occur in the form of solid nests, adenomatoid structures, or cysts (Fig. 221). They are composed of conjunctival epithelium containing mucous cells which may continue to grow and secrete. The secreted mucus is retained within the inclusions and accounts for the large cystoid or pseudoglandular spaces. Enlargement of these cysts may create the illusion of growth of the nevus. These non-neoplastic cells from the surface epithelium sometimes have been mistaken for the epithelioid cells of malignant melanoma and at other times the formation of epithelium-lined cysts has led to the diagnosis of adenocarcinoma. Pigmentation of conjunctival nevi varies greatly. Many are salmon pink amelanotic masses while an equal number are heavily pigmented.

Melanoma. Melanomas derived from nevi occur in the conjunctiva. The histologic properties of these conjunctival melanomas are similar to those described in Chapter IV. They usually occur in the bulbar conjunctiva or at the limbus; they are unusual in the caruncle and rare in the palpebral conjunctiva. The degree of pigmentation may vary, but they usually appear as black or gray tumors. They are richly vascularized and bleed easily. Those malignant melanomas

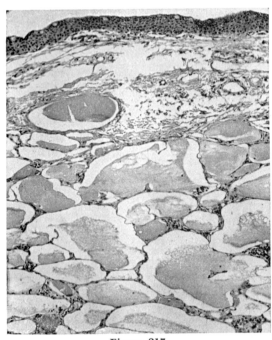

Figure 217.

Lymphangioma, bulbar conjunctiva. ×125. AFIP Acc. 193871.

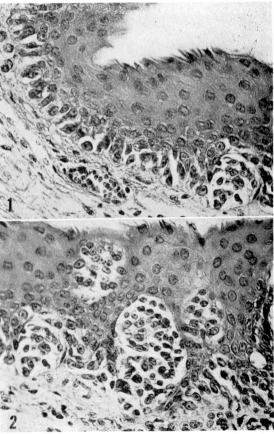

Figure 218. Junctional Nevus of Bulbar Conjunctiva

The nevus cells, occurring individually and in clusters, are within the epithelium. ×305. AFIP Acc. 819328.

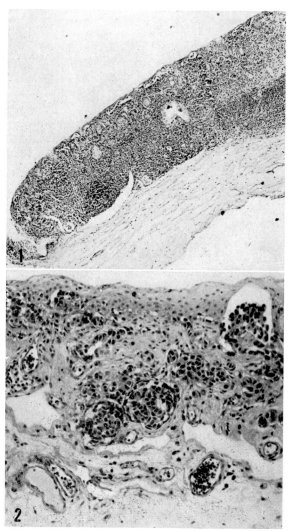

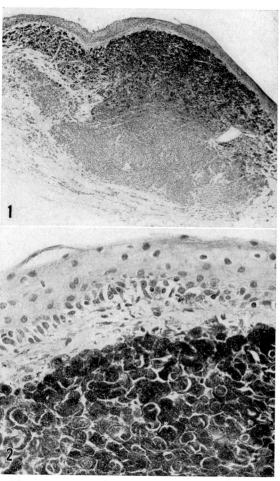

Figure 219.   Compound Nevi, Bulbar Conjunctiva

1. ×50. AFIP Acc. 139483.

2. ×145. AFIP Acc. 283131. The nevus cells are found beneath the epithelium as well as within it.

Figure 220.   Subepithelial Nevus of Conjunctiva

As in dermal nevi of the skin, the nevus cells are confined to the subepithelial tissues.

1. ×48.   2. ×300. AFIP Acc. 741084.

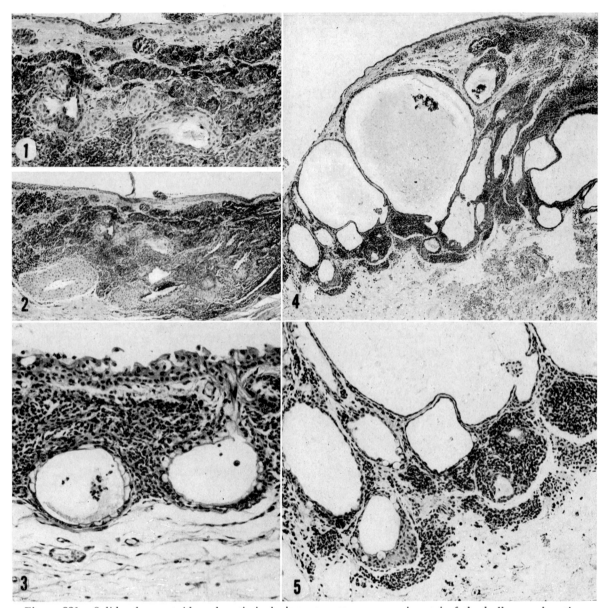

Figure 221. Solid, adenomatoid, and cystic inclusions are very common in nevi of the bulbar conjunctiva.

1. ×115. AFIP Acc. 705722.
2. ×35. AFIP Acc. 705722.
3. ×180. AFIP Acc. 174218.
4. ×48. AFIP Acc. 713602.
5. ×120. AFIP Acc. 713602.

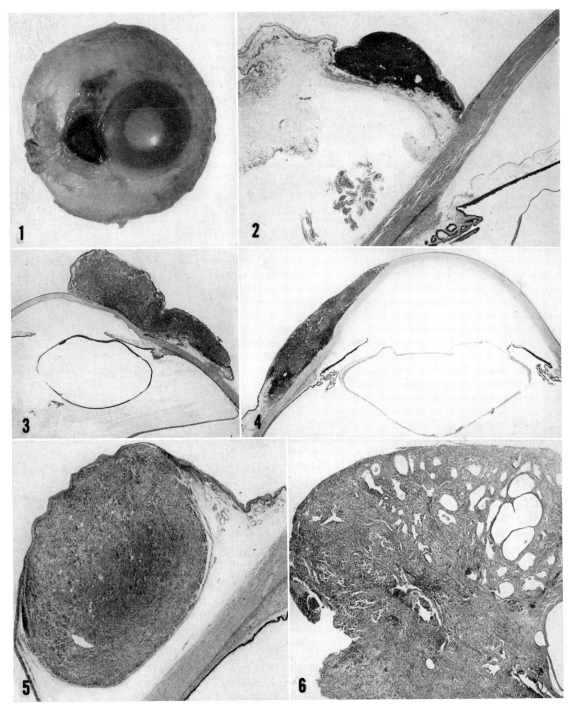

Figure 222. Malignant Melanoma, Bulbar Conjunctiva

1 and 2. Heavily pigmented malignant melanoma of bulbar conjunctiva. Rapid growth of black tumor in 50 year old white man who had had a lesion removed from same site 36 years earlier. ×2 and ×15. AFIP Acc. 231176.

3. Lightly pigmented polypoid malignant melanoma of bulbar conjunctiva and cornea in a 74 year old white man who had always had a brown spot on the nasal side of the conjunctiva. ×5. AFIP Acc. 138757.

4 and 5. Infiltrative and polypoid malignant melanoma in a 59 year old white man who had previously had lesions removed from the same area at ages 5 and 52 (see 6). ×7 and ×15. AFIP Acc. 501247.

6. Malignant melanoma arising in a cystic nevus of bulbar conjunctiva excised at age 52 (same case shown in 4 and 5). ×24.

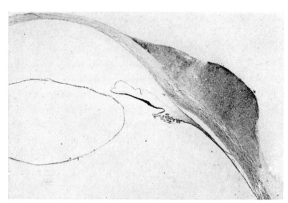

Figure 223.   Infiltrative malignant melanoma, limbus.
×6. AFIP Acc. 554064.

arising from nevi near the limbus tend to form bulky pedunculated tumors which do not invade the underlying sclera (Fig. 222). Others, however, may invade the cornea or orbit (Fig. 223). Small, flat areas of pigmentation in other parts of the conjunctiva frequently accompany a melanoma. Histologically they are quite often epithelioid in character, but a mixture of epithelioid and spindle cell types may also be seen (Figs. 224, 225). The natural behavior of these melanomas is not predictable but there is reason to believe they are considerably less malignant than similar melanomas of the eyelids and skin (Lewis and Zimmerman, 1958).

Precancerous and cancerous melanosis. According to Reese, precancerous melanosis is a flat, widespread pigmented epithelial lesion which may in the beginning show spontaneous variations in the degree and extent of pigmentation.

Histologically the pigmentation begins in the basal cell layer and first exhibits an intraepithelial type of growth which can not be distinguished microscopically from a junctional nevus, except for the absence of epithelial inclusions (Fig. 221). With increasing activity the hydropic cells and the cell clusters extend into the epithelium toward the surface. Nuclear anaplasia may become apparent. In the stroma there develops a subepithelial inflammatory infiltration with pigment phagocytosis (Fig. 226).

Quite frequently a very malignant neoplasm develops from this precancerous stage. The epithelial involvement spreads and localized melanomas form. Anaplastic tumor cells involve the epithelial layer, and invade the stroma. Multiple nodular tumors may form (Figs. 227, 228).

Lymphomas. Lymphomas of the conjunctiva may appear independently, be associated with generalized lymphosarcoma, or be due to one of the leukemias. The most frequent type of "lymphoma" is a smooth, slightly fleshy

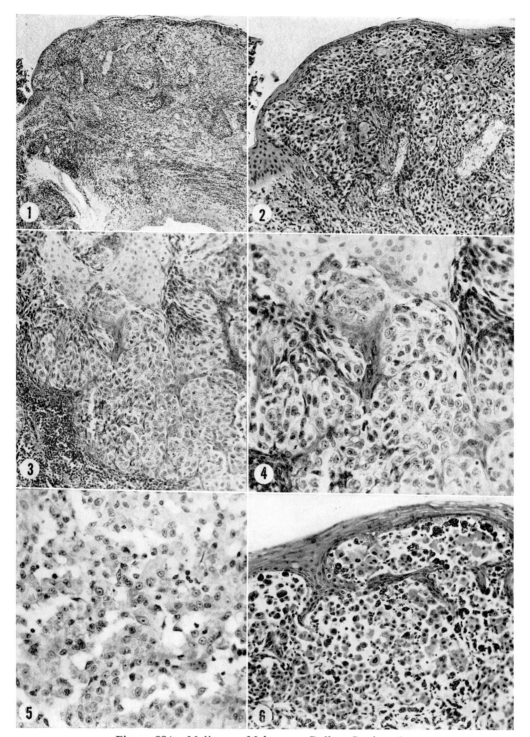

Figure 224. Malignant Melanoma, Bulbar Conjunctiva

1 and 2. Malignant melanoma arising in a compound nevus of bulbar conjunctiva that had been present since early childhood. The tumor began to grow rapidly at age 59. ×48 and ×135, respectively. AFIP Acc. 643700.

3 and 4. Malignant melanoma, limbus. ×140 and ×275, respectively. AFIP Acc. 543991.

5. Malignant melanoma, limbus. This tumor which was composed almost entirely of large epithelioid cells was removed by simple excision when the patient was 70 years old. Fifteen years later there was no evidence of recurrence or metastasis. ×305. AFIP Acc. 710505.

6. Malignant melanoma, epithelioid cell type, limbus, in 79 year old man who had noted slow growth of lesion for 5 years. × 125. AFIP Acc. 182300.

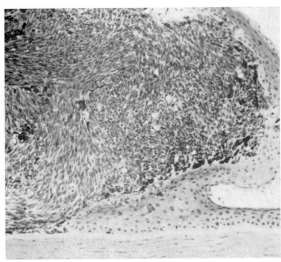

Figure 225. Spindle cell type of malignant melanoma of limbus. A small pigmented birthmark on bulbar conjunctiva near limbus had remained unchanged until the patient was 31 years old. The eye was enucleated one year later when the tumor had extended onto the cornea. ×240. AFIP Acc. 67345.

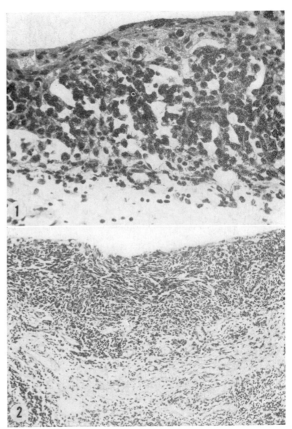

Figure 226. Cancerous Melanosis, Bulbar Conjunctiva

1. In this area there is diffuse intraepithelial invasion by the malignant melanoma. Elsewhere there was stromal invasion and formation of an elevated tumor nodule. ×305. AFIP Acc. 749632.

2. Associated inflammatory changes are frequently present. ×130. AFIP Acc. 596399.

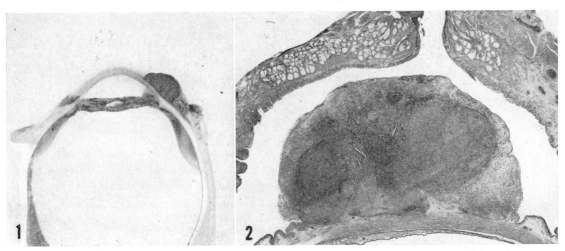

Figure 227. Malignant Melanoma of Conjunctiva Derived from Precancerous Melanosis

1. AFIP Acc. 763871.
2. ×6. AFIP Acc. 897677.

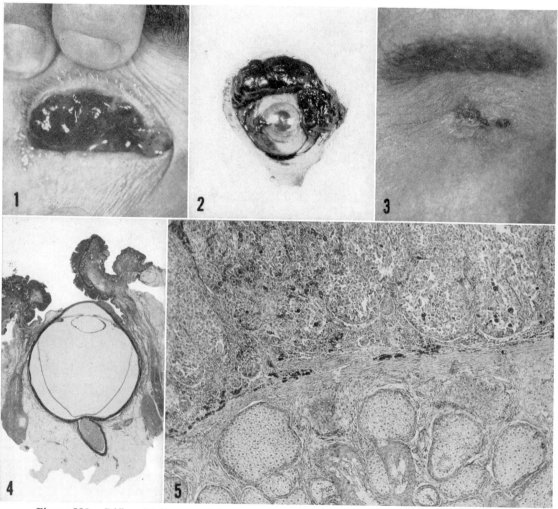

Figure 228. Diffuse Malignant Melanoma (Cancerous Melanosis) of Conjunctiva and Cornea

1. Preoperative appearance. AFIP Acc. 161980.
2. Exenterated orbital contents. Same case.
3. Postoperative recurrence. Same case.
4. Extensive involvement of cornea, bulbar and palpebral conjunctiva. AFIP Acc. 281650.
5. Involvement of tarsal conjunctiva. ×62. Same specimen.

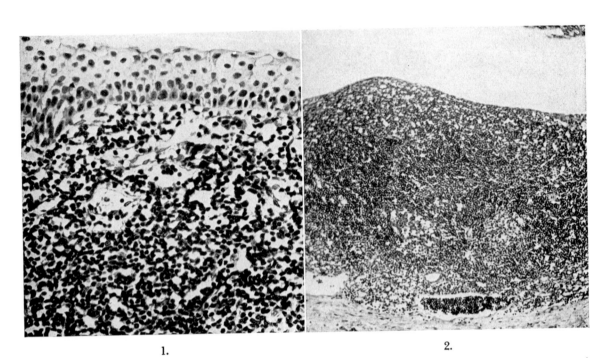

1.   2.

Figure 229. Lymphocytic Hyperplasia, Conjunctiva

1. ×275. AFIP Acc. 187647.
2. ×35. AFIP Acc. 187647.

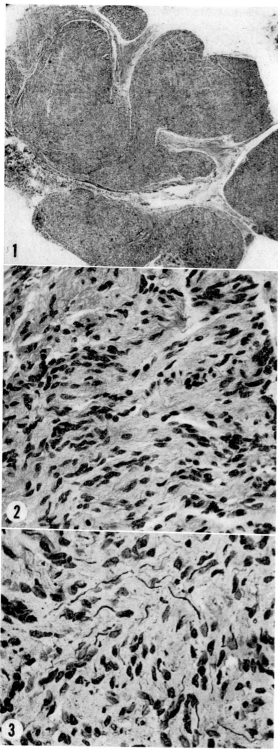

Figure 230. Recurrent plexiform neurofibroma of bulbar conjunctiva. The patient did not show evidence of von Recklinghausen's disease. Case reported by Dabezies and Penner.

1. ×13.
2. ×305.
3. Axis cylinders demonstrated by Bodian's stain. ×500. AFIP Acc. 962489.

elevated tumor which forms in the region of the caruncle or in the fornix and gradually spreads over a wide area. Biopsy often reveals masses of mature lymphocytes in a delicate vascular stroma sometimes accompanied by numerous reticulum cells and plasma cells. This is considered to be a benign lymphocytic hyperplasia and it is rarely associated with generalized lymph node involvement or other evidence of lymphomatous disease (Fig. 229). It responds well to small doses of x-ray.

Connective tissue tumors. Fibroma and neurofibroma rarely occur in the conjunctiva. Fibromas often are firm and consist mainly of a dense connective tissue. Most fibrous lesions here represent reactive hyperplasias and therefore fall into the category of inflammatory pseudotumors.

Neurofibroma of the conjunctiva (Fig. 230) is usually but not always a manifestation of von Recklinghausen's disease. Conjunctival neurofibromas may appear as one or more small localized tumors 1 to 3 mm. in diameter, and elevated 1 to 2 mm. They are firm, nontender, fixed in position, and are covered by normal epithelium. In diffuse orbital neurofibromatosis numbers of enlarged tortuous nerves may appear under the conjunctiva. The histology of these tumors has been described in Chapter IV. These may be difficult or impossible to distinguish from Axenfeld's nerve loops (Fig. 59) except for the characteristic position of the latter.

REFERENCES

Anderson, B., and Oglesby, F.: Corneal Changes from Quinone-Hydroquinone Exposure. A.M.A. Arch. Ophthal. *59*:459–501, 1958.
Ash, J. E., and Wilder, H. C.: Epithelial Tumors of Limbus. Trans. Amer. Acad. Ophthal. Otolaryng. *46*:215–222, (May-June), 1942.
Ashton, N., and Rey, A.: Hyaline Infiltration of Eyelid. Brit. J. Ophthal. *35*:125–133, (March), 1951.
Beigelman, M. N.: Vernal Conjunctivitis. Los Angeles, Univ. of S. Calif. Press, 1950.
Braendstrup, P.: Infantile Cystinosis with Cystine Crystals in Cornea and Conjunctiva. Acta Ophthal. *30*:365–377, 1952.
Busacca, A.: Biomicroscopie et Histopathologie de l'oeil. Vol. I, Zurich, Schweizer Druck- und Verlagshaus A. G., 1952.
Cogan, D. G., Kuwabara, T., and Howard, J.: The Nonelastic Nature of Pingueculas. A.M.A. Arch. Ophthal. *61*:388–389, 1959.
Cogan, D. G., et al.: Ocular Manifestations of

Systemic Cystinosis. A.M.A. Arch. Ophthal. *55*:36–41, 1956.

Custodis, E.: Die essentielle Bindehautschrumpfung des menschlichen Auges. Arch. f. Ophthal. *137*:364–418, 1937.

Dabezies, O. H., and Penner, R.: Neurofibroma of the Bulbar Conjunctiva. In press.

Duggan, J. W., and Gaines, S. R.: Ocular Complications of Erythema Exudativum Multiforme. Amer. J. Ophthal. *34*:189–197, (Feb.), 1951.

François, J.: Les Ectodermoses Erosives Pluriorificielles. Acta Ophthal. *32*:5–36, 1954.

François, J., and Rabaey, M.: Adenoma of Limbal Conjunctiva. Brit. J. Ophthal. *35*:237–241, (April), 1951.

François, J., Rabaey, M., and Evens, L.: Tumeurs Epitheliales de la Conjonctive Bulbaire. Boll. d'ocul. *35*:615–641, 1956.

Hogan, M. J.: Atopic Keratoconjunctivitis. Amer. J. Ophthal. *36*:937–947 (July), 1953.

Kennedy, R. J., and Sullivan, J. V.: Epithelial Plaques of Conjunctiva. Amer. J. Ophthal. *35*:843–847, (June), 1952.

Landing, B. H., and Farber, S.: Tumors of the Cardiovascular System, Fascicle 7. Atlas of Tumor Pathology, 1956, Armed Forces Institute of Pathology, Washington, D. C.

Lever, W. F.: Pemphigus: Histopathologic Study. A.M.A. Arch. Dermat. and Syph. *64*:727–753, (Dec.), 1951.

Lewis, P. M., and Zimmerman, L. E.: Delayed Recurrences of Malignant Melanomas of the Bulbar Conjunctiva. Amer. J. Ophthal. *45*:536–543, 1958.

Long, J. C., and Danielson, R. W.: Mercurial Discoloration of Eyelids. Amer. J. Ophthal. *34*:753–756, (May), 1951.

MacCallan, A. F.: The Epidemiology of Trachoma. Brit. J. Ophthal. *15*:369–411, 1931.

McGavic, J. S.: Intraepithelial Epithelioma of Cornea and Conjunctiva (Bowen's Disease). Amer. J. Ophthal. *25*:167–176, (Feb.), 1942.

Margileth, A. M.: Cat Scratch Disease as a Cause of the Oculoglandular Syndrome of Parinaud. Pediatrics *20*:1000–1005, 1957.

Mohamed, A. F. M.: Schistosomiasis of the Conjunctiva. Bull. ophthal. Soc. Egypt *49*:120, 1956.

Patz, A.: Ocular Involvement in Erythema Multiforme. A.M.A. Arch. Ophthal. *43*:244–256, (Feb.), 1950.

Pico, G.: Chronic Pseudotumoral Edema of the Conjunctiva of Possible Myxedematous and Amyloid Origin. Trans. Amer. Ophthal. Soc. *58*:132–154, 1960.

Reese, A. B.: Precancerous and Cancerous Melanosis of Conjunctiva. Amer. J. Ophthal. *39*:96–100, (April), 1955.

Reese, A. B.: Tumors of the Eye. New York, Paul B. Hoeber, 1951.

Roberts, W. H., and Wolter, J. R.: Ocular Chrysiasis. A.M.A. Arch. Ophthal. *56*:48–52, 1956.

Rones, B.: Ochronosis Oculi in Alkaptonuria. Amer. J. Ophthal. *49*:440–446, 1960.

Scuderi, G.: Istopatologia del Tracoma. Torino, Edizione Minerva Medica, 1957.

Seitz, R.: Über die Ochronotischen Pigmentierungen am Auge. Klin. Monatsbl. Augenh. *125*:432–440, 1954.

Sjögren, H.: Zur Kenntnis der Keratoconjunctivitis sicca (Keratitis Filiformes bei Hypofunktion der Tränendrüsen). Acta Ophthal. Suppl. *2*:1–151, 1933.

Sugar, H. S., Reazi, A., and Schaffner, R.: The Bulbar Conjunctival Lymphatics and Their Clinical Significance. Trans. Amer. Acad. Ophthal. Otolaryng. *61*:212–223, 1957.

T'ang, F. F., Chang, H. L., Huang, Y. T., and Wang, K. C.: Studies on the Etiology of Trachoma with Special Reference to Isolation of the Virus in Chick Embryo. Chin. Med. J. *75*:429–466, 1957.

Walsh, F. B., and Howard, J. E.: Conjunctival and Corneal Lesions in Hypercalcemia. J. Clin. Endocr. *7*:644–652, (Sept.), 1947.

Chapter VI

The Cornea and Sclera

THE CORNEA

ANATOMY

The cornea forms the anterior one-sixth of the circumference of the outer coat of the eye. It is somewhat oval and has an average diameter of approximately 11 mm. vertically and 12 mm. horizontally. The radius of curvature is slightly greater on the outer than on the inner surface. Von Bahr reports that the thickness varies from about 0.56 mm. in the center to about 1.0 mm. at the periphery. It is more sharply curved than the sclera, with which it is continuous (Fig. 60). At the corneoscleral junction there is a shallow furrow, the scleral sulcus, which indicates the position of the limbus in surgical procedures.

The cornea can be divided into five layers, proceeding from without inwards: epithelium, Bowman's membrane, substantia propria or stroma, Descemet's membrane, and the endothelium (Fig. 231).

The epithelium consists of five or six layers of stratified squamous epithelium resting on a very delicate argyrophilic basement membrane. The latter is very difficult to identify in routine hematoxylin-eosin–stained sections of normal eyes and should not be confused with Bowman's membrane which is very prominent. In certain pathologic states the basement membrane becomes thickened and

it is then easy to identify. The basal layer consists of plump cylindrical cells containing rounded, anteriorly placed nuclei. Resting on this layer are three layers of polyhedral cells which have a wing-shaped appearance in ordinary histologic preparations, because of both their convex anterior and concave posterior surfaces and of edges that taper. The outermost layer of "wing cells" is more flat. Finally, there are two layers of surface cells which are very large in surface expanse, but are very thin (4 microns in the region of the nucleus). The nuclei are exceedingly flat and stain less densely than those of the cells in the deeper layers. The normal surface cells exhibit no tendency for keratinization but are joined together by cell bridges, as in the epidermis. As the bridges shrink, intercellular spaces develop; when inflammation supervenes, leukocytes are found in these spaces. These superficial cells normally are exfoliated and constantly are replaced by cells from the next deeper layers of the epithelium.

Bowman's membrane is a uniformly thick (10 to 16 microns), homogeneous sheet beneath the basement membrane of the epithelium from which it is sharply defined. The posterior surface of the membrane does not have a clear contour, but merges with the superficial lamellas of the stroma, to which it

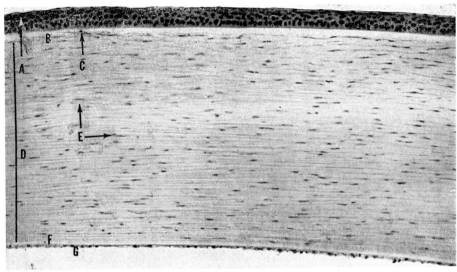

Figure 231. Normal Cornea

A, epithelium. B, Bowman's membrane. C, "pore" in Bowman's membrane. D, substantia propria. E, corneal corpuscles. F, Descemet's membrane. G, endothelial layer. ×165. AFIP Acc. 51854.

is firmly attached. In fact, it is a modified layer of the stroma, differing only in its homogeneity and in the orientation of its fibrils by the electron microscope. Numerous perforations or pores in the membrane provide for the passage of the terminal branches of the corneal nerves. The periphery of Bowman's membrane marks the inner boundary of the limbus.

The substantia propria or stroma forms 90 per cent of the thickness of the cornea. It is avascular, consisting of two elements, lamellas and cells. The lamellas are broad bands of interlacing collagenous fibrils extending over the entire width of the cornea, arranged parallel to its surface. The fixed corneal cells (corpuscles) are ordinary connective tissue cells lying in the lamellar interspaces, where they are flattened and compressed. They have thin nuclei, ill-defined borders, and delicate cell membranes. Wandering leukocytes which are distorted into long spindle shapes are seen in the lamellar interspaces.

The cornea is richly supplied with unmyelinated nerves, derived from the ciliary nerves, which are end branches of the ophthalmic division of the fifth cranial nerve. They enter the stroma in the middle layers from a plexus in the suprachoroidal space and run forward in a radial fashion toward the center of the cornea, dividing dichotomously. The nerve fibers, 30 to 60 in number, are

visible biomicroscopically as whitish threads crossing the limbus but are not seen in tissue sections unless special stains are used. The nerves emerge from the deeper part of the cornea, pass through canals in Bowman's membrane, and terminate by forming a plexus beneath the epithelium. Free nerve endings run between the epithelial cells.

The nerve endings are plexiform ramifications with free nerve terminals, except around the sclerocorneal junction where both Krause's end-bulbs and endings for cold sensation are present. Tower has shown that one afferent fiber is represented by ramifying terminal endings which extend over a quadrant or more of the cornea and may spread into the adjacent sclera and conjunctiva.

Descemet's membrane is a homogeneous, sometimes laminated, acellular eosinophilic membrane resembling the lens capsule and lamina vitrea of the choroid. This membrane lies on the posterior aspect of the stroma and can be stripped from it easily. Descemet's membrane differs from Bowman's membrane both in its staining reaction and in its behavior. It is not modified stroma but appears to be a product of the endothelium. Recent studies by Jakus with the electron microscope in animals and humans and by Garron et al. in humans show that this membrane is composed of a regularly arranged lattice work of fine fibers having a periodicity mostly of 1000 angstroms (probably collagen), and that it is not "structureless," as was formerly believed. Peripherally, Descemet's membrane splits to partially envelope the anterior border-ring of Schwalbe at the apex of the trabecular area (Figs. 232, 233). Schwalbe's ring, when prominent, is composed of closely packed collagen fibers and variable amounts of elastic tissue, arranged in bundles and coursing circumferentially about the periphery of Descemet's membrane (Fig. 245). Burian et al. have found it to be prominent in about 12 to 15 per cent of normal eyes.

The endothelium is a single layer of cells

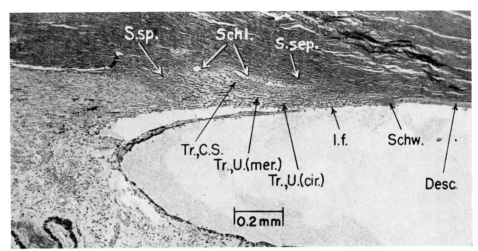

Figure 232. Inner surface of peripheral cornea, corneoscleral trabecula, and angle of anterior chamber: Desc.. Descemet's membrane; Schw., ring of Schwalbe; S. sep., scleral septum; Schl., canal of Schlemm; Tr., C. S., corneoscleral trabecula; Tr., U. (mer.), uveal trabecular fibers related to the meridional ciliary muscle fibers; Tr., U. (cir.), uveal trabecular fibers related to the radial and circular ciliary muscle fibers; S. sp., scleral spur. From **Burian, Braley, and Allen (1955).**

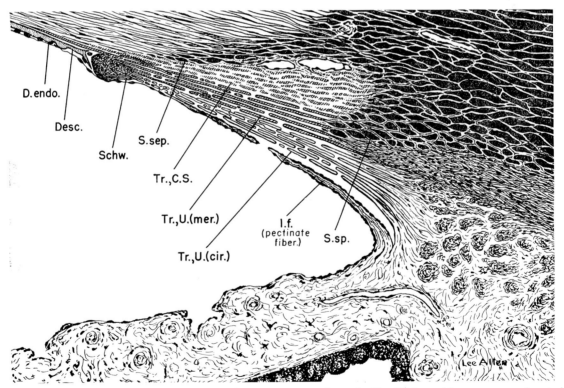

Figure 233. Semischematic representation of same structures shown in Fig. 232 but with a more prominent **ring of Schwalbe.** From Burian, Braley, and Allen (1955).

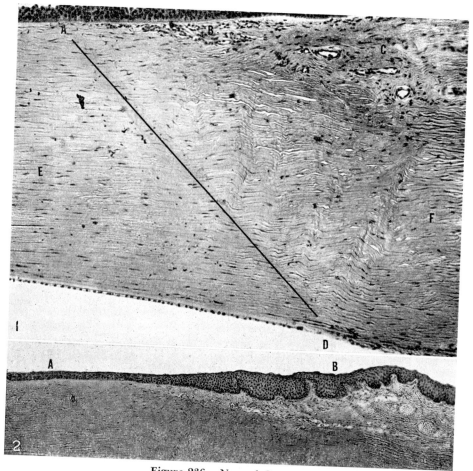

Figure 236. Normal Cornea

1. Limbus. A, end of Bowman's membrane. B, vascular loops. C, conjunctival stroma. D, end of Descemet's membrane. The diagonal line represents the limbus, or transition from cornea (E) to sclera (F). ×165. AFIP Acc. 42453.

2. Limbus. Transition from corneal (A) to conjunctival (B) epithelium. ×75. AFIP Neg. 103951.

extending over the inner surface of Descemet's membrane. In ordinary sections the cells appear almost rectangular, with a rich granular cytoplasm and a rather pale staining flattened nucleus. Morphologically this layer resembles mesothelium rather than endothelium. Electron microscopy has demonstrated that each cell is anchored to its neighbor (Fig. 234) by extensive interdigitations of the cell surfaces. This permits the endothelium to be stripped off in sheets.

The *limbus* is a transition zone, about 1 mm. wide, which is found at the periphery of the cornea. Its landmarks are ill-defined histologically except for the terminations of Bowman's membrane and Descemet's membrane which indicate the anterior and posterior extremities of its inner aspect. Clear corneal stroma extends further to the periphery

than would be indicated by a straight line drawn between the ends of Bowman's membrane and Descemet's membrane (Figs. 235, 236). This is especially true of the middle layers of the corneal stroma. More superficially the limbal capillary network extends inward close to the end of Bowman's membrane, while in the deeper layers there are the trabeculas, Schlemm's canal, its collector channels, and the deep scleral plexus. At the termination of the cornea the conjunctival epithelium increases rather rapidly to ten or more layers, with the greatest change in the basal layer, where the cells are more numerous and closely packed, and are smaller, with a scanty cytoplasm. The limbus contains numerous arterial channels from the anterior conjunctival and anterior ciliary vessels, and venous channels from the region of the ciliary body (anterior ciliary veins). The limbal stroma lacks the orderly arrangement which is characteristic of cornea and resembles ordinary connective tissue.

PHYSIOLOGY

Transparency of the cornea. The cornea is transparent, but the mechanism whereby corneal transparency is maintained is not known. The factors believed to contribute to its clarity may be divided into two categories: (1) the physical arrangement of the fibers and cells, and (2) their state of hydration.

The anterior surface of the cornea is extremely smooth because of the wetting effect of the thin film of tears with which it is covered, the regularity of the epithelium, and the absence of cornified cells. There are no blood vessels or lymphatics in the cornea and the cell membranes are in such excellent apposition that there is scarcely any intercellular fluid. There also is considerable regularity in the stromal fibers and it has been suggested by Maurice (1957) that transparency is effected by a means analogous to a diffraction grating.

The state of hydration of the cornea and sclera has been shown by Fischer and by Cogan and Kinsey to be of the utmost importance for their optical properties. The cornea normally is maintained in an extreme state of deturgescence and as such it is transparent, whereas the sclera is normally hydrated and is in consequence opaque. If the cornea is hydrated experimentally it may become as opaque as the sclera and, conversely, if the sclera is dehydrated experimentally it may become quite transparent. Under various clinical conditions, such as endothelial dystrophy and bullous keratopathy, it is the hydration or swelling of the cornea which accounts for much of its opacification.

The maintained deturgescence of the cornea distinguishes this tissue from most other tissues. The mechanism by which this is accomplished does not depend on the osmotic pressure of the interstitial fluid nor on the hydrogen ion concentration. It is only partially effected by the hydrostatic pressure. Rather, the chief factor appears to be a "pumping out" of fluid from the cornea either by an osmotic gradient across the semipermeable endothelium and epithelium, as postulated by Cogan and Kinsey, or by an active secretion, as postulated by Maurice, by Langham and Taylor, and by Harris. Whatever the mechanism, the result is a removal of the interstitial fluid and consequent optical homogeneity of the cornea. The sclera, on the other hand, has no pump-like mechanism and the accumulation of interstitial fluid results in multiple reflecting surfaces with consequent opacity.

According to Meyer and Chaffee, a further factor of probable significance for the optical properties of the cornea is the presence of sulfated polysaccharides that are absent from the sclera, but as yet the role of these constituents has not been elucidated.

Permeability of the cornea. The epithelium and endothelium are semipermeable membranes that do not permit the passive transfer of purely water-soluble substances but are freely permeable to fat-soluble substances. The corneal stroma, on the other hand, is freely permeable to water-soluble substances but not to purely fat-soluble substances. Therefore, only those substances will traverse the entire cornea which have both lipoid and water solubilities at neutral hydrogen ion concentration. This applies to most alkaloids and other weak electrolytes which are used in ophthalmic therapy.

The only exception to the foregoing generalization is water itself, for water as studied with D_2O will pass readily through the surface membranes despite the lack of lipid solubility.

Metabolism of the cornea. The cornea is avascular and normally blood vessels do not penetrate the peripheral stroma more than 0.75 to 1.0 mm. Metabolites reach the tissue by diffusional processes from the limbal capillaries, the aqueous humor and the tears. The oxygen uptake of the cornea, when computed per milligram wet weight, is small compared to that of many active tissues. Nine-tenths of the oxygen uptake of the cornea, however, is by the epithelium, and when the respiration of the corneal epithelium alone is computed, it is similar to that of liver. The relatively high consumption of oxygen indicates that the corneal epithelium is the site of the active aerobic metabolism. It appears that the cytochrome system is functioning since the oxygen uptake is sensitive to cyanide. The corneal epithelium is capable of consuming glucose, glycogen, lactate, and pyruvate. Under anaerobic conditions, lactate is produced in amounts equivalent to the glucose and glycogen lost. Glycolysis is inhibited by fluoride and iodo-acetate, and under these circumstances phosphate esters accumulate, indicating that the glycolytic system follows the usual pathways. Under aerobic conditions the pattern of glucose metabolism in corneal epithelium is usually different in that 35 per cent of the glucose metabolized is by the hexose monophosphate shunt pathway and 65 per cent by the conventional glycolytic mechanism. According to Kinoshita et al., it appears that the corneal epithelium has one of the most active shunt mechanisms ever observed.

In contrast to the active aerobic metabolism of the epithelium, the stroma has no oxygen uptake and can utilize neither lactate nor pyruvate. Nevertheless, it is capable of utilizing glucose at a rate per cell of about twice that of the epithelium. Lactate is produced by the stroma but cannot be consumed by it. In the isolated cornea the lactate produced by the stroma is thought to be utilized by the epithelium and constitutes an appreciable fraction (perhaps 25 per cent) of the total carbohydrate supply of the epithelium. Moreover, the aerobic glucose consumption of the stroma with the epithelium in place appears to be somewhat less than in the freshly denuded stroma, indicating a control of glycolysis in the stroma by the oxidative metabolism of the adjacent epithelium. This is analogous to the familiar intracellular Pasteur effect.

The denuded corneal stroma, however, rapidly loses its ability to utilize glucose, and an examination of the distribution of phosphate esters in the tissues suggests that the failure in glucose consumption is due to an exhaustion of the capacity of the tissue to transfer phosphate from glycerophosphate to hexoses. It may be concluded, therefore, that the epithelium normally assists the stroma in maintaining a supply of carriers for energy-rich phosphate transfers.

There is, then, a complex metabolic exchange between the corneal stroma and epithelium. It seems most likely that the cornea is not unique in this respect, and that complex metabolic interactions may be present in many tissues where adjacent cells of different structural and functional types are components of a highly organized integrated structure. Studies in this field have been carried further in respect to the cornea than to many other tissues. The significance of such interactions is obvious in pathologic processes in which the death or disease of some cells results in changes in their neighbors.

The origin of the nutritional fluid in the cornea has received considerable attention. It is probable that this fluid enters the cornea from several sources. Gruber, in 1894, produced rust spots in the corneas of cats with pieces of iron wire and, by subsequently injecting potassium ferrocyanide into the circulation, caused the spots to turn blue from the periphery to the center while the aqueous remained uncolored. This diffusion from the vessels had been previously observed by Leber in 1873. Laqueur, in 1872, had demonstrated that a similar passage of substances from the aqueous, entering the periphery and diffusing towards the center of the cornea, could occur when ferrocyanide was injected into the anterior chamber. The work of Cogan and his co-workers strengthened the evidence that the cornea probably receives the greater part of its nutritional fluid from the limbal vascular plexus. The tears, which contain approximately 50 milligrams of glucose per 100 cc., also may contribute to the nutrition of the cornea. Herrmann and Hickman have shown that in vitro the cornea is capable of imbibing glucose when the epithelial surface is irrigated with a solution of this material. It is possible also that the cornea, at least under unusual circumstances, may receive some nutritional components from the aqueous. Evidence for this is the continued viability of corneal grafts, with over half of the cornea replaced, when the donor cornea is connected with the recipient only by a fibrinous clot for two or three days after operation. Further indirect evidence of the continued survival of the stromal cells has been supplied by the experiments of Gunderson with free-floating implants of the cornea in the anterior chamber.

Fischer has shown that the cornea takes up oxygen from the outside air and discharges carbon dioxide. Friedenwald and Pierce confirmed his finding that carbon dioxide normally escapes from the aqueous via the cornea, but they were unable to show that the oxygen passed from the outside air through the cornea into the aqueous at the normally existing partial pressures of oxygen in the aqueous and in air. This in no way contradicts the evidence for direct uptake of oxygen by the corneal epithelium for its own endogenous respiration. It would seem that the corneal epithelium normally utilizes the oxygen from the air but may be able to accommodate itself to a diminished oxygen supply for periods of many hours.

ANATOMIC LANDMARKS*

"The limbus generally is used as the anatomic landmark for the placement of incisions for glaucoma surgery. But a review of the literature reveals that the limbus as a surgical landmark has a different meaning for different authors. Yet one finds such explicit statements as 'The incision for iridectomy should be started one millimeter behind the limbus.' From where should such a crucial millimeter be measured? The limbus is not a sharp linear junction but a zone of transition which itself may be more than a millimeter wide.

"Anterior border of the limbus. Published diagrams indicate that many authors when referring to the limbus as a landmark mean the junction of the limbal and corneal epithelium; that is, the anterior border of the limbus. The vague terminology evolved from the time when prepared flaps of conjunctiva and Tenon's capsule were seldom used in the performance of iridectomy or cataract extraction. Instead, the keratome or Graefe-knife incision was made through the conjunctiva and stroma with a single stroke.

"The posterior stromal border of the true limbus often could not be used as a landmark with such techniques because it was covered by the limbal epithelium and forward extension of Tenon's capsule. Therefore, it is understandable that the junction of the limbal and corneal epithelium became the landmark designated by surgeons as the limbus.

"Anterior border as a landmark. Even if

---

* Quoted from: Swan, K.: Surgical Anatomy in Relation to Glaucoma: In: Symposium on Glaucoma, edited by Clark, W. B., St. Louis, C. V. Mosby Co., 1959, pp. 41–43.

this terminology were not confusing to beginning surgeons, the anterior border of the limbus still is not an ideal landmark for determining the position of the structures of the chamber angle. It varies markedly in different persons. Also, it extends further onto the surface of clear corneal stroma superiorly and inferiorly than it does medially and laterally. The surface outline of clear cornea is a horizontal oval; the internal border of the cornea at Schwalbe's line forms an almost perfect circle.

"The junction of limbal stroma and sclera, once it is exposed, is a more constant and trustworthy surgical landmark for localizing the structures of the chamber angle.

"Inclination of anterior border. By definition the limbus is the peripheral transitional zone of the cornea. Under the microscope the anterior border corresponds to a line drawn from the end of Bowman's membrane to the end of Descemet's membrane. At the superior limbus of most eyes, this line will be almost parallel to the visual axis rather than perpendicular to the corneal surface."

Swan has shown that if an incision is made perpendicular to the surface of the globe at the junction of corneal and limbal epithelium, it actually is entirely in clear corneal stroma and enters the anterior chamber through Descemet's membrane and the endothelium anterior to the trabecula (Fig. 237).

"Posterior border of the limbus. Often the posterior border of the limbus cannot be seen through the conjunctiva and Tenon's capsule in the normal young adult. It is readily visible, however, in patients of all ages when the conjunctiva and Tenon's capsule are reflected. Then it appears as a relatively sharp line of demarcation between the bluish semitransparent limbal stroma and the opaque white scleral fibers. In my opinion this junction is an important landmark in the anterior segment relative to placement of incisions for glaucoma and cataract surgery. If this is to be appreciated, it is necessary to return to microscopic sections.

"The posterior border of the limbus is difficult to recognize under the microscope. It is delineated by variations in the size and direction of the stromal fibers. Some fibers appear in cross section as they pass in a circular direction around the cornea. It can be seen that

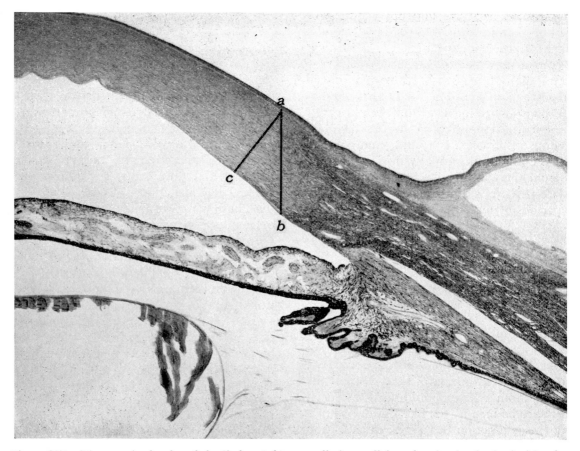

Figure 237. The anterior border of the limbus (a-b) generally is parallel to the visual axis. An incision begun at the anterior border of the limbus superiorly (point a) and made perpendicular to the surface will be entirely corneal and will enter the anterior chamber (point c), a considerable distance anterior to Schwalbe's line (point b) (modified from Swan, 1959). ×26. AFIP Acc. 630832.

on the outer surface of the globe the scleral fibers extend further forward than they do on the inside of the globe. In most eyes, the posterior border of the limbus runs, as does the anterior border, roughly parallel to the visual axis rather than perpendicular to the surface of the globe.

"Incision from the posterior limbal border. In most eyes an incision made perpendicular to the surface of the stroma at the junction of the limbus and sclera will be entirely in the avascular limbal stroma. It will enter the anterior chamber just in front of Schlemm's canal and just behind the posterior determination of Descemet's membrane. That is, it will pass through the anterior, nonfunctional part of the trabecula (Fig. 238). I believe this to be the ideal point of entry of incisions for iridectomy and cataract extractions."

GROWTH AND AGING

During growth, little change is seen in the corneal epithelium and endothelium. The stroma, which contains many nuclei at birth (Fig. 239), shows a moderate thickening and increased density of the fibers during early growth and a proportionate decrease in the number of nuclei.

With advancing age the cornea becomes thinner and flatter. The refractive index increases due to condensation of the stroma. Small localized exaggerations of this phenomenon produce scattered dust-like opacities in the deep stroma known biomicroscopically as cornea farinata. A specific histologic counterpart of this change has not been described.

The eyes of older people may show small basophilic or calcific deposits histologically just peripheral to the termination of Bowman's membrane (Fig. 240). A condition called crocodile shagreen in which a faint geographical or mosaic pattern appears either in Bowman's or in Descemet's membrane may appear clinically and is thought to be due to a variation in the thickness and transparency of these membranes in old age. Vision rarely is affected and Müller has described a case of anterior crocodile shagreen following trauma in which there were ruptures in Bowman's membrane. Histopathologic studies apparently have not been made in cases of posterior crocodile shagreen.

Arcus senilis is the most common of all senile changes in the cornea. Clinically it first appears as an opaque zone of lipoid infiltration near the corneal periphery superiorly and inferiorly and eventually forms a complete ring around the corneal periphery. The arcus is separated from the limbus by a narrow band of comparatively clear cornea. It shows a sharp edge on its limbal margin and a fading edge on the corneal margin.

Arcus senilis cannot be recognized in ordinary hematoxylin and eosin sections, but with such a fat stain as Sudan III, the presence mainly of intracellular and lesser amounts of extracellular fat globules can be shown. This lipoid material is concentrated in two wedge-shaped portions of the corneal stroma, the apices of which are directed toward the midstroma. One is adjacent to Bowman's membrane (Fig. 241), the other near Descemet's membrane. Both of these corneal membranes show a heavy concentration of stainable fat. Large and small globules are seen anteriorly, in and between the lamellas, in the corneal cells, and in macrophages.

The relation of hypercholesteremia to arcus

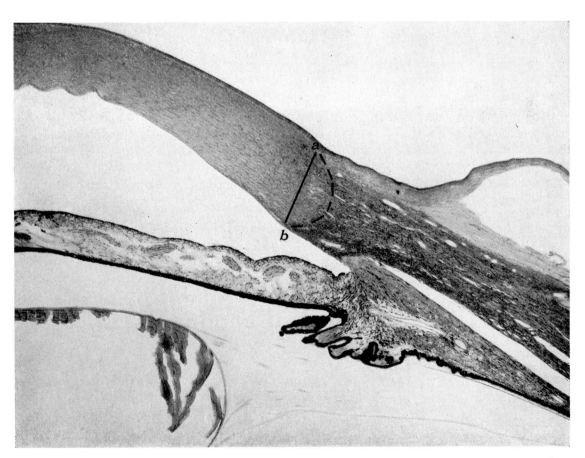

Figure 238. The posterior border of the limbus (broken line) varies, but in most eyes an incision started at the junction of semitransparent limbal stroma and opaque sclera (point a) will pass through the anterior end of the trabecula (point b) in front of Schlemm's canal and the deep scleral plexus to enter the anterior chamber at its narrowest part (modified from Swan, 1959). ×26. AFIP Acc. 630832.

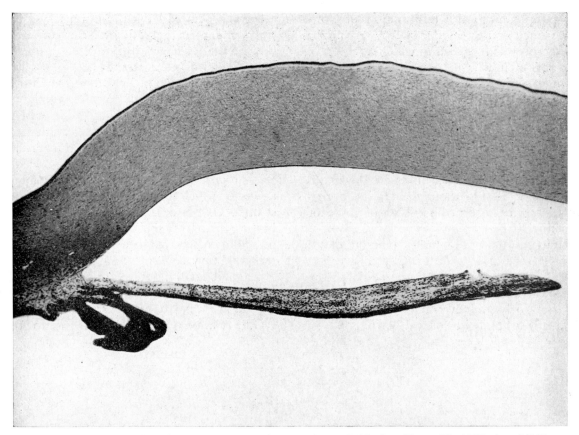

Figure 239. Cornea in infancy: many corneal corpuscles and thin lamellas. ×55. AFIP Acc. 74538.

senilis is not a direct one. In rabbits a high cholesterol diet will produce histologic lesions which are similar to arcus senilis, but analyses of the lipids present in the corneas of these animals as well as in human disease shows that cholesterol makes up only a small fraction of the lipids present. Patients with juvenile arcus may show a high blood cholesterol or evidence of disturbance in fat metabolism, whereas those with arcus senilis have a normal fat metabolism.

Another change due to aging is the presence of small hyaline excrescences, Hassall-Henle warts, in the periphery of Descemet's membrane (Fig. 242). These localized nodular thickenings are comparable to drusen of the lamina vitrea of the choroid. Garron and Feeney have shown these warts to contain a 1000A banded material, probably collagen, which shows numerous cracks and fissures containing extrusions or extensions of the corneal endothelium. They are rarely seen be-

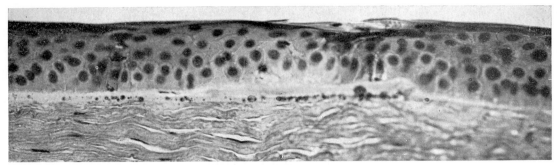

Figure 240. Aging: Cornea

Basophilic deposits about periphery of Bowman's membrane may be associated with aging. ×230. AFIP Acc. 103975.

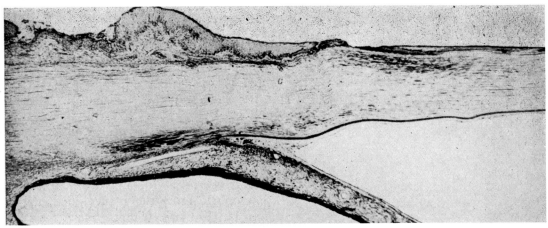

Figure 241. Aging: Cornea

Deposits of fat (dark areas) in limbal tissues and in Descemet's membrane in arcus senilis. Eye was enucleated because of secondary glaucoma. Frozen section stained for fat. ×51. AFIP Acc. 28911.

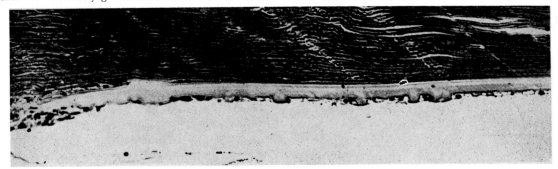

Figure 242. Aging: Cornea

Hassall-Henle warts: focal thickenings of Descemet's membrane. ×230. AFIP Acc. 103975

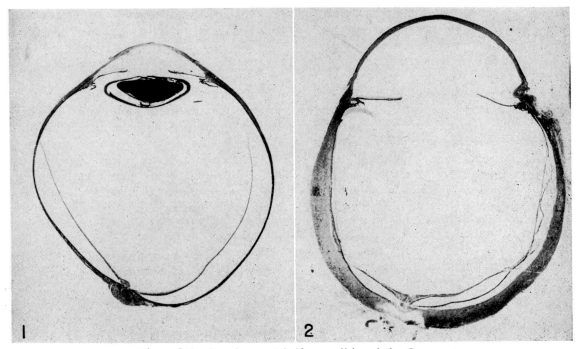

Figure 243. Developmental Abnormalities of the Cornea

1. Microcornea. ×4. AFIP Acc. 53045.
2. Megalocornea. ×3. AFIP Acc. 139158.

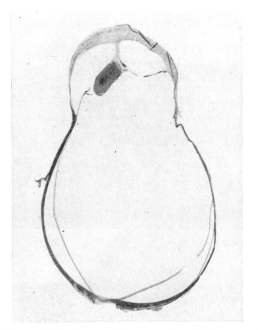

Figure 244. Congenital corneal staphyloma. ×2. AFIP Acc. 133050.

fore the age of twenty and increase in number with advancing age.

CONGENITAL ABNORMALITIES

Megalocornea. Megalocornea (anterior megalophthalmos) is a nonprogressive congenital enlargement of the anterior segment of the eye (Fig. 243–2). It is more common in males, and its inheritance is recessive and sex-linked. It usually is bilateral. The corneal diameter usually measures between 13 and 18 mm. The cornea is clear and is normal histologically. The anterior chamber is deep and there are no tears in Descemet's membrane. Occasionally posterior embryotoxon or a Krukenberg spindle may be present. The ciliary region is enlarged; the zonular fibers often are stretched and lax, and a subluxation or dislocation of the lens with a tremulous iris frequently is present. The findings of arachnodactyly may be present. In the early stage the intraocular pressure is normal but glaucoma or cataract may develop. Megalocornea probably is due to enlargement of the ciliary region due to temporary changes in the growth rates of the various parts of the optic cup.

The relationship between megalocornea and keratoconus on the one hand and megalo-cornea and keratoglobus on the other has been discussed by many, some believing that keratoglobus is but an exaggerated form of megalocornea, and others that keratoconus may become diffuse, with peripheral thinning and stretching, producing the picture of keratoglobus. It may be that all these conditions are closely related, and merely represent variants of a common hereditary defect. The association with arachnodactyly would suggest this.

Microcornea. In microcornea (anterior microphthalmus) the corneal diameter usually is less than 10 mm., but the cornea is transparent and has a normal histologic structure (Fig. 243–1). It is the result of an arrest of development after the fifth month. The anterior segment of the eye frequently is shortened, and there is a tendency to develop glaucoma. True microcornea is unassociated with other ocular deformities and seems to have a recessive type of inheritance.

Congenital corneal opacities. Congenital corneal opacities may be localized or diffuse and involve the superficial or deep cornea. They may occur in association with microphthalmus, anterior synechias, persistence of the vascular pupillary membrane, coloboma of the iris or anterior choroid, or with teratomatous changes.

Some congenital *leukomas* are dense, and situated deep in the central cornea, with an adherent iris. Descemet's membrane usually is defective in the region of the opacity. In some the leukoma seems to be due to a defect in development; in others the findings suggest an intrauterine inflammation. The exact embryologic basis for the development of these opacities is not known. Birth injuries of the cornea can lead to scarring which may be indistinguishable from true congenital leukoma. A defect which is closely related to congenital leukoma is congenital anterior staphyloma. This is characterized by a conical or spherical protrusion of a diffusely scarred cornea which is lined by iris. Bowman's and Descemet's membranes and the stroma are missing or are severely damaged; the iris is atrophic and adherent to the cornea; the lens may be deformed and cataractous, and the ciliary body is atrophic (Fig. 244).

Embryotoxon. Posterior embryotoxon (Axenfeld, 1920) is a congenital opacity at the

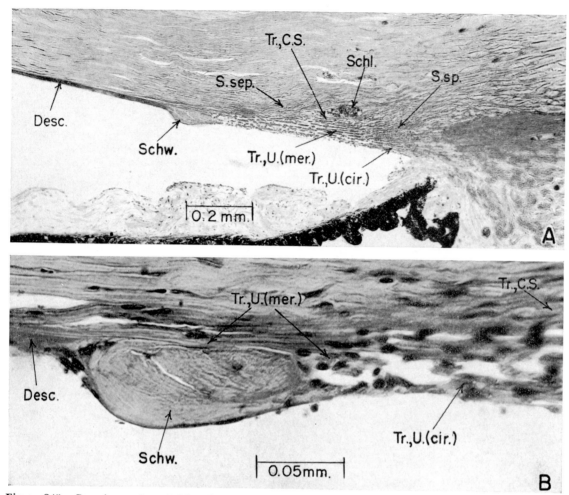

Figure 245. Prominent ring of Schwalbe without anomalous development of anterior chamber angle may be found in 15 per cent of eyes. Desc., Descemet's membrane; Schw., ring of Schwalbe; S. sep., scleral septum; Schl., Schlemm's canal; Tr., C. S., corneoscleral trabecula; Tr., U. (mer.), uveal trabecular fibers related to the meridional ciliary muscle fibers; Tr., U. (cir.), uveal trabecular fibers related to the radial and circular ciliary muscle fibers; S. sp., scleral spur. From Burian, Braley, and Allen (1955).

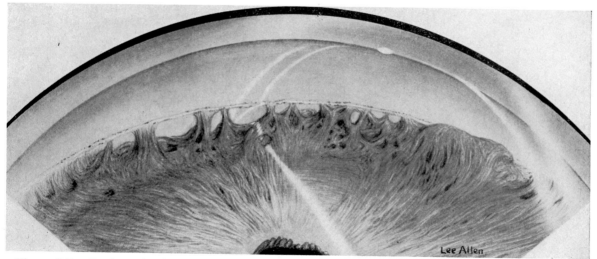

Figure 246. Gonioscopic view of lower quadrant of left eye of a 25 year old woman who had posterior embryotoxon and massive iris processes with an associated congenital glaucoma. From Burian, Braley, and Allen (1955).

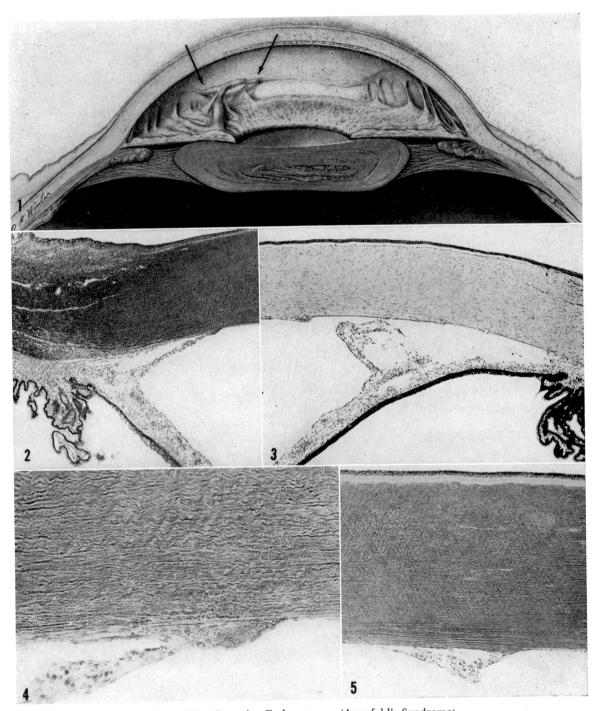

Figure 247. Posterior Embryotoxon (Axenfeld's Syndrome)

1. There is irregular thickening of Schwalbe's ring which is located more centrally than normal. Thick ropy cords of iris stroma cross the anterior chamber to become inserted into this structure. A portion of Schwalbe's ring is separated from the cornea (arrows).

2, 3, 4 and 5. Photomicrographs prepared from same eye shown in 1. ×56, ×50, ×305, and ×115, respectively AFIP Acc. 83124.

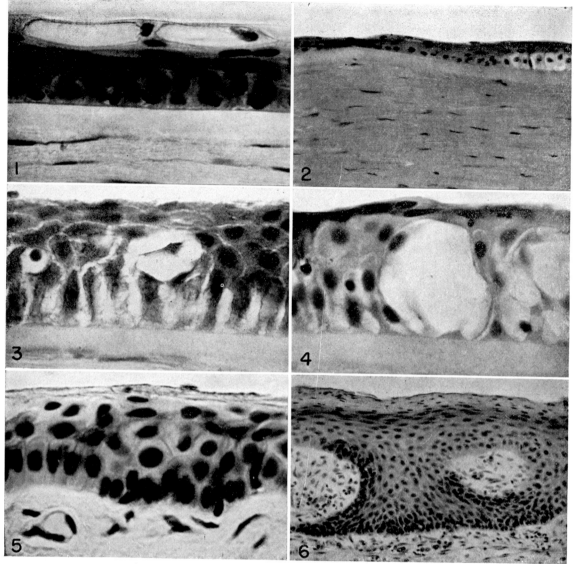

Figure 248.   Edema and Hyperplasia of Corneal Epithelium

1. Intracellular edema of superficial cells. Polymorphonuclear leukocytes in basal layer. ×700. AFIP Acc. 50449.

2. Intracellular edema of basal layer, right. Pitting of epithelium resulting from edema, left. ×175. AFIP Acc. 55491.

3. Intracellular edema of polyhedral cells. Intercellular edema of cells of basal layer. ×600. AFIP Acc. 59128.

4. Vesicle formation. ×600. AFIP Acc. 56558.

5. Irregularities and early hyperplasia in area of destruction of Bowman's membrane in old syphilitic keratitis. Note blood vessel in substantia. ×765. AFIP Acc. 42996.

6. Hyperplasia of epithelium in chronic keratitis with destruction of Bowman's membrane. ×220. AFIP Acc. 59579.

level of Descemet's membrane arising as a congenital variation or anomaly of the size and position of the anterior border ring of Schwalbe (Fig. 245). A number of variants have been described. Usually the anterior border ring is thickened and displaced axially so that when the observer views the cornea from in front, clear cornea is seen peripheral to the opacity. Frequently large abnormal iris processes or broad sheets of tissue of varying distribution and size extend from the iris to the cornea (Fig. 246, 247). Microscopically there most often is hypertrophy of the collagenous tissue which constitutes the anterior border ring. A veil-like tissue may be present between Schwalbe's ring and the periphery of

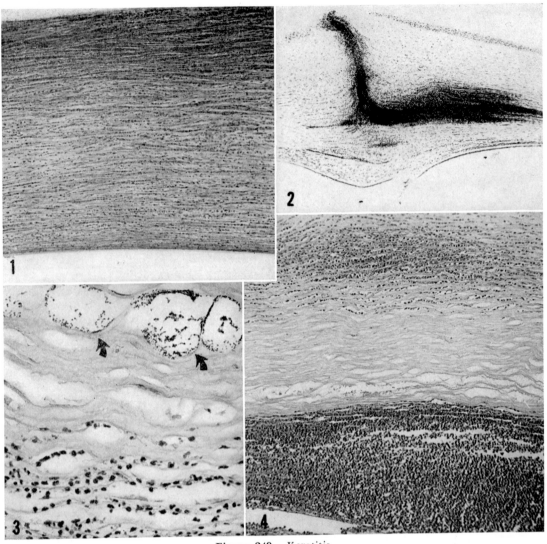

Figure 249. Keratitis

1. Acute diffuse keratitis with necrosis of superficial lamellas. Infiltration of all layers by polymorphonuclear leukocytes. ×125. AFIP Acc. 194376.

2. Abscess in infected corneal wound. ×100. AFIP Acc. 24075.

3. Colonies of gram-positive cocci (arrows) deep in corneal stroma (same case shown in 4). ×305.

4. Acute bacterial keratitis with pus in anterior chamber (hypopyon). ×100. AFIP Acc. 956284.

the cornea. This tissue consists of partially differentiated trabecular fibers. Strands of pigmented connective tissue extend backward a short distance to become continuous with the iris stroma. In some cases the angle structures and trabecular area are relatively normal. In others there is defective development of these structures and glaucoma is present (see Chapter XII).

Dermoid tumors have been considered in the previous chapter.

INFLAMMATIONS OF THE CORNEA

General. The transparency and lack of vessels in the cornea modify the symptoms due to inflammation and the evolution of clinical changes. Epithelial edema almost always is present in corneal inflammation and varies from mild edema to frank vesicle formation (Fig. 248).

The edema produces a loss of corneal transparency. In superficial lesions edema is due to the absorption of relatively hypotonic tears, and in deep stromal lesions it may be due to endothelial injury. Edema of the epithelium appears clinically as fine vesicles and edema of the stroma produces a diffuse haziness.

In most corneal inflammations hyperemia of the limbal vessels occurs. The continuity of the episcleral vessels with those of the iris leads to reflex dilatation and inflammation of the iris. Some severe corneal inflammations cause an outpouring of leukocytes from the iris into the anterior chamber, producing a hypopyon.

Polymorphonuclear leukocytes migrate into the area of corneal injury from the dilated limbal vessels within eight to twelve hours. Because of the laminated structure of the corneal stroma superficial lesions in the cornea attract cells from the superficial limbal vessels and deep lesions attract cells from vessels of the deep limbal plexus. Thus, in some inflammations, either the superficial or deep layers or all layers of the cornea may be involved and if the lamellas have not become too disturbed, the invading cells remain between the layers where they gained entrance (Fig. 249). Within twelve to twenty-four hours following the onset macrophages which originate from the limbus and from the corneal stromal cells appear at the site of the injury. These cells ingest the invading organisms, the dying polymorphonuclear leukocytes, and the destroyed corneal tissue. During the healing phase the corneal stroma contains many lymphocytes and plasma cells (Fig. 250).

Vascularization of the cornea occurs if the inflammation is severe and accompanied by necrosis. The agent responsible for budding and migration of the limbal blood vessels into the corneal tissue is not known. Edema certainly is a factor and in some instances capillary tufts can be seen at the limbus near a swollen stroma but not in more normal adjacent areas.

Vascularization of the cornea proceeds in one of two ways: (1) small aneurysms form on the capillaries and burst, the endothelium migrating to surround the hemorrhage; (2) the endothelial cells may proliferate to form buds or sprouts which lengthen into the stromal tissue and become canalized. The capillaries, like the inflammatory cells, have little tendency to migrate beyond the area of injured corneal tissue. In epithelial lesions or in superficial stromal lesions, therefore, the vascularization is superficial, whereas in deeper corneal inflammations the vessels extend into the deeper layers of the stroma. Once vascularization of the cornea has occurred, the inflammatory reaction is essentially similar to that of other vascularized tissue (Fig. 251).

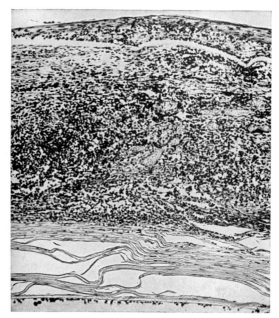

Figure 250. Keratitis

Chronic active keratitis, involving outer and middle layers. Keratic precipitates. ×50. AFIP Acc. 163398.

Bowman's membrane is not an effective barrier to bacterial invasion, but Descemet's membrane is an excellent one. Ulcers of the cornea may destroy the stroma down to the level of Descemet's membrane. This membrane may be effective in preventing perforation of the cornea for a number of days but it often bulges, forming a descemetocele. Descemet's membrane does not form an effective barrier to diffusion of toxic substances, for in many corneal ulcers a sterile anterior chamber hypopyon appears as a result of irritation of the iris.

Nonulcerative Corneal Inflammation

Nonulcerative corneal inflammations may be divided into a number of types:
1. Epithelial
2. Subepithelial
3. Stromal

Epithelial keratitis. Epithelial keratitis without ulceration is uncommon, and occurs in viral diseases such as superficial punctate keratitis, and the occasional keratitis associated with adenovirus type III infections.

SUPERFICIAL PUNCTATE KERATITIS. The epithelial infiltrates in *superficial punctate keratitis* are discrete, scattered over the central

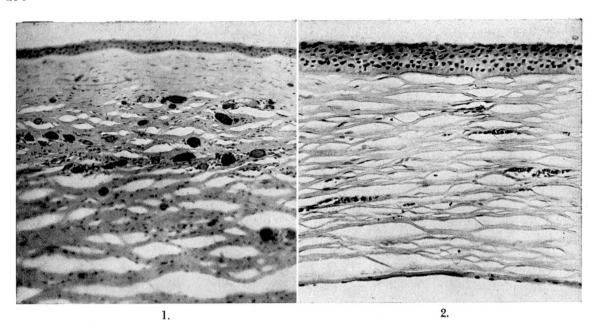

1.　　　　　　　　　　　　　　　　　　　　　　2.

Figure 251. Keratitis, Old

1. Vascularization of outer corneal lamellas in chronic keratitis. Bowman's membrane intact. Epithelial atrophy. ×125. AFIP Acc. 68569.

2. Vascularization of substantia following interstitial keratitis. Destruction of Bowman's membrane. Slight irregularities in arrangement of epithelial cells. ×275. AFIP Acc. 331369.

two-thirds of the cornea, and approximately 0.5 mm. in diameter. Microscopic examination of these infiltrates shows edema and swelling of the corneal epithelial cells, intercellular edema, and exudate under the epithelium. Polymorphonuclear leukocytes are seen in moderate numbers, depending on the degree of inflammation, but after the first one or two days the cellular infiltrate is of the lymphocytic type.

SUPERFICIAL EPITHELIAL EROSIONS. Superficial epithelial erosions often have been called superficial punctate keratitis. These erosions show small areas of edema and degeneration of the superficial cells and the changes are secondary to any type of inflammation of the conjunctiva. The eroded areas stain with fluorescein in a diffuse punctate pattern.

Subepithelial keratitis. EPIDEMIC KERATOCONJUNCTIVITIS. Subepithelial keratitis is typified by the infiltrates which occur in epidemic keratoconjunctivitis, in peripheral marginal infiltration, and in leprosy. The infiltrates of epidemic keratoconjunctivitis are 0.5 to 1.5 mm. in diameter and usually are located in the central two-thirds of the cornea. During the acute stage there is edema of the stromal fibers close to the region of Bowman's membrane with splitting of the collagen fibers, and secondary degeneration. Edema and swelling also occur in Bowman's membrane. After a few days some lymphocytic infiltration occurs. Healing is accompanied by proliferation of the fixed corneal cells to replace the defect, leaving a macular scar which persists for two to four years.

PERIPHERAL MARGINAL INFILTRATION. The infiltrates in *peripheral marginal infiltration* often lie close to the epithelium, but may be deeper. They are 1 to 2 mm. in diameter, and microscopic examination shows necrosis of the corneal tissue and infiltration by polymorphonuclear leukocytes. Healing occurs by fibroblastic proliferation. Occasional infiltrates extend toward the surface and rupture through the epithelium.

LEPROSY. *Leprotic* superficial punctate keratitis is characterized by infiltration of groups of lepra bacilli between the lamellas of the cornea under Bowman's membrane. They are surrounded by necrotic lamellas and an accumulation of polymorphonuclear leukocytes. Bowman's membrane may be eroded, and the nodules of bacilli then involve the epithelium. Healing is accompanied by scar formation.

TRACHOMA FOLLICLES. The virus of trachoma can affect the cornea and limbus, as well as the conjunctiva. With a loupe, and with the slit lamp microscope the upper limbus often shows follicles in the active stage. The follicles are composed of masses of lymphocytes, which surround a germinal center of reticuloendothelial cells. They may rupture or persist for months, following which they regress, leaving depressed, round scars (Herbert's pits).

TRACHOMA PANNUS. Vascularization and infiltration of the limbus and cornea superiorly produces the typical *corneal pannus*, which appears in stage two of the disease. The early lesions consist of edema and desquamation of the corneal epithelial cells, polymorphonuclear and lymphocytic infiltration beneath the epithelium in the region of Bowman's membrane, gradual destruction of the periphery of this membrane, and vascularization of the affected area, including the ad-

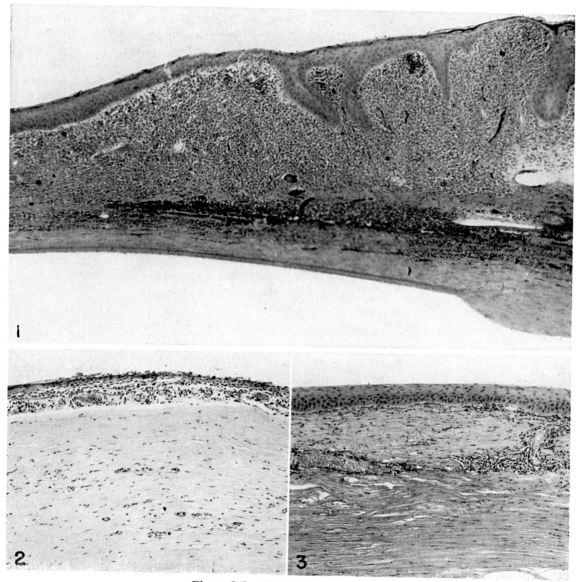

Figure 252. Trachomatous Pannus

1. Dense chronic inflammatory cell infiltration of conjunctiva. Inflammatory tissue extending beneath corneal epithelium and outer corneal lamellas. ×105. AFIP Acc. 28910.

2. Vascular inflammatory membrane between corneal epithelium and Bowman's membrane. Vascularization of substantia. ×75. AFIP Acc. 204432.

3. Dense, vascular inflammatory membrane infiltrated by lymphocytes between corneal epithelium and outer lamellas of substantia. ×125. AFIP Acc. 306211.

jacent superficial lamellas. Healing is accompanied by replacement of the vascular granulation tissue by fibroblasts, with gradual disappearance of all but the larger vessels (Fig. 252).

Stromal keratitis. Stromal keratitis occurs as a result of the extension of conjunctival and superficial corneal infections to the stroma. Also, it may occur in systemic diseases, such as syphilis, tuberculosis, and sarcoidosis. The inflammation may occur primarily in the cornea, or may develop as a result of extension from the limbus, or by spread from the uveal tract. Disciform keratitis often is produced by viruses, but it may follow trauma.

HERPES ZOSTER. The virus of herpes zoster has not as yet been recovered from affected ocular tissues although it has from skin vesicles. It causes peripheral and central nervous system lesions. Involvement of the gasserian ganglion and ophthalmic division of the fifth cranial nerve are common. It is typical for vesicles to appear on the skin over the distribution of the branches of this nerve. When the nasociliary branch is affected, keratitis, scleritis, and iridocyclitis may occur. The corneal lesions are accompanied by severe pain and conjunctival hyperemia, and consist of one or more subepithelial infiltrates measuring about 0.5 mm. As the condition progresses, similar infiltrations may appear in the deeper layers of the stroma. The lesions in the superficial and deep layers may coalesce to produce a disciform keratitis. Perforation of a disciform lesion occurs at times. The primary opacities of the cornea tend to clear over a number of months, leaving only nebulous changes in the corneal tissue.

Histologically, the small opacities show edema of the stroma and a slight polymorphonuclear leukocytic infiltration. The larger opacities have a pathologic picture which is similar to that described for disciform keratitis except that the cellular infiltration is more prominent. The inflammation characteristically persists for eight months to two years and is followed by scarring (Fig. 253).

HERPES SIMPLEX. Disciform keratitis at times is a complication of dendritic keratitis, especially since the advent of steroid therapy of ocular inflammations. The evolution of the inflammation is slow and progressive, the process eventually occupying an area of 5 to 8 mm., and extending from the region of Bowman's membrane into the deeper stroma. Vessels do not invade the cornea for a considerable period, unless necrosis occurs. In the initial stages there is edema of the lamellas with accumulation of fluid within the cells and the fibers. The lamellas swell and become fragmented, and following this there is migration of polymorphonuclear leukocytes and macrophages from the limbus. This reaction soon is replaced by a lymphocytic cellular infiltrate, and in more advanced lesions one usually sees considerable destruction of the lamellas, with replacement by large numbers of lymphocytes and scattered macrophages. By this time vessels have invaded toward the necrotic foci, and typical inflammatory granulation tissue appears. Healing is very slow in such lesions, and even after the eye apparently is completely over the effects of the infection, microscopic examination shows considerable residual inflammation and repair (Fig. 253–1, 2). Examination of sections removed even one to two years after subsidence of the disease shows considerable residual inflammation. It has been postulated that recurrences of the dendritic keratitis may be favored by the reactivation of inflammation in the damaged corneal stroma.

Milder cases of disciform keratitis which are due to epidemic keratoconjunctivitis, herpes simplex, and vaccinia often subside slowly over a period of months, leaving a relatively clear and avascular cornea. There is little corneal necrosis in such cases, and repair is minimal.

SYPHILITIC INTERSTITIAL KERATITIS. Interstitial keratitis in congenital syphilis rarely is evident at birth. It usually appears between the ages of five and fifteen years as an acute inflammation, in one eye first, then in the other, of the middle stromal layers and anterior uveal tract. Only in a few instances has histologic study been possible during the active stage and organisms have not been demonstrated in the lesions. The entire cornea is thickened and edematous, with diffuse and localized lymphocytic infiltration in the middle and deeper layers of the stroma (Fig. 254). The lamellas are separated from each other by the exudation, and often show necro-

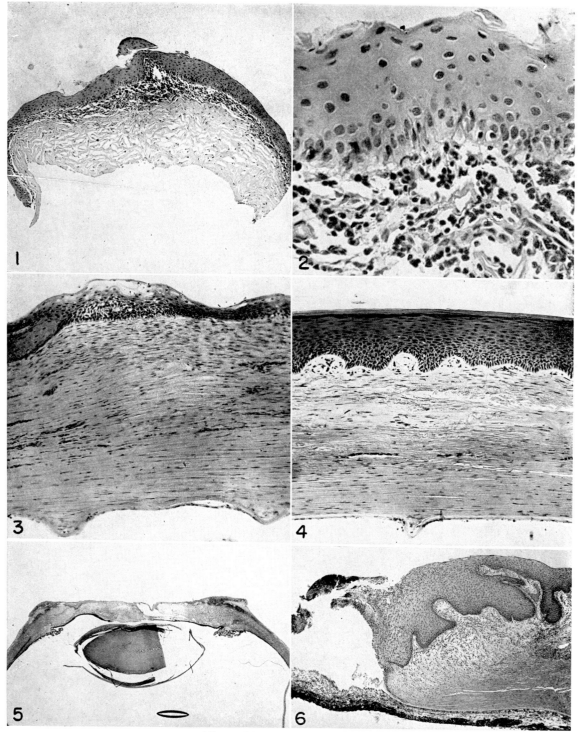

Figure 253. Herpetic Keratitis

1. Focal subepithelial lymphocytic infiltration. ×75. AFIP Acc. 66171.

2. Degenerative changes in nuclei of epithelial cells. ×400. AFIP Acc. 66171.

3. Herpes zoster ophthalmicus. Onset 6 months before enucleation. Edema of corneal epithelium. Scarring and vascularization of substantia. ×125. AFIP Acc. 73411.

4. Herpes zoster ophthalmicus. Onset 2 years before enucleation. Epidermidalization of corneal epithelium. Scarring and vascularization of substantia. Fold in Descemet's membrane. ×12. AFIP Acc. 210793.

5. Perforated corneal ulcer, sequela of herpes zoster ophthalmicus. Crater bridged by epithelium. ×5. AFIP Acc. 45518.

6. Hyperplasia of corneal epithelium at margin of perforated ulcer, sequela of herpes zoster ophthalmicus. Minimal inflammatory cell infiltration. ×48. AFIP Acc. 190716.

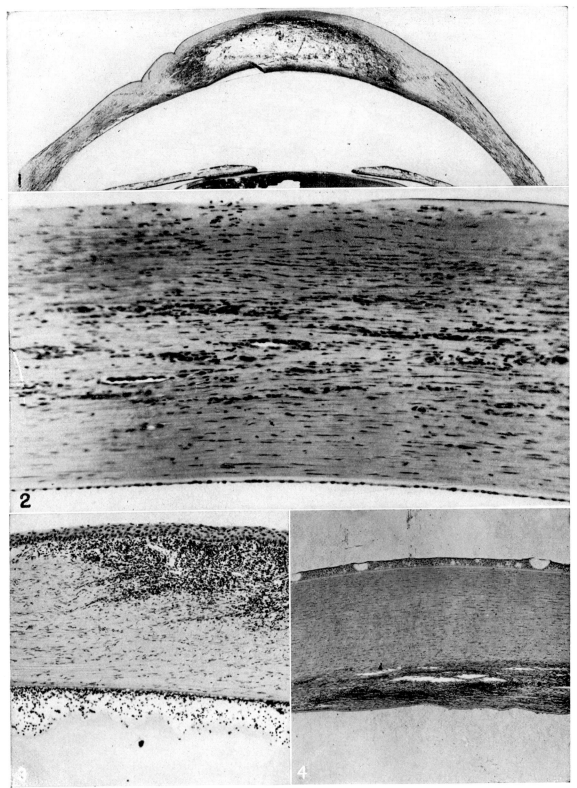

Figure 254. Syphilis

1. Interstitial keratitis. Necrosis of middle corneal lamellas. Peripheral vascularization of substantia. ×15. AFIP Acc. 42760.

2. Interstitial keratitis. Lymphocytic infiltration and vascularization of substantia. ×280. AFIP Acc. 39694.

3. Chronic keratitis. Large confluent keratic precipitates composed of lymphocytes, plasma cells and monocytes. ×125. AFIP Acc. 28905.

4. Keratitis profunda pustuliformis. Chronic inflammatory cells infiltrating deep area of necrosis. ×35. AFIP Acc. 56558.

sis. Vascularization of the cornea appears early in the deeper layers, especially in the areas of intense inflammation and necrosis. Much of the inflammatory process soon is concentrated around the newly-formed vessels. Miliary gummas occasionally are seen in the deeper layers of the cornea, in the limbal tissues, and at the root of the iris. In severe cases, necrosis of the infiltrate occurs.

At the periphery in the deeper layers the infiltration of cells and new vessels may be so intense it resembles granulation tissue (epaulet). The infiltration produces folding of Descemet's membrane, and may result in necrosis of this layer and the underlying endothelium. Newly formed connective tissue may develop deep to such damaged areas, and line the cornea. Bowman's membrane may be subjected to the same type of destruction.

Healing occurs by the phagocytosis and removal of debris by macrophages and polymorphonuclear leukocytes, proliferation of corneal fibroblasts, and gradual conversion of the damaged areas to vascularized scar. Bowman's membrane often shows large areas of destruction with fibrous replacement.

Widespread inflammation of the eye most often occurs at the time of the corneal inflammation. There is inflammation in the iris, ciliary body, trabecular area, and peripheral choroid, all leading to scarring and atrophy. At times even the posterior choroid and retina are affected. The damage to the iris and angle structures often leads to chronic secondary glaucoma, or, if this complication is not present, frequently it is precipitated later by a keratoplasty.

In healed lesions the vascular channels laid down in the cornea often persist for many years, even though they may be devoid of circulating blood. Local injury and local nonspecific inflammation may suffice to cause a reopening of these old vascular channels, leading to an apparent late relapse which may, in fact, be only a nonspecific local vasomotor reaction.

EXPERIMENTAL SYPHILITIC KERATITIS. In experimental syphilis of the rabbit, keratitis is very common and closely resembles the human lesion both clinically and histologically. It is, however, a milder disease than that of the human eye and generally heals with little or no residual scarring. The causative

organisms are readily demonstrable in the rabbit cornea by the Levaditi technique, by dark field preparations of tissue juice, and by animal inoculation.

The role of allergy in syphilitic interstitial keratitis has been studied by Rich, Chesney and Turner. Treponema pallidum produces neither an exotoxin nor an endotoxin, and can live and multiply in a nonallergic host without eliciting an inflammatory reaction. A lesion develops only after the appropriate incubation period, when the host has become allergic to the treponemal material.

PATHOGENESIS IN HUMANS. The varying course of the human disease, with its characteristically long incubation period, its primary, secondary and tertiary stages, reflects the course of the allergic and immune reactions toward the infecting organism. The mechanism of the corneal involvement in humans further is complicated by the fact that local injuries, even minor nonpenetrating injuries of the eye, appear capable of precipitating the attack of keratitis in a subject with congenital syphilis.

TUBERCULOUS INTERSTITIAL KERATITIS. It has not been clearly established that actual infection of the cornea by tubercle bacilli occurs. Interstitial inflammation does occur in tuberculous patients, but organisms never have been identified or isolated from the corneal tissue. A hypersensitivity to tuberculoprotein has been postulated as a cause for this type of inflammation. The corneal lesions of tuberculous keratitis begin in the deeper layers of the cornea, most often near the limbus. They are grayish or gray-white, of triangular shape, with the base at the limbus, and may invade the cornea 2 to 3 mm. Initially they are avascular, but cases which persist lead to vascularization. Eventually densely opaque scars form which are wedge-shaped. Exacerbations and remissions are common, and new lesions develop which either are independent foci or are extensions from an old lesion. Limbal lesions extend not only into the cornea, but also to the sclera and episclera. Anterior uveitis commonly is associated with the corneal inflammation.

LEPROSY. Interstitial keratitis may occur in lepromatous leprosy. Often it is associated with involvement of the iris and ciliary body (Fig. 255). The infiltration develops slowly

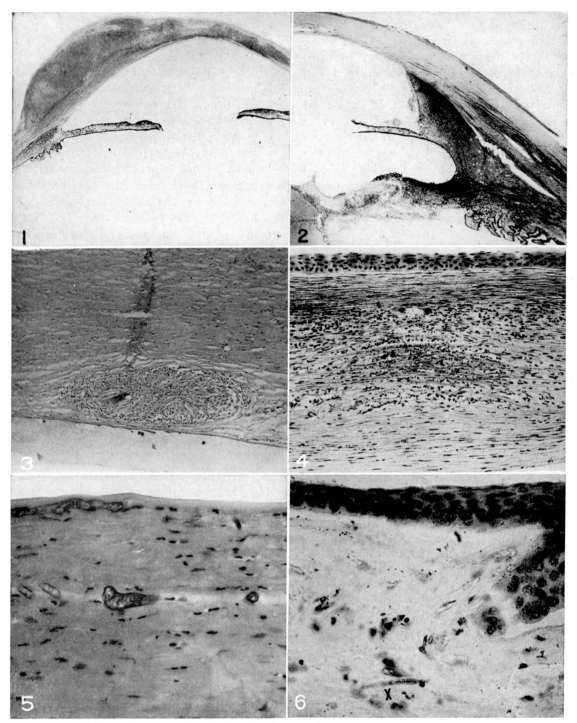

Figure 255. Specific Infections of Cornea

1. Leproma of cornea. ×7. AFIP Acc. 90780.
2. Lepromatous iridocyclitis and keratitis. ×20. AFIP Acc. 123164.
3. Miliary tubercle. ×75. AFIP Acc. 28930.
4. Interstitial keratitis, possibly tuberculous. ×125. AFIP Acc. 160975.
5. Mucormycosis. ×300. AFIP Acc. 87679.
6. Onchocerciasis with microfilaria (X) in cornea. ×400. AFIP Acc. 192365.

at the periphery as a result of extension from the deeper tissues, and gradually extends toward the center. Vascularization of the infiltrates subsequently occurs.

Keratitis also may be produced by parasites such as the filarias in onchocerciasis (Fig. 255–6).

Corneal Ulceration

Classification. Corneal ulceration due to organisms may be of bacterial, viral, or fungal origin.

BACTERIAL. Most corneal ulcers of the infectious type are caused by *bacteria*, which are introduced into the tissues following trauma (Fig. 74). With the exception of the diphtheria bacillus, gonococcus, and some Koch-Weeks organisms, bacteria cannot penetrate the intact corneal epithelium to cause ulceration. Bacterial corneal ulcers can result from infection by almost all virulent pyogenic organisms, but the most frequent offenders are the pneumococcus, beta hemolytic streptococcus, pseudomonas, Friedlander's bacillus, the diplobacillus of Petit, and the gram negative coliform organisms. Characteristically these organisms affect the central *two-thirds* of the cornea, whereas most *peripheral* corneal ulcerations are due to the staphylococcus, influenza bacillus, and the diplobacillus of Morax-Axenfeld.

VIRAL. Viral corneal ulcers are less common, because these organisms most often cause keratitis without ulceration. Herpes simplex virus produces the typical dendritic ulcer of the epithelium, and chronic disciform ulcers.

FUNGAL. Fungal corneal ulcers most often follow injury, particularly foreign bodies (Fig. 88). They may develop as a complication of treatment of a wound, a bacterial or viral ulcer, or other corneal lesions with antibiotics or corticosteroids for prolonged periods (Figs. 255–5 and 256). Ley and others have shown the enhancing effect of corticosteroids in fungal infections of the cornea in experimental animals. Open corneal wounds which receive continuous topical therapy with these drugs are likely to develop fungal infections.

A group of interesting corneal ulcers appear following injuries or such infections as dendritic keratitis. In such cases the cultures and scrapings are negative for bacteria, fungi,

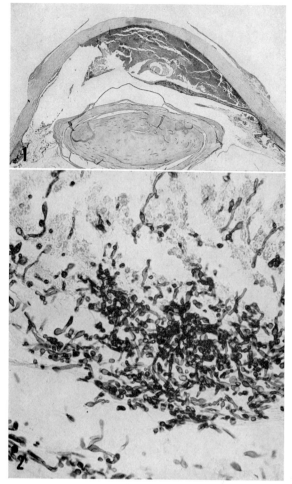

Figure 256.

Mycotic keratitis probably due to Candida sp., a complication of bullous keratopathy in a diabetic patient who had secondary glaucoma. 1. ×5. 2. ×350. Gridley fungus stain. AFIP Acc. 687652. From Haggerty and Zimmerman (1958).

or a virus. It is assumed in this group, which is typified by the chronic disciform ulcer following herpes simplex infection, that the persistence of the ulcer is due to the action of the products of the necrotic corneal lamellas.

General histopathology. Classically, three stages of corneal ulceration are described; the progressive stage, the regressive stage and the healing stage (Figs. 74, 257, 258). In the *progressive stage,* there is edema and a polymorphonuclear cellular infiltrate in the stroma. The ulcer often begins following an injury with secondary infection. The cells of the epithelium and the stroma in the area of the infection swell and undergo necrosis. The lamellas around the ulcer are infiltrated by

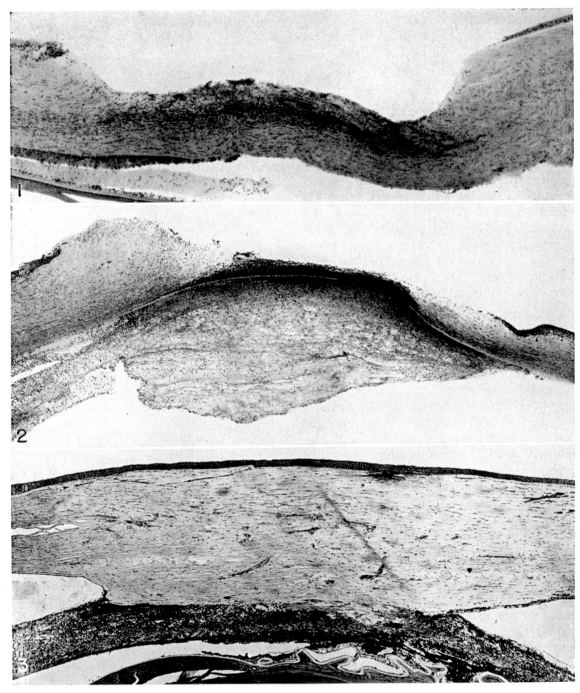

Figure 257. Corneal Ulcer

1. Purulent ulcer with deep crater. ×70. AFIP Acc. 68257.

2. Perforated purulent hypopyon ulcer. Break in Descemet's membrane. ×35. AFIP Acc. 57941.

3. Healed central perforated ulcer. Vascularization of corneal scar, adhesion of iris to cornea at site of perforation. ×40. AFIP Acc. 47276.

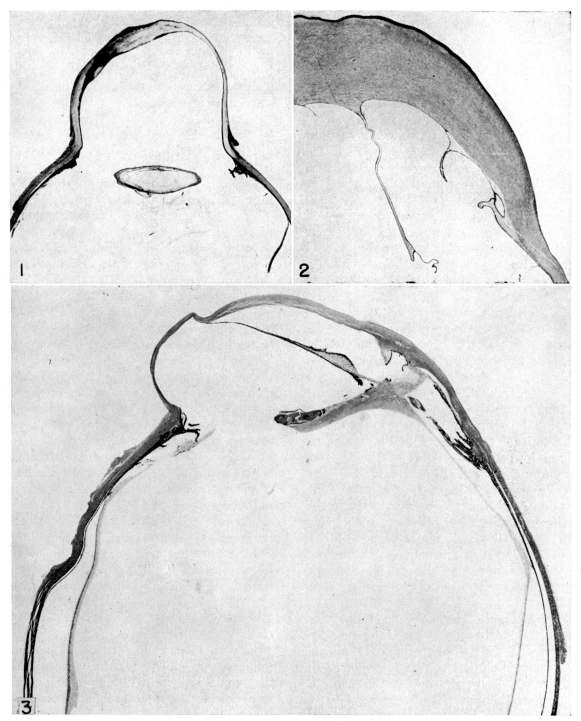

Figure 258. Corneal Staphyloma

1. Corneal staphyloma following perforated gonorrheal ulcer in newborn. Anterior chamber obliterated by bulging kerato-iridic scar. AFIP Acc. 28106.

2. Strands of iris pigment epithelium extending into posterior chamber. ×16. AFIP Acc. 37394.

3. A large staphyloma may be observed on the left while an adherent leukoma is present on the right. ×7. Univ. of Calif. Acc. 56–644.

polymorphonuclear leukocytes and soon show necrosis. Polymorphonuclear leukocytes, lymphocytes and plasma cells are seen to infiltrate the limbal tissues.

Toxins and inflammatory products diffuse toward Descemet's membrane where they are retarded, and produce a deep area of inflammation and necrosis (posterior abscess) under the ulcer. Hypopyon forms as a result of diffusion of some products into the aqueous to produce a sterile iritis.

If the superficial ulcer and deep abscess meet, the cornea is reduced to extreme thinness and Descemet's may bulge (descemetocele; keratocele) or become necrotic and rupture. Healing often is rapid following such a rupture, possibly because the lowered pressure leads to more rapid diffusion of antibodies and cells through the cornea and from the aqueous.

In the *regressive stage*, a line of demarcation forms between normal cornea and infected area and the necrotic tissue sloughs away. In the *healing stage* epithelium covers the crater, vessels migrate into the area from the limbus and the corneal cells proliferate to form connective tissue. Histiocytes also are converted to fibroblasts to assist in the repair. The entire depression eventually may be replaced by connective tissue to the level of the normal cornea. The stroma, however, usually remains thinned in the area of ulceration. With the passage of time the nuclei of the connective tissue cells tend to disappear and the small vessels gradually are obliterated. The larger vessels may remain as ghost vessels, and not carry blood. Hyaline and calcareous degeneration of the scar are common.

Specific types of corneal ulceration. DENDRITIC. Dendritic ulceration is the most frequent virus infection of the cornea. The characteristic clinical picture is produced by the growth of herpes simplex virus in the corneal epithelium. Histologically there is ulceration and Bowman's membrane may show only slight edema. The epithelial cells adjacent to the ulcer are edematous and may show the typical intranuclear inclusion bodies of Lipschutz, which are acidophilic masses occupying most of the nuclear area and surrounded by a clear zone or halo. The basophilic chromatin of the nucleus is clumped

on the nuclear membrane. Scrapings of the corneal epithelium may show multinucleated giant cells in a large number of cases. In some severe cases moderate polymorphonuclear and lymphocytic infiltration occurs beneath the epithelium in the superficial stroma. If damage to the lamellas occurs slight scarring may result.

In certain instances dendritic keratitis may be associated with development of a chronic disciform keratitis, which has been discussed (page 200).

Longstanding dendritic ulceration may be followed by stromal inflammation (Fig. 259). This type is known as a chronic postherpetic ulcer. The ulceration varies from a torpid superficial central ulcer which persists for months to a progressive enlarging ulcer which invades the deeper lamellas. Perforation is not uncommon in the latter form, and severe iritis is the rule. Microscopic examination of these chronic ulcers has been possible because they are often managed by therapeutic keratoplasty. Chronic superficial ulcers show the typical crater which is filled with fibrin, cellular debris, and epithelium in various stages of degeneration and regeneration. The adjacent lamellas show a remarkable separation by inflammatory exudate, which is composed of edema fluid, albuminous material, cellular debris, polymorphonuclear leukocytes in various stages of disintegration, and macrophages (Fig. 259). Vascularization is common. Deeper ulcers show extensive necrosis of the lamellas with massive infiltration by inflammatory cells and blood vessels. Organisms rarely, if ever, can be demonstrated in sections or cultures from the buttons obtained from such ulcers. Herpes virus cannot be demonstrated in HeLa cells or in embryonated eggs after inoculation with ground-up tissue from such ulcers. It can be assumed that either: (1) the virus produces the stromal lesion, then becomes incorporated into the nucleoprotein of the stromal cells from which it cannot be readily released, or (2) the virus does not invade the stroma, but initiates a progressive inflammation with stromal necrosis, and the products of the corneal tissue keep the disease process active. The course of the inflammation in many cases suggests that a trophic disturbance prolongs the disease.

CATARRHAL OR MARGINAL CORNEAL ULCER. Catarrhal or marginal corneal ulcer is a rather shallow and benign condition which begins either as an epithelial ulcer or as a subepithelial abscess which ulcerates. There is no tendency to spread centrally, and the ulcer usually is circumscribed. There is a strong tendency to recur. The condition is most frequently seen in association with blepharoconjunctivitis, and is due to the action of staphylococcal toxin on hypersensitive tissues. Histologically these small ulcers have the same appearance as larger central ulcers. Small scars result after healing.

RING ULCER. Ring ulcer is a more destructive and invasive corneal lesion than the simple catarrhal ulcer. Clinically the ulcer results from coalescence of separate infiltrates or ulcers at the corneal periphery and it advances circumferentially either to form a complete ring or to involve the central area. It usually is thought to be of endogenous origin,

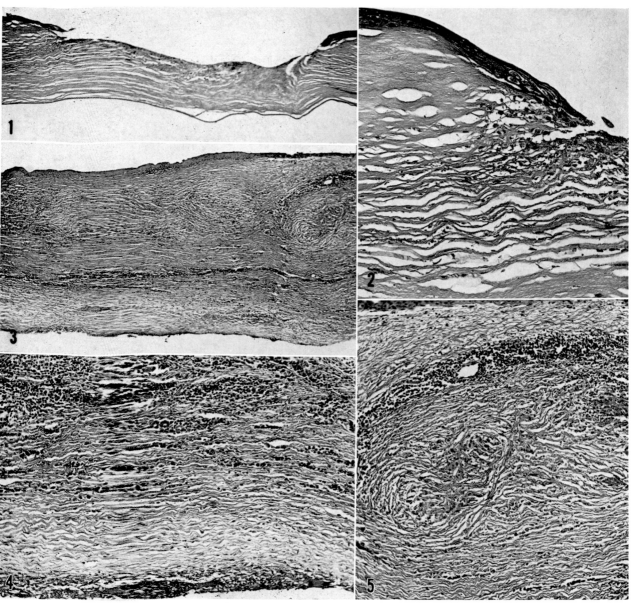

Figure 259. Chronic Herpetic Keratitis

1 and 2. Recurrent herpetic ulceration of the cornea (metaherpetic keratitis) of 17 years' duration. Univ. of Calif. Acc. 58–637. ×35 and ×165, respectively.

3, 4 and 5. Disciform keratitis 18 years after typical dendritic keratitis. Univ. of Calif. Acc. 58–9. ×40, ×115, and ×115, respectively.

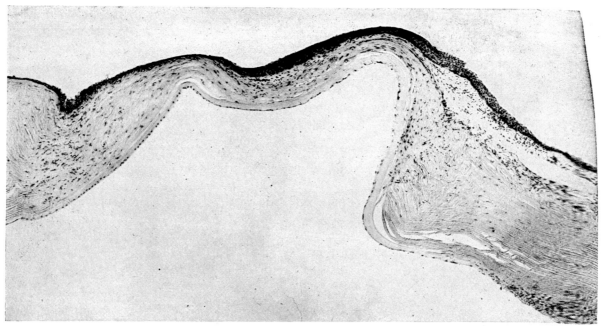

Figure 265. Dystrophy, Corneal

Fuchs' marginal degeneration. ×55. AFIP Acc. 202621.

brane also contributes to its formation. Eventually thick hyaline plaques elevate the epithelium and separate it from Bowman's membrane. The histologic appearance of this type of pannus differs from that associated with inflammatory processes (see page 311) mainly in a much lesser degree of lymphocytic and plasma cell proliferation and the minimal destruction of Bowman's membrane.

Band keratopathy. Band keratopathy, known also as zonular dystrophy and band keratitis, may be secondary to intraocular disease such as iridocyclitis, absolute glaucoma or phthisis bulbi, or may occur as a primary form in certain systemic metabolic disorders. Band keratopathy occurs in a plane corresponding to the interpalpebral tissue. It begins near the termination of Bowman's membrane, leaving a clear zone of cornea in the periphery. The condition then gradually extends across the cornea in the horizontal plane from each side and merges centrally.

Cogan, Albright, and Bartter reported nineteen cases of band keratopathy and calcification in the cornea in patients with hypercalcemia. Four of these patients had hyperparathyroidism, five had vitamin D poisoning, two had sarcoidosis, and eight had severe renal damage.

The earliest histologic change is a fine basophilic stippling in Bowman's membrane representing the deposition of calcium salts. The superficial corneal lamellas become fragmented and degenerated and are replaced by a relatively avascular fibrous tissue interspersed with areas of hyaline degeneration. There often is an extensive degenerative pannus accompanying the changes in Bowman's membrane. Deposition of calcium salts and refractile hyalin material also occurs in this pannus. The affected cornea may become greatly thickened (Fig. 264).

Senile marginal degeneration. Senile marginal degeneration is a very rare, usually bilateral, condition mostly appearing in the aged but occasionally occurring in young persons. Seventy-five per cent of cases occur in men. The condition may begin peripheral to, coincident with, or central to an accompanying arcus senilis and usually starts in the upper cornea. It is a slowly progressive, painless, noninflammatory condition which begins with a fibrillar degeneration of the peripheral lamellas just beneath Bowman's membrane which, like the epithelium, remains intact initially. This process leads to the formation of a gutter-like furrow. A relatively clear zone may be present between it and the limbus. As the furrow deepens, the floor becomes thinner and eventually bulges. The de-

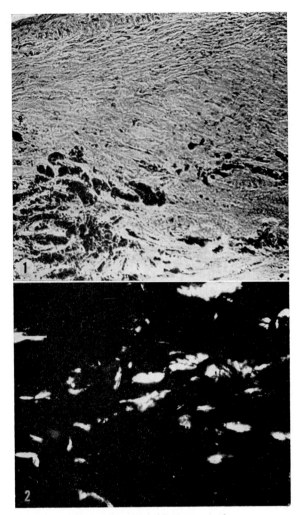

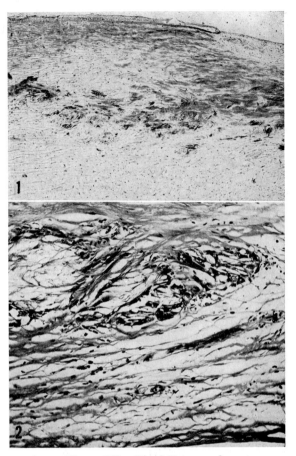

Figure 266. Lipid Keratopathy

1. Frozen section of cornea stained with Sudan IV. The coarse sudanophilic globules (black deposits) are chiefly intracellular in areas of fibrocytosis while the more finely dispersed droplets are extracellular in relatively acellular areas.

2. Birefringent crystals (white areas) demonstrated by photography with polarized light. From Cogan and Kuwabara (1958).

Figure 267. Lipid Keratopathy

1. Frozen section of cornea stained with oil red O. Finely dispersed lipid droplets account for the grey discoloration of the necrotic acellular superficial stroma observed at top of field and on the right. The coarse black deposits across center of field are associated with a foreign body reaction as shown in 2. ×50. AFIP Acc. 913910.

2. Paraffin section stained with H and E; same case shown in 1. ×130.

generated lamellas become replaced by a vascular connective tissue.

Later, when the cornea is weakened and ectatic, cracks appear in Descemet's membrane, the lamellas and Bowman's membrane in the affected area are almost completely gone, and the abnormal epithelium is separated from Descemet's membrane only by a thin layer of vascular connective tissue (Fig. 265).

Central Stromal Conditions

Lipid keratopathy. Lipid keratopathy, also called lipoid dystrophy, is characterized by the appearance of a fatty plaque in, or adjacent to an area of the cornea which is becoming or has been previously vascularized. According to Cogan and Kuwabara, these plaques occur predominantly but not exclusively in patients with higher than average blood cholesterol levels. These authors induced similar plaques in hypercholesteremic rabbits by producing vascularization of the cornea. The fatty plaques of the human and rabbit corneas are similar to those of blood vessels with atheromatosis. The lipid deposits affect all portions of the cornea, but mainly the stroma. The fat stained by Sudan is more abundant than that stained by osmic acid, showing that there is more fat of the cholesterol and fatty acid type than of the neutral

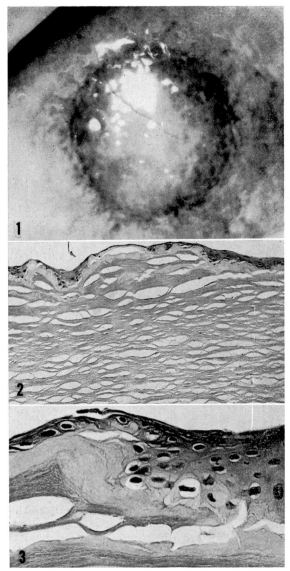

Figure 268. Superficial Corneal Dystrophy, Probably Bücklers Type IV.

1. Clinically the corneal surface presents a pitted appearance resembling beaten metal.

2 and 3. Irregular thickening and marked degeneration of Bowman's membrane; atrophy of epithelium. 2. ×115. 3. ×440.

All from AFIP Acc. 838190. (Courtesy of Doctor S. T. Jones.)

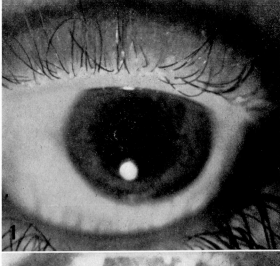

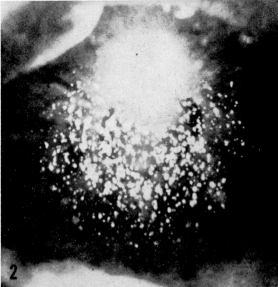

Figure 269. Granular Dystrophy

1. Granular and ring-shaped opacities are present in the axial part of the cornea, a very early case. AFIP Acc. 918257.

2. A more advanced case with larger and more numerous opacities. Between the granules and about the periphery the stroma is clear. AFIP Neg. 60–6049.

type. Histologically the plaques and diffuse deposits of fat in the cornea contain two types of sudanophilic lipid: bright red globules, often as large as 20 μ in diameter, predominantly located within cells, and fine extracellular granules (Fig. 266–1). The latter, located mainly in the acellular hyalinized areas, may be derived from necrosis of cells containing the bright red globules. Viewed with low-power the material gives the appearance of diffuse sudanophilia. Associated with the diffuse granular sudanophilic deposits are unstained birefringent crystals (Fig. 266–2).

With hematoxylin and eosin stains the cornea with lipid keratopathy shows an increased cellularity in some areas and a decrease or hyalinization in others (Fig. 267). The corneal stromal cells show degeneration

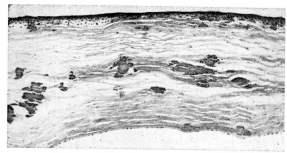

Figure 270. Granular Dystrophy

There are many sharply delineated focal areas of hyaline degeneration involving all levels of the corneal stroma in the axial region. Trephine specimen. Masson trichrome stain. ×90. AFIP Acc. 907066. From Jones and Zimmerman (1961).

and areas of hyalinization with deposition of fat within cells and between the lamellas. Macrophages in large numbers and foreign body giant cells may be seen between the lamellas and around the blood vessels. In older lesions the macrophages and vessels are markedly diminished and hyalinization and calcification occur.

Although associated with abnormal vascularity, the development of the fatty plaque is not necessarily associated with reactivation of the initial inflammatory process and therefore often is interpreted as a dystrophy. Cases of central fatty plaques do occur in the absence of any previous inflammatory disease, but it is still doubtful whether there is such a thing as a primary "lipid dystrophy," unless it be arcus senilis.

Heredofamilial dystrophies. Many different clinical types of heredofamilial corneal dystrophy have been reported, and histopathologic studies have been performed on a number of them by Franceschetti and coworkers. Hereditary dystrophies may affect primarily the epithelium and its basement membrane (Stocker and Holt), Bowman's membrane (Verdi and Filippone; Bücklers type IV) (Fig. 268), the stroma (Bücklers), or Descemet's membrane and the endothelium (Theodore; McGee and Falls; Snell and Irwin). Our knowledge of the pathologic anatomy of these disorders has increased greatly as a result of the study of tissue removed at the time of keratoplasty.

The three classical forms of hereditary corneal dystrophy (granular, macular, and lattice) appear to involve primarily the cor-

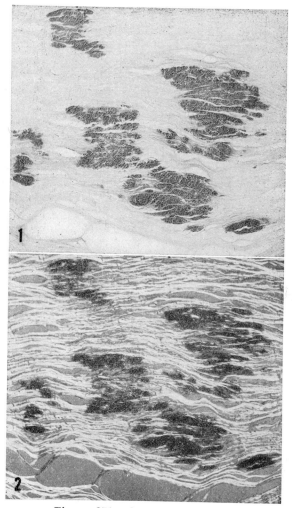

Figure 271. Granular Dystrophy

The focal areas of hyaline degeneration often appear irregularly rectangular and they characteristically exhibit a loss of the normal birefringence of corneal lamellas.

1. Hematoxylin and eosin-stained section photographed with ordinary illumination. ×165.

2. Same field photographed with polarized light. AFIP Acc. 943178. From Jones and Zimmerman (1961).

neal stroma, and Jones and Zimmerman have shown that each of these dystrophies has distinctive clinical and histopathologic characteristics.

Granular dystrophy. Granular dystrophy (Groenouw I or Bücklers I) is inherited as a dominant characteristic. The stromal opacities are discrete grayish granules or rings located in the central (axial) portion of the cornea (Fig. 269). The peripheral portion of the cornea is always free of opacities. In some cases only the superficial stroma appears to

PLATE I

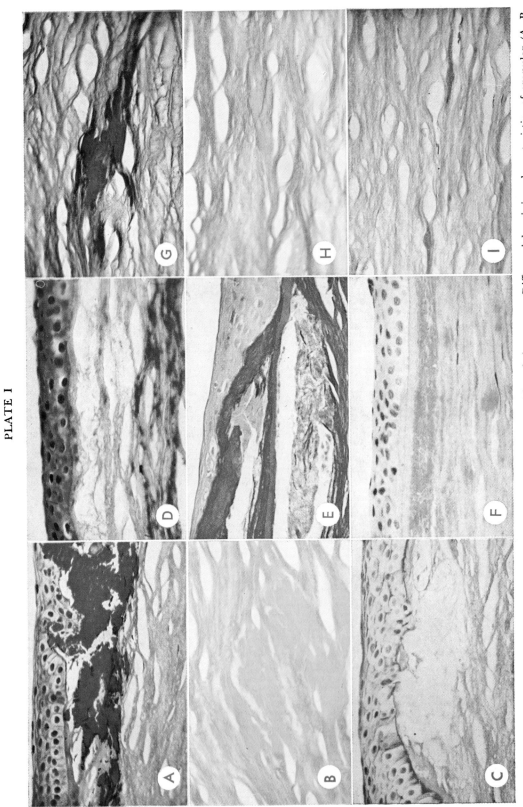

Histopathologic differentiation of granular, macular and lattice dystrophies of the cornea. Differential staining characteristics of granular (A, B, and C), macular (D, E, and F), and lattice dystrophies (G, H, and I) observed in paraffin sections: The sections shown in the top row (A, D, and G) have been stained with Masson's trichrome, those in the middle row (B, E, and H) have been prepared by the colloidal iron method for acid mucopolysaccharides and counterstained with van Gieson's solution, while those in the bottom row (C, F, and I) have been subjected to the periodic acid-Schiff reaction. The Masson stain and colloidal iron reaction serve to differentiate macular dystrophy from granular and lattice dystrophies, while the periodic acid-Schiff reaction is helpful in separating granular dystrophy from macular and lattice dystrophies. (A, B and C: AFIP Acc. 929101, ×265. D and F: AFIP Acc. 847253, ×325. E: AFIP Acc. 840032, ×325. G, H, and I: AFIP Acc. 220210, ×220.) (From Jones & Zimmerman, 1961; reprinted with the permission of the authors and of the American Journal of Ophthalmology.)

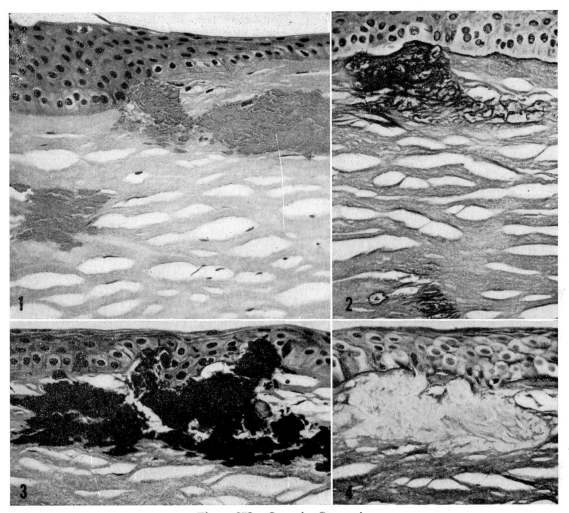

Figure 272. Granular Dystrophy

1. The lesions are composed of eosinophilic granules. H and E. ×305.

2. The collagenous lamellas appear to be transformed into tangled masses of argyrophilic fibrils. Wilder's reticulum stain. ×305.

3. The lesions are brilliant red with Masson's trichrome stain. ×305.

4. The affected corneal lamellas give a much less intense periodic acid-Schiff reaction than does the normal stroma. ×305.

AFIP Acc. 929101. From Jones and Zimmerman (1961).

be involved while in others the lesions may be found at all levels of the stroma (Fig. 270). The stroma between the granules remains clear, and the visual acuity is usually normal or affected only moderately until late in life. Because the visual impairment is usually mild, keratoplasty is infrequently performed, and material for pathologic study is relatively difficult to obtain. Microscopically the opacities consist of focal areas of hyaline degeneration in which the stromal fibers appear finely granulated (Figs. 271, 272). The affected areas stain a brilliant red with the Masson tri-

chrome stain (Color Plate I). They are less PAS-positive and less birefringent than the uninvolved stroma. These latter two features, together with the fine granularity of the lesions, serve to differentiate granular from lattice dystrophy.

Macular dystrophy. Macular dystrophy (Groenouw II or Bücklers II) is a much more disabling disease, characterized by a recessive inheritance, the presence of irregular grayish opacities with indistinct borders, and diffuse cloudiness of the stroma between the opacities (Fig. 273). Although the axial portion of

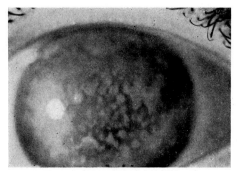

Figure 273. Macular Dystrophy

There are large irregular macular opacities between which the corneal stroma is diffusely cloudy. The peripheral cornea is also involved. AFIP Acc. 840032. From Jones and Zimmerman (1959).

the cornea is most severely affected, the periphery is also involved. There is usually a severe impairment of vision relatively early in life. When keratoplasty is performed, a full-thickness graft is generally indicated because all levels of the stroma are usually involved. Microscopically there is mucoid degeneration of the corneal lamellas (Figs. 274, 275). As the collagenous fibers disintegrate they are replaced by pools of mucoid material which stains with Alcian blue or colloidal iron (Color Plate I). This material is not sensitive to hyaluronidase. The corneal corpuscles and even the endothelial cells contain similar bluestaining material. Nonspecific degenerative changes may be observed in the epithelium, basement membrane, Bowman's membrane, and Descemet's membrane. The latter sometimes exhibits changes similar to those of guttate keratopathy (Fig. 276).

Lattice dystrophy. Lattice dystrophy (Biber-Haab-Dimmer or Bücklers III) has a dominant hereditary pattern. Linear lesions, which usually branch and are translucent by retroillumination, occur in the stroma, while the intervening tissue remains relatively clear. The stromal lesions may spare the deeper layers; usually the periphery of the cornea is clear. The visual acuity may be reduced early in life. On clinical examination, nonspecific epithelial and subepithelial changes may be severe enough to obscure the typical linear lesions in the stroma. The epithelial and subepithelial alterations probably cause much of the visual disturbance. Both

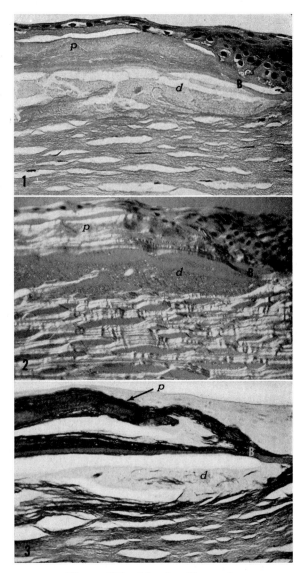

Figure 274. Macular Dystrophy

There is a large area of mucoid degeneration (d) involving the superficial stroma just beneath Bowman's membrane (B). The hyaline plaque (p) that has formed between the markedly attenuated epithelium and Bowman's membrane is the product of a secondary pathologic process. The primary lesion (d) is characterized by destruction of corneal lamellas loss of normal birefringence, and an accumulation of hyaluronidase-resistant mucoid while the plaque (p) above Bowman's membrane contains a large number of newly formed birefringent collagen fibers From same case shown in Fig. 273.

1. H and E, ordinary illumination. ×305.

2. Same as 1 but photographed with polarized light.

3. Colloidal iron with van Gieson counterstain. The stromal lesion (d) is pale blue while the plaque (p) is bright red. ×325.

AFIP Acc. 840032.

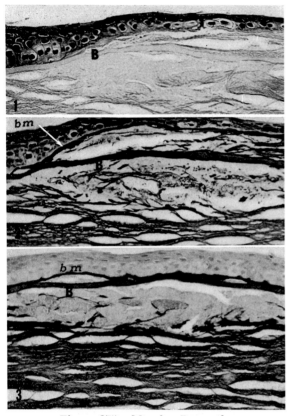

Figure 275. Macular Dystrophy

There is advanced destruction of the stromal collagen and accumulation of mucoid material beneath Bowman's membrane (B). Some mucoid material has also seeped into the space between the irregularly thickened basement membrane of the epithelium (b.m.) and Bowman's membrane.

1. H and E. ×305.
2. Wilder's reticulum stain. ×305.
3. Colloidal iron with van Gieson counterstain. ×305.

AFIP Acc. 840032. From Jones and Zimmerman (1959).

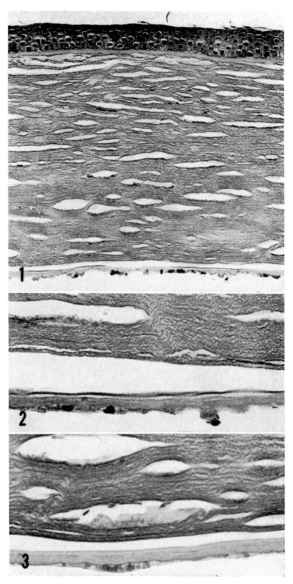

Figure 276. Macular Dystrophy

There is marked degeneration of the corneal endothelium. Descemet's membrane exhibits both diffuse and wart-like thickening. AFIP Acc. 840032. 1. ×165. 2. ×440. 3. ×440.

lamellar and penetrating keratoplasty have been performed in many cases of lattice dystrophy with excellent results. Microscopically, the characteristic stromal lesions are fusiform areas of hyaline degeneration which lack the granular character of the lesions seen in granular dystrophy. They are also typically PAS-positive, and are more birefringent than the normal corneal tissue when examined with polarized light (Fig. 277 and Color Plate I). Dense accumulations of hyalin are usually observed between the extremely irregular epithelium and Bowman's membrane (Fig. 278). While these are of no significance

in differential diagnosis, they are of paramount importance clinically because of their effect on vision.

Salzman's nodular dystrophy. This is a rather rare nonfamilial corneal condition which is more common in women and is unilateral at the onset, but often becomes bilateral. Its etiology is unknown but it occurs in eyes previously affected by phlyctenular keratitis. Clinically, there are one to eight bluish-white nodules which project above

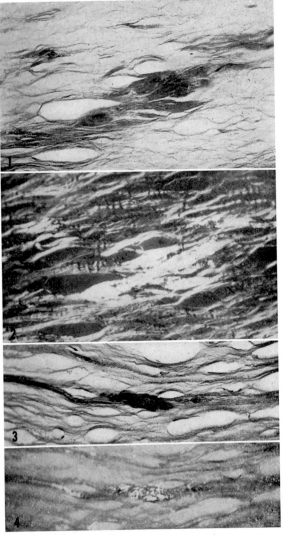

Figure 277. Lattice Dystrophy

The specific stromal lesions consist of fusiform areas of hyaline degeneration of the corneal lamellas in which the affected collagen fibers become more birefringent than the unaffected lamellas. AFIP Acc. 220210.

1. H and E, ordinary light. ×305.

2. Same field as 1 but photographed with polarized light.

3. Masson trichrome stain. The affected lamellas stain brilliant red. Ordinary light, ×305.

4. Same field as in 3 but photographed with polarized light. From Jones and Zimmerman (1959).

the corneal surface. In some instances there is no corneal vascularization and in others the nodules are formed at the ends of vessel loops.

Histopathologically the early nodule is a hypertrophic lesion involving the anterior stroma, Bowman's membrane and epithelium.

The epithelium may be atrophic or hyperplastic with some areas of vacuolation of cells and nuclear pyknosis. Thick acellular plaques of hyalin form between the epithelium and Bowman's membrane (Fig. 279). The latter may become frayed and degenerated, and the adjacent lamellas are affected similarly. Later the epithelium becomes thinned, Bowman's membrane is lost, and the stromal lamellas and cells are markedly degenerated.

Hurler's disease. Hurler's disease (gargoylism) is a congenital heredofamilial systemic disturbance characterized clinically by dwarfism, mental retardation, facies resembling that of cretinism, thickening of the skin and periarticular structures, and cloudy corneas. The clouding of the corneas may be present at birth but often begins near the end of the first year of life, gradually increases and becomes stationary at the fourth or fifth year. Progression may be observed during adolescence. Biomicroscopy shows diffuse fine refractile dots, chiefly in the stroma, and tending to become more macular beneath Bowman's membrane with increasing age. Vascularization does not occur. According to Lindsay et al., the basic lesion of this disease is the intracellular and extracellular deposition and storage of a substance giving the histochemical reaction for glycogen. Certain data presented by these authors suggest that the glycogen may be combined with a protein.

Uzman studied the chemistry of substances deposited in the tissues in this disease by isolation of fractions from spleens which were removed surgically from two patients with gargoylism, and from spleens and livers which were obtained at autopsy from two other patients. Two fractions were found; one (Fraction S) belonged to a class of water-soluble glycolipids and the other (Fraction P) belonged to the group of sulfonated polysaccharides or mucopolysaccharides. The proportion in which these two substances occurred varied in different organs. Along this line Dawson showed that the solubility characteristics of the material found in the nervous system differed from that in visceral organs, the former behaving histochemically like the cerebrosides.

Meyer et al. studied the urine of five pa-

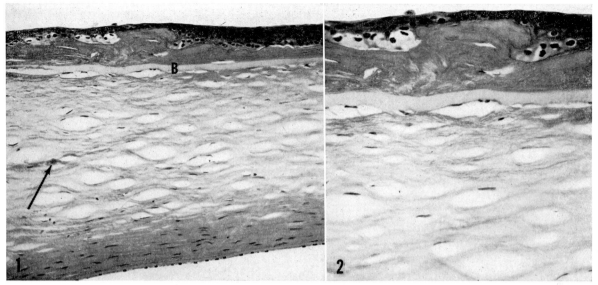

Figure 278. Lattice Dystrophy

There is an extensive deposit of hyalin between the very irregular and markedly degenerated epithelium and Bowman's membrane (B). One of the specific stromal lesions which has been cut almost transversely is indicated by the arrow (compare with other stromal lesions from same case shown in Fig. 277). AFIP Acc. 220210.

1. H and E, ×150.
2. H and E, ×300.

tients and the liver of another patient, all of whom had gargoylism. The urine of four of the five patients contained a mixture of mucopolysaccharide which could be demonstrated to be chondroitin sulfate-B and heparitin sulfate, with the former predominating. The urine of one patient, and the liver of another, yielded only heparitin sulfate. There was no correlation between the type of polysaccharide excreted and the severity of the disease or the postulated mode of inheritance.

These two papers indicate that gargoylism results from a disturbance in mucopolysaccharide metabolism, and Meyer et al. suggested that gargoylism results from the overproduction of certain mucopolysaccharides due to a genetically determined error of differentiation.

The condition is not a fat storage disease as had once been assumed. The characteristic cellular lesion is a swelling of the cytoplasm resulting in enlargement of the cell. The widespread involvement of most tissues of the body explains the protean clinical manifestations.

Microscopic examination of the cornea reveals swelling of the cytoplasm of the fixed corneal corpuscles. Some infiltration of macrophages containing glycoprotein and acid

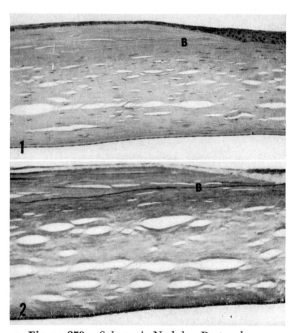

Figure 279. Salzman's Nodular Dystrophy

A dense collagenized acellular plaque is interposed between the atrophic epithelium and Bowman's membrane (B).

1. H and E. ×115.
2. PAS. ×130. AFIP Acc. 941176.
Courtesy of Dr. D. G. Cogan.

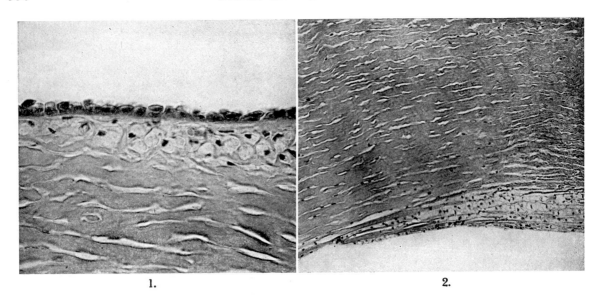

1.   2.

Figure 280.   Gargoylism

1. Swollen cells beneath peripheral corneal epithelium. The appearance of these cells is accounted for on the basis of storage or ingestion of glycoprotein and acid mucopolysaccharide. ×400. AFIP Acc. 87437.

2. Similar cells in intertrabecular spaces of corneoscleral meshwork. ×125. AFIP Acc. 87437.

mucopolysaccharide occurs between the lamellas and especially at the edges of Bowman's and Descemet's membrane (Fig. 280). The trabecular and corneal endothelial cells also are involved. According to Hogan et al., in the late stages there is thinning and loss of Bowman's membrane, and an infiltration into Bowman's zone by large cells containing finely granular material. Fresh frozen sections show no staining with Sudan or osmium. This observation together with the reports by Lindsay and co-workers that affected cells stain positively for glycogen and for acid mucopolysaccharides supports the present belief that Hurler's syndrome is due to a disturbance in carbohydrate metabolism and is not a fat storage disease.

Cystinosis. Cystinosis is described in detail in Chapter V. In this disease the cystine crystals in the cornea are characteristically deposited in the anterior stroma except at the limbus where they extend throughout the entire thickness of the stroma (Figs. 189, 281).

Keratoconus. This condition is a noninflammatory ectasia of the axial portion of the cornea usually beginning in youth or adolescence (Fig. 282). It is almost always bilateral and its etiology is unknown. It progresses for five to six years after onset, then ordinarily remains quiescent. Acute relapses are not uncommon, even in the 35 to 45 year age group. The well-developed ectasia of keratoconus is confined to the central part of the cornea, rarely occupying more than the central half, the apex of the cone displaced somewhat down and nasally.

Microscopically, Chi et al. have shown there is fragmentation of the basement membrane of the corneal epithelium, as well as fibrillation of Bowman's membrane and the anterior stroma in the early stages (Fig. 283). Later Bowman's membrane appears wavy and contains many gaps which are filled in with either connective tissue or epithelium. There is marked thinning of the central cornea. The lamellas later show further degenerative changes, especially at the apex of the cone. Descemet's membrane may be folded or torn. As a result of this there is a disturbance in corneal hydration, and acute or chronic edema of the cone may develop.

Endothelial Disturbances

Cornea guttata and Fuchs' dystrophy. Fuchs in 1910 described a bilateral epithelial dystrophy, mainly in women, unassociated with inflammation, and characterized by loss of sensation, superficial corneal cloudiness

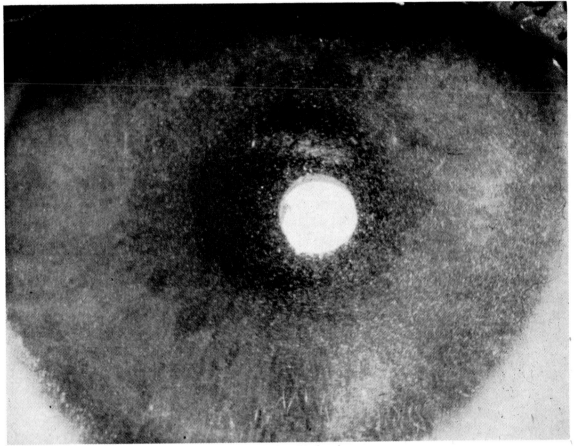

Figure 281. Cystinosis

Fine scintillating polychromatic cystine crystals are dispersed throughout the corneal stroma. See also Fig. 189. From Garron (1959).

and epithelial edema mainly affecting the central cornea (Fig. 284). He later speculated that the endothelium might be involved in production of this lesion. Subsequent observers showed that the stromal and epithelial changes were preceded by a disturbance of the corneal endothelium which led to thickening of Descemet's membrane and wart-formation in the central portion of the cornea, eventually causing a disturbance in hydration of the cornea with epithelial edema. These changes in Descemet's membrane eventually came to be known as cornea guttata. They resemble Hassall-Henle warts, but differ in that the latter remain in the peripheral portion of Descemet's membrane, are not associated with epithelial edema, and are found in almost all eyes beyond age forty as a manifestation of aging.

That cornea guttata leads to Fuchs' epi-

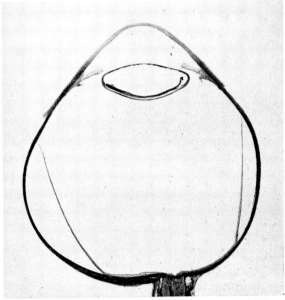

Figure 282. Keratoconus. ×3. AFIP Acc. 88459.

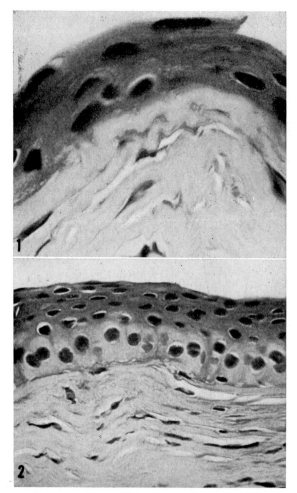

Figure 283. Keratoconus

Fragmentation and interruption of Bowman's membrane and degenerative changes in the superficial stroma are observed in the early stages.

1. ×1107. AFIP Acc. 840033.
2. ×575. AFIP Acc. 840033.

thelial dystrophy is supported by the following observations: (1) cases have been reported in which the endothelial changes were present in both eyes, and epithelial changes were present in one eye; (2) cases have been observed in which, after long observation of an eye with cornea guttata, epithelial edema has developed; (3) histopathologic study of keratoplasty buttons removed from patients with typical Fuchs' epithelial dystrophy usually show similar degenerative changes in the endothelium and diffuse or nodular thickening of Descemet's membrane with wart formation.

The changes in cornea guttata commence

in the axial cornea but gradually spread toward the periphery.

According to Chi et al., histologically there are conspicuous alterations in the corneal endothelium and in Descemet's membrane. The endothelial cells are unevenly distributed, flattened, and distorted by globular intracytoplasmic bodies of varying size. The endothelial nuclei exhibit great pleomorphism and degenerative changes. There is marked thickening of Descemet's membrane, which may appear laminated (Fig. 284–4). Hemispherical and flat-topped excrescences or warts are found irregularly throughout Descemet's membrane (Fig. 284–2, 5). Usually the corneal endothelium appears to be extremely thin or absent over these warts. Fine pigment granules are often present in the endothelium.

The progression of cornea guttata upsets the corneal physiology and leads to the overhydration of stroma and epithelium. Thus in advanced cases we find epithelial edema, bulla formation, thickening of the basement membrane, and formation of a degenerative pannus (Fig. 284–3).

Bullous keratopathy. Bullous keratopathy resembles cornea guttata and Fuchs' dystrophy in that the disturbed corneal hydration with formation of vesicles and bullae and the ensuing degenerative pannus are due primarily to pathologic changes in the endothelium. The surface changes may occur following surgical injury to the endothelium, with adherence of lens or anterior hyaloid membrane to the back of the cornea, after epithelialization of the anterior chamber, but most often it is observed following the endothelial damage produced by long-standing glaucoma. The bullae may be large or small, localized or diffuse, depending on the cause. Chronic bullae often are in contact with Bowman's membrane and are lined by a thin connective tissue derived from the nerve canals in Bowman's membrane.

PIGMENTATION OF THE CORNEA

Blood staining of the cornea. When anterior chamber hemorrhage is associated with increased intraocular pressure, blood pigment may pass into the cornea. For this to occur, damage to the corneal endothelium usually

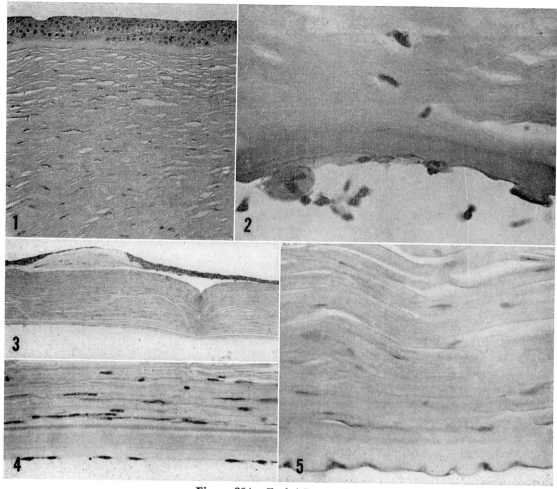

Figure 284. Fuchs' Dystrophy

1. Edema of corneal epithelium and stroma. ×120. Univ. of Cal. 60–80.
2. Diffuse and wart-like thickening of Descemet's membrane from same case shown in 1. ×480.
3. Bullous separation of corneal epithelium and pannus-formation. ×75. AFIP Acc. 139507.
4. Marked thickening and lamination of Descemet's membrane. ×400. AFIP Acc. 44597.
5. Diffuse and nodular thickening of Descemet's membrane. ×400. AFIP Acc. 238575.

is necessary, and, if the endothelium is sufficiently damaged, blood staining of the cornea may occur even without increased intraocular pressure. Histologically, reddish granules of hemoglobin are observed diffusely throughout the stromal fibers (Fig. 285-1). Later, when the pigment is phagocytized by the corneal corpuscles or wandering cells, it is converted into hemosiderin (Fig. 285-2). Clinically, this causes the corneal color to vary from rusty to greenish-black to greenish-yellow. Clearing is slow and begins at the periphery, proceeding toward the center.

Melanosis. Melanin pigment may be found in the limbus and cornea in several conditions which are discussed elsewhere (see Chapters I, II, V).

Argyrosis, siderosis and chalcosis. Various foreign substances such as silver (argyrosis), iron (siderosis) and copper (chalcosis) produce pigmentation of the cornea. In the case of argyrosis, the silver granules accumulate principally around the connective tissue fibers in front of Descemet's membrane. Iron and copper pigments have a similar distribution, and also involve the endothelium.

Kayser-Fleischer ring. The Kayser-Fleischer ring is seen in patients with the familial disease known as hepatolenticular degeneration (Wilson's disease). The ring occurs as a ruby-red or bright green band of

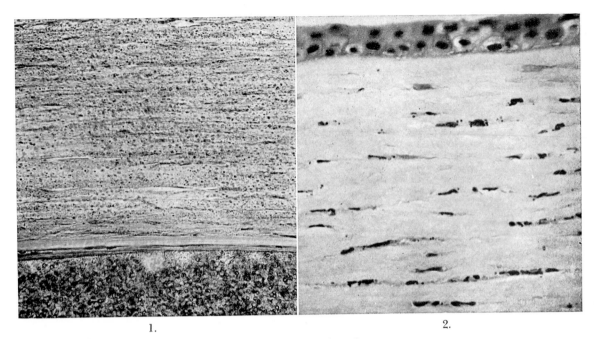

Figure 285. Pigmentation, Cornea

1. Blood staining of cornea, recent. Hemorrhage in anterior chamber. ×275. AFIP Acc. 493955.
2. Blood staining of cornea, old. Hemosiderin in corneal corpuscles. ×765. AFIP Acc. 69770.

pigmentation about 2 mm. wide in the posterior cornea around the limbus. It extends varying degrees around the peripheral circumference of the cornea. Histologically, it appears as a deposit of greenish-black pigment in the posterior half of Descemet's membrane at the periphery (Fig. 286). It is not removed by oxidation or reduction, but it is soluble in Lugol's solution and sodium cyanide. The pigment remains after ashing and presumably is the sulfide of an inorganic heavy metal which spectroscopically appears to be copper.

Hudson's or Stahli's line. In certain persons over fifty years of age, and in others with intraocular or corneal disease a linear horizontal yellow, brown, or green line, Hudson's or Stahli's line, crosses the cornea at the junction of the middle and lower thirds. It has been shown to be a deposit of hemosiderin in the corneal epithelium. Breaks in Bowman's membrane are usually not present. In corneal leukomas and in keratoconus (Fleischer's ring) the iron pigment also has been shown to be in the epithelium.

Krukenberg's spindle. In a number of ocular diseases, especially in pigmentary glaucoma and in those with damage to uveal pigment a vertical spindle-shaped deposit of pigment accumulates on the posterior surface of the central cornea (Krukenberg's spindle). The pigment is deposited on and is phagocytized by the endothelial cells. About 90 per cent of cases are bilateral. Krukenberg's spindle is common in the aged and in high myopia.

Corneal tattooing. Tattooing of the cornea with India ink, gold, platinum and silver

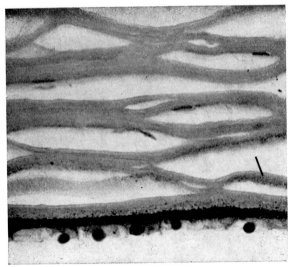

Figure 286

Kayser-Fleischer ring. Pigment in and around Descemet's membrane. ×600. AFIP Acc. 264768.

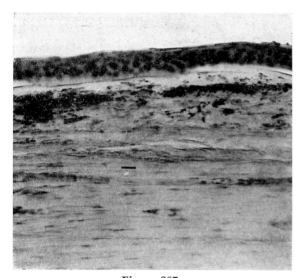

Figure 287.

Tattooing of cornea. ×175. AFIP Acc. 27229.

produces pigmentation of the stroma in the region of the tattooing. This is due to deposition of the pigment or the metallic granules between the corneal lamellas. Phagocytosis of the material by the corneal cells is observed. The epithelium contains no pigment (Fig. 287).

TUMORS OF THE CORNEA

Neoplasms. Since neoplasms of the cornea almost always represent secondary extensions of lesions which are primary in the bulbar conjunctiva and limbus, they are considered in Chapter V. A few rare primary carcinomas and malignant melanomas have been observed, but they are so similar to those which are primary in the conjunctiva that they will not be discussed at this time. It should be mentioned, however, that when the cornea is involved, either by an extension from the limbus or as a primary cancer, the process characteristically remains superficial to Bowman's membrane. Even when a large fungating mass is present, Bowman's membrane restricts the growth and prevents extension into the stroma. Typically in cases of long duration, particularly with ulceration and inflammation or after repeated surgical excisions, a pannus develops between the neoplasm and Bowman's membrane. There also may be slight vascularization of the superficial corneal stroma, but characteristically the middle and deeper layers are spared.

Fibrous tumors. These usually arise in the areas of previous inflammation, injury or surgery. Such tumors are similar to keloids and are not true neoplasms.

Dermoids. These are choristomatous tumors of the cornea, usually occurring at the lower outer limbus. Since they are congenital lesions, they have already been mentioned in this chapter.

THE SCLERA

ANATOMIC AND PHYSIOLOGIC CONSIDERATIONS

The sclera comprises five-sixths of the fibrous outer tunic of the eye. It is interrupted posteriorly by the optic nerve, and by the emissaria, or canals for the perforating nerves, arteries and veins. The sclera is perforated posteriorly by the long and short posterior ciliary vessels and nerves, by the vortex veins near the equator, and by the anterior ciliary vessels in front of the rectus muscles. Melanocytes frequently are present in the emissaria, especially in the Negro. A long posterior ciliary nerve may traverse the sclera and loop back to the ciliary body. When it is associated with neurilemmal or connective tissue proliferation, the loop may form a prominent elevation 4 to 7 mm. posterior to the limbus (intrascleral nerve loop of Axenfeld) (Fig. 59). Biopsy of such a nodule may lead to an erroneous diagnosis of neurofibroma. When pigmented, the nerve loop may be mistaken for a melanotic tumor or foreign body. Except for the perforating vessels, the sclera is relatively avascular and does not contain lymphatics. The episcleral tissue contains many blood vessels, and these frequently participate actively in inflammatory reactions.

Histology

The sclera is a dense, tough, fibrous structure, consisting mainly of collagen and elastic fibers imbedded in a mucopolysaccharide

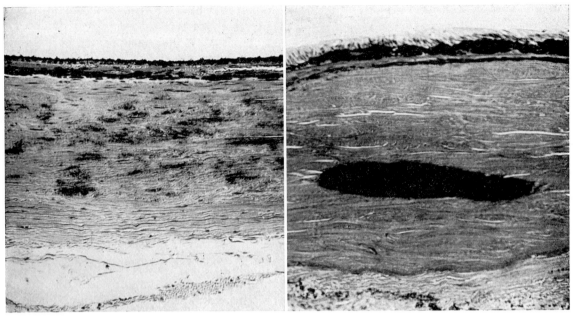

Figure 288. Aging: Sclera

1. Granular calcium deposits in sclera. ×115. AFIP Acc. 130793.
2. Calcareous plaque in degenerated scleral fibers. ×130. AFIP Acc. 95102.

matrix. Anteriorly it blends into the regularly arranged lamellas of the cornea, while posteriorly it is interrupted by a foramen through which the optic nerve passes. The thin bands of scleral tissue stretched across this opening are known as the lamina cribrosa. The scleral thickness is greatest at the posterior pole, where it measures approximately 1 mm.; it gradually decreases towards the equator, the thinnest portion lying beneath the tendons of the rectus muscles.

The superficial layers of the sclera, called the episcleral tissue, are made up of loosely arranged bundles of connective tissue with relatively numerous blood vessels. In the deeper layers the bundles become firmer and thicker until the transition to the dense fibrous tissue of the sclera proper is complete. The bundles of collagenous fibers, together with the numerous elastic fibers, form complicated patterns. Adjacent to the cornea and about the posterior foramen, the bundles run in concentric circles. Elsewhere they form a pattern of loops running backward, mainly in a meridional direction. Between the bundles of collagenous fibrils are the fixed cells, which resemble those in the cornea. The innermost layer of the sclera, the lamina fusca, is distinguished by its brownish color which is due to the large number of branching melanocytes. The connective tissue bundles in this layer are smaller and flatter and the elastic fibers more numerous. The outer sclera blends with Tenon's capsule.

GROWTH AND AGING

In the young, the sclera is thin and relatively transparent. With increasing age and thickening of its fibers, the sclera develops an acellular appearance.

In the aged, fat deposits may appear, giving the sclera a yellowish color. Finely granular calcium deposits are sometimes seen (Fig. 288–1). Cogan and Kuwabara have recently described the condition known as scleral plaques as focal senile translucency of the sclera. This condition is common in the elderly. The involved areas are almost invariably located in front of the tendinous insertion of the lateral and medial recti. Initially, the translucent areas are characterized by a loss of cellularity and later by calcification (Fig. 288–2). Hyalinization, contrary to general belief, is not found. According to Cogan et al., these calcific plaques are unique in biologic tissue in that they may contain large amounts of calcium sulfate.

CONGENITAL ANOMALIES OF THE SCLERA

Scleral cysts. Scleral cysts have been noted at the limbus in very young infants. Originally the cysts are small, immovable, sessile elevations lined by flat cells resembling squamous epithelium, arranged in one or more layers. Occasional cysts communicate with the anterior chamber.

Blue scleras. A light blue sclera, usually associated with brittle bones, dislocation of the joints, and deafness, constitutes a heredofamilial complex known as the syndrome of van der Hoeve and de Kleyn. There is delayed condensation of the sclera from about the third month of development. The sclera is not pigmented but is abnormally thin and translucent, permitting the uveal pigment to form a blue background. The collagen fibers are sparse and immature. Occasional associated ocular abnormalities are retrobulbar neuritis, zonular cataract, posterior embryotoxon, megalocornea and keratoconus. Other abnormalities recorded are maculas of the skin, delayed dental development, spina bifida, cleft palate, congenital heart disease and hemophilia.

Ochronosis. In ochronosis, a recessive inbred disorder of phenylalanine and tyrosine metabolism, homogentisic acid is excreted in the urine (alkaptonuria) and many tissues, especially cartilages, are discolored by yellow or "ochre" pigment (hence the term, ochronosis). The eyes may exhibit symmetrical pigmentary deposits in the corneal periphery and diffuse scleral and episcleral pigmentation in the region of insertion of the rectus muscles (Fig. 190). The pigment cannot be distinguished histologically or chemically from melanin. In one tragic case reported by Skinsnes enucleation was performed because of the erroneous diagnosis of malignant melanoma. Microscopically, the pigment appears to be absorbed by swollen and degenerated collagenous and elastic tissue fibers in the sclera and episclera (Fig. 289). Homogeneous, irregularly spheroidal, yellow deposits are also present in the stroma of the peripheral cornea (Figs. 190, 289–1).

INFLAMMATION OF THE SCLERA

Because of the comparatively uninterrupted course and density of its connective tissue, the sclera is infiltrated only with great difficulty by inflammatory and neoplastic cells. Those cells that make their way into or out of the eye generally do so either through the blood stream or along the perivascular and perineural spaces about the perforating vessels and nerves. It is not unusual in cases of focal infection within the eye to find the perivascular spaces at some distance from the lesion choked with cells.

Because it is an almost avascular inert fibrous structure, diseases affecting the sclera are comparatively rare and their pathology relatively simple. The etiologic and pathogenetic factors and general pattern of the inflammatory reactions are essentially the same as those affecting tendons and tendon sheaths elsewhere in the body (e.g., rheumatoid diseases, tuberculosis and syphilis).

Episcleritis. Episcleritis occurs in a *diffuse* form in toxic, allergic and infectious conditions. Also, it occurs spontaneously due to unknown causes. It is seen in primary coccidioidomycosis, erythema multiforme, erythema nodosum, and in infectious diseases. The inflammation is a recurrent nongranulomatous process with widespread hyperemia, edema, and lymphocytic infiltration. Healing occurs without scarring.

Circumscribed or *nodular* episcleritis occurs in granulomatous diseases and in the diffuse connective tissue and vascular diseases, such as periarteritis nodosa and cranial arteritis. The nodules are composed of a mass of large mononuclear cells and some giant cells, with or without central necrosis. Surrounding this is a zone of lymphocytic and plasma cell infiltration.

Rheumatoid scleritis. Characteristic "rheumatoid" lesions occur in the sclera and cornea, but in about one-half the cases there is no history of rheumatoid arthritis or related diseases. Clinically, the scleral lesions fall into two groups, diffuse and circumscribed, but intermediate forms have been noted and the histologic features of both are similar. In the diffuse scleral lesions the involvement extends over a large area of the sclera, which may become thickened several times the normal (brawny scleritis) or so thinned that the uvea herniates through

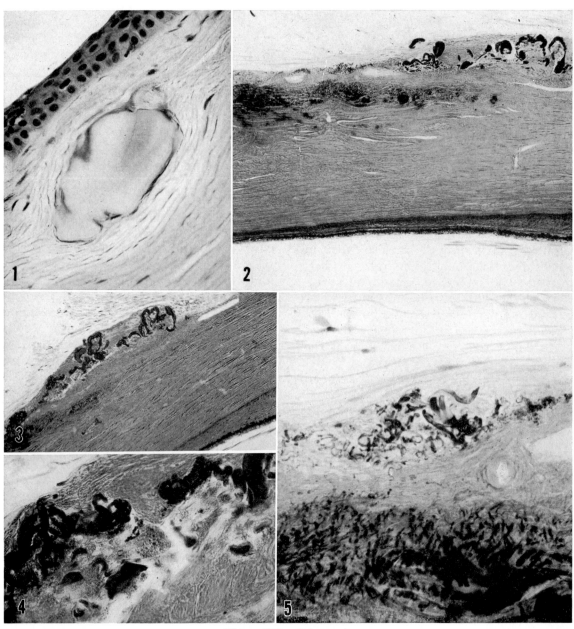

Figure 289. Ochronosis

Same case shown in Fig. 190.

1. Irregularly spheroidal deposits of homogeneous yellow-brown material are found in the superficial stromal layers of the peripheral cornea. H and E. ×350.

2. Much melanotic pigment stains the outer scleral lamellas and impregnates swollen elastic tissue fibers in the episclera. Verhoeff's elastic tissue stain. ×70.

3. Weil's myelin stain. ×50.

4. Weil's myelin stain. ×300.

5. Swollen elastic tissue fibers in sclera and episclera. Verhoeff's stain. ×400.

AFIP Acc. 871509. From Rones (1960).

(scleromalacia perforans). The characteristic lesion consists of a central area of necrosis surrounded by a palisade of epithelioid and giant cells (Fig. 28). A broad zone of non-specific chronic inflammatory reaction extends into the underlying choroid or ciliary body and involves the overlying episclera. Damage and inflammatory infiltration of the intraocular tissues may become widespread. Extension into the loose tissues of the orbit is generally less conspicuous. These cases run a prolonged course with frequent exacerbations.

In the cases characterized by discrete scleral lesions (rheumatoid nodules), isolated foci of necrosis occur in the sclera. These are surrounded by the typical granulomatous inflammatory infiltrate, but there may be very little congestion of the tissues, and minimal damage to the intraocular structures. When these discrete foci of scleral necrosis occur in the anterior half of the sclera, necrosis of the overlying conjunctiva may produce a punched-out defect into which uveal tissue may bulge (focal scleromalacia perforans). Healing may follow, leaving a slate-blue spot where the uveal tissue is covered only by a thin scar, but perforation of the uveal prolapse and secondary intraocular infection are not uncommon.

Similar discrete, punched-out areas of necrosis have been observed in the cornea, usually near the limbus. Loosening and sloughing of the necrotic tissue may permit prolapse of the iris with loss of the eye as the usual outcome. Less severe nonperforating lesions of the cornea also occur in rheumatoid arthritis, but these have not been subjected to histologic study.

Sparganosis. In certain parts of the Far East where animal flesh is applied to the skin or eyes as poultices, larvae (spargana) of tapeworms related to Diphyllobothrium latum may emigrate and become encysted in the patient's tissues (Hunter et al., 1960). Any part of the body surface to which the poultices are applied may become infected. Ocular sparganosis is a well recognized entity, lesions occurring in the lids, conjunctiva, episclera (Fig. 290), and orbit. The encysted larvae are surrounded by a wall of epithelioid cells about which the blood vessels exhibit cuffing

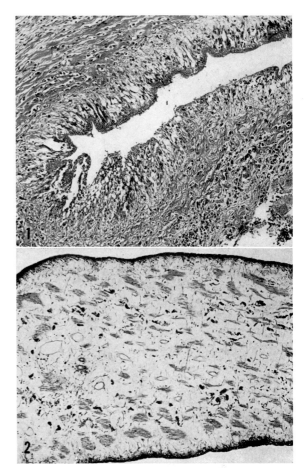

Figure 290. Sparganosis

1. Cystoid granuloma excised from episclera. The sparganum which measured 63 mm. in length was contained in the lumen of this lesion. ×115. AFIP Acc. 953047.

2. A portion of the larva removed from the lesion shown in 1. ×115.

by lymphocytes and plasma cells (Fig. 290).

SCLERAL HEALING

Scleral healing differs from that of the cornea in that the influence of the overlying epithelium is absent. Mainly there is an ingrowth of vessels from the episcleral and uveal tissues with the formation of a simple fibrous scar. The scleral cells, themselves, seem to participate little, if at all.

INJURIES

Injuries of the anterior and posterior sclera have been discussed in some detail in Chapter III. The avascularity and relative acellularity of the sclera make it relatively

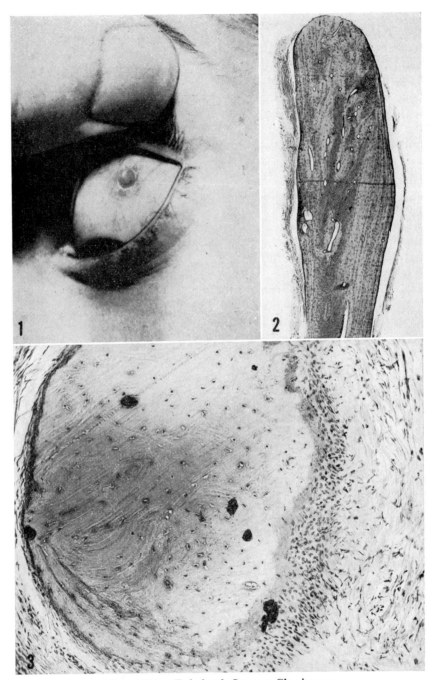

Figure 291. Episcleral Osseous Choristoma

1. Occurrence in upper temporal quadrant is typical. AFIP Acc. 868475.
2. ×16. AFIP Acc. 92770.
3. ×115. AFIP Acc. 93512.
From Boniuk and Zimmerman (1961).

unreacitive, and it plays a passive role in the healing of wounds. Anterior perforating injuries involve the adjacent ciliary body, vitreous and even the lens. The intraocular pressure is lowered, and the wound lips become inverted and fixed by a clot. The clot organizes from the episclera and uvea, and dense connective tissue bands extend into the eye from the wound region. Atrophy of the eye with disorganization often results. Posterior perforating injuries involve the choroid, vitreous, and retina. Vitreous usually is lost. Infolding of the scleral lips, organization of a clot or prolapsed vitreous, and formation of fibrous bands which extend into the vitreous occur. Retinal and choroidal detachment may follow.

Contusions may lead to scleral rupture at the equator, beneath a rectus muscle, or posteriorly around the optic nerve. The vitreous usually escapes through such a tear, and considerable hemorrhage occurs. Healing is similar to that of perforating wounds.

TUMORS

Fibromas may appear on the anterior sclera around the limbus. They usually are firm, fixed, of variable size, and are composed of fairly mature, densely packed fibroblasts.

Hemangiomas of the uveal tract may, on rare occasions, involve the adjacent sclera.

Neurofibromas affect the anterior perforating nerves at times, and appear as localized small tumors.

Conjunctival carcinomas rarely invade the sclera, but if the inflammation around the tumor is marked, softening occurs and the sclera is affected. More often the sclera shows localized tumors around the emissarium where the tumor is extending into the eye.

Osseous choristomas occur in the episclera, typically in the upper temporal quadrant, 5–10 mm. from the limbus (Boniuk and Zimmerman). These are relatively rare tumor-like malformations composed of mature compact bone (Fig. 291). The solitary nodules are freely moveable, being nonadherent to the bulbar conjunctiva or sclera. They vary in size and shape from that of a small pea to that of an almond. Clinically, these tumors are usually believed to be conjunctival dermoids though their bony texture

and the absence of hairs and fat should help make the proper differential diagnosis.

Dermoid tumors of the episclera are similar to, but much less common than, those of the limbus (see Chapter V and Fig. 168). While the limbal dermoids occur mainly in the lower temporal quadrant, those in the episclera away from the limbus have a more random distribution.

REFERENCES

Axenfeld, Th.: Embryotoxon Corneae Posterius. Ber. deutsch. Ophth. Gesellsch. *42*:301–302, 1920.

Boniuk, M., and Zimmerman, L. E.: Episcleral Osseous Choristoma. Amer. J. Ophthal. 53:290–296, 1961.

Bücklers, M.: Die erblichen Hornhautdystrophien. Dystrophiae corneae hereditariae. Bücherei des Augenarztes, 3 Heft, Stuttgart, Ferdinand Enke, 1938.

Burian, H. M., Braley, A. E., and Allen, L.: External and Gonioscopic Visibility of the Ring of Schwalbe and the Trabecular Zone; Interpretation of the Posterior Corneal Embryotoxon and the So-called Congenital Hyaline Membranes on the Posterior Corneal Surface. Trans. Amer. Ophthal. Soc. *52*: 389–428, 1955.

Buschke, W., Friedenwald, J. S., and Moses, S. G.: Effect of Ultraviolet Irradiation on Corneal Epithelium: Mitosis, Nuclear Fragmentation, Posttraumatic Cell Movements, Loss of Tissue Cohesion. J. Cell. Comp. Physiol. 26:147–164, 1945.

Chi, H. H., Katzin, H. M., and Teng, C. C.: Histopathology of Keratoconus. Amer. J. Ophthal. *42*:847–860, 1956.

Chi, H. H., Teng, C. C., and Katzin, H. M.: Histopathology of Primary Endothelial-epithelial Dystrophy of the Cornea. Amer. J. Ophthal. *45*:518–535, 1958.

Clark, William, B.: Hereditary and Constitutional Dystrophies of the Cornea. Amer. J. Ophthal. *33*: 692–703, (May), 1950.

Cogan, D. G., Albright, F., and Bartter, F. C.: Hypercalcemia and Band Keratopathy: Report of Nineteen Cases. A.M.A. Arch. Ophthal. *40*:624–638, (Dec.), 1948.

Cogan, D. G., and Kinsey, V. E.: The Cornea. I. Transfer of Water and Sodium Chloride by Osmosis and Diffusion through Excised Cornea. A.M.A. Arch. Ophthal. 27:466–476, 1942.

(*b*) Cogan, D. G., and Kinsey, V. E.: The Cornea. II. Transfer of Water and Sodium Chloride by Hydrostatic Pressure through Excised Cornea. *Ibid.* 696–70*.

(*c*) Kinsey, V. E., and Cogan, D. G.: The Cornea III. Hydration Properties of Excised Corneal Pieces. A.M.A. Arch. Ophthal. 28:272–284, 1942.

(*d*) Kinsey, V. E., and Cogan, D. G.: The Cornea. IV. Hydration Properties of the Whole Cornea. *Ibid.* 449–463.

(*e*) Cogan, D. G., and Kinsey, V. E.: The Cornea. V. Physiological Aspects. *Ibid.* 661–669.

(f) Cogan, D. G., Hirsch, E. O., and Kinsey, V. E.: The Cornea. VI. Permeability Characteristics of Excised Cornea. A.M.A. Arch. Ophthal. *31*:408–412, 1944.

(g) Cogan, D. G., and Hirsch, E. O.: The Cornea. VII. Permeability to Weak Electrolytes. A.M.A. Arch. Ophthal. *32*:276–282, 1944.

(h) Holt, M., and Cogan, D. G.: The Cornea. VIII. Permeability of Excised Cornea to Ions, as Determined by Measurements of Impedance. A.M.A. Arch. Ophthal. *35*:292–298, 1946.

Cogan, D. G., and Kuwabara, T.: Lipid Keratopathy and Atheroma. Circulation *18*:519–525, (Oct.), 1958.

Cogan, D. G., and Kuwabara, T.: Focal Senile Translucency of the Sclera. A.M.A. Arch. Ophthal. *62*: 604–610, 1959.

Cogan, D. G., and Kuwabara, T.: Ocular Changes in Experimental Hypercholesterolemia. A.M.A. Arch. Ophthal. *61*:219–225, 1959.

Dawson, I.M.P.: Histology and Histochemistry of Gargoylism. J. Path. Bact. *67*:587–604, 1954.

Dunnington, J. A., and Weimar, V. L.: Influence of the Epithelium on the Healing of Corneal Incisions. Amer. J. Ophthal. *45*:89–95, 1958.

Fischer, F. P.: The Biochemistry and Metabolism of the Eye. In Ridley, F., and Sorbsby, A., eds., Modern Trends in Ophthalmology. London, Butterworth and Co., 1940, Chapter 33, pp. 348–360.

Fischer, F. P.: Über die Permeabilität der Hornhaut und über Vitalfärbungen des Vorderen Bulbusabschnittes mit Bemerkungen über die Vitalfärbung des Plexus Chorioideus. Arch. f. Augenh. *100–101*: 480–555, 1929.

Franceschetti, A., and Babel, J.: II. The Heredofamilial Degenerations of the Cornea: B. Pathological Anatomy. Acta XVI Concilium Ophthalmologicum (Britannia), 245–283, 1951.

Friedenwald, J. S., and Buschke, W.: Mitotic and Wound-healing Activities of the Corneal Epithelium. A.M.A. Arch. Ophthal. *32*:410–413, (Nov.), 1944.

Friedenwald, J. S., and Buschke, W.: The Influence of Some Experimental Variables on the Epithelial Movements in the Healing of Corneal Wounds. J. Cell. Comp. Physiol. *23*:95–107, (April), 1944.

Friedenwald, J. S., Buschke, W., and Corwell, J. E.: Exudate from Injured Cells in Its Relation to the Healing of Wounds of the Corneal Epithelium. J. Cell Comp. Physiol. *25*:45–52, (Feb.), 1945.

Friedenwald, J. S., Hughes, W. F., Jr., and Herrmann, H.: Acid-base Tolerance of the Cornea. A.M.A. Arch. Ophthal. *31*:279–283, 1944.

Friedenwald, J. S., and Pierce, H. F.: Circulation of the Aqueous. VI. Intraocular Gas Exchange. A.M.A. Arch. Ophthal. *17*:477–485, (March), 1937.

Fuchs, E.: Dystrophia Epithelialis Cornea. Arch. f. Ophth. *76*:478–508, 1910.

Fuchs, E.: Zur Anatomie der Pinguecula. Arch. f. Ophth. *37*(3):143, 1891.

Garron, L. K.: Cystinosis. Trans. Amer. Acad. Ophthal. Otolaryng. *63*:99–108, 1959.

Garron, L. K., and Feeney, M. L.: Personal Communication.

Goar, E. L.: Dystrophies of the Cornea. Amer. J. Ophthal. *33*:674–692, (May), 1950.

Grant, W. M., and Kern, H. L.: Action of Alkalis on the Corneal Stroma. A.M.A. Arch. Ophthal. *54*:931–939, 1955.

Gruber, R.: Beiträge zur Kenntnis der Hornhaut-Circulation. Arch. f. Ophth. *40*:25–64, 1894.

Gundersen, T.: Results of Autotransplantation of Cornea into Anterior Chamber; Their Significance Regarding Corneal Nutrition. A.M.A. Arch. Ophthal. *20*:645–650, 1938.

Haggerty, T. E., and Zimmerman, L. E.: Mycotic Keratitis. Southern Med. J. *51*:153–159, 1958.

Harris, J. E.: The Physiologic Control of Corneal Hydration. Amer. J. Ophthal. *44*:262–280, (Nov.), 1957.

Herrmann, H., and Hickman, F. H.: Studies on the Physiology, Biochemistry, and Cytopathology of the Cornea in Relation to Injury by Mustard Gas and Allied Toxic Agents. X. Exploratory Studies on Corneal Metabolism. Bull. Johns Hopkins Hosp. *82*: 225–250, 1948.

(b) Herrmann, H., and Hickman, F. H.: XII. Further Experiments on Corneal Metabolism in Respect to Glucose and Lactic Acid. *Ibid.* 260–272.

(c) Herrmann, H., and Hickman, F. H. XIII. The Consumption of Pyruvate, Acetoin, Acetate and Butyrate by the Cornea. *Ibid.* 273–286.

(d) Herrmann, H., and Hickman, F. H.: XIV. The Utilization of Ribose and Other Pentoses by the Cornea. *Ibid.* 287–294.

(e) Herrmann, H., and Moses, S. G.: XV. Studies on Non-protein Nitrogen in the Cornea. *Ibid.* 295–311.

Hogan, M. J., and Cordes, F. C.: Lipochondrodystrophy (Dysostosis Multiplex; Hurler's Disease); Pathologic Changes in Cornea in Three Cases. A.M.A. Arch. Ophthal. *32*:287–295, (Oct.), 1944.

Hughes, W. F., Jr.: Alkali Burns of the Eye. I. Review of Literature and Summary of Present Knowledge. A.M.A. Arch. Ophthal. *35*:423–449, 1946.

Hughes, W. F., Jr.: Alkali Burns of the Eye. II. Clinical and Pathologic Course. A.M.A. Arch. Ophthal. *36*: 189–214, 1946.

Hunter, G. W. III, Frye, W. W., and Swartzwelder, J. C.: A Manual of Tropical Medicine. Philadelphia, W. B. Saunders Co., 1960.

Jakus, M. A.: Studies on the Cornea. II. The Fine Structure of Descemet's Membrane. J. Biophys. Biochem. Cytol. *2*:243–252, (Part II, Supplement), 1956.

Jones, S. T., and Zimmerman, L. E.: Histopathologic Differentiation of Granular, Macular, and Lattice Dystrophies of the Cornea. Amer. J. Ophthal. *51*: 394–410, 1961.

Jones, S. T., and Zimmerman, L. E.: Macular Dystrophy of the Cornea (Groenouw type II). Amer. J. Ophthal. *47*:1–16, 1959.

Kinoshita, J. H., Masurat, T. and Helfant, M.: Pathways of Glucose Metabolism in Corneal Epithelium. Science *122*:72–73, 1955.

Langham, M. E., and Taylor, I. S.: Factors Influencing the Hydration of the Cornea in the Excised Eye and the Living Animal. Brit. J. Ophthal. *40*:321–340, 1956.

Laqueur, L.: Uber die Durchgangigkeit der Hornhaut

für Flüssigkeiten. Centralb. f. d. med. Wissensch. *10*:577–579, 1872.

Leber, T.: Studien über den Flüssigkeitswechsel im Auge. Arch. f. Ophth. *19*:87–185, 1873.

Ley, A. P.: Experimental Fungus Infections of the Cornea, Proc. Assoc. Research Ophth. Amer. J. Ophthal. *42*:59, 1956.

Ley, A. P., and Sanders, T. E.: Fungus Keratitis. A.M.A. Arch. Ophthal. *56*:257, 1956.

Lindsay, S., Reilly, W. A., Gotham, T. J., and Skahin, R.: Gargoylism. Am. J. Dis. Child. *76*:239–306, 1958.

McDonald, J. E.: Early Components of Corneal Wound Closure. A.M.A. Arch. Ophthal. *58*:202–216, 1957.

McDonald, J. E., and Wilder, H. C.: The Effect of Beta Radiation on Corneal Healing. Amer. J. Ophthal. *40*:170–180, (Nov.), 1955.

McGee, H. B., and Falls, H. F.: Hereditary Polymorphous Deep Degeneration of the Cornea. A.M.A. Arch. Ophthal. *50*:462–467, 1953.

Maurice, D. M.: The Permeability to Sodium Ions of the Living Rabbit's Cornea. J. Physiol. *112*:367–391, 1951.

Maurice, D. M.: The Structure and Transparency of the Cornea. J. Physiol. *136*:263–286, 1957.

Merriam, G. R., Jr.: Late Effects of Beta Radiation on the Eye. A.M.A. Arch. Ophthal. *53*:708–717, (May), 1955.

Meyer, K., and Chaffee, E.: The Mucopolysaccharide Acid of the Cornea and Its Enzymatic Hydrolysis. Amer. J. Ophthal. *23*:1320–1325, (Dec.), 1940.

Meyer, K., Grunbauch, M. M., Linker, A., and Hoffman, P.: Excretion of Sulfated Mucopolysaccharides in Gargoylism (Hurler's Syndrome). Proc. Soc. Exp. Biol. Med. *97*:275–279, 1958.

Müller, P.: Degenerescence en Mosaique ("Chagrin de Crocodile" Vogt) de la Membrane de Bowman à la suite d'une Keratite Traumatique avec Hypopyon. Ann. Oculist *182*:122–127, (Feb.), 1949.

Rich, A. R., Chesney, A. M., and Turner, T. B.: Experiments Demonstrating That Acquired Immunity in Syphilis Is Not Dependent upon Allergic Inflammation. Bull. Johns Hopkins Hosp. *52*:179–202, (March), 1933.

Rones, B.: Ochronosis Oculi in Alkaptonuria. Amer. J. Ophthal. *49*:440–446, 1960.

Schoninger, Leni: Uber Pterygium. Klin. Monatsbl. f. Augenh. *77*:805–813, 1926.

Sigelman, S., and Friedenwald, J. S.: Mitotic and Wound-healing Activities of the Corneal Epithelium. Effect on Sensory Denervation. A.M.A. Arch. Ophthal. *52*:46–57, 1954.

Skinsnes, O. K.: Generalized Ochronosis. A.M.A. Arch. Path. *45*:552, 1948.

Smelser, G. K.: The Influence of Vehicles and Form of Penicillin and Sulfonamides on Mitosis and Healing of Corneal Burns. Amer. J. Ophthal. *29*:541–551, (May), 1946.

Smelser, G. K., and Ozanics, V.: The Effect of Chemotherapeutic Agents on Cell Division and Healing of Corneal Burns and Abrasions in the Rat. Amer. J. Ophthal. *27*:1063–1073, (Oct.), 1944.

Smelser, G. K., and Ozanics, V.: The Effect of Local Anesthetics on Cell Division and Migration following Thermal Burns of the Cornea. A.M.A. Arch. Ophthal. *34*:271–277, (Oct.), 1945.

Smelser, G. K., and Pfeiffer, R. L.: The Influence of Grenz Rays on Cell Division and Wound Healing in the Corneal Epithelium. A.M.A. Arch. Ophthal. *39*:1–8, (Jan.), 1948.

Snell, A. C., and Irwin, E. S.: Hereditary Deep Dystrophy of the Cornea. Amer. J. Ophthal. *45*:636–638, 1958.

Stocker, F. W., and Holt, L. B.: Rare Form of Hereditary Epithelial Dystrophy; Genetic, Clinical, and Pathologic Study. A.M.A. Arch. Ophthal. *53*:536–541, 1955.

Swan, K.: Modification in the Technique of Filtration Operation: In: Symposium on Glaucoma, edited by Clark, W. B., St. Louis, C. V. Mosby Co. 1959, pp. 191–203.

Theodore, F. H.: Congenital Type of Endothelial Dystrophy. A.M.A. Arch. Ophthal. *21*:626–638, 1939.

Tower, S. S.: Unit for Sensory Reception in Cornea, with Notes on Nerve Impulses from Sclera, Iris and Lens. J. Neurophysiol. *3*:486–500, 1940.

Tower, S. S.: Pain: Definition and Properties of the Unit for Sensory Reception. Assn. Research Nerv. and Ment. Dis. Proc. *23*:16–43, 1943.

Uzman, L. L.: Chemical Nature of the Storage Substance in Gargoylism. A.M.A. Arch. Path. *60*:308–318, 1955.

Verdi, G. P., and Filippone, A.: A Case of Heredofamilial Corneal Degeneration of Reis-Bücklers Type. Boll. d'ocul. *37*:410–430, 1958.

Von Bahr, G.: Corneal Thickness: Its Measurements and Changes. Amer. J. Ophthal. *42*:251–265, (Aug.), 1956.

Weimar, V. L.: The Sources of Fibroblasts in Corneal Wound Repair. A.M.A. Arch. Ophthal. *60*:93–109, 1958.

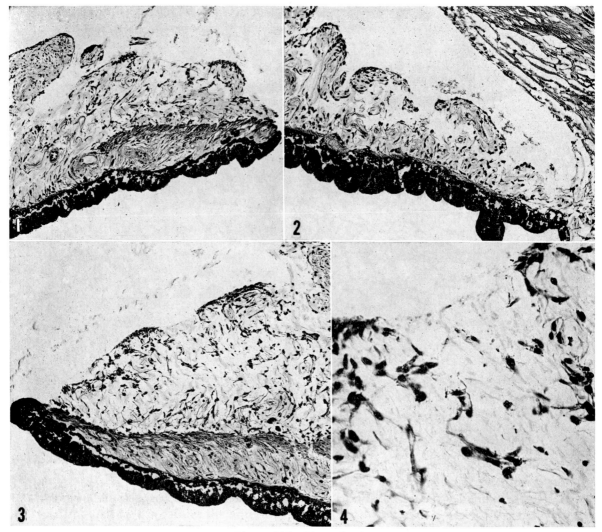

Figure 293. Normal Iris

The cells on the anterior surface of the iris do not form a continuous delimiting membrane. The crypts are especially free of lining cells. AFIP Acc. 850915.

1. Pupillary zone. ×85.
2. Peripheral iris. ×115.
3. Pupillary zone. ×115.
4. Same crypt shown in center of 3, enlarged to ×400.

Plate II). The character of the connective tissue of the stroma permits rapid expansion and contraction. The blood vessels, which comprise a substantial portion of the volume of the iris, generally run radially in a sinuous manner. They enter the iris root and pass through the ciliary zone in several layers. At the junction of the ciliary and pupillary zones, they anastomose to form the minor circle of the iris which consists of both arteries and veins. The vessels, which frequently appear thick-walled, have been shown by electron microscopy to consist of an endothelial lining and a thick collar of collagen

fibrils (Figs. 295, 296). This thick adventitia may account for the remarkably low permeability of iris vessels. The veins of the iris have perivascular sheaths. The nerve fibers are sensory, vasomotor and motor, the latter supplying the iris muscles. They are not visible by ordinary staining methods. There are many branching pigment-bearing melanocytes scattered through the stroma. Clump cells are rounded epithelial cells, derived from the posterior pigment epithelium, which have migrated into the stroma in the region of the sphincter (Fig. 292–3).

The dilator muscle of the pupil or posterior

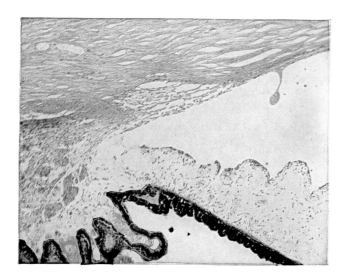

COLOR PLATE II. This eye from a 66-year-old white woman was enucleated because of a small choroidal melanoma. The tension was 16.9 mm. Hg and the other eye was completely normal. (AFIP Acc. 758543. All illustrations magnified ×65.)

(A) The routine hematoxylin-eosin-stained section gives the impression that the intertrabecular spaces are empty. Observe also that the iris stroma and the uveal tissue in the chamber angle appear to contain an abundance of nonstaining ground substance.

(B) An adjacent section stained for acid mucopolysaccharides by the Rhinehart-Abul-Haj technic reveals much stainable material in the intertrabecular spaces and in the iris stroma. Acid mucopolysaccharides appear blue; collagen fibers stain red and the smooth muscles of the iris and ciliary body are pale yellow-green because of the picrofucsin counterstain employed.

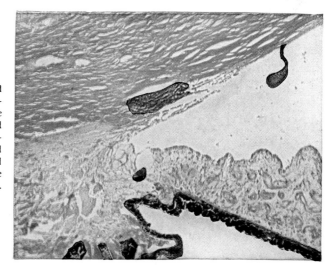

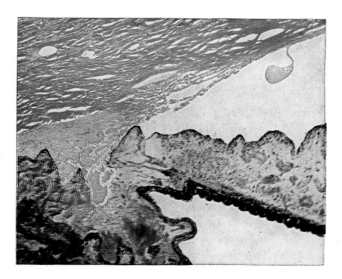

(C) Another adjacent section has been stained by the same technic employed in B but the section was first treated with bovine testicular hyaluronidase. Now only a trace of the acid mucopolysaccharide remains in the intertrabecular spaces and none is observed in the iris stroma. This is histochemical evidence that an hyaluronidase-sensitive acid mucopolysaccharide is present in the trabecula and iris stroma.

(From: Zimmerman, L. E.: Am. J. Ophth. 44, 1, 1957.)

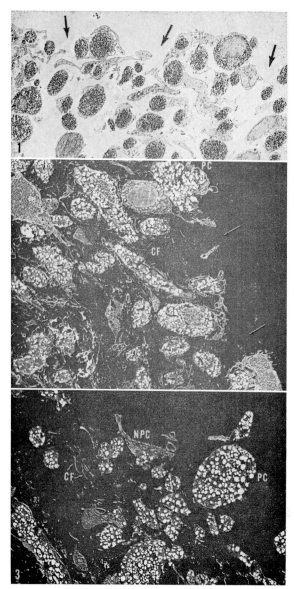

Figure 294. Normal Iris

Electron micrographs reveal many apertures (arrows) measuring 1–2 microns in width between the pigmented (PC) and nonpigmented (NPC) stromal cells which are concentrated along the anterior iris surface. These cells exhibit no specialized orientation and they are not intimately interdigitated. No true endothelial membrane covers the iris. Many collagenous filaments (CF) may be observed between the stromal cells.

1. Rhesus monkey. ×2,650.

2. Two year old human. Shadow-cast with uranium. ×2,830.

3. Adult human. Shadow-cast with uranium. ×2,830. (From Tousimis and Fine, 1959.)

membrane (Fig. 297) is a smooth muscle and extends from the region of the sphincter muscle to the base of the iris. It is fused to the sphincter near the edge of the pupil and sends off prolongations into the ciliary body at its peripheral end. Fuchs' spur consists of a few dilator fibers and pigment cells which project into the sphincter muscle near its mid-portion. Michel's spur is a similar projection at the peripheral edge of the sphincter muscle. The dilator and the sphincter muscles of the pupil are derived from the pigment epithelium of the iris and therefore are neuroectodermal muscles. The sphincter muscle of the pupil is a smooth muscle which lies in the posterior iris stroma next to the pupil (Figs. 293, 298). It has attachments to the stromal fibers which permit it to function even after removal of a segment of the pupillary portion of the iris.

The epithelium of the iris consists of two layers of densely pigmented cells, distinguishable as separate layers after bleaching (Fig. 297) and by electron microscopy. The anterior layer contains the nuclei of the dilator muscle fibers (Fig. 297). The epithelium forms the posterior surface of the iris and provides a lining for the anterior part of the posterior chamber. The melanin pigment granules in these cells usually are uniform in amount and distribution. At the pupillary margin the two layers of pigment epithelium are continuous and they form the pigment seam.

THE CILIARY BODY

Anatomy. The ciliary body is approximately 6 to 6.5 mm. wide and extends from the base of the iris to become continuous with the anterior choroid at the ora serrata (Fig. 60). On sagittal section it appears as a right triangle, the short side or face forming the lateral boundary of the anterior chamber (Fig. 299). It is composed of two parts: (1) The corona ciliaris (pars plicata) which forms the anterior 2 mm. and contains the ciliary processes, which are irregular radial ridges 2 mm. long, 0.8 mm. high, and approximately 70 in number. Because of their irregularity the ordinary meridional sections of the eye reveal segments of several processes projecting into the posterior chamber. (2) The orbiculus ciliaris (pars plana) which is the posterior or flat part of the ciliary body; it measures 4 to 4.5 mm. in length. Posteriorly the stroma of the pars plana merges with the choroid while the ciliary epithelium abruptly unites with the retina. The union presents a scalloped outline (the ora serrata), the convex projections of which are directed posteriorly. On the nasal side the serrations are more prominent. The vitreous base and the strongest of the zonular fibers are attached to the posterior half of the pars plana along the ora serrata and somewhat back on the retina. On the temporal side in the region of the vitreous base the two layers of ciliary epithelium are more firmly attached to each other, and the pigment epithelium is thicker. Therefore, according to Schepens, the ora serrata characteristically presents distinctive differences on the temporal and nasal sides, the serrations being less prominent but more deeply pigmented on the temporal side.

Histology. The ciliary body consists of six layers: the outermost lamina fusca or suprachoroidal tissue plane, the ciliary muscle, the layer of vessels, the lamina vitrea, the epithelium, and the internal limiting membrane. The lamina fusca or suprachoroidal tissue plane is a potential space between the sclera and the ciliary body. The ciliary muscle is separable into three groups of fibers (Fig. 299). The outermost, Brücke's muscle, forms the *longitudinal portion* which attaches anteriorly to the scleral spur and trabecular fibers. The innermost, Müller's muscle, forms the *circular portion.* The *radial portion* is formed by some of the anterior fibers of the longitudinal muscle which run obliquely to become continuous with the circular fibers. Posteriorly the fibers end in branched stellate figures (muscle stars) in the suprachoroid at the equator or beyond. The major vascular circle of the iris lies in the ciliary body in front of the circular muscle. The connective tissue stroma of the ciliary muscle layer contains blood vessels, nerves and melanocytes.

The vessel layer is a direct continuation of the vessel layer of the choroid. The stroma of this layer resembles that of the choroid but has fewer melanocytes and a denser connective tissue (Fig. 300). Each ciliary process is a fold of connective tissue with a vascular

(*Continued on p. 354.*)

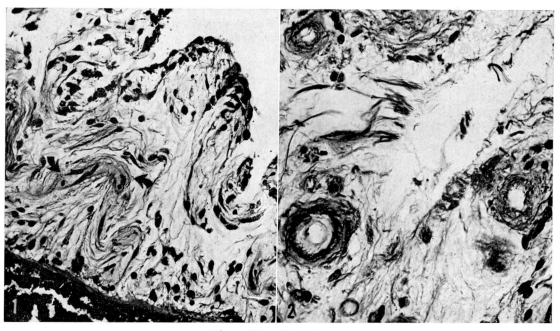

Figure 295. Normal Iris

Stromal cells and fibrils are oriented about the vessels, giving them the appearance of being thick-walled. AFIP Acc. 850915.

1. A capillary (arrow) and its ensheathing stromal fibrils are shown in semilongitudinal section. ×280.
2. Three similar capillaries are observed in cross-section. Wilder's stain for reticulum. ×450.

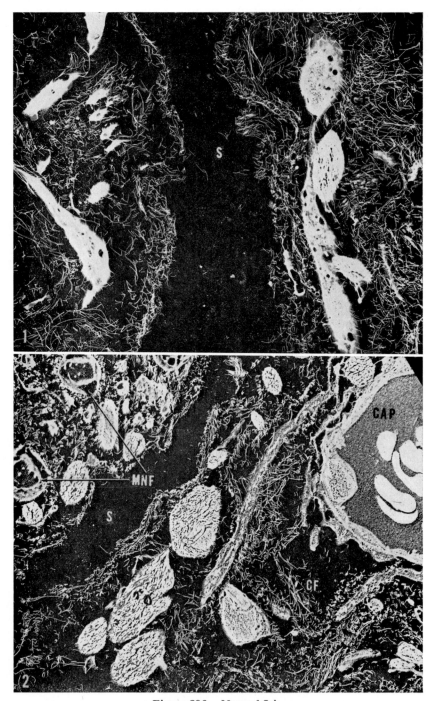

Figure 296.   Normal Iris

Electron micrographs of iris stroma reveal linear spaces (S) or canals passing between aggregates of stromal tissue—collagenous filaments (CF), pigmented and nonpigmented cells, capillaries (CAP), and myelinated nerve fibers (MNF).

1. Adult human. Shadow cast with uranium. ×2,830.

2. Rhesus monkey. Shadow cast with uranium. ×2,830. (From Tousimis and Fine, 1959.)

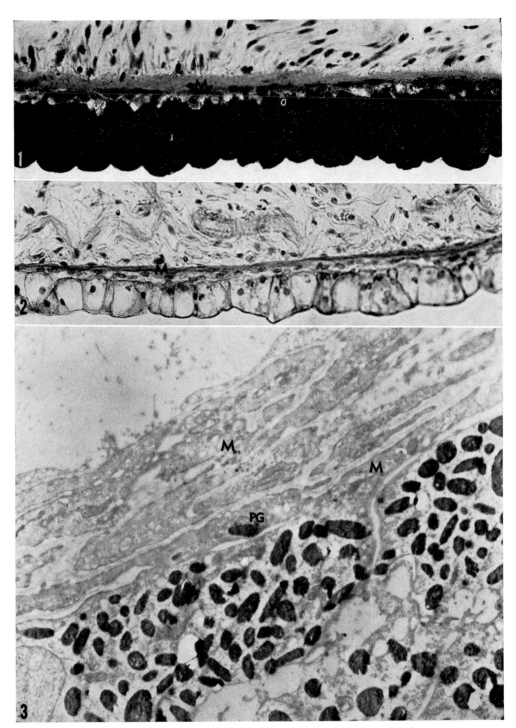

Figure 297. Pigment Epithelium and Dilator Muscle of Iris

1. The dilator muscle (M) of the iris lies just anterior to the double-layered pigment epithelium. ×250. AFIP Acc. 84029.

2. Bleached section reveals the double-layered pigment epithelium, the anterior layer of which gives rise to the dilator muscle. ×250. AFIP Acc. 118267.

3. Electron micrograph demonstrates the continuity that exists between the dilator muscle cells (M) and the anterior row of pigmented epithelial cells. An occasional pigment granule (PG) may be seen in the elongated protoplasmic extension of these smooth muscle cells. Rhesus monkey. ×12,270. (From Tousimis and Fine, 1959.)

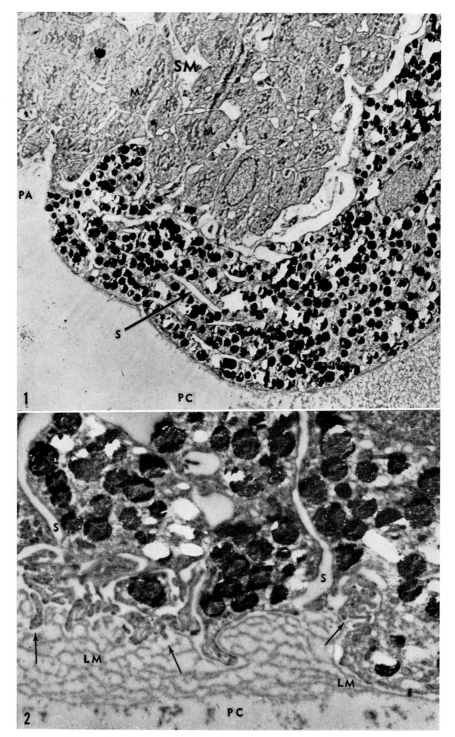

Figure 298.

1. Electron micrograph of pupillary margin of rhesus monkey iris. Mitochondria (M) may be seen in the sphincter muscle cells (SM). The pupillary area (PA) is to the left and the posterior chamber (PC) is at the bottom of the picture. Large intercellular spaces (S) are present between the two layers of cells forming the pigmented epithelium. ×4,500. (From Tousimis and Fine, 1959.)

2. Electron micrograph of the posterior surface of the rhesus monkey iris. There is marked infolding of the cytoplasmic membrane as a result of which the cell surface appears to have a myriad of microvilli (arrows) projecting toward the posterior chamber (PC). A multi-layered limiting membrane (LM) covers the surface of these cells and the openings of the intercellular spaces (S). ×16,000. (From Tousimis and Fine, in Smelser, 1961.)

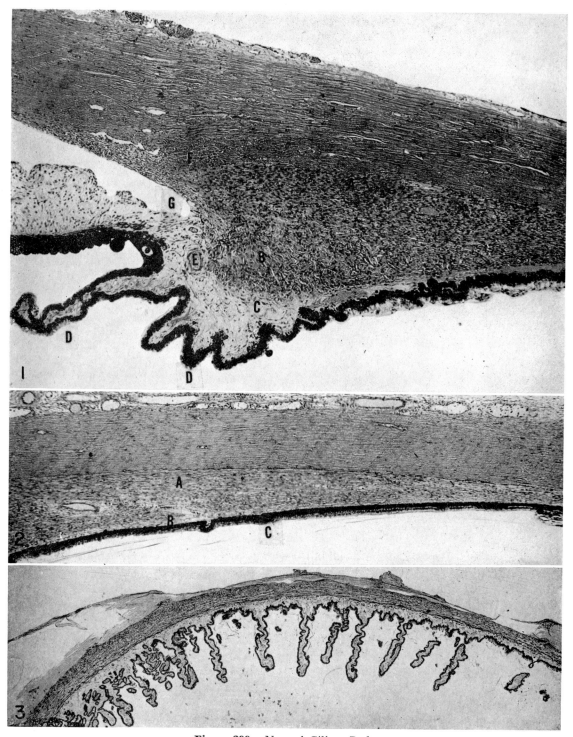

Figure 299. Normal Ciliary Body

1. Corona ciliaris. A, longitudinal muscle. B, radiating and circular muscles. C, vascular layer. D, ciliary processes. E, circulus arteriosus major. F, scleral spur. G, anterior chamber angle. ×75. AFIP Acc. 84029.

2. Orbiculus ciliaris (pars plana). A, longitudinal muscle. B, vascular layer. C, epithelial layers. ×55. AFIP Acc. 82691.

3. Flat section of ciliary processes. ×20. AFIP Acc. 38096.

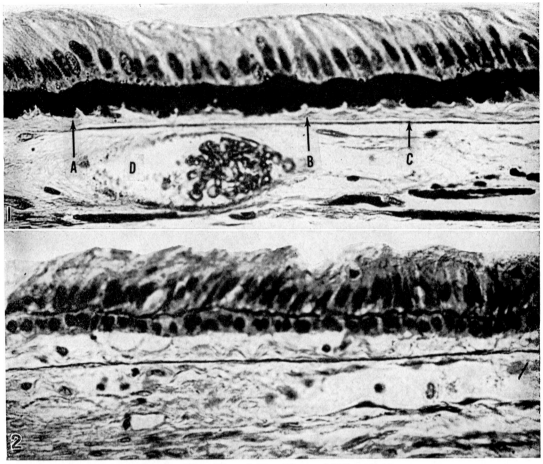

Figure 300.   Normal Pars Plana of Ciliary Body

1. Columnar epithelium of pars ciliaris retinae near ora serrata, and cuboidal pigment epithelium. A, cuticular layer of Bruch's membrane. B, avascular connective tissue layer. C, elastic layer of Bruch's membrane. D, vascular layer of ciliary body. ×515. AFIP Acc. 47846.

2. The same, bleached section. ×515. AFIP Acc. 118267.

core and covered by ciliary epithelium. (Fig. 299–3). The posterior ciliary arteries traverse the suprachoroidal space to supply the major circle of the iris, from which branches pass to enter the anterior ciliary processes. Each process is supplied by a small arterial branch which breaks up into large capillaries, 20 to 30 microns in diameter (Fig. 301), all of which are drained by a single vein. According to Friedenwald and Stiehler, the walls of these capillaries are much more permeable than those elsewhere in the eye, and recently Holmberg has demonstrated by electron microscopy that these capillaries have very thin walls which contain exceedingly large pores measuring 200 to 1000 angstroms (Fig. 302).

Bruch's membrane splits at the ora serrata into an outer elastic and an inner cuticular layer which are separated by a layer of avascular collagenous connective tissue (Fig. 300). The elastic lamina gradually vanishes in the anterior part of the corona ciliaris but the cuticular lamina reaches the iris root.

The epithelium consists of two layers of cells, the outermost of which is pigmented (Figs. 300, 303). In the adult the two layers are firmly united at the ora serrata so that most retinal separations stop at this site. According to Schepens (1954), the union of these two layers of ciliary epithelium is strongest on the temporal side along a hyperpigmented bandshaped area adjacent to the ora serrata (Fig. 303). At times, particularly in infants,

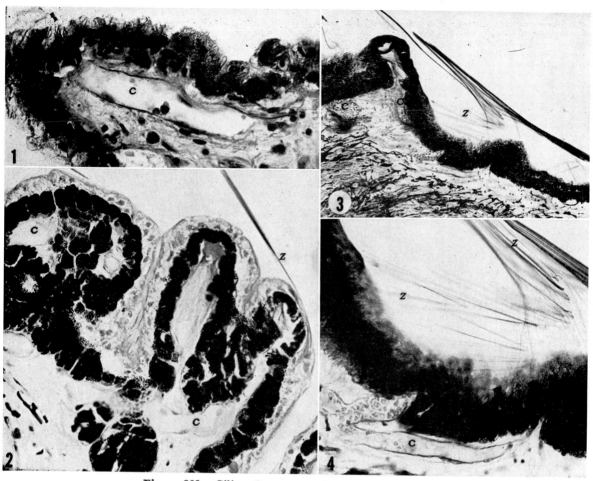

Figure 301. Ciliary Processes and Zonular Attachments

Large capillaries (c) lie in close apposition to the pigmented epithelium. Zonular fibers (z) attach to the surface of the nonpigmented epithelium. AFIP Acc. 630832.
1. ×380. Verhoeff's stain.
2. ×305. Periodic acid-Schiff reaction
3. ×115. Periodic acid-Schiff reaction.
4. ×305. Periodic acid-Schiff reaction.

and in choroidal tumors, retinal separation extends into the pars plana up to the ciliary processes. The innermost layer of ciliary epithelium acquires pigment as it approaches the iris root. Both Holmberg and Pappas have presented evidence, obtained by electron microscopy, that the ciliary epithelium has secretory activity.

The internal limiting membrane is a complicated meshwork (Fig. 304) which, according to Holmberg, on electron microscopy contains homogeneous material of low density within its meshes. The membrane which dips down to fill cleft-like spaces between adjacent epithelial cells, appears to contain a homogeneous material (Holmberg, 1960). The

zonular fibers of the lens are attached to this membrane.

In accommodation, contraction of the ciliary muscle allows a change in the form of the crystalline lens, changing the dioptric power of the eye. According to Rones, contraction and relaxation of the ciliary muscle are believed to influence the outflow of aqueous through the trabecula, some of the muscle fibers attaching to the wall of the canal (color plate). Anatomic studies by Flocks et al. have shown that pilocarpine, by its action on the ciliary muscle, scleral spur, and trabecula, enlarges the openings in the corneoscleral trabecula and decreases the resistance to aqueous outflow.

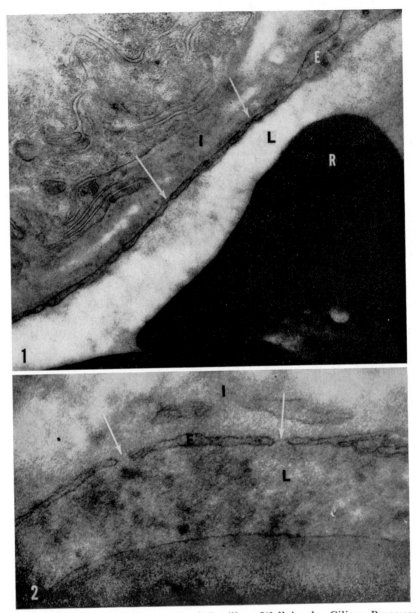

Figure 302. Electron Micrograph of Capillary Wall in the Ciliary Processes

I, interstitial space between pigment epithelium and capillary; E, endothelium of capillary; L, lumen of capillary; R, red blood cell in lumen.

1. Many focal areas of extreme attenuation of the capillary wall are seen (arrows). Rhesus monkey, ×27,400. (Courtesy of Dr. B. S. Fine, unpublished work.)

2. Pores (arrows) in capillary wall. ×84,000. (Courtesy of Dr. A. S. Holmberg, 1959.)

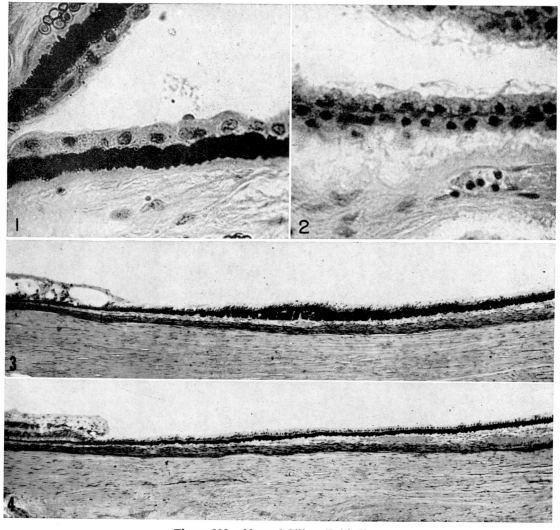

Figure 303. Normal Ciliary Epithelium

1. Cuboidal epithelium of pigment layer and pars ciliaris retinae, over ciliary process. ×515. AFIP Acc. 47846

2. The same, bleached section. ×515. AFIP Acc. 118267

3. The pigment epithelium of the pars plana on the temporal side often appears hyperplastic as compared with the corresponding layer on the nasal side (see 4). Cystoid degeneration of the oral retina is also more frequent and extensive on the temporal side. ×60. AFIP Acc. 45119.

4. Nasal side of same section of eye shown in 3 reveals the pigment epithelium to be thinner. There is no cystoid degeneration of the peripheral retina. ×60.

THE CHOROID

Anatomy. The choroid forms the middle coat of the posterior eye and extends from the ora serrata to the optic nerve. It is attached to the sclera, chiefly by the perforating vessels and nerves. It varies in thickness from 0.1 mm. anteriorly to 0.22 mm. posteriorly. Small amounts of choroidal tissue, including melanocytes in some heavily pigmented persons, extend across the optic nerve canal as a loose meshwork which is perforated by the nerve bundles.

Histology. The choroid consists of five layers. From without inward there are the suprachoroid, a layer of large vessels (Haller's layer), a layer of vessels of medium caliber (Sattler's layer), the choriocapillaris, and Bruch's membrane (lamina vitrea) (Fig. 305). The suprachoroid (lamina suprachoroidea, or lamina fusca) consists of branching collagenous and elastic fibers containing fibroblasts,

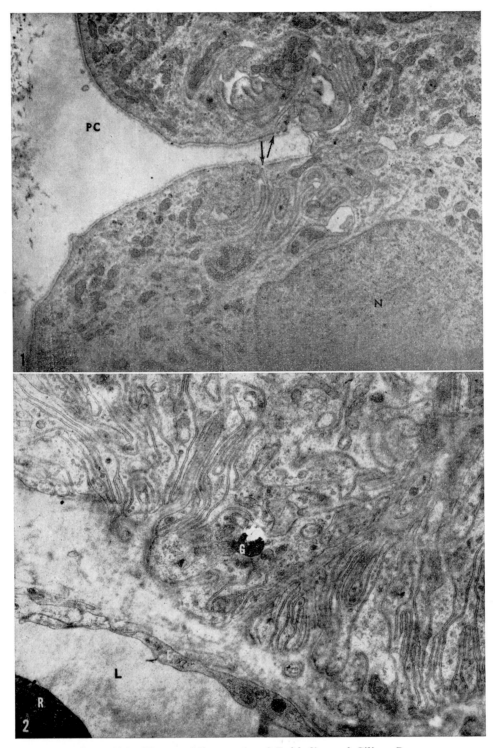

Figure 304. Electron Micrographs of Epithelium of Ciliary Process

1. Inner surface of nonpigmented ciliary epithelium presents many deep, tortuous infoldings (arrows). The posterior chamber (PC) is to the left; a portion of the cell nucleus (N) is shown. Rhesus monkey. ×12,400.

2. Outer surface of pigmented epithelium also presents a very complex series of deep infoldings. Most of the pigment granules are found at the other end of the cell (not shown in this field) but one granule (G) is present. Only ground substance is observed between the cell and the capillary shown at lower left. E, endothelium of capillary; L, lumen of capillary; R, red blood cell in capillary. Rhesus monkey. ×16,000. (Courtesy of Dr. B. S. Fine, unpublished work.)

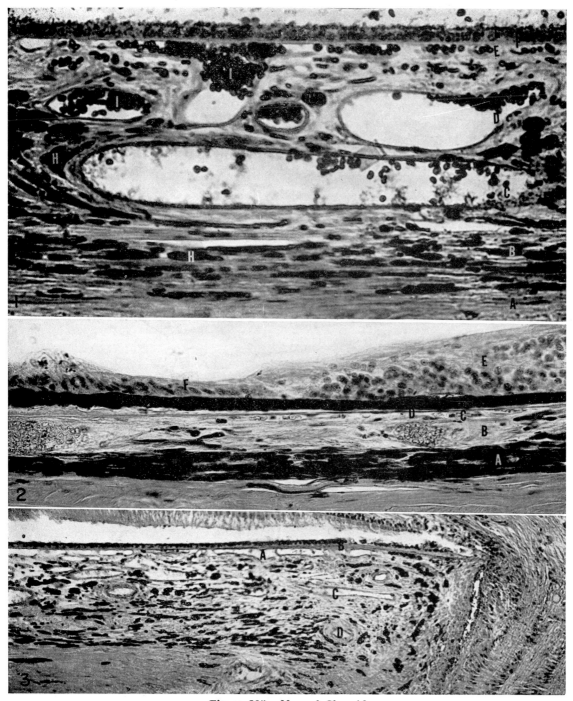

Figure 305. Normal Choroid

1. A, lamina fusca of sclera. B, suprachoroid. C, vascular layer, large vein in outer portion. D, vascular layer, medium-sized vein in inner portion. E, choriocapillaris. F, Bruch's membrane. G, retinal pigment epithelium. H, melanocytes. I, red blood cells. ×425. AFIP Acc. 47846.

2. Choroid at ora serrata. A, suprachoroid with melanocytes. B, vascular layer. C, choriocapillaris. D, Bruch's membrane. E, retina. F, pars ciliaris retinae. ×360. AFIP Acc. 47846.

3. Choroid at margin of optic disk; layers are less well defined with exception of choriocapillaris (A) and Bruch's membrane (B). Stroma is more dense, veins (C) smaller, arteries (D) more prominent. ×150. AFIP Acc. 47846.

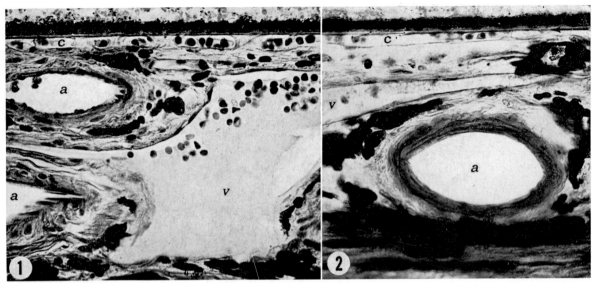

Figure 306. Normal Choroid

Arteries (a), veins (v), choriocapillaris (c), and Bruch's membrane (arrows). 30 year old man. AFIP Acc. 630832.
1. ×380. Verhoeff's stain.
2. ×380. Periodic acid-Schiff reaction.

melanocytes, and smooth muscle fibers. The laminas are more tightly adherent to each other in the posterior choroid and where the vessels pass through them; hence, choroidal detachment rarely occurs posteriorly. The vascular layers consist of arteries and veins, the latter predominating. The arteries decrease in caliber as they approach the choriocapillaris. From this point the veins eventually drain into the vortex system. According to Ashton, the vessels anastomose freely but there are no arteriovenous anastomoses. Wybar (1954) demonstrated free anastomoses between the anterior and posterior vessels of the choroid, suggesting that several of the posterior ciliary vessels probably could supply the entire choroid. He also (1955) found definite anastomoses between the retinal and uveal veins about the optic nerve, which might explain the variable course following occlusion of the central retinal vein. The stroma of the vessel layers consists of collagenous and elastic tissue with variable numbers of melanocytes, depending on the genetic make-up of the individual. The choriocapillaris is a single layer of capillaries, extending from the disk to the ora serrata. They are among the largest in the body, and have a greater size in the macular region than elsewhere.

The lamina vitrea, or Bruch's membrane, is a thin membrane which lines the entire inner choroid. It consists of an extremely thin external elastic lamina derived from the network of delicate fibrils which invests the choriocapillaris, and an inner cuticular layer

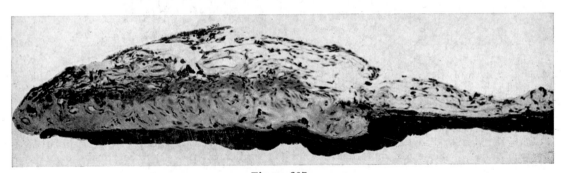

Figure 307.

Senile hyalinization of pupillary zone of iris, particularly behind sphincter. ×120. AFIP Acc. 103975.

produced by the retinal pigment epithelium (Figs. 305, 306). The choroid is abundantly supplied with nerves, most of which come from short ciliary nerves, and it is traversed by the long posterior ciliary nerves which run forward to supply the ciliary body and iris. Ganglion cells are scattered through the choroid.

The choroid is essentially a network of blood vessels which supplies nutriments to the outer retina and the anterior ocular structures. The degree of pigmentation of the fundus, which often varies with the complexion of the individual, is determined by the amount of pigment in the choroid. The amount of pigment in the retinal epithelium by contrast does not show comparable variations except in albinism.

GROWTH AND AGING

Iris. The melanocytes of the iris contain little or no pigment at birth. Within the first few months the pigment increases and the iris color deepens. In the newborn, the pupils are small and the iris crypts are absent, but they become more apparent during the first year or two. The stroma of the infant iris appears more cellular than in the adult because the nuclei of the connective tissue cells are closer, there is less ground substance, and there are fewer fibers between the stromal cells (Fig. 239). With growth, the entire tissue becomes thicker and a greater amount of intercellular matrix is seen in proportion to the number of nuclei. During childhood and adolescence, the pupils attain their maximum size.

In advanced age, there is flattening of the iris surface with a tendency toward obliteration of the crypts and surface markings because of stromal atrophy (Fig. 307). This may expose the posterior pigment epithelium to view. The sphincter muscle of the pupil becomes sclerotic with age, and the pupil is smaller and less mobile. The pigment epithelium may become hyperplastic (Fig. 308) or atrophic and lose some of its pigment. The liberated pigment granules are deposited on

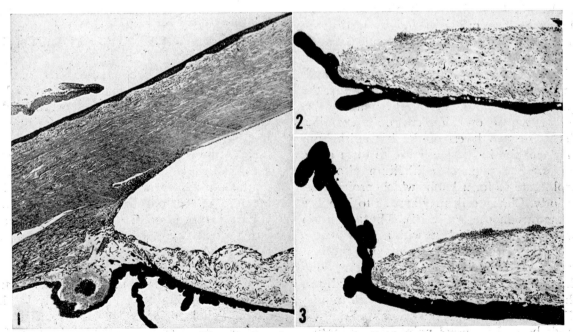

Figure 308. Proliferative Reactions of Pigment Epithelium of Iris

1. Senile hyperplasia is observed most frequently near the iris root. ×100. AFIP Acc. 249015.

2 and 3. Excrescences of hyperplastic pigment epithelium in the pupil are observed most often in children who have been on miotics. ×60. AFIP Acc. 769145. (From case reported by Christensen, Swan, and Huggins, 1956.)

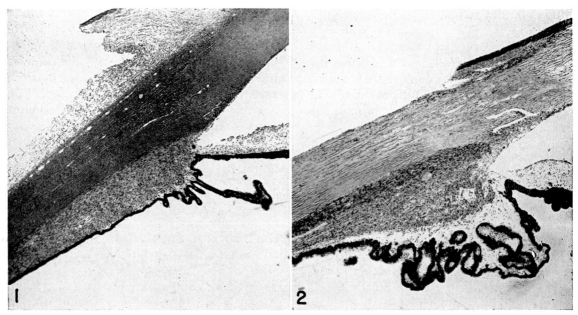

Figure 309. Growth and Aging of Ciliary Body

1. Ciliary body, age 10 months. Flat corona, thin vascular layer and long narrow processes. ×45. AFIP Acc. 186179.

2. Ciliary body, age 68. Prominent corona, thick vascular layer and broad processes. ×45. AFIP Acc. 206642.

the posterior cornea, occasionally in a vertical line (Krukenberg's spindle), on the anterior surface of the iris, on the lens, in the anterior chamber angle, and in the corneoscleral meshwork. Free pigment is phagocytosed by the corneal endothelium and by histiocytes. If the stroma in the pupillary zone becomes atrophic simultaneously, the condition is usually termed senile hyalinization of the pupillary zone. Owing to the stromal atrophy, the sphincter muscle of the pupil frequently becomes visible on biomicroscopic examination. The two layers of the iris epithelium may separate in the senile eye to form cystic spaces. The pigment epithelium also may proliferate to form knobs which project posteriorly. Clump cells may appear to be more numerous in the senile iris. The adventitia of the iris vessels thickens with age.

Nodular excrescences composed of proliferated pigment epithelium may appear along the pupillary border of the iris, especially in children who have been treated with miotics (Fig. 308–2). The pigment epithelium extends beyond its usual point of termination to form two-layered membranes, minute nodules, and small epithelial cysts in the pupillary aperture. Christensen, Swan, and Huggins have suggested that while the pathogenesis of this reaction remains unknown, it may represent a specific tissue response to parasympathetic stimulation. The resultant lesions, except for their occurrence in the pupillary zone, resemble the "senile proliferations" observed near the iris root (**Fig. 308–1**).

Ciliary body. The ciliary body of the young eye appears to contain more nuclei because the muscle fibers are not fully developed and very little connective tissue is present (Fig. 309). The corona of the ciliary body of the young eye is flat. The prominent corona of the adult results from hypertrophy of the muscle fibers and an increase in the amount of surrounding connective tissue. Ciliary processes on the posterior peripheral iris, present in fetal life and seen in many animals, normally are displaced backward at or soon after birth.

In advanced age, the processes of the ciliary body become hyalinized, particularly in the subepithelial region (Fig. 310–1, 2). These changes are accompanied by thickening of a basement membrane, demonstrable with the periodic acid fuchsin stain. Eventually fine basophilic granules (calcium salts) may be

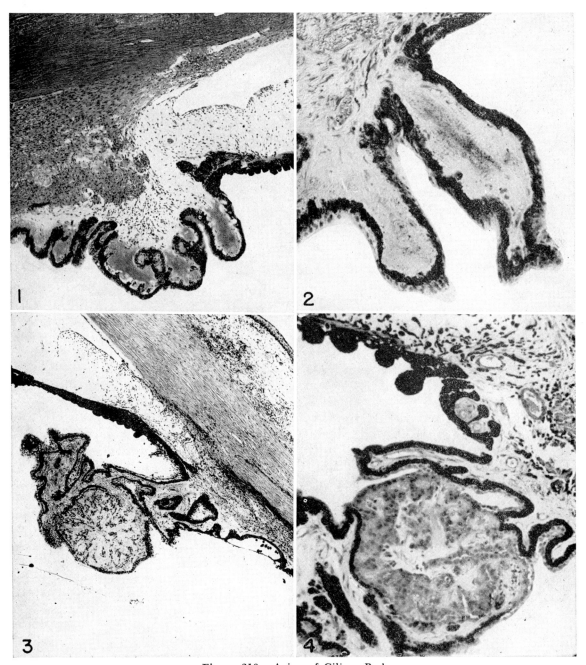

Figure 310.   Aging of Ciliary Body

1. Ciliary body. Thick vascular layer and hyalinized processes. ×70. AFIP Acc. 84029.
2. Granular calcium deposits in hyalinized ciliary processes. ×115. AFIP Acc. 160972.
3. Pseudoadenomatous hyperplasia of ciliary epithelium. ×48. AFIP Acc. 190350.
4. Pseudoadenomatous hyperplasia of ciliary epithelium. Nodular hyperplasia of ciliary pigment epithelium ×175. AFIP Acc. 28134.

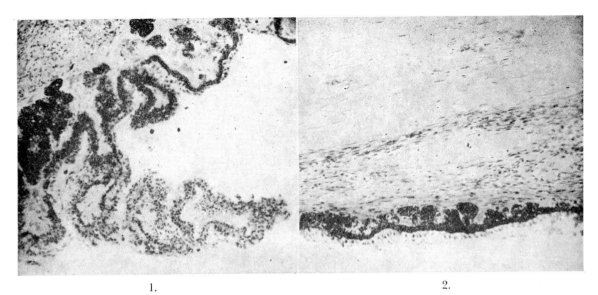

1.   2.

Figure 311.

1. Loss of pigment from layer of ciliary pigment epithelium. Proliferation of ciliary epithelium. ×120. **AFIP** Acc. 69605.

2. Proliferation of ciliary pigment epithelium of pars plana. ×125. AFIP Acc. 130793.

seen in sharp contrast to the smooth eosinophilic background. Associated with this is a progressive sclerosis and obliteration of the blood vessels in the ciliary processes. The ciliary muscle becomes very atrophic and hyalinized in the aged.

The two epithelial layers over the processes may proliferate, forming a mass which protrudes into the posterior chamber. Excessive tubular hyperplasia, chiefly of the nonpigmented epithelium, may produce a mass with an adenomatous appearance (Fig. 310–3, 4). Proliferation of the pigmented layer may be associated with a loss of pigment (Fig. 311–1). In the pars plana, proliferated pigment epithelium may form numerous small knobs extending into the vascular layer (Fig. 311–2).

Choroid. Nuclei are relatively numerous in the choroid of the young and the neophyte in eye pathology may interpret them as infiltrating inflammatory cells (Fig. 312). According to Reese and Blodi, extramedullary hematopoiesis occurs in and around the eye, especially in the choroid, both in prematurely born and full term infants.

In the aged, small focal thickenings (excrescences or drusen) may develop in the cuticular portion of the lamina vitrea. They are dome-shaped, homogeneous, sometimes calcified, and are covered by degenerated pigment epithelium (Fig. 313). Drusen are be-

lieved to be formed by activity of the senescent retinal pigment epithelium but they also may be seen in youth. They are more common, more numerous, and more variable in size and shape when they develop as a result of a pathologic process. The senile eye also may reveal granular deposits on Bruch's membrane which result from lipoidal degeneration of the retinal pigment epithelium (Fig. 313–3). These deposits are less rounded than drusen and contain calcium granules more frequently. Atrophy and depigmentation of the choroid in the extreme periphery of the fundus are common in the aged. Similar atrophic changes also are frequently seen in the peripapillary region. In both areas the lesion is associated with, and perhaps caused by, fibrosis, hyalinization and occlusion of the choroidal vessels, particularly of the choriocapillaris. Lipoid infiltration of the deeper layers of the choroid may be associated with arcus senilis, and Bruch's membrane also may contain lipids. A common degenerative change is one which results in diffuse thickening and basophilic staining of Bruch's membrane. It begins around the disk and extends peripherally (Fig. 313–1). Sometimes actual breaks occur in this membrane and the clinical and microscopic picture resembles that seen in angioid streaks. In advanced cases there may be extensive calcification.

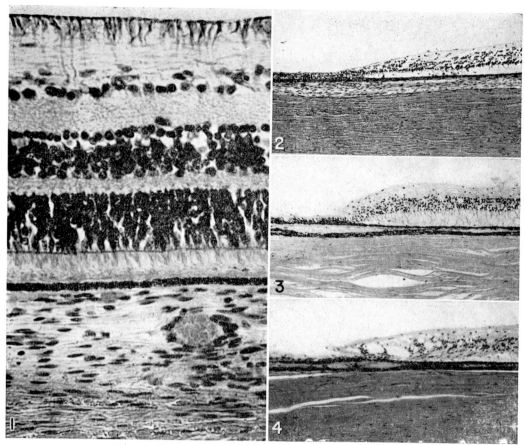

Figure 312. Growth and Aging of Choroid and Retina

1. Choroid and retina in an infant. Abundant nuclei, inconspicuous vessels and absence of pigment in choroid Narrow outer plexiform layer in retina. ×425. AFIP Acc. 74538.
2. Ora serrata in infant. ×90. AFIP Acc. 186179.
3. Ora serrata in adolescent. ×90. AFIP Acc. 192373.
4. Ora serrata in adult. Early cystoid degeneration. ×90. AFIP Acc. 36099.

CONGENITAL AND DEVELOPMENTAL ABNORMALITIES

Aniridia. Aniridia probably is due to an arrest in the differentiation of the optic cup at the 70 to 80 mm. stage. Complete absence of the iris (aniridia) is rare. It usually is incomplete, a narrow rim of rudimentary iris being present at the periphery. Usually both eyes are affected but the disease may be more severe in one eye than in the other. Associated defects are cataract, microphakia, poor development of the fovea and extensive retinal aplasia.

Histologically, the rudimentary iris consists of undeveloped ectodermal and mesodermal elements. It may be in contact with the trabecular meshwork (Fig. 314). Glaucoma frequently is associated with this condition.

Coloboma of the iris. Congenital coloboma of the iris is characterized by an absence of a sector of the iris. The remainder of the iris is normal. *Typical* colobomas are situated in the position of the fetal fissure (down and nasally) and often extend through the entire uveal tract. *Atypical* colobomas involve other iris sectors. The defect may extend from the pupil to the periphery or involve only a part of the iris.

Histologic examination of the base of a typical coloboma reveals changes similar to those seen in aniridia (Fig. 315–1). The edge of the coloboma is formed by rounded mesodermal stroma as well as by folded pigment epithelium. The remains of the pupil-

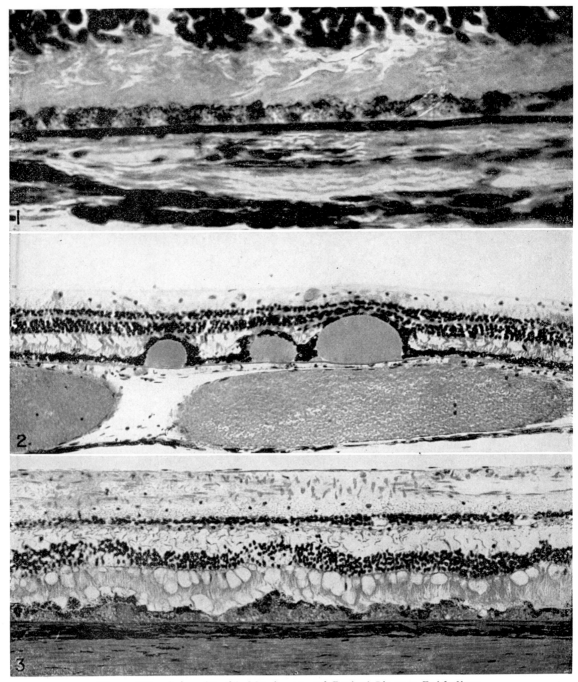

Figure 313.   Aging: Bruch's Membrane and Retinal Pigment Epithelium

1. Basophilic staining of Bruch's membrane. ×400. AFIP Acc. 117252.
2. Drusen on Bruch's membrane. ×130. AFIP Acc. 87481.
3. Lipoidal degeneration of retinal pigment epithelium. ×215. AFIP Acc. 78025.

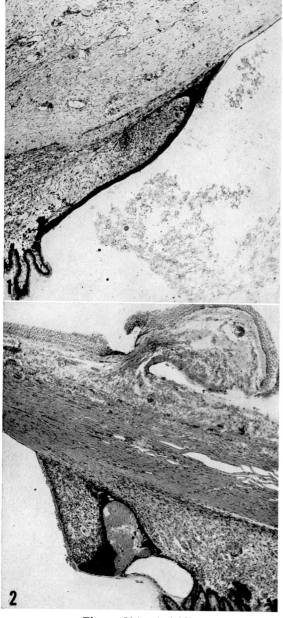

Figure 314. Aniridia

The rudimentary iris is adherent to the trabeculas and peripheral cornea; the anterior chamber angle is obliterated.

1. ×50. AFIP Acc. 54300.
2. ×50. AFIP Acc. 97493.

lary membrane and a few anomalous connective tissue strands may be present.

Typical colobomas of the iris occur in a position consistent with the line of closure of the fetal fissure (Fig. 318). Atypical colobomas of the iris seem to result from a persistence of vessels at the edge of the optic cup which

prevent development of the neuroectodermal iris.

Persistent pupillary membrane. Complete or incomplete persistence of the vascular pupillary membrane is a common congenital anomaly. All such membranes are attached to the lesser iris circle, and differ thereby from acquired posterior synechias (Fig. 315–4, 5). Persistence of the entire vascular membrane is rare, and may be associated with microphthalmos.

Incomplete pupillary membranes may have a few vascular and connective tissue strands arising from the lesser circle which do not adhere to the lens capsule. Others attach to the anterior surface of the lens with or without cataract formation.

The failure of complete atrophy and absorption of the mesoderm and vessels accounts for persistence of the membrane. Extensive membranes often are seen when there is an arrest in the development of the entire eye or if there is a temporary arrest at the five months stage, causing persistence of the vessels beyond the time they usually atrophy.

Hyperplasia of the anterior tunica vasculosa lentis. Hyperplasia of the anterior part of the tunica vasculosa lentis produces a thick layer of tissue on the anterior iris and in the pupil. A thick pupillary membrane of vascular, densely nucleated connective tissue results, which extends over the iris. A cataract may be formed if this tissue adheres to the lens.

Cysts of the iris and ciliary body. Congenital ectodermal iris cysts occasionally occur on the anterior surface. They are lined by stratified or irregular layers of cylindrical and cuboidal cells, and vary from 1 mm. in diameter to a size sufficient to fill the anterior chamber.

Neuroectodermal cysts may occur in the posterior iris and ciliary body (Fig. 316), and produce an interesting series of findings. The two neuroectodermal layers which form the ciliary and iris epithelium are poorly united in fetal life. According to Vail and Merz faulty union may lead to subsequent separation with an accumulation of fluid between the two layers to produce these cysts. It is not known whether they are always congenital. They often are bilateral and may occur in

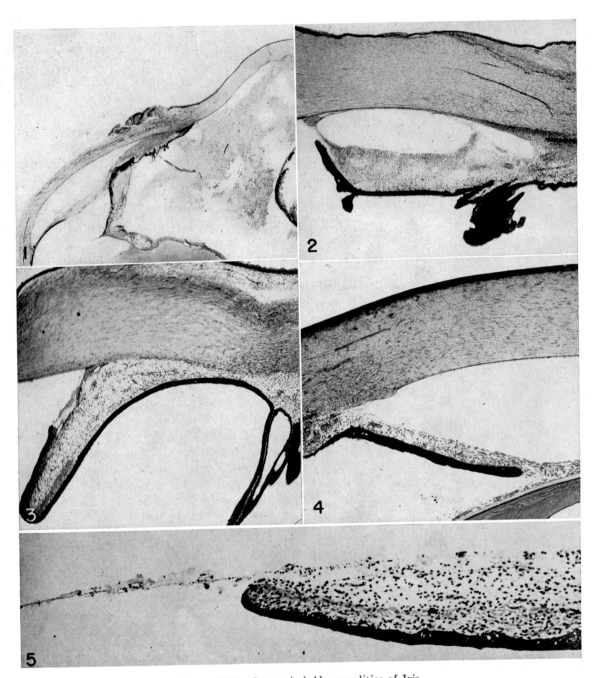

Figure 315.   Congenital Abnormalities of Iris

1. Coloboma of iris. ×5. AFIP Acc. 54300.
2. Incomplete separation of iris. Absence of sphincter and dilator muscles. ×40. AFIP Acc. 25934.
3. Incomplete separation of iris. Absence of canal of Schlemm. Congenital ectropion uveae. ×45. AFIP Acc. 28625.
4. Persistent pupillary membrane adherent to lens. ×60. AFIP Acc. 53033.
5. Persistent pupillary membrane. ×130. AFIP Acc. 104617.

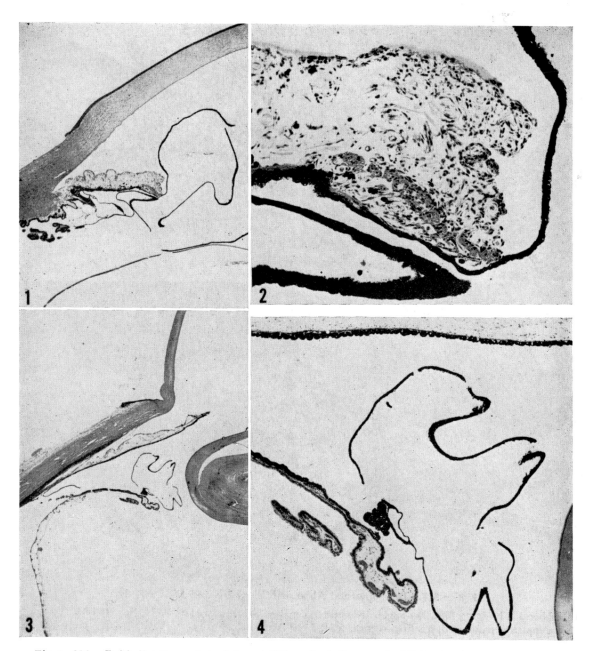

Figure 316. Epithelial Cysts of the Iris and Ciliary Body Suspected of Being Malignant Melanomas

1 and 2. Huge cysts arise from the posterior surface of the iris and from the adjacent ciliary processes and project through the pupil into the anterior chamber. This eye was otherwise normal. ×14 and ×115, respectively. AFIP Acc. 120891.

3 and 4. There are multiple malformations of the anterior uveal tract localized to the nasal side of this eye: The iris root arises much farther back on the ciliary body than is normal; the pars plicata has not developed; the ora serrata extends into the one large malformed ciliary process; and a large cyst which fills much of the posterior chamber is associated with subluxation of the lens toward the opposite side. ×11 and ×50, respectively. AFIP Acc. 765506.

forms of purulent endophthalmitis. There is pain, congestion and edema of the bulbar conjunctiva. A purulent exudate may accumulate either in the anterior chamber or in the vitreous cavity.

The microscopic picture of acute purulent uveitis as it occurs when merely part of a purulent endophthalmitis or panophthalmitis has been described in Chapter II. However, certain aspects of the changes in the uveal tract in purulent uveitis warrant emphasis. The exudate in the anterior chamber (the hypopyon) consists of fibrin and polymorphonuclear leukocytes (Fig. 73–1). Exudate also fills the trabecular meshwork and may be present in the posterior chamber. Polymorphonuclear leukocytes adhere to the posterior surface of the cornea but do not form large aggregates. The vessels of the uveal tract in the involved area are dilated and frequently plugged by polymorphonuclear leukocytes or fibrinous thrombi. The uveal stroma is edematous and infiltrated by polymorphonuclear leukocytes. The entire iris is involved. The ciliary muscle is usually little affected but the ciliary processes and epithelium are intensely inflamed. In the choroid, the reaction begins in the inner vessel layers but spreads toward the retina and suprachoroidea. The cellular infiltration may be diffuse, or focal, with abscess formation (Fig. 72–2). However, portions of the uveal tract more remote from the acute process may contain lymphocytes and plasma cells instead of polymorphonuclear leukocytes. A similar mononuclear reaction may be seen in the choroid in association with a purulent iridocyclitis. The cellular infiltrate even may vary in different layers in the same area of the uvea. Polymorphonuclear leukocytes may predominate in the choriocapillaris while lymphocytes and plasma cells are present in the adjacent large vessel layers.

Necrosis of the inflamed uveal tissue occurs and pigment from the disrupted melanocytes is scattered and phagocytosed by macrophages. These phagocytes also pick up other cellular debris, including the remains of disintegrated polymorphonuclears. Hence, in the older abscesses macrophages may replace the polymorphonuclear leukocytes.

During the healing phase there is organization of the inflammatory exudate. Vascularized connective tissue containing lymphocytes and plasma cells (granulation tissue) form about the abscesses, walling them off. Similar membranes form on the anterior surface of the iris, covering the pupil, and sometimes binding the pupil to the lens (occlusion and seclusion of the pupil). Membranes called *cyclitic membranes* form along the plane of the anterior vitreous face, anchored on each side at the pars plana. These originate from cells in the adjacent ciliary body and retina. Posteriorly, the retinal pigment epithelium and visual cells may be destroyed and adhesions form between the choroid and retina in the areas of scarring. Such widespread degeneration of the uvea often is associated with the eventual picture of atrophy of the eyeball with shrinkage (see Chapter II).

Exogenous nongranulomatous uveitis. Some types of exogenous uveitis may be milder than either purulent or granulomatous uveitis. Clinically the inflammation may be acute, subacute or chronic. The bulbar conjunctiva is congested, the aqueous is turbid, and there are small keratic precipitates composed of clusters of lymphocytes and plasma cells. The iris is edematous and its markings are indistinct. Posterior synechias and vitreous opacities occur. Such inflammations occur after trauma, either accidental or surgical, and are produced by relatively mild irritants (e.g., blood, injured tissues, antigenic proteins, etc.). The introduction of bacteria of low virulence into the eye either through injury or operation also may cause a nongranulomatous uveitis instead of a purulent uveitis, especially if prophylactic antibiotics have been administered and the acute inflammation suppressed. Practically all intraocular surgery is followed by a benign form of iridocyclitis as a result of trauma. Complications during or after surgery, such as the incarceration of portions of lens, uveal tissue, and vitreous in the wound, may cause such inflammation. Lens capsule incarcerated in a wound is not absorbed and may cause prolonged iridocyclitis. Absorbing lens material may do the same, and the degree of inflammation of the iris and ciliary body depends upon the amount of lens cortex in the eye and the rapidity with which it dissolves. Lens-induced inflammation is discussed more thoroughly in Chapter III. Intraocular hem-

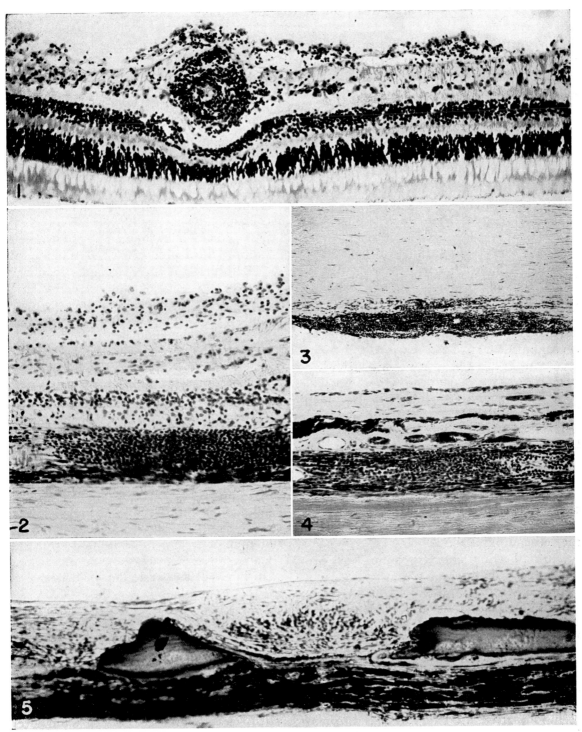

Figure 321 Chronic Chorioretinitis

1. Lymphocytic periphlebitis and diffuse inflammatory cell infiltration in retina. ×160. AFIP Acc. 39429.

2. Lymphocytic infiltration in choroid. Loss of retinal architecture. Clumps of mononuclear cells on inner surface of retina. ×185. AFIP Acc. 118803.

3. Lymphocytic infiltration in episclera (chronic episcleritis). ×145. AFIP Acc. 168768.

4. Lymphocytic infiltration in choroid. Fibrous membrane and proliferated pigment epithelium between choroid and completely atrophic retina. ×125. AFIP Acc. 186127.

5. Chorioretinal scar and calcified drusen from Bruch's membrane projecting into retina. ×76. AFIP Acc. 30571.

orrhage is followed by an irritative iridocyclitis or choroiditis.

The microscopic findings differ from those of purulent uveitis. The early cellular infiltrate which may be diffuse or focal is predominantly lymphocytic and monocytic; subsequently an increasing number of plasma cells appear and associated with them are plasmacytoid cells and Russell's bodies, especially in iris lesions (Figs. 33, 34, 35, 36). There is a fibrinous exudate in the anterior chamber, pupil, posterior chamber, and vitreous. Because of the relatively high protein content of the exudate, it stains pink with eosin (Figs. 3–3, 4). The choroidal inflammatory exudate is similar to that in the anterior uvea and is associated with perivascular infiltration ("cuffing") of the retinal vessels (Fig. 321–1) by lymphocytes and proliferation of the vascular endothelium. Although tissue destruction is mild compared with that in acute purulent uveitis, necrosis sometimes occurs in the areas of intense cellular infiltration, especially in inflammatory nodules. The stromal melanocytes disintegrate, lose their branching processes, and become rounded. The pigment epithelium of the iris, ciliary body and retina may be destroyed or it may proliferate to form nodules, tubules and plaques. The epithelial cells also migrate, those of the ciliary body extending into the posterior chamber or into cyclitic membranes. The pigmented epithelial cells migrate into the retina around the vessels.

During healing the inflammatory cells and fibrinous exudate may be absorbed without connective tissue proliferation but a certain amount of scarring most often results. Adhesions often form between the iris and trabecula, occluding the angle (peripheral anterior synechia), or between the iris and lens (posterior synechia) (Fig. 36). Inflammatory membranes form on the anterior iris surface and may extend across the pupil producing occlusion and seclusion. Adhesions also may form between the choroid and retina (Fig. 321).

Exogenous granulomatous uveitis. The only important examples of granulomatous uveitis following trauma are sympathetic ophthalmia and those due to foreign bodies. Other causes of post-traumatic and postoper-ative granulomatous inflammation such as phaco-anaphylaxis, and intraocular hemorrhage usually produce an endophthalmitis rather than a uveitis and are therefore considered in other chapters. Retained intraocular foreign bodies also more often produce an endophthalmitis and have been considered in Chapter III.

Sympathetic ophthalmia. Sympathetic ophthalmia practically always follows ocular injuries with prolapse of iris or ciliary body. This condition also may follow surgical procedures such as those for glaucoma (iridencleisis), and cataract in which a postoperative iris prolapse is produced. After surgical wounds the incidence is less frequent than after injuries; occurrences at a frequency of one to two per thousand were reported in the past following cataract and trephine operations. The incidence has been reported as five to ten per thousand following iris inclusion operations. Following perforating wounds with untreated iris or ciliary body prolapse, in which enucleation is not carried out soon after injury, the disease develops in as many as 3 to 5 per cent of cases. Enucleation of the injured eye within two weeks of the injury provides almost complete protection; if enucleation is performed within a week, protection is complete. The frequency of traumatic and postoperative sympathetic ophthalmia has diminished tremendously in many countries during recent years because of prompt treatment of injured eyes, particularly those with damage to uveal tissue. During World War II the incidence of sympathetic ophthalmia in the United States Armed Forces was extremely low because of the prompt attention given to ocular injuries.

The clinical picture of the disease differs little from that of other forms of granulomatous ublitis, except for the constant bilaterality of the typical fully developed disease. A definite incubation period of two weeks seems to be necessary for development of the disease. The injured eye (exciting eye) develops a post-traumatic inflammation of variable severity and nondescript character which persists. The character of this inflammation often changes toward the end of the second week after the injury, so that light perception becomes defective, and examination shows heavy mutton-fat K.P. on the cornea, in the angle, and on the iris and pupil (Fig. 322). The aqueous is very turbid, with fibrin and many cells. At any time after the beginning of the third week after the injury up to many years later the disease develops in the uninjured (sympathizing) eye, photophobia being the initial symptom. This is followed by rapid evolution of a diffuse uveitis having the same characteristics as that seen in the exciting eye. In untreated cases the disease follows a prolonged, severe course (1 to 2 years), leading to loss of useful vision in 50 per cent of cases. The remaining cases have more or less reduced vision. Some reports indicate that if the disease has recently commenced in the sympathizing eye very little benefit results from enucleating the exciting eye; other reports show the reverse to be true. Corticosteroid and corticotropin therapy have a remarkable ability to amelioriate the signs of many cases of sympathetic ophthalmia, a fact which may be of some significance from a pathogenetic standpoint.

While most cases of sympathetic ophthalmia occur in obvious relationship to perforating wounds of the eyeball, a few present an apparently identical clinical and histologic picture in the absence of perforating trauma. One case at the Armed Forces Institute of Pathology is known to have occurred in relation to an intraocular malignant melanoma. It should be pointed out that occasionally there are clinical resemblances to the Vogt-Koyanagi-Harada syndrome including auditory defects, and cutaneous changes. In many instances the histologic picture in both these diseases is identical.

Pathology. The characteristic morphologic features of the disease were established with great clarity by the classic studies of Ernst Fuchs. There are few contributions to the ophthalmic literature which compare with his in the clarity and comprehensiveness of their presentation. Little, if anything, has been added to the description of the disease in the half century since Fuchs wrote.

In sympathetic ophthalmia there typically is a diffuse and often massive lymphocytic infiltration of the uveal tissues (Fig. 17). The inflammation is granulomatous and is characterized by nests or areas of epithelioid cell

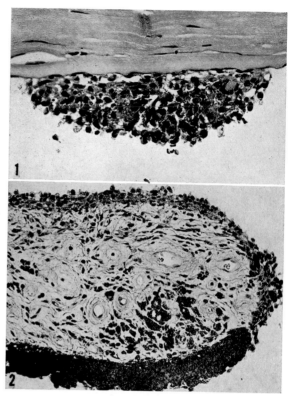

Figure 322. Sympathetic Uveitis

1. Agglutinated large mononuclear cells adherent to corneal endothelium (mutton fat K.P.'s). ×305. AFIP Acc. 273515.

2. Similar cells adhere to anterior surface and pupillary margin of iris. ×200. AFIP Acc. 273515.

infiltration superimposed on the lymphocytic infiltrate. Giant cells are commonly present among the epithelioid cells (Fig. 12). Caseation or necrosis is rare. When seen it is minimal and inconspicuous. In the early stages the epithelioid cell nests are small and widely scattered, and eosinophilic polymorphonuclear cells often are observed in the surrounding lymphocytic zones. Later the lesions grow and merge, giving the uveal tract a mottled or marbled appearance in which pale-staining areas of epithelioid cell infiltration alternate with darker staining areas of lymphocytic infiltration. In more than half the cases the whole uveal tract is evenly and diffusely involved, but in a limited number of cases either the choroid or the anterior uveal tissues may be relatively unaffected. Tissue destruction in the choroid is generally inconspicuous. The infiltrate characteristically extends from the choroid into the sclera along the sheaths of the perforating vessels and

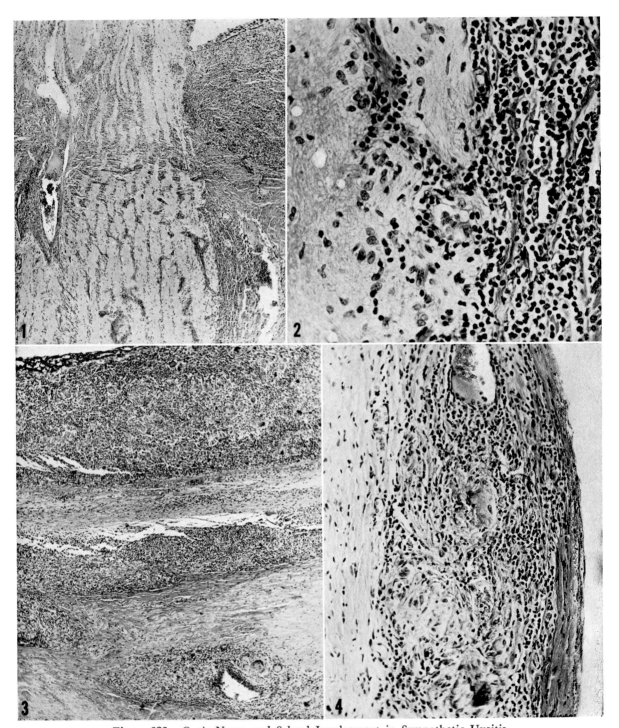

Figure 323. Optic Nerve and Scleral Involvement in Sympathetic Uveitis

1 and 2. The inflammatory reaction involves the meninges and extends into the optic nerve via the pial septum. ×42 and ×330, respectively. AFIP Acc. 724889.

3. The scleral canals are thickened by the granulomatous inflammatory tissue. ×55. AFP Acc. 724889.

4. The reaction reaches the episcleral surface along the emissary vessels and nerves. ×410. AFIP Acc. 724889

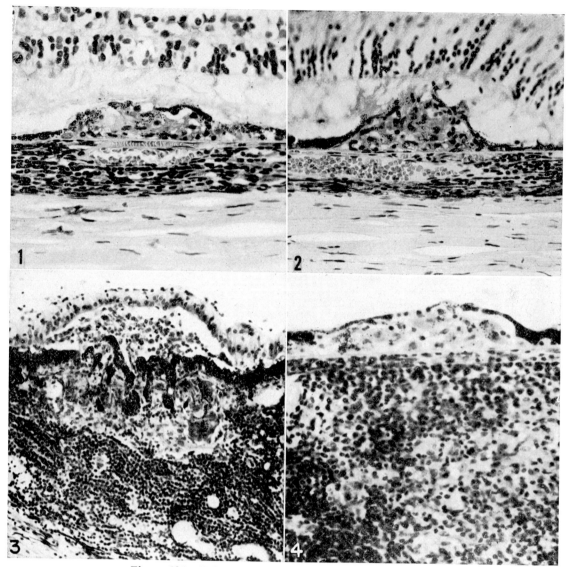

Figure 324. Dálen-Fuchs Nodules in Sympathetic Uveitis

1. ×305. AFIP Acc. 909319.
2. ×265. AFIP Acc. 909319.
3. ×145. AFIP Acc. 183508.
4. ×300. AFIP Acc. 53309.

nerves, and nodular lesions often are to be found in the episcleral tissues at the points of emergence of these channels (Fig. 323). Similar nodular lesions are more rarely seen in the meninges of the optic nerve. These epibulbar lesions are regularly related to local accumulations of melanocytes in the episclera and meninges.

In many instances the choroidal inflammation is sharply limited by Bruch's membrane and the choriocapillaris, while the overlying pigment epithelium and retina are unaffected (Fig. 17). This is a feature that distinguishes sympathetic ophthalmia morphologically from other forms of granulomatous endophthalmitis, since similarly extensive lesions in the choroid, caused, for instance, by tuberculosis or syphilis, are regularly associated with massive destruction of the overlying pigment epithelium and retina. Isolated small nodular lesions do, however, occur in the pigment epithelium. They usually take the form of small hemispherical mounds consisting chiefly of epithelioid cells and scattered

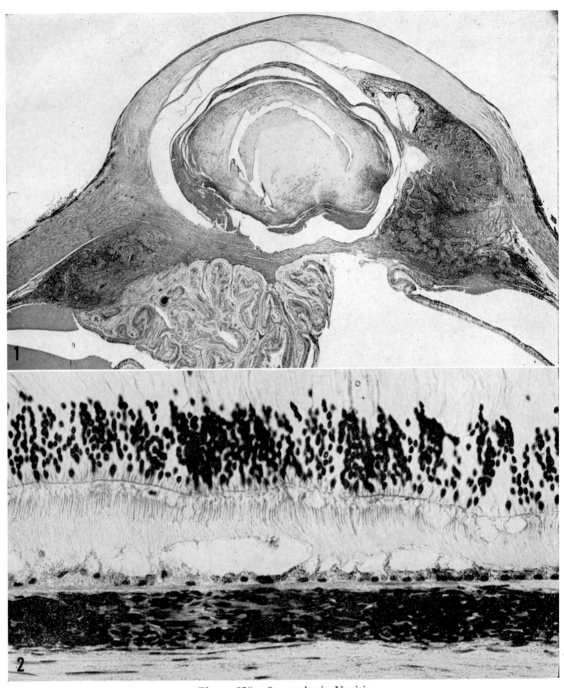

Figure 325. Sympathetic Uveitis

1. The exuberant proliferation of chronic granulomatous inflammatory tissue has filled the posterior chamber. While often most massive, these anterior segment lesions are less diagnostic of sympathetic uveitis than are the posterior lesions (see Figs. 17, 323, and 324). ×12. AFIP Acc. 891154.

2. Choroidal infiltrate in sympathizing eye. ×400. AFIP Acc. 195025.

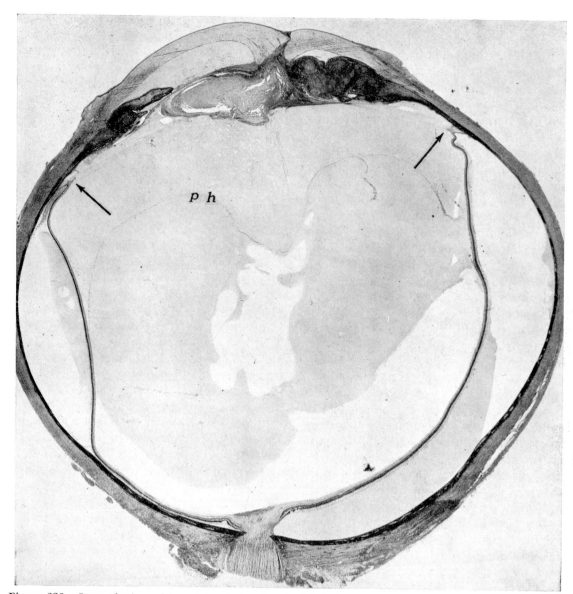

p h

Figure 326. Sympathetic uveitis and lens-induced endophthalmitis following perforating wound of cornea and lens. There is a massive granulomatous inflammatory reaction centered about the site of lens perforation while on the opposite side the iris and ciliary body are much less extensively involved. The endophthalmitis has produced inflammatory traction bands in the vitreous. These have tented (arrows) and detached the retina. Posteriorly, the vitreous has become separated from the retina and serous exudate has accumulated behind the posterior hyaloid surface (p h). In a complicated case such as this the diagnosis of sympathetic uveitis is difficult to make from the anterior segment reaction alone; the choroid, however, reveals the diagnostic alterations (see text for description). ×6. AFIP Acc. 28571.

cells of the pigment epithelium. These nodules were first described by Dálen and later by Fuchs (Fig. 324). In cases in which useful vision is ultimately recovered, small round areas of depigmentation often can be seen ophthalmoscopically in the periphery of the fundus, presumably representing the scars left by Dálen-Fuchs nodules. Friedenwald has pointed out that the nodules occur most

frequently when the retina has been detached. He has suggested that the Dálen-Fuchs nodule develops in relation to local foci of hyperplasia of the pigment epithelium.

In the ciliary body and iris, where the lamina vitrea either is absent or forms a poor boundary, destruction of the epithelial layers is common, and a massive exudate of epithelioid cells and lymphocytes usually forms on the surface of the ciliary processes and in the space between the iris and the lens (Fig. 325–1). The pattern of this exudate, including scattered cells and cell fragments from the pigment epithelial layer, is one of the characteristic morphologic features of the disease. Frequently, however, the diagnosis of sympathetic uveitis is difficult to establish from examination of the anterior segment alone (Fig. 326). Often the iris and ciliary body are so badly injured, incarcerated in the wound, involved in a reaction to foreign bodies, or affected by an associated phaco-anaphylactic response that it is impossible to be certain whether sympathetic uveitis is or is not present. As Blodi has recently shown, phaco-anaphylaxis and sympathetic uveitis are frequently co-existent. Therefore, the pathologist must rely primarily on the choroidal changes in establishing a diagnosis of sympathetic uveitis.

In most of the cases of sympathetic ophthalmia that have become available for histologic study, only the exciting eye has been subjected to examination. In some instances in which the sympathizing eye has been enucleated, the lesion has shown the same characteristics (Fig. 325–2) as those of the exciting eye. However, Greeves, in a study of thirteen supposedly sympathizing eyes, observed iridocyclitis, but no particular tendency for the inflammatory reaction to be situated in the posterior portion of the uveal tract. Rupture of the lens capsule without trauma or operation had occurred in three cases. He concluded that no special characteristic of the sympathetic process is invariably found in the sympathizing eye. Proof that these cases were examples of sympathetic ophthalmia is lacking.

Fuchs observed that, especially in the early stages of the disease, the infiltrating epithelioid cells regularly contain scattered melanin granules and show no tendency for necrosis. In contrast with this, in other forms of uveal disease the melanin granules which are liberated by the death or injury of the melanocytes generally are picked up by macrophages, which become so heavily laden that they appear solid, their nuclei being obscured by the cytoplasmic masses of melanin. They also frequently show necrosis. The distinction in regard to pigment phagocytosis is not absolute, for in tuberculous or syphilitic uveal lesions melanin granules may be found in an occasional epithelioid cell. However, in sympathetic ophthalmia, especially in the early stages of the disease, pigment phagocytosis by epithelioid cells rather than by macrophages is so striking that Fuchs was led to suggest uveal pigmented cells as the possible origin of the epithelioid cells in sympathetic ophthalmia. This idea is not in accord with modern concepts of the cytogenesis of epithelioid cells, but nevertheless it serves to underscore the characteristic prominence of this morphologic feature of the disease.

Relatively few cases of sympathetic ophthalmia have been studied histologically in the late stages when the inflammatory process has finally burned itself out. In the few that have been examined the uveal tract shows widespread interstitial scarring and a marked reduction in the number of melanocytes.

Pathogenesis. Bilateral symmetry of lesions involving paired organs has been noted in many endogenous infections. The frequent bilaterality of renal tuberculosis and of mumps orchitis may be cited as examples. The cutaneous lesions in syphilis and the exanthems often exhibit a bilateral symmetry. The high incidence of bilateral lesions in endogenous endophthalmitis conforms to this general pattern. What is remarkable about sympathetic ophthalmia, therefore, is not its bilaterality but the bilaterality of the lesion in paired organs following an injury to only one of the pair. No similar "sympathetic" inflammations following unilateral injury are known to occur in organs other than the eye.

Two paths have been followed in the attempts to explain this unique phenomenon. One group of workers has sought for a specific organism which might be the causative agent. As the result of extensive studies a variety of different bacteria have been isolated from the exciting eye. Most of these organisms are of relatively avirulent types, and their wide variety suggests that they may represent accidental contaminants, entering the eye at the time of the original injury, or at the time of the bacteriologic study. Verhoeff found thread-like, presumably mycotic, structures in the ocular abscesses of both eyes in one case that had the clinical features of sympathetic ophthalmia. In this case, lesions in the choroid were indistinguishable from those of sympathetic uveitis, but these lesions contained no organisms.

Von Szily inoculated herpes virus into the uveal tissues of one eye of rabbits and produced bilateral choroiditis. The choroidal lesions, however, were not granulomatous in type, and von Szily himself did not regard his experiments as indicating that the herpes virus was the cause of sympathetic ophthalmia. He concluded merely that bilateral uveitis could be caused by unilateral inoculation of a virus and hence that a virus could not be excluded as the possible cause of sympathetic ophthalmia. The herpes virus would not be the one implicated, however, for efforts to transmit the herpes virus to rabbits from human cases of sympathetic ophthalmia have been consistently unsuccessful.

Marchesani suggested that ordinary pyogenic organisms might in some indirect fashion be related to the disease. By inoculating staphylococci into one eye of rabbits he produced a choroidal infiltrate in the opposite eye. Von Szily, however, showed that similar choroidal infiltrates could result from the production of staphylococcal abscesses anywhere in the body. Clarification of this peculiar phenomenon was furnished by Friedenwald and Rones who observed diffuse choroidal infiltrates of this type in all forms of sepsis, along with generalized lymph node enlargement, acute splenic tumor and other constitutional symptoms of febrile disease. It seems most unlikely that these nonspecific reactions have anything whatever to do with sympathetic ophthalmia.

Recent experimental work by Schreck, who claimed to have demonstrated a causative microorganism, apparently related to the Rickettsia group, has not been verified by other workers, and it now is considered that he was dealing with the causative agent of leukosis or "gray eye" in chickens.

Elschnig was the first to suggest that sympathetic ophthalmia might be connected with allergy to some autogenous substance. He gave this novel concept the picturesque name "horror autotoxicus." This hypothesis was later extensively explored by Woods, who was able to show that the ocular tissues of sensitized animals can manifest allergic reactions to the local or systemic administration of the

antigen, and that uveal tissue can act as antigen for sensitization. The degree of sensitization produced by homologous uveal antigen was negligible, but animals sensitized to heterologous uveal tissue gave a slight but definite reaction to homologous uveal material. The ocular reactions produced in these animals were very slight and did not resemble sympathetic ophthalmia.

Woods next attempted to discover whether patients with sympathetic ophthalmia showed evidence of specific reactions to uveal tissue. Complement fixation and opsonic index studies gave equivocal results, but Woods found that the intradermal injection of a uveal pigment suspension in patients with sympathetic ophthalmia generally resulted in the slow development of an indurated nodule, while those without sympathetic ophthalmia seldom reacted in this manner.

Histologic examination of these cutaneous reactions was undertaken by Friedenwald, who found that a granulomatous reaction to the uveal pigment developed in most cases of sympathetic ophthalmia and that this cutaneous reaction was strikingly similar to the granulomatous lesion in the uveal tissues (Fig. 327). The characteristic cutaneous reaction is not always present at the onset of the disease, and the skin test is not a reliable guide for the decision as to whether a suspicious eye should or should not be enucleated. In almost all cases in which the test was made several months after the onset of the disease, the reaction in the skin was found to be positive. In a few cases in which the disease had finally subsided the test became negative. In patients not suffering from sympathetic ophthalmia the cutaneous reaction to uveal pigment was very rarely granulomatous in type. Some of these false positive reactions occurred in cases of Vogt-Koyanagi syndrome, a few others in cases of uveitis not related to sympathetic ophthalmia, and a very small number in the absence of uveitis. Taken together with Woods' preceding studies the evidence seems very strong that patients with sympathetic ophthalmia have an abnormal reaction to uveal tissue components. Friedenwald was able to elicit the typical granulomatous reaction in cases of sympathetic ophthalmia by a suspension of uveal tissue from albino animals and con-

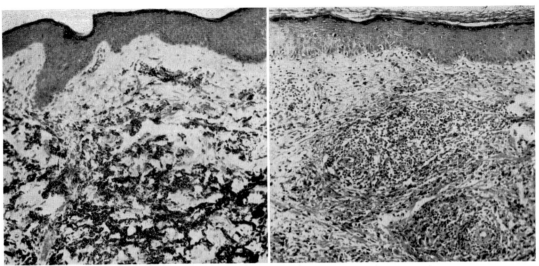

Figure 327. Skin Test for Sympathetic Uveitis

1. Negative uveal pigment skin test. Undisturbed injected melanin pigment in dermis. ×120. AFIP Acc. 55994.

2. Positive uveal pigment skin test in a case of sympathetic uveitis. Granulomatous reaction similar to that seen in uveal tract. The injected melanin pigment has been phagocytized by epithelioid cells. ×120. AFIP Acc. 176476.

cluded that melanin was not the specific antigen.

Since the effort to sensitize animals even with heterologous uveal tissue produces only a feeble reaction, an effort has been made to enhance the antigenicity of such material with the aid of some adjuvant. Lucic and Gifford injected staphylococcus toxin mixed with heterologous or homologous uveal tissue emulsion into rabbits, and obtained slightly higher degrees of sensitization but no intraocular reaction similar to sympathetic ophthalmia. Collins, using guinea pigs as the test animal, injected homologous uveal tissue suspension together with an adjuvant consisting of heat-killed tubercle bacilli suspended in oil with a detergent. This same adjuvant had previously been shown by Le Moignic and Pinoy to sensitize guinea pigs homologously to brain and to kidney, though the precise nature of this autosensitization still remains obscure. In Collins' animals there was a diffuse mononuclear infiltration of the choroid without any cellular reaction in the ocular fluids. The histologic picture which he described resembles more closely that of septic choroiditis than that of sympathetic ophthalmia, but the issue still remains uncertain.

In summary, it would appear that allergy to uveal tissue components plays a significant role in sympathetic ophthalmia but that this alone is not sufficient to elicit the disease.

Endogenous uveitis. Endogenous uveitis may be secondary to a systemic disease but most often is due to unknown causes. *Suppurative* endogenous uveal inflammations are more uncommon than in previous years. They may occur during a septicemic disease or be induced by metastasis of organisms from remote infections. Most pyogenic bacteria and fungi may produce such an infection. The findings are similar to those which are due to exogenous infection.

Endogenous nongranulomatous uveitis. Endogenous *nonsuppurative* uveal inflammations are the most common types of uveitis. The nongranulomatous form is characterized by an unspecific type of inflammatory reaction and frequently is of completely obscure origin. It may be associated at times with numerous and diverse conditions, e.g., bacterial, food protein, and pollen allergies, lens hypersensitivity, Behçet's syndrome, heterochromic iridocyclitis, rheumatoid arthritis, and such viral diseases as herpes simplex, herpes zoster, measles, mumps, whooping cough, chickenpox, and influenza, etc.

Nongranulomatous uveitis may affect any part of the uvea. Typically, the onset is usually acute rather than insidious, and ciliary congestion is marked, with pronounced pho-

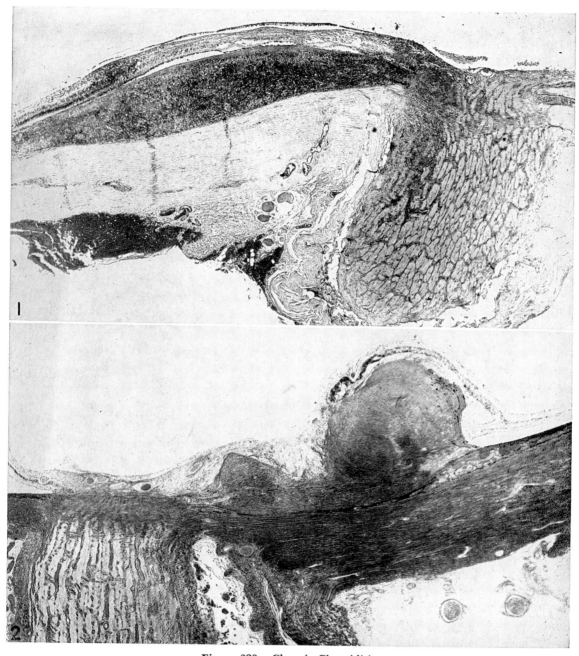

Figure 328. Chronic Choroiditis

1. Massive lymphocytic infiltration in choroid adjacent to and involving optic nerve (choroiditis juxta-papillaris) ×36. AFIP Acc. 28149.

2. Massive fibrous chorioretinal adhesion and atrophy of both coats resulting from old choroiditis juxta-papillaris. ×30. AFIP Acc. 118218.

tophobia and lacrimation. The inflammatory reaction in the iris usually is slight and is limited to a loss of luster, blurring of the iris pattern, and dilatation of the capillaries. There are no nodules and the tendency for formation of posterior synechias varies with the amount of exudation. The aqueous flare usually is intense and there may be a heavy gelatinous or fibrinous exudate in the anterior chamber. The deposits on the posterior cornea are small and pin-point, and are chiefly composed of lymphocytes. The course of the iritis usually is short (2 to 3 weeks) and recovery may be followed by amazingly few

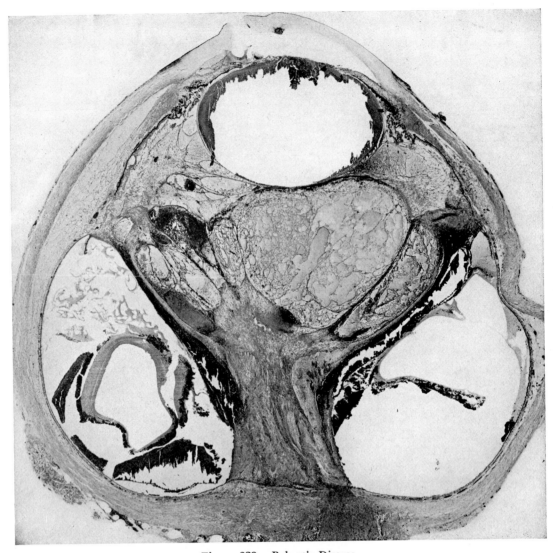

Figure 329. Behçet's Disease

Most of the cases in which enucleation has been performed have had extensive areas of hemorrhagic and coagulative necrosis of the retina. ×6. AFIP Acc. 220085. (Case report by Braley, 1958.)

residua. Only after repeated attacks in some cases is organic damage done to the eye.

The histologic findings are identical with those of exogenous nongranulomatous uveitis (Figs. 33, 34, 35, 36, 321, 328). Recurrent episodes of uveitis always cause scarring and atrophy. Plasma cells commonly predominate and plasmacytoid cells and Russell's bodies quite often are numerous. These cell types are particularly characteristic of nongranulomatous iritis and since they are believed to be concerned with antibody production, this form of uveitis may represent a local tissue response to antigenic stimulation.

Relapsing iridocyclitis with mucocutaneous lesions. Behçet's syndrome is characterized by retinal vasculitis, recurrent bilateral iridocyclitis with hypopyon, aphthous ulcers of the mouth and genitalia, dermatitis, arthralgia, thrombophlebitis, and neurologic disturbances. The disease affects both men and women, especially between the ages of 20 and 30 years. The lesions of the skin and mucous membranes most often appear before those of the eyes. The skin lesions may consist of dermatitis herpetiformis, erythema nodosum, and nondescript painful subcutaneous nodules. The etiology is obscure, and the disease appears to be more common in the Mediterranean countries. Among the causative factors which have been described are a hypersensitivity to an avirulent bacterium, a Streptococcus viridans infection, and a Staphylococcus albus infection. Behçet (1940) believed the disease was caused by a virus, and has found intracellular and extracellular elementary bodies in scrapings from the aphthas of his patients. Sezar (1953) reported the isolation of a virus from the vitreous and subretinal fluid in three cases and claimed to have produced an experimental disease similar to that of the human in rabbit eyes. This has not been verified, and the results are open to question. Others consider the syndrome to be due to a retinal vasculitis and several cases with infarctions in the retina with hemorrhage are on record.

Pathological examination of the eyes shows a serohemorrhagic exudate containing polymorphonuclear leukocytes in the vitreous and in the anterior and posterior chambers (Fig. 329). There are extensive areas of retinal necrosis. Mononuclear and polymorphonuclear leukocytes are found in the iris,

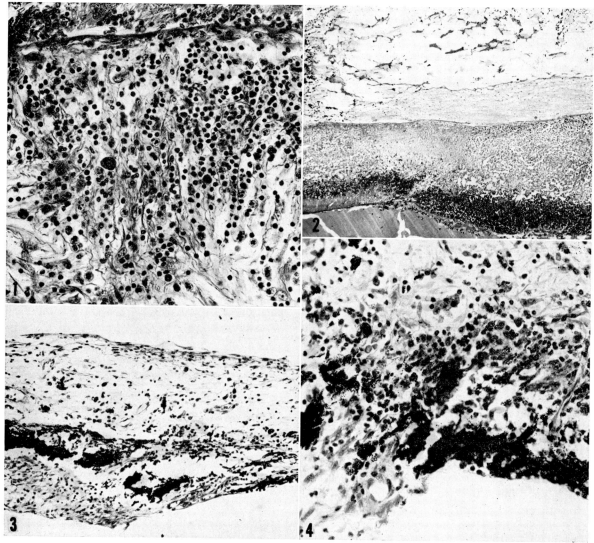

Figure 330.   Behçet's Disease

1. Mononuclear and polymorphonuclear leukocytes infiltrate the choroid. Same case shown in Fig. 329. ×305.
2. Extensive coagulative and hemorrhagic necrosis of the retina. ×35. AFIP Acc. 840404.
3 and 4. Chronic nongranulomatous iritis with destruction of pigment epithelium and proliferation of granulation tissue into posterior chambers. ×130 and ×305, respectively. AFIP Acc. 840404.

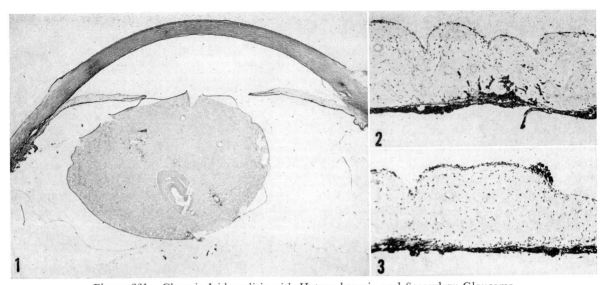

Figure 331. Chronic Iridocyclitis with Heterochromia and Secondary Glaucoma

The patient had experienced intermittent attacks of unilateral uveitis for more than 20 years.

1. Peripheral anterior synechia is present on one side and the lens reveals hypermature cataractous changes. ×7. AFIP Acc. 751122.

2 and 3. The iris contains minute focal areas of necrosis involving the pigment epithelium and dilator muscle but there is virtually no inflammatory reaction. ×80. AFIP Acc. 751122.

ciliary body, and choroid, depending on the stage of the disease. Braley (1958) found unusual cells in the retina and the extraocular muscles of one of his cases (Fig. 330); these appeared to be either immature lymphocytes or reticulum cells.

Heterochromic iridocyclitis. Heterochromic iridocyclitis is a disease of the iris and ciliary body of one eye; this condition is most common in young adults and leads to depigmentation of the affected iris. It is not associated with ocular inflammation, and is characterized by small, round, white keratic precipitates, constant cells and flare in the aqueous; absence of synechias; fine anterior vitreous opacities; occasional peripheral foci of choroiditis and a posterior subcapsular cataract. Glaucoma occurs in about twenty per cent of cases.

Very few eyes with this condition have been studied microscopically except those which have been removed following surgical procedures for cataract or glaucoma. A very mild nonspecific lymphocytic infiltration of the iris and ciliary body is seen in uncomplicated cases. The iris changes appear to be of degenerative rather than of inflammatory origin (Fig. 331). Vascular sclerosis, stromal atrophy, and pigmentary degeneration are characteristic of this condition. The etiology

and pathogenesis are unknown, but the condition may be the result of trophic changes in the ocular tissues produced by a disturbance in sympathetic innervation.

Ocular involvement is rare in acute rheumatic fever but may occur with rheumatoid arthritis. Band keratopathy, chronic iridocyclitis, and cataract develop in approximately 20 per cent of cases of rheumatoid arthritis in children (Still's disease). The keratopathy probably is secondary to the iridocyclitis but is not characteristic of this disease alone.

Rheumatoid arthritis occurs in approximately 5 per cent of the population in the United States; iridocyclitis may appear in such a group but not in higher incidence than in the nonrheumatoid population. There is a much higher incidence of acute recurrent iridocyclitis in patients with *spondylitis* (10 to 15 per cent); however, posterior uveitis is rare in this condition.

Herpes zoster. Iritis or iridocyclitis often appears with the corneal involvement in herpes zoster; occasionally it precedes the corneal disease or does not appear until later. The iridocyclitis may be mild and produce miosis of the pupil and hyperemia of the iris; or it may be severe and prolonged.

An extremely severe, and fortunately rare,

complication of herpes zoster was described under the name of "herpes iridis" by Machek in 1895, and subsequently verified by others. In this type vesicles form in the iris stroma, and there is intense, almost uncontrollable pain. The disease lasts for months, and frequently is complicated by a hyphema which is believed to result from necrosis of the iris vessels. The vesicles finally absorb and leave focal areas of atrophy with depigmented scars.

Gilbert (1921) described the histologic changes produced in the eye in herpes zoster. He found a lymphocytic infiltration of the endoneurium and perineurium of the ciliary nerves, and a periarteritis which led to complete necrosis and bleeding. The prolonged inflammation seen in herpes iridis is thought to be due to tissue necrosis rather than a result of specific action of the virus.

Systemic diseases. A nongranulomatous uveitis may be associated with numerous febrile illnesses, such as measles, mumps, chickenpox, influenza and whooping cough. The uveitis usually is bilateral, mild, and self-limited and either an iridocyclitis or choroiditis may occur.

Hypersensitivity. Hypersensitivity to various proteins appears to play a definite role in certain types of uveitis. Toxins from a focus of infection may create a state of hypersensitivity and produce nongranulomatous uveitis. According to Woods (1956), many cases of nongranulomatous uveitis show a specific streptococcal hypersensitivity. Other bacteria such as the gonococcus, pseudomonas and staphylococcus produce an occasional case of nongranulomatous uveitis. This type of uveitis also has been shown to occur in serum sickness, and drug, pollen, and food hypersensitivities.

Lens-induced uveitis. Lens substance can elicit a severe inflammatory response (Fig. 100). This has been discussed in Chapter III, because such phacogenic inflammations are usually post-traumatic. In nontraumatic cases the liquid cortex of a hypermature cataract may escape through the altered capsule and provoke a bland outpouring of macrophages which cause secondary glaucoma. Ordinarily in these cases the uveal tract shows no lymphocytic or plasma cell reaction, but the characteristic macrophages, filled with finely granular pale eosinophilic particles of lens substance, may accumulate and fill the iris crypts (see Phacolytic Glaucoma, Chapter XII). According to Flocks et al., in contrast to the well-defined clinicopathologic complex of phacolytic glaucoma, other forms of lens-induced inflammation form a broad spectrum with phaco-anaphylaxis (see Chapter III) at one extreme and phacolytic glaucoma at the other. Phaco-anaphylaxis usually follows accidental perforation of the lens capsule or extracapsular extraction and is characterized by a granulomatous reaction centered about masses of lens matter (Fig. 100). Associated with it is a diffuse nongranulomatous iridocyclitis. Plasmacytosis is often conspicuous in the iris. In many of the intermediate forms of lens-induced uveitis a well-developed granulomatous reaction is not observed about the lens, but varying degrees of nongranulomatous inflammatory reaction are seen. When these inflammations follow injury, the reaction is most intense at the site of perforation of the lens capsule and the iris is typically bound down to the lens by the inflammatory tissue. A similar process may be seen in association with mature (not Morgagnian) cataracts in which there is no evidence of a ruptured capsule. Presumably escape of lens protein from these cataractous lenses is capable of provoking a uveitis. The resultant picture of nongranulomatous uveitis has been called phacotoxic uveitis by Irvine and Irvine although there is a growing belief that it is merely a variant of phaco-anaphylaxis (Woods, 1959).

Endogenous granulomatous uveitis. The etiology of endogenous granulomatous uveitis is much the same as for endogenous granulomatous endophthalmitis. Infectious causes include bacterial, viral, mycotic and parasitic agents.

The etiology of most cases cannot be determined by clinical study. Positive diagnosis rests on the demonstration of the causative agent in cultures of uveal tissue and by identification of organisms in tissue sections. The organisms which cause leprosy, tuberculosis, syphilis, actinomycosis, coccidioidomycosis, candidiasis, cryptococcosis, blastomycosis, toxoplasmosis, visceral larva migrans, cysticercosis, and inclusion body virus disease have

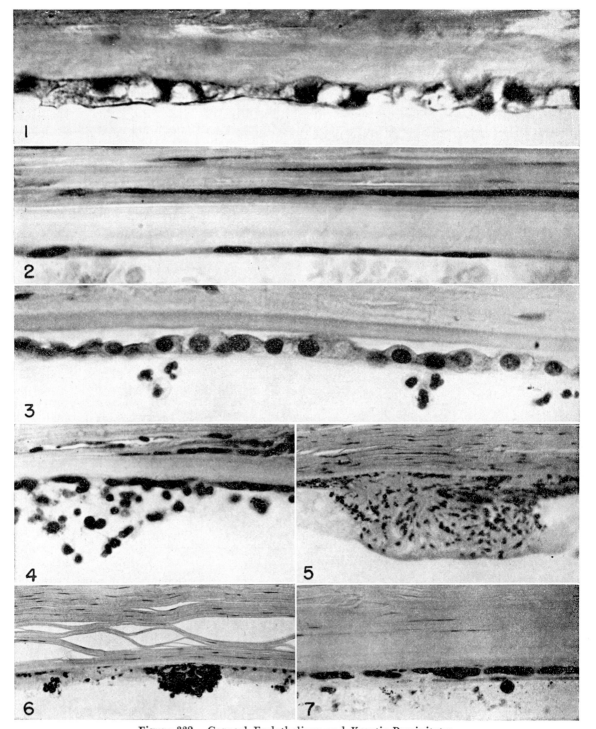

Figure 332.   Corneal Endothelium and Keratic Precipitates

1. Edema of corneal endothelium. ×1000. AFIP Acc. 60104.

2. Degeneration of corneal endothelium. Flattening of cells and disappearance of some nuclei. ×765. AFIP Acc. 45242.

3. Small keratic precipitates in acute inflammation. Polymorphonuclear leukocytes and occasional mononuclear cells clinging to posterior surface of cornea. ×680. AFIP Acc. 63267.

4. Large mononuclear cell keratic precipitates in granulomatous inflammation. ×330. AFIP Acc. 37670.

5. Organizing keratic precipitates in granulomatous inflammation. ×150. AFIP Acc. 44596.

6. Keratic precipitates composed of mononuclear cells containing melanin granules. ×125. AFIP Acc. 190352

7. Melanin granules phagocytized by endothelial cells. ×400. AFIP Acc. 141466.

been found in uveal granulomas and therefore are known causes of granulomatous uveitis. Although these ocular infections are often characterized by granulomatous uveitis, the initial infection quite often is in the retina rather than in the uveal tract. This is particularly true of toxoplasmosis; in this disease the causative agent almost always is found in the necrotic retina while the granulomatous inflammatory reaction is observed in the choroid. A granulomatous or nongranulomatous uveitis may occur in other infectious diseases such as brucellosis, leptospirosis, and histoplasmosis but the causative organisms have rarely if ever been demonstrated in the human eye. Sarcoidosis, sympathetic ophthalmia, Vogt-Koyanagi-Harada disease, and juvenile xanthogranuloma (nevoxanthoendothelioma) are characterized by granulomatous uveitis but the etiology of these conditions is not known.

Despite the diverse causes of granulomatous uveitis, there are many similarities in the basic clinical picture. The onset usually is insidious, the cellular reaction in the tissue is greater than the vascular reaction, and the ciliary congestion usually is not severe. Organic changes occur in the iris with thickening due to cellular infiltration, and loss of the normal surface pattern. Nodules or tubercles on the surface and diffuse or localized infiltrates which suggest nodules deep in the iris stroma sometimes are present. Synechia formation is common and mutton-fat precipitates occur on the cornea, in the angle, on the iris and on the anterior capsule of the lens. These greasy precipitates microscopically consist chiefly of epithelioid cells with a few lymphocytes. Nodules of epithelioid cells are common at the pupillary border of the iris (Koeppe nodules) or on the anterior iris surface near the pupil (Busacca nodules).

It should be mentioned that the terms granulomatous and nongranulomatous are pathologic concepts, and that the clinical pictures have been fitted to them on the basis of the pathologic studies. It is not always possible to correlate the clinical with the pathologic findings, however.

If the disease is localized in the choroid, it takes several forms. There may be the acute onset of a large, circumscribed exudative choroidal lesion with some vitreous haze.

Such lesions often remain as solitary foci, frequently recur, remain active for from one to several months, then heal leaving a large area of atrophy and scarring. Similar lesions may be multiple and widespread in the fundus, but there is a tendency for such lesions to occupy a sector of the uvea. Toxoplasmic infections tend to recur adjacent to an old focus. Other choroidal lesions are small, circumscribed, nonexudative, involve the posterior choroid, and are about 1 mm. in diameter. Small hemorrhages commonly occur at their margin. They have a prolonged course and healing is characterized by a sharply outlined, depressed scar. Relapses are common, but the new lesions usually are independent of the old scars. Very commonly both eyes are involved, either simultaneously or successively. The whole picture in these indolent cases is so different from that of the exudative lesions that one might be inclined to believe the two have little or nothing in common. Unfortunately no clear-cut distinction is possible.

There are many histologic findings common to all forms of granulomatous uveitis, regardless of etiology. The perilimbal blood vessels are dilated and lymphocytes and plasma cells are present in the conjunctiva and episclera. So-called precipitates, variously consisting of polymorphonuclear leukocytes, lymphocytes, epithelioid cells, and an occasional giant cell, form on the edematous corneal endothelium (Fig. 332). The aqueous contains an eosinophilic proteinaceous material. Granulomatous foci are seen in small areas or are diffuse in the iris, ciliary body and choroid and are accompanied by tissue damage and necrosis. They consist of lymphocytes, plasma cells and epithelioid cells. The epithelium of the iris, ciliary body and retina eventually shows atrophy in some areas and proliferates in other areas to form nodules and tubules. The retina overlying the inflammatory lesions in the choroid generally shows considerable degeneration and there is perivascular lymphocytic infiltration in the adjacent more normal areas (Figs. 321, 328). The underlying sclera may be infiltrated by lymphocytes, and often is softened and slightly ectatic. Macrophages are found scattered throughout the vitreous. In severe cases they collect on the surface of the retina at a

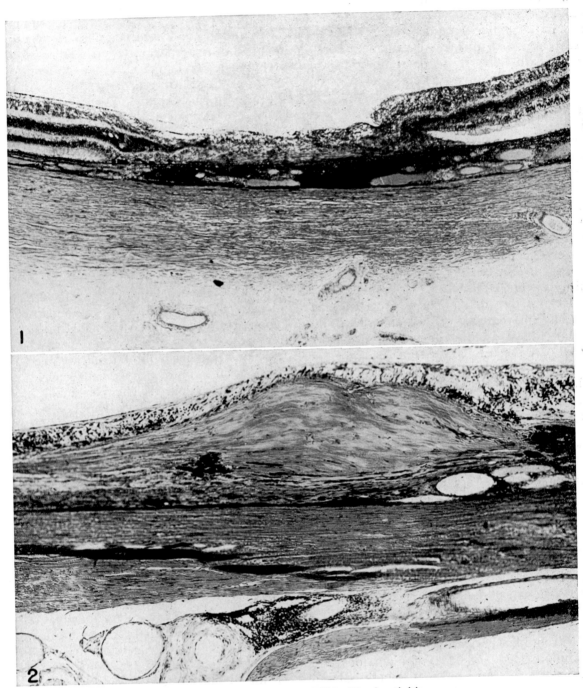

Figure 333.   Possible syphilitic Chorioretinitis

1. Active chorioretinitis. Focal lesion at macula in patient with positive Wassermann reaction. ×70. AFIP Acc. 63839.

2. Chorioretinal scar in patient with positive Wassermann reaction. Fibrous chorioretinal adhesions with proliferated retinal pigment epithelium at macula. Lymphocytic periphlebitis in episclera. ×130. AFIP Acc. 102840.

distance from the chief lesion and may even enter the retina along the retinal veins.

After the inflammation subsides, the eye whitens and the precipitates become crenated and slightly pigmented, and either may persist or finally disappear. Small nodules in the iris, ciliary body and choroid may either absorb without residua, or leave atrophic or hyalinized scars. Large granulomas are replaced by connective tissue and massive scars (Fig. 333).

A number of conditions which produce granulomatous uveitis will be discussed briefly and characteristic microscopic and clinical signs will be noted. They are not listed in order of importance. The frequency with which any one of these conditions is listed as the cause of granulomatous uveitis seems to vary in different studies and areas of the world. It often is possible in active granulomatous infections to demonstrate the causative organism in tissue sections, but when the eyes are examined only after the active phase of the disease it may not even be possible to make a presumptive diagnosis. Often, however, the reaction pattern may suggest a specific disease. Many active cases, however, which are studied early by histologic methods and cultures remain undiagnosed.

Sarcoid. Boeck (1899) described the lesions of skin, mucous membrane and lymph nodes to which he gave the name sarcoid. According to Longcope (1941), in this disease involvement of the uvea, eyelids, conjunctiva or orbital tissues occurs in more than half of the cases. Intraocular involvement is most commonly seen in the anterior uvea but almost any other portion of the eye may also be affected. Heerfordt, in 1909, described a syndrome of bilateral uveitis, fever and swelling of the lacrimal and parotid glands to which he gave the name uveoparotid fever. In 1936, Bruins Slot demonstrated that uveoparotid fever was a manifestation of sarcoidosis, a conclusion which soon was confirmed by others.

Uveal sarcoid lesions most often occur in the ciliary body. Sarcoid lesions of the iris and ciliary body occasionally present such a characteristic clinical picture that the diagnosis may be suspected strongly on inspection (Fig. 21). Opaque pinkish-yellow nod-

ules occur which are more vascular than tuberculous lesions, and there is less hyperemia and infiltration of the surrounding tissues in sarcoidosis. Ciliary body sarcoid lesions usually involve the corona ciliaris, and may fill the angle and the posterior chamber.

The characteristic histologic lesions described by Boeck consist of densely packed masses of epithelioid cells, often associated with many giant cells of the Langhans type (Figs. 18, 21, 119), and surrounded by layers of lymphocytes. Curious asteroid inclusions and laminated basophilic bodies, Schaumann bodies (Figs. 119–3, 4), occasionally are seen in the cytoplasm of the giant cells, but these are rare in the intraocular lesions. These bodies are not pathognomonic of sarcoidosis, since they occur in other granulomatous lesions. Sarcoid nodules have little tendency to caseate, but the occurrence of small central foci of fibrinoid necrosis do not rule out the diagnosis of this condition. There is much less tissue destruction with sarcoid nodules than with other granulomatous lesions, and healing may take place with negligible scar formation. Lymphocytic infiltration surrounding the epithelioid cell nodule is also very scanty compared to that seen in other granulomas. The intraocular sarcoid lesions are often small, usually not more than 1 mm. in diameter, but many small lesions may coalesce into large conglomerate masses consisting of closely packed epithelioid cells and giant cells. This is especially true of those lesions in the ciliary body and iris which may also fill the anterior and posterior chambers.

The diagnosis of intraocular sarcoid cannot be made from microscopic tissue sections alone. Other clinical and laboratory data are required. These include a negative or feeble reaction to the usual intradermal injection of tuberculoprotein; elevation of the serum proteins; a rise in serum globulin with reversal of the albumin-globulin ratio; radiographically demonstrable changes in the lungs and long bones; and nodular skin lesions. Biopsy of other tissues may be necessary to assist in confirmation of the diagnosis.

Leprosy. The lesions of leprosy are of two kinds: lepromatous or nodular and tuberculoid or neural. The ocular manifestations are among the most important complications of the disease. In lepromatous leprosy the

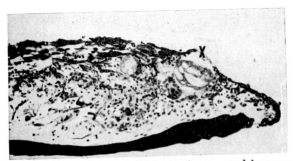

Figure 334. Leprous iritis. X, degenerated leprous giant cells in pupillary zone. ×125. AFIP Acc. 217657.

cornea, conjunctiva, iris and ciliary body may be extensively involved, but the posterior segment rarely is affected and even then the lesions are minute. Interstitial keratitis and scleritis are fairly common. Tuberculoid leprosy involves the trigeminal nerve and causes corneal anesthesia but rarely affects the eye itself.

Keratic precipitates, anterior and posterior synechias, and occlusion of the pupil occur in the lepromatous form. The iris vessels are congested. The stroma of the iris and ciliary body are infiltrated with chronic inflammatory cells, foam cells and giant cells (Figs. 10, 16, 255, 334). The anterior uvea, cornea and sclera may reveal the fully developed leproma, a granulomatous lesion consisting of densely packed masses of epithelioid cells, with some giant cells. The surrounding zone of lymphocytes, commonly seen in granulomas of other types, is scanty or absent. Caseation and necrosis do not occur in the uncomplicated leproma, but ulceration and secondary infection may lead to some necrosis. Fibrosis and scarring also are relatively insignificant and the individual leproma may heal with minor residual damage. The histiocytes, epithelioid cells and giant cells of the leproma contain vast numbers of acid-fast Mycobacterium leprae, and often the cytoplasm of these cells has a foamy appearance in hematoxylin and eosin preparations, due presumably to the large amount of lipoid material derived from the bacilli in these cells. Lepromas may be miliary or conglomerate. The organisms are found chiefly in foam cells, although they often occur extracellularly in the cornea, iris, ciliary body and even in the retina.

Tuberculosis. Miliary tubercles of the iris, ciliary body and especially the choroid may appear during the terminal stages of generalized miliary tuberculosis and in tuberculous meningitis, especially in children. Progressive and massive ocular tuberculosis may result.

Miliary tubercles of the choroid clinically appear as ill-defined, pale yellow, round or oval areas in the fundus. They often are multiple and are more common at the posterior pole.

As in other organs, miliary tubercles of two types are to be seen on histologic examination: (1) the so-called hard tubercle consisting of a mass of epithelioid and giant cells with little or no caseation (Fig. 19), and (2) the so-called soft tubercle in which necrosis and caseation are conspicuous (Fig. 24).

The occurrence of miliary tubercles of the choroid in cases of generalized miliary tuberculosis (Fig. 335), although relatively rare, demonstrates the possibility of blood-borne metastasis of the tuberculous infection to the eye. Such blood-borne metastases may occur in a number of organs in the absence of generalized miliary tuberculosis or a progressive tuberculosis of the organ of primary infection, such as the lung or gastrointestinal tract.

According to Verhoeff (1913), in chronic tuberculous iridocyclitis the primary intraocular focus of the disease may be in the

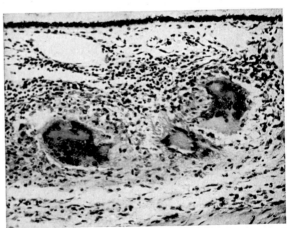

Figure 335. Miliary tubercle in choroid in case of generalized miliary tuberculosis. ×135. AFIP Acc. 30637.

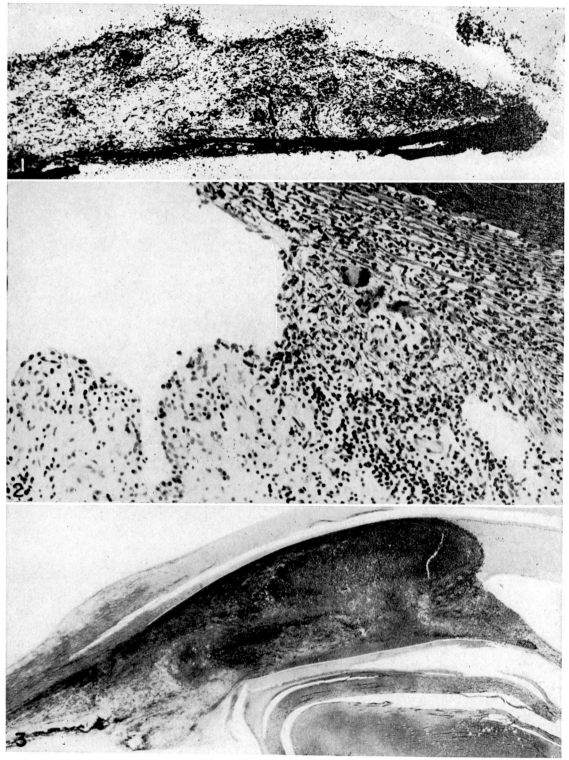

Figure 336. Syphilitic Uveitis

1. Dense lymphocytic and plasma cell infiltration of iris with escape of inflammatory cells into anterior and posterior chambers. ×110. AFIP Acc. 28905.

2. Granulomatous adhesion with giant cells between iris and corneoscleral meshwork. ×35. AFIP Acc. 88459.

3. Gummatous iridocyclitis. ×22. AFIP Acc. 107413.

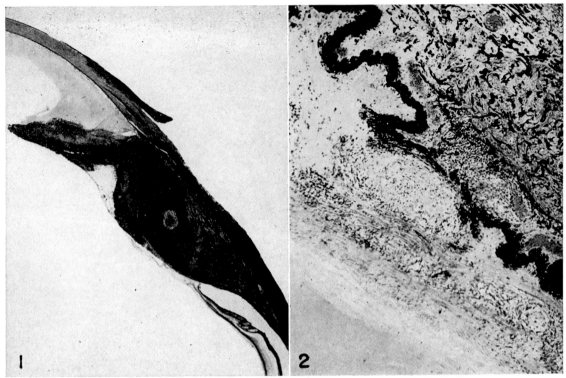

Figure 337. Syphilitic Uveitis

1. Gummatous iridocyclitis. AFIP Acc. 28905.

2. Granulomatous lesion in vascular layer of ciliary body, involving ciliary epithelium and vitreous. ×95 AFIP Acc. 117900.

ciliary body with rupture of the granuloma into the posterior chamber, and spread to adjacent structures. Chronic anterior ocular tuberculous inflammations have an insidious onset with tubercles which appear as grayish avascular nodules about 2 mm. in size in the iris stroma, surrounded by a zone of congestion. After healing there is a somewhat depressed scar. It should be emphasized that most diagnoses of chronic or recurrent anterior ocular tuberculosis are made on clinical evidence, and that it is extremely rare for this diagnosis to be made microscopically. According to Woods, organismal metastasis is responsible for the infection but by the time the eye is enucleated the organisms have long since disappeared. This entire problem awaits solution. Necrotizing granulomas may lead to perforation of the cornea, limbus, or sclera (Figs. 23, 24).

In early childhood these lesions are characterized by massive exudation and caseation with relatively little fibrosis. In the adult the fibrotic changes are prominent and the local disease tends to run a much more chronic course with less caseation. Tubercle bacilli are demonstrable in the lesions in some organs; thus histologic differentiation from other forms of granuloma rarely presents difficulties. In the eye this rarely is true.

The course of ocular tuberculosis depends on the site of metastasis. Lesions originating in the choroid tend to spread both forward into the retina and vitreous and backward into the sclera and orbital tissues. Occasional patients with active pulmonary tuberculosis develop metastatic retinal tuberculosis which progresses rapidly to panophthalmitis (Fig 23). Other patients may have unsuspected tuberculous lung infections and when given corticosteroid treatment they suddenly develop severe ocular tuberculosis. Organisms may be found in large numbers in the infected tissue. This is especially characteristic of retinal tuberculosis and in certain cases the bacilli are most numerous in the necrotic pigment epithelium.

Syphilis. Ocular lesions occur in the late

secondary and tertiary stages of syphilis, but microscopic and other laboratory proof in such cases is extremely rare. Iritis occurring in the late secondary stage of the infection is the most frequent ocular complication of syphilis. Diffuse congestion of the iris, with formation of fleshy, pink inflammatory nodules, occurs most often near the pupillary margin. On microscopic examination these nodules present the appearance of miliary gummas (Figs. 336, 337).

Iritis in tertiary syphilis closely resembles that seen in tuberculous disease. The infiltrates, however, usually are more vascularized and fleshy in syphilis. Corneal, scleral and episcleral lesions may appear in both types of iritis, and secondary glaucoma is a frequent complication.

Miliary gummas often are difficult to differentiate from tubercles, therefore it is useless to make attempts to separate these entities on the basis of fine histologic detail. In the late stages of the disease scar formation and nonspecific chronic inflammatory infiltration dominate the scene and the picture is indistinguishable from the late stages of other infectious processes.

Gummas of the iris and choroid are usually miliary in size, but those in the ciliary body sometimes attain considerable proportions, filling a large part of the anterior eye, and causing massive necrosis of the involved tissues including the sclera, limbus, and adjacent structures (Figs. 336, 337, 338).

Histologically, the gumma shows a central eosinophilic, homogeneous area of necrosis surrounded by actively proliferating vascularized connective tissue containing numerous lymphocytes, plasma cells, epithelioid cells, and an occasional multinucleated giant cell. Treponema pallidum has been demonstrated in the inflamed uveal and retinal tissues in a few instances. Occasionally the presence of characteristic syphilitic endarteritis in the environs of an inflammatory focus provides a useful diagnostic feature.

Syphilitic choroiditis resembles tuberculous choroiditis. The lesions generally are small, about 1 to 2 mm. in diameter, and usually are multiple. Like many other syphilitic manifestations, syphilitic choroiditis may present a pleomorphic pattern. A number of rare fundus lesions have in the past been attributed to syphilis on evidence that now appears rather questionable. Many of these rare forms have not been examined histologically during their active stages. The more common lesions show a granulomatous

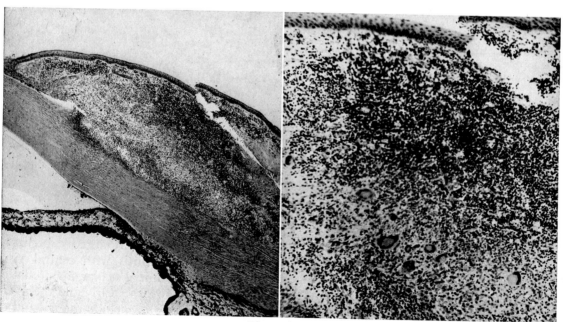

Figure 338.
1. Granulomatous conjunctivitis in patient with positive Wassermann. ×48. AFIP Acc. 293579.
2. Giant cells in granulomatous conjunctivitis, same eye. ×125.

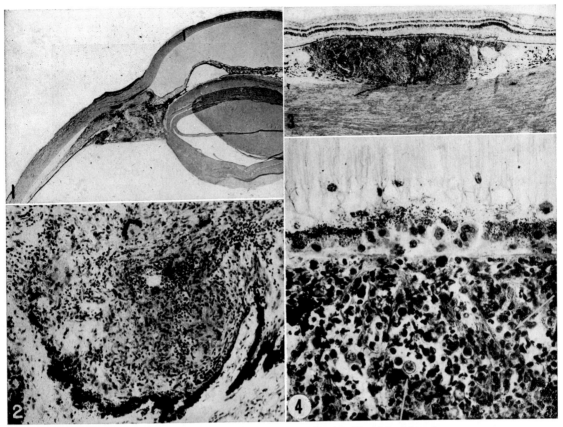

Figure 341. Disseminated Blastomycosis with Uveal Involvement

1 and 2. Granulomatous iridocyclitis. ×7 and ×125, respectively. AFIP Acc. 87260. (See Fig. 11 for organisms in this lesion.)

3 and 4. Granulomatous choroiditis. Arrows indicate some of the numerous blastomycetes. ×16 and ×220, respectively. AFIP Acc. 736114. (Case reported by Sinskey and Anderson, 1955.)

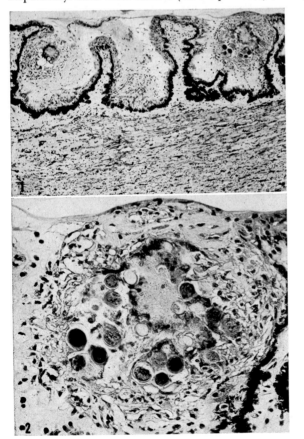

lateral exudative choroiditis with retinal detachment and little or no involvement of the anterior uvea. Some or all of the cutaneous, meningeal, and auditory manifestations of the Vogt-Koyanagi syndrome may occur. The retinal detachment may subside spontaneously in two to three months in the Harada form. Today these two syndromes are considered to be different manifestations of the same disease, intermediate types having been described. Various components of these syndromes may also be seen in sympathetic uveitis.

Figure 342. Disseminated Coccidioidomycosis with Intraocular Involvement

1. Granulomas containing spherules of C. immitis on inner surface of ciliary body. ×80. AFIP Acc. 818810.

2. Same lesion shown in upper right corner of 1. ×305. (Case reported by Brown, Kellenberger, and Hudson, 1958.)

body. E᷂
edly sh᷂
tached.
aqueous
with shr
Iris
membra᷂
terior su᷂
ization ᷂
layer of ᷂
Ectro᷂
eversion
iris, is ᷂
membra᷂
(Fig. 34–
ter musc᷂
all are ᷂
exposed
rior surf
clinical ᷂
ation of
terior su᷂
eversion
Entro᷂
character
margin ᷂
the lens ᷂
Atroph᷂
of inflam᷂
replaced
become
atrophy ᷂
entire str᷂
in the ir᷂
thicker. ᷂
and flatte᷂
alinized ᷂
ciliary ᷂
atrophy ᷂
focal. Wh᷂
ing chorc᷂

1.   2.

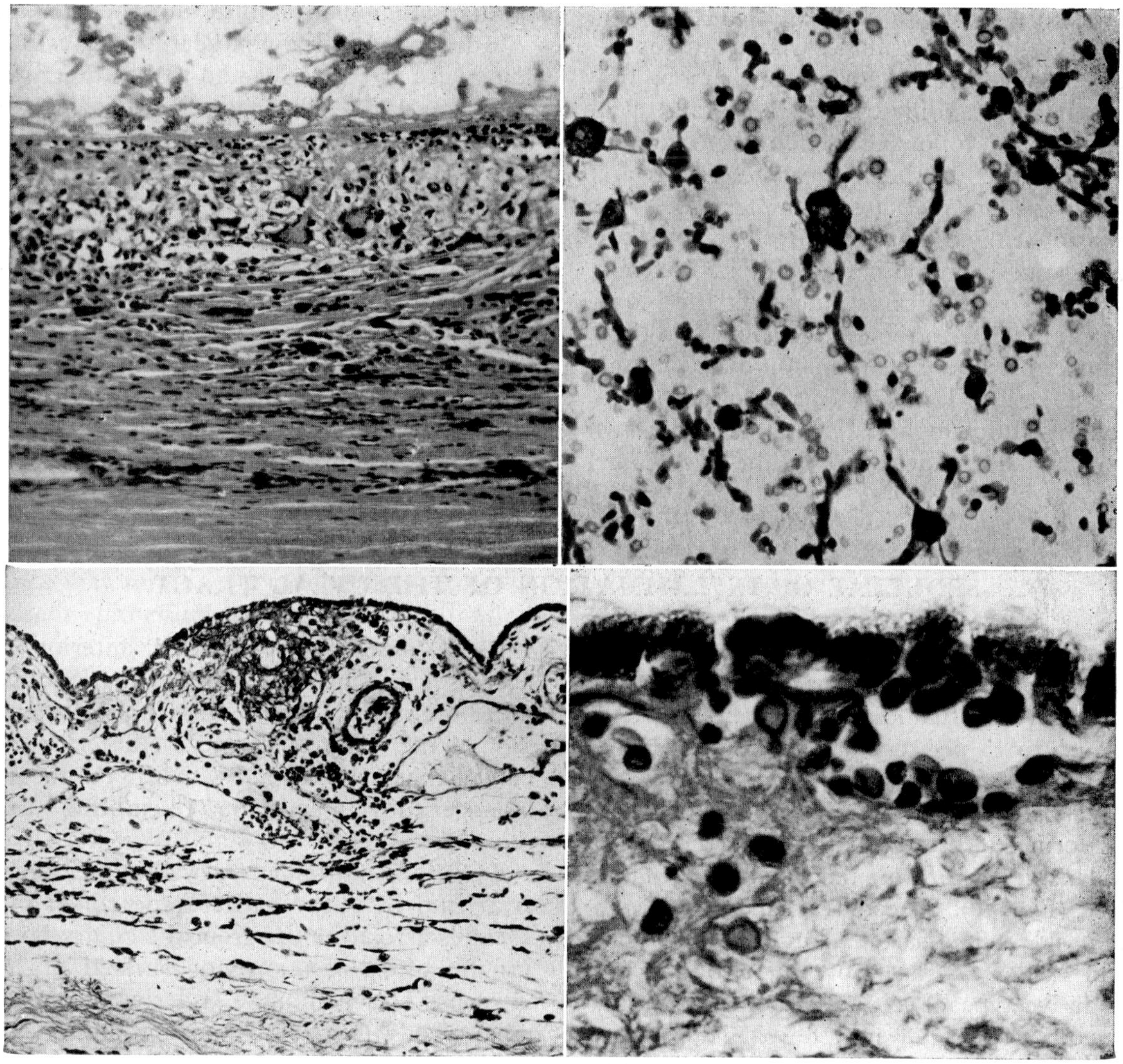

3.   4.

Figure 343.   Ocular Involvement in Cryptococcosis

1 and 2. Granulomatous chorioretinitis in an elderly woman who showed no other manifestations of cryptococcosis at the time of enucleation. ×225 and ×355, respectively. AFIP Acc. 161194.

3 and 4. Choroidal lesions in a widely disseminated infection that was superimposed on a malignant lymphoma. Bauer's stain. ×125 and ×900. AFIP Acc. 262406.

While the histopathologic changes observed in these diseases may be similar to those found in sympathetic uveitis, the inflammatory process tends to be more focalized and is associated with marked proliferation of the retinal pigment epithelium and chorioretinal scarring (Fig. 340).

Brucellosis.   Uveitis is a rare complication of brucellosis. Among 413 patients with Brucella melitensis infections Puig Solanes and coworkers found two cases of iridocyclitis, one bilateral and one unilateral, which

they believed were related to the brucellar infection. They also found four cases of iridocyclitis and one choroiditis in which the etiology was questionable.

Fungal and parasitic infections.   Granulomatous lesions may be seen in the uvea in actinomycosis, aspergillosis, blastomycosis (Fig. 341), coccidioidomycosis (Fig. 342), candidiasis, and cryptococcosis (Fig. 343), usually in the form of an endophthalmitis (Fig. 78) or panophthalmitis; these have been described in Chapter II. Ocular involvement

injuries often are associated with such iris foreign bodies. In such cases the iris often seals the lens capsule tear by fibrous proliferation.

Perforating injuries of the limbus and anterior sclera produce severe damage to the ciliary body, with hemorrhage, detachment and prolapse into the wound (Figs. 86, 345–4). Sympathetic ophthalmia may follow untreated incarcerations of the ciliary body in open wounds. Such injuries usually produce a marked endophthalmitis and eventually lead to the sequelae of this condition. Subsequently the intraocular scar tissue may give rise to recurrent intraocular hemorrhages and the eventual loss of the eye.

Perforating wounds of the choroid often produce extensive hemorrhage and endophthalmitis (Fig. 101). During absorption of the clot granulation tissue gradually forms and eventually the injured tissues are converted into an atrophic scar. A connective tissue overgrowth may extend into the vitreous, and lead to choroidal and retinal detachment.

Damage to the uveal tract is produced intentionally during a number of surgical procedures such as iridectomy, iridencleisis, cyclodialysis and cyclodiathermy. Occasionally as a result of more radical operations in which several rectus muscles are detached, scleral tissue resected, and excessive diathermy applied, the vascular supply to the anterior uvea is compromised. In such cases the resultant widespread necrosis leads to rapid deterioration of the eye and consequent blindness (Fig. 346).

METABOLIC DISEASES

Diabetes. Several characteristic changes may be observed in the iris of the diabetic. The pigment epithelium often is vacuolated and presents a lacy appearance (Fig. 347–1, 2). Each cell appears markedly enlarged by the vacuoles which distend the cytoplasm. This vacuolization is due to the accumulation of glycogen. The intensity and frequency of this change is not correlated with that of the diabetic retinopathy. A delicate vascular membrane (rubeosis iridis) may appear on the anterior surface of the iris in late diabetes. The membrane is derived from the iris stroma, and its contraction may produce ectropion. At times even in the absence of retinal vein occlusion hemorrhagic glaucoma appears. This suggests that the iris capillaries may participate in the capillary disease of the chronic diabetic.

CIRCULATORY DISTURBANCES OF THE UVEAL TRACT

CHOROIDAL VESSELS

The choroidal arteries and arterioles share with those of the spleen the remarkable property of showing hyaline thickening and sclerosis of their media in the absence of generalized vascular disease. This change makes its appearance in the choroid in the fifth decade of life and increases progressively thereafter. No functional changes in the choroid have been correlated with this phenomenon, but it would seem possible that some of the senile and presenile chorioretinal degenerations, which not infrequently have been observed in the absence of generalized vascular sclerosis, may be related to this local vascular change. This arteriolar and arterial hyalinization morphologically is indistinguishable from the arterial and arteriolar changes characteristic of malignant hypertension and nephrosclerosis. In evaluating the ocular lesions associated with hypertension, therefore, due allowance must be made for this "normal" aging process of the choroidal arterial tree.

The choroidal vascular system is remarkable also for the anatomic segregation of the capillaries into a single layer. Precapillary arterioles pass to this layer from the deeper

tures, major infarcts and ap
rhages are extremely rare.

Atherosclerotic lesions of t
teries are extremely common.
matous plaques are to be fou
choroidal arteries near the p
the eyeball in almost every c
generalized atherosclerosis. 1
frequency of these lesions sug
sions of the affected arteries
should be much more comm
sclerotic occlusions of the
Nevertheless, infarct and apop
roid are relatively rare. Pres
lateral anastomotic connectic
roidal arterial tree are suffici
to protect the choroid from n
the result of an isolated art
Atherosclerotic choroidal h
however, occur and may on o
massive. The expulsive hem
are rare complications of intr
procedures represent extrem
lesions of this type.

The choroidal veins show
atherosclerotic changes. Occ
vortex veins have been obsen
hemorrhagic glaucoma, but t
the atherosclerotic process i
choroidal capillary layer in
sclerotic individuals often she
hyaline changes. It is difficu
whether this is to be classifie
an atherosclerotic manifesta
general participation of the c
atherosclerotic process has,
adequate analysis. The possib
tween these lesions and those
ular tuft have already been d

MALIGNANT HYPERTEN
ARTERIOLAR SCLE

The most characteristi
change in the blood vessel
hypertension is a hyaline sul
posit in the terminal arteriol
severe and fulminating form
the hyaline subendothelial
companied by necrosis of th
converting the whole arterio
almost structureless cord. Cap
show this necrotic reaction

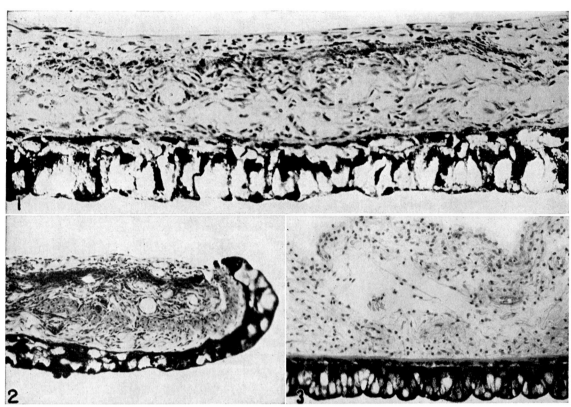

Figure 347. Vacuolation of Iris Pigment Epithelium in Diabetes Mellitus and in Gargoylism.

1. Diabetic iridopathy. Vascularization of anterior surface of iris. Vacuolation of iris pigment epithelium. ×205. AFIP Acc. 100161.

2. Diabetic iridopathy. Vascularization of pupillary zone of iris. Ectropion uveae. Vacuolation of iris pigment epithelium. ×120. AFIP Acc. 186024.

3. Gargoylism. ×125. AFIP Acc. 87437.

regions of the choroid and break up into numerous capillaries all in the same plane. The venules are similarly oriented. The whole structure resembles a set of interconnected umbrella skeletons with the capillaries representing ribs and the arterioles and venules representing shafts. This anatomic relationship can be seen in exaggerated form in the tapetum fibrosum of the choroid of cattle, where the shafts, the arterioles and venules, are greatly elongated in traversing the fibrous layer of the tapetum.

Segregation of the capillaries into a single layer makes the choroid an especially favorable structure in which to study capillary fibrosis and hyalinization. In the kidney the glomerular tuft presents a similar segregation of capillaries from other grosser structures, and in the glomerulus, also, capillary hyalinization and sclerosis are well recognized. In other organs where the capillaries

are not anatomically segregated, it is difficult to distinguish a hyalinized capillary from a hyalinized collagen fiber. Considerations of this nature must be kept in mind in evaluating the significance of hyaline and fibrotic changes in the choriocapillaris.

The major collecting veins of the choroid, the vortex veins, pass through rigidly fixed channels in the sclera. Venous occlusions at the sites of scleral perforations, while not as common as venous occlusions at the retinal arteriovenous crossings, are much more frequent than similar lesions in small veins elsewhere in the body.

ATHEROSCLEROSIS

Atherosclerosis of the ciliary body and iris vessels has been inadequately studied. Because of the elaborate anastomotic connections of the arterial tree in each of these struc-

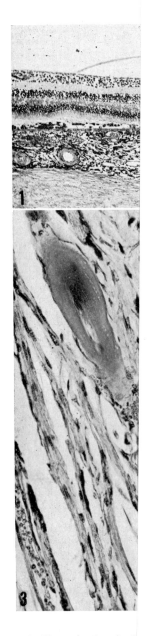

1. Necrosis of retinal
a patient with malignar
2. Thrombosis of chc
3. Arteriolar necrosis
×305. AFIP Acc. 98188
4. Detachment of cili
75 year old woman whc
was suspected. ×8. AF

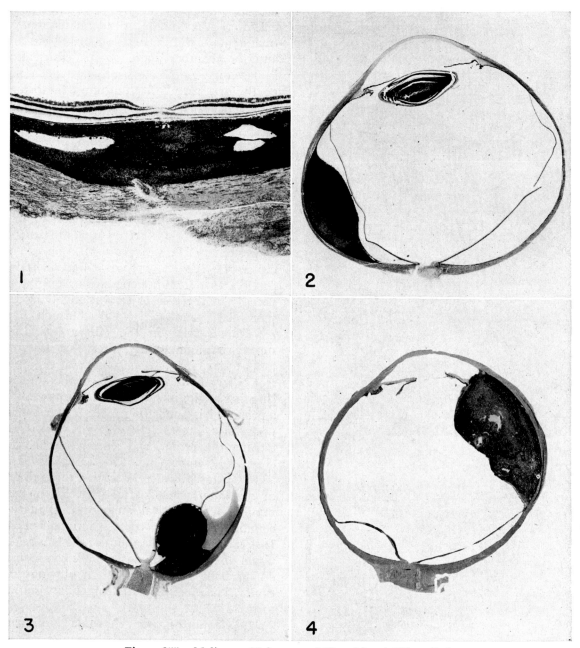

Figure 355.   Malignant Melanoma of Choroid and Ciliary Body

1. Flat malignant melanoma of choroid beneath macula. AFIP Acc. 282868.
2. Malignant melanoma of choroid confined by Bruch's membrane. Note pigment variation. AFIP Acc. 79372.
3. Malignant melanoma of choroid which has broken through Bruch's membrane and spread to form characteristic mushroom shape. Invasion of overlying retina by tumor. Serous separation of adjacent retina. AFIP Acc. 106356.
4. Malignant melanoma of ciliary body invading filtration angle and peripheral choroid. AFIP Acc. 273944.

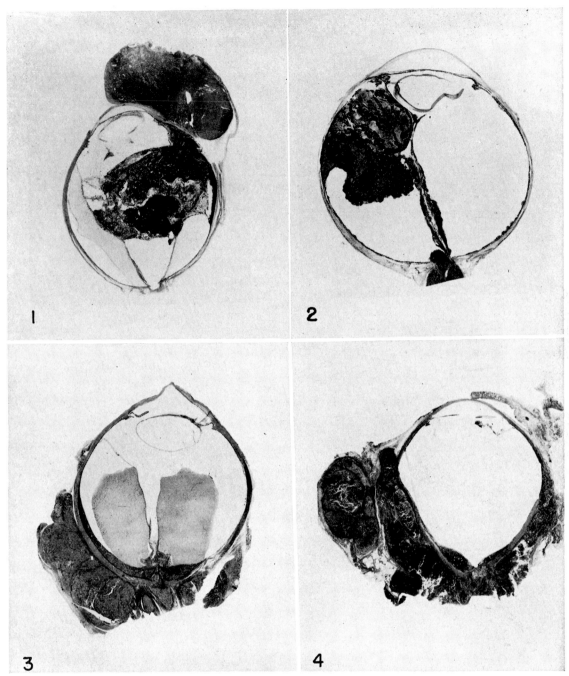

Figure 356. Malignant Melanoma of Choroid and Ciliary Body

1. Malignant melanoma of ciliary body invading iris and choroid. Pale necrotic areas in intraocular mass. Extension through sclera at limbus, forming large epibulbar mass. Secondary glaucoma evidenced by excavation of optic disk. Serous detachment of retina. AFIP Acc. 187850.

2. Partially necrotic malignant melanoma of ciliary body and peripheral choroid. Seeding of tumor along inner surface of choroid. Diffuse invasion of retina seen only in tumors in which extensive necrosis has allowed dissemination of tumor cells. Detachment of retina. Invasion of optic nerve secondary to that of retina. AFIP Acc. 288264.

3. Flat malignant melanoma of choroid invading optic disk to lamina cribrosa. Massive extrabulbar extension through sclera. Subretinal serous exudate. Retinal detachment. AFIP Acc. 175013.

4. Massive extrabulbar extension from small malignant melanoma of choroid around optic disk. AFIP Acc. 159090.

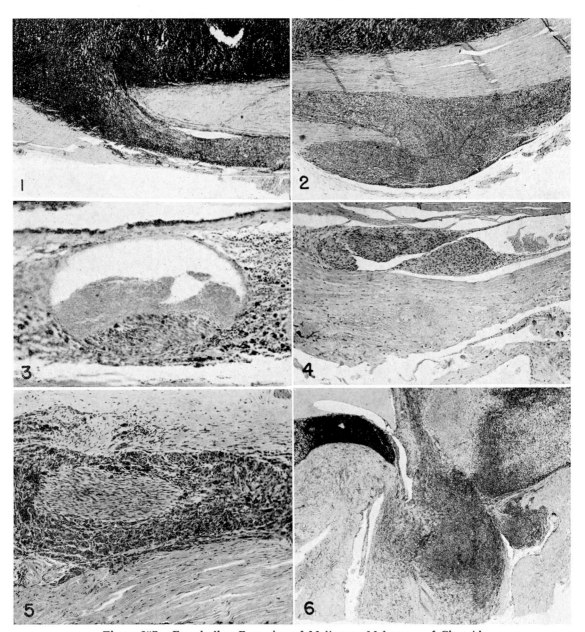

Figure 357. Extrabulbar Extension of Malignant Melanoma of Choroid

1. Extension of tumor into long posterior scleral canal. ×48. AFIP Acc. 39090.

2. Epibulbar nodule resulting from extension through sclera in long posterior canal. ×48. AFIP Acc. 109307.

3. Tumor cells in vortex vein at entrance into choroid. ×125. AFIP Acc. 204090.

4. Tumor cells in vortex vein in scleral canal. ×75. AFIP Acc. 198121.

5. Tumor in scleral canal, in close association with long posterior ciliary nerve. ×75. AFIP Acc. 61136.

6. Invasion of retina and optic nerve by partially necrotic malignant melanoma of choroid. Tumor cells are seen in nerve beyond depressed lamina cribosa. ×24. AFIP Acc. 234621.

breaks through Bruch's membrane and spreads out to form a mushroom-shaped mass, elevating and detaching the retina (Fig. 355–3). The summit of the tumor usually becomes adherent to the overlying retina, but rarely infiltrates this tissue. If the tumor should penetrate the retina it is recognized easily with the ophthalmoscope. According to Rones and Linger (1954), ordinarily the retina over the tumor shows edema with microcystic degeneration, and this may be an early sign with small tumors, but similar retinal changes are observed over hemangiomas of the choroid (MacLean and Maumenee, 1960). The pigment epithelium of the retina exhibits degenerative and proliferative changes. There usually is proteinaceous exudate beneath the detached retina adjacent to the tumor; occasionally the entire retina becomes detached. It is common for a small melanoma in the upper eye, or at the level of the equator to cause extensive serous detachment inferiorly. The sclera beneath the tumor may be thinned. The tumor often extends out of the eye along the ciliary nerves and vessels (Fig. 357). This type of epibulbar extension typically produces small, well encapsulated nodules. These ordinarily are completely removed with the globe when the eye is enucleated. Necrosis of the melanoma and adjacent sclera allows direct access to the orbit with the formation of epibulbar nodules within Tenon's capsule. According to Leopold (1958), if there is diffuse invasion of the orbit (Fig. 356–3, 4), or if the extrabulbar nodule is necrotic or incised during enucleation, exenteration should be performed. Occasionally tumor cells are seen in blood vessels, particularly the vortex veins (Fig. 357–3, 4). Invasion of the optic nerve occurs from juxtapapillary choroidal melanomas (Fig. 357–6). These may simulate primary melanomas of the disk. Extension posteriorly through the nerve and into the meninges may occur but is unusual.

Classification of melanomas of the uveal tract.

Malignant melanomas of the uveal tract have been classified according to their cell type, argyrophil fiber content, and pigment content (Callender, 1931; Wilder and Callender, 1939). The Callender classification includes the following histopathologic types listed in the order of increasing malignancy.

Callender's classification.

SPINDLE A. These tumors are composed almost exclusively of slender spindle-shaped cells containing very small inconspicuous flattened nuclei. The nuclear chromatin is frequently arranged as a line extending through the center of the nucleus in its long axis (Fig. 358–1). Spindle A tumors are often completely amelanotic.

SPINDLE B. These melanomas are also composed of spindle-shaped cells. The nuclei of these tumors are larger and they contain a more prominent nucleolus (Figs. 358–2; 359–2). The entire cell is also larger than those in spindle A tumors. Pigmentation is variable.

FASCICULAR. In this type, the palisaded arrangement of the spindle cells (mainly of the spindle B type) suggests that of neurilemmoma. Palisading may be predominantly perivascular or in ribbon form (Fig. 358–3, 4). The arrangement rather than cytologic characteristics determined the degree of malignancy.

NECROTIC. Tumors of this type contain so few viable areas that it is impossible to classify them properly by cytologic and histologic characteristics.

EPITHELIOID. Tumors of this group are composed almost exclusively of the large epithelioid cells which are irregularly polygonal and very variable in size and shape. Their nuclei are large, hyperchromatic and conspicuously nucleolated. Multinucleated forms are seen frequently. The cytoplasm is abundant, usually homogenous and, in amelanotic cells, definitely acidophilic. The cell walls, unlike those of the spindle types, usually are well defined and the cells frequently appear to be separated from one another. Mitoses generally are more common in this type (Fig. 358–5). The degree of pigmentation varies markedly.

MIXED. This is the most common type of melanoma, accounting for more than half of all malignant melanomas of the ciliary body and choroid. It is characterized by a combination of spindle and epithelioid cell types. These tumors, therefore, exhibit all of the combined variations encountered in those melanomas.

Occasional tumors contain as a prominent element deeply pigmented branching cells, resembling the normal choroidal melanocytes

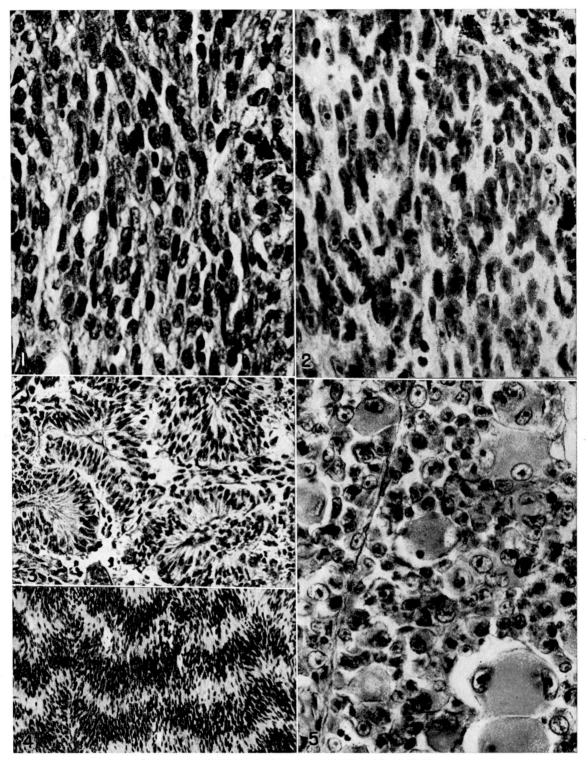

Figure 358. Malignant Melanoma of Choroid: Cell Types

1. Spindle cell, subtype A. Nucleoli absent or ill-defined. Line or fold in long axis of nucleus. ×650. AFIP Acc. 168852.

2. Spindle cell, subtype B. Prominent nucleoli. ×705. AFIP Acc. 48420.

3. Fascicular type. Palisading of tumor cells around blood vessels. ×250. AFIP Acc. 231963.

4. Fascicular type. Palisading of tumor cells in ribbon form. ×125. AFIP Acc. 289600.

5. Epithelioid cell type. Large round cells. Lack of cohesiveness between individual cells. Bizarre and multinucleated forms. ×500. AFIP Acc. 65901.

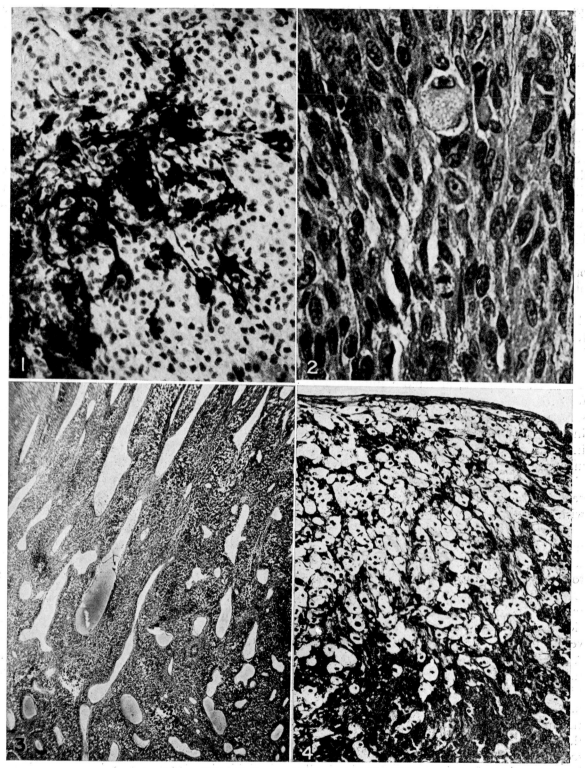

Figure 359. Malignant Melanoma of Choroid

1. Branching pigmented cells in mixed cell type, choroid. ×255. AFIP Acc. 55899.
2. Activity in predominantly spindle B type evidenced by mitosis and epithelioid cell. ×650. AFIP Acc. 129215.
3. Tumor blood vessels in malignant melanoma. ×24. AFIP Acc. 74029.
4. Foamy cells: histiocytes which have ingested lipids from degenerating tumor cells. ×125. AFIP Acc. 306782.

(Fig. 359–1) (Friedenwald, 1932 and Reese, 1947). Reese was impressed by the high degree of malignancy of tumors containing these cells in large numbers. In the series reported by Wilder and Paul (1951), the branching pigmented cell invariably was associated with the epithelioid type and it seems reasonable to assume that the poor prognosis of these tumors is due, not to the normal appearing melanocytic cells, but to their epithelioid cells. It is for this reason that the Registry of Ophthalmic Pathology has not employed a separate designation for tumors containing large numbers of branching melanocytes.

Cytogenesis. Since each of the cell types often exists in combination with any of the others, it is unlikely that they have different derivations. The distinctive characteristics of the various types probably result from a different mode of growth of tumor cells which have the same origin. Separation of these cell types into various groups is useful for descriptive purposes, and more importantly, for prognostic reasons, as will be shown. The same mixture of cell types frequently is seen in metastatic lesions. Intraocular melanomas in which epithelioid cells are not identified may give rise to metastases in which they are abundant. The highly malignant epithelioid cell type probably is present in most cases with metastasis.

Prognosis according to cell type. The most recent follow-up study of the large series of intraocular melanomas (1624 cases followed at least 5 years) in the Registry of Ophthalmic Pathology has reconfirmed the previous reports that Callender's classification is of great prognostic value. The five-year mortality rate of patients with spindle A melanomas is so low (5 per cent) that these tumors have been considered virtually benign. This low incidence of tumor deaths may be within the "experimental error" of the method, for the tumors are classified on the basis of random sampling of a few microscopic slides. It is possible that if a much larger number of sections were examined, all of those lethal spindle A tumors would be found to contain significant numbers of spindle B or epithelioid cells that had been missed in the original sections. The five-year mortality rate rises to 14 per cent for spindle B and fascicular tumors, 51 per cent for the necrotic and mixed cell types, and 69 per cent for the pure epithelioid melanomas.

For prognostic purposes the Callender classification can be simplified to good advantage. Since there is a striking difference in the prognosis depending upon the presence or absence of epithelioid cells, the tumors can be divided accordingly into two groups. Pure spindle cell tumors (spindle A, spindle B, and fascicular) have an overall ten-year mortality of only 33 per cent while the remainder (mixed, necrotic, and epithelioid) have a much higher mortality rate of 82 per cent.

Flocks et al. found an interesting relationship of cell type to the size of choroidal melanomas. Small tumors, e.g., those less than 1 sq. cm., carrying a favorable prognosis have been found to consist predominantly of spindle A and B cells, while large tumors have a poor prognosis and more often contain a significant proportion of epithelioid cells. This is taken as further evidence to support the belief that malignant melanomas probably arise from nevi. Spindle A and B melanomas apparently represent stages in the transition of nevi to malignant melanomas containing epithelioid cells.

Stromal tissue, reticulin content. Melanomas have relatively little stromal tissue but argyrophilic reticulin fibers are often deposited about individual tumor cells or about nests or lobules of the neoplasm. The amount of reticulin deposited in melanomas varies considerably. There may be a dense network in some areas, while others are devoid of fibers (Fig. 360). In general, the tumors which have a heavy reticulin fiber content are more benign than are those with a lower fiber content (Wilder and Paul, 1951; Zimmerman, Paul and Parnell, 1958). This is taken as evidence of a favorable host response since the reticulin fibers are believed to be derived from the stroma, not from the tumor cells. A heavy deposit of reticulin fibers may simply be a reflection of slow growth which affords the stroma an opportunity to envelop individual cells more completely than is possible when the neoplastic cells are growing and dividing more rapidly.

Pigmentation. Most melanomas are pigmented but the degree of pigmentation varies greatly. The pigment melanin is derived from

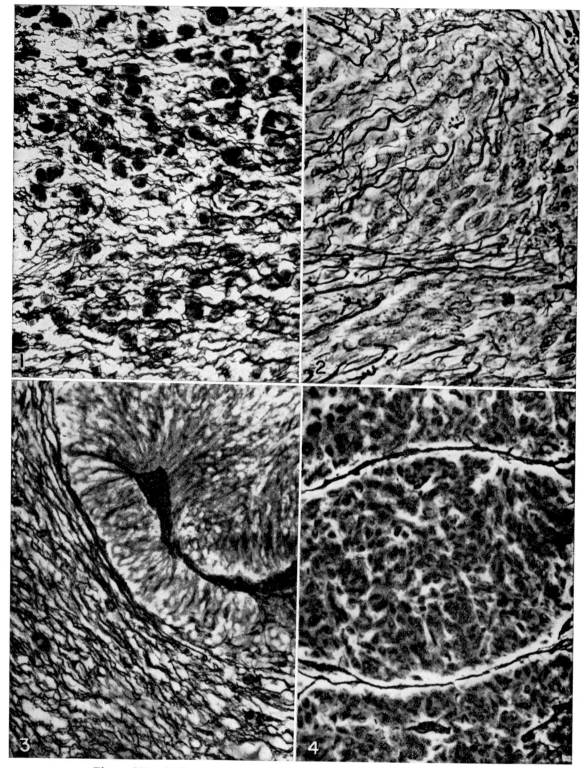

Figure 360. Malignant Melanoma of Choroid, Argyrophil Fiber Content

1. Heavy argyrophil fiber content. Wilder reticulum stain. ×330. AFIP Acc. 34822.

2. Marked fiber content. Not all tumor cells are surrounded by argyrophil fibers. Wilder reticulum stain. ×650. AFIP Acc. 168852.

3. Heavily fibered and unfibered areas in same field. Wilder reticulum stain. ×410. AFIP Acc. 54107.

4. Fibers absent except in interlobular stroma; none surrounding individual tumor cells. Wilder reticulum stain. ×348. AFIP Acc. 54017.

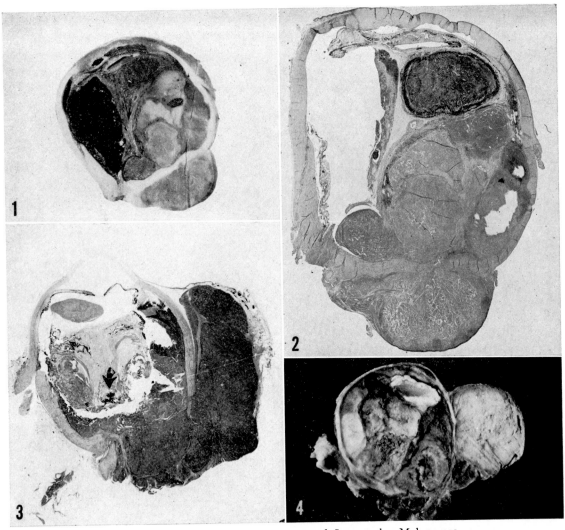

Figure 361. Necrotic and Unsuspected Intraocular Melanomas

1. Eye removed at autopsy in the case of a 32 year old white man who had been treated medically for endophthalmitis 6 months before admission. He died 4 days later, markedly jaundiced. At autopsy the liver was found massively enlarged by metastatic melanoma. AFIP Acc. 612166.

2. Same eye shown in Fig. 1. The intraocular tumor, microscopically as well as grossly, was almost entirely necrotic. ×5.

3. This phthisical eye had been blind for 22 years following injury (arrow indicates retained metallic foreign body in vitreous). The melanoma which arose in the choroid posteriorly was unsuspected until extraocular extension led to proptosis. ×2¼. AFIP Acc. 24068.

4. This eye of a 69 year old woman had been blind from glaucoma and cataract for over 10 years. The intraocular neoplasm remained asymptomatic; preoperatively the extraocular extension was thought to be a primary rhabdomyosarcoma of the internal rectus muscle. AFIP Acc. 805502.

the cytoplasm of the tumor cells but it is not confined to them. It may also be contained in macrophages or free in the tissues in areas of necrosis. Usually, pigmentation is dense in some areas and may obscure cell detail whereas in other areas the tumor is almost devoid of pigment. In general, heavily pigmented tumors are more malignant than amelanotic melanomas (Wright, 1949). Mil-

ares (1940) has observed that metastases almost never contain more pigment than the primary tumor and usually contain considerably less. Study of material in the Registry of Ophthalmic Pathology indicates that metastases may contain either more or less pigment than the primary tumor, although very deeply pigmented secondary tumors usually originate from primary tumors with a rather high melanin content. Pigmented and non-pigmented metastatic nodules may appear in the same organ.

Necrosis of melanoma. Areas of necrosis are seen in almost all melanomas, and occasionally necrosis may be too extensive to permit accurate classification on the basis of cell type (Fig. 361). Necrosis occurs if the tumor outgrows its blood supply. It is in association with the necrotic tumors that massive hemorrhage, uveitis and panophthalmitis are most often seen. Relatively small areas of necrosis in ciliary body tumors may produce an iridocyclitis at an early stage before a large tumor mass can be seen. Absorption of larger necrotic areas may lead to the formation of cystic spaces in the tumor. Large foamy cells, histiocytes which have ingested lipoidal material from degenerating tumor cells, are sometimes present in malignant melanomas, usually peripherally (Fig. 359–4).

Glaucoma. Uveal melanomas cause glaucoma in several ways. Tumors of the anterior segment invade the anterior chamber angle. Posterior tumors produce retinal detachment and forward displacement of the peripheral iris, blocking the anterior chamber angle. A large necrotic tumor of the choroid may cause glaucoma as a result of a complicating hemorrhage, uveitis, or panophthalmitis.

Unsuspected melanomas. In a study of 1000 malignant melanomas of the ciliary body and choroid on file in the Registry of Ophthalmic Pathology, Makley and Teed found that in 21 per cent of the affected eyes the media were opaque at the time of enucleation. Thus the tumor in these cases could not be visualized, and in more than one-half, even the possibility of a malignant melanoma was not suspected before enucleation. Other studies have also shown that about 10 per cent of melanomas are discovered only after the enucleated eye is examined in the pathology laboratory (Kirk and Petty, 1956). In more than 90 per cent of such unsuspected melanomas the eye is glaucomatous and in about one-fourth the tumor is markedly necrotic. Occasionally the tumor arises in a phthisical eye that has long been blind from an old injury (Fig. 361–3).

Fatal cases. Death usually results from blood stream metastasis; the liver is the organ most frequently involved (Fig. 362). An in-teresting but poorly understood observation that has been made frequently is the late occurrence of massive hepatic metastasis with enlargement of the liver to five or more times its normal size and the complete absence of metastases in other organs. However, in other cases, metastases may be present in almost every organ of the body including the gastrointestinal tract, skin, subcutaneous tissue, spine, lungs, and lymph nodes. Such metastases may appear more than ten years after enucleation and when isolated they may seem to represent a new primary tumor. Approximately 15 per cent of all patients with uveal melanomas die within one year, and about 45 per cent die of metastasis within five years after enucleation. In succeeding five-year periods deaths from generalized malignant melanoma continue, but at a markedly declining rate. Metastatic deaths have been reported as long as 35 years after enucleation, and even in these cases there has been little or no evidence of recurrence of the primary neoplasm or development from a new primary. The prognosis is worse in large tumors than in small ones. When tumors of the very malignant diffuse types are excluded, prognosis does not appear to be influenced by shape or by perforation of Bruch's membrane. High mortality is associated with extraocular extension and lethality is increased in the older age groups.

Melanocytosis. Ocular melanocytosis has been discussed in Chapter II. The uveal tract shows diffuse heavy pigmentation due to infiltration by melanocytes. Malignancy occasionally occurs, either as a diffuse process, or as a localized tumor. Microscopically the uvea contains large numbers of pigmented cells, which appear foamy after bleaching (Fig. 67).

Hemangioma

The only primary intraocular tumors which are certainly not of neuroectodermal derivation are the angiomatous lesions of the uveal tract and retina. These properly belong in the group of hamartomas and are not true neoplasms. Frequently they are components of syndromes (e.g., the Sturge-Weber syndrome and Von Hippel-Lindau disease) and are regarded as phakomatoses. The latter

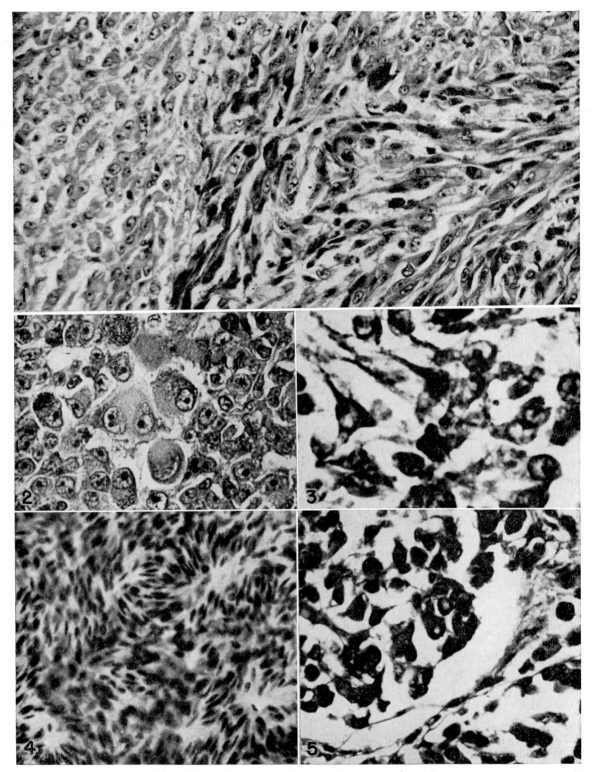

Figure 362. Malignant Melanoma, Metastases from Eye

1. Epithelioid and spindle B cells in liver metastasis. ×280. AFIP Acc. 61087.
2. Epithelioid cells in brain metastasis. ×545. AFIP Acc. 52550.
3. Branching pigmented cells in same brain metastasis. ×965. AFIP Acc. 52550.
4. Fascicular type in liver metastasis. ×375. AFIP Acc. 56238.
5. Epithelioid type in same liver metastasis. ×375. AFIP Acc. 56238.

term has been almost exclusively used in the ophthalmic literature to designate a group of heredofamilial disorders characterized by the widespread formation of hamartomas.

Incidence of hemangioma of uveal tract. Hemangiomas do occur in the iris and ciliary body but most frequently they are located in the choroid. A review by Stokes of the uveal hemangiomas which appear in the Registry of Ophthalmic Pathology revealed 36 cases of hemangioma of the choroid, one hemangioma of the ciliary body, and two hemangiomas of the iris.

Hemangioma of the iris. Hemangiomas of the iris are observable clinically and are seldom excised. Therefore, laboratory specimens of these lesions are not numerous. Glaucoma results if the anterior chamber angle is extensively blocked by the tumor or if blood or cellular debris accumulates in the anterior chamber angle.

Hemangioma of the choroid. Hemangioma of the choroid, when unaccompanied by the other constituents of the Sturge-Weber syndrome, seldom is diagnosed correctly prior to enucleation. In about half the cases found in laboratory collections the lesion had been mistaken for a malignant melanoma. In the others the vascular tumors were found after the removal of the eye because of absolute glaucoma of unknown cause. The tumors usually are referred to as cavernous hemangiomas, but they probably are simple angiomas, representing an abnormal development of choroidal vessels into arteries, veins, and capillaries.

Clinical appearance. The vascular anomaly in the choroid typically involves the posterior pole, adjacent to the optic disk, although it may extend to the equator or beyond, usually on the temporal side (Fig. 363). The apparently solid elevation of the retina seldom is marked except, perhaps, in the macular region. The involved part of the fundus overlying the tumor is usually slightly darker than elsewhere and the retinal vessels may be tortuous. Extensive microcystoid degeneration of the retina overlying the tumor may be observed. The borders of the hemangioma are irregular. These tumors can be diagnosed with greater certainty if the possibility of hemangioma is kept in mind. They *never* are pigmented, whereas melanomas

usually are. The pigment can be seen best with indirect ophthalmoscopy and by use of a contact lens and slit lamp microscope. The retina may detach at a remote point from the hemangioma, in contrast to melanoma. Hemangiomas produce either an arcuate field defect or a localized scotoma, whereas melanomas produce large scotomas which involve the periphery, depending on the amount of retinal detachment they produce.

Histologic appearance. These tumors most often produce great thickening of the choroid on the temporal side of the disk and consist of endothelial-lined spaces of varying sizes which are engorged with blood and separated by almost no connective tissue stroma. There is no capsule and the tumor merges imperceptibly with normal choroid peripherally. Bruch's membrane is intact over the tumor. Proliferation and metaplasia of the pigment epithelium of the retina over the tumor may form a mass of connective tissue frequently containing bone. Degeneration of the retina with extensive microcyst formation is commonly present over the tumor.

Glaucoma. The intraocular pressure in an eye which contains a choroidal hemangioma frequently is slightly lower than that of the fellow eye. The possible explanations for development of glaucoma associated with choroidal hemangioma are numerous and have been summarized by Anderson (1939). Congenital malformation of the anterior chamber angle similar to that found in hydrophthalmos (primary congenital glaucoma) may be responsible. A hemangioma of the choroid may cause glaucoma in a manner similar to that of other intraocular tumors by increasing the bulk of the intraocular contents, by compression and interference with the drainage of one or more of the vortex veins, or by blocking the venous return from the ciliary body. Glaucoma also may be caused by vascular stasis, resulting from slowing of the choroidal circulation due to the great increase in the number of choroidal vessels, to pressure, or to interference with the choroidal drainage by a coexisting orbital hemangioma, or through interference with drainage from the cavernous sinus by a coexisting meningeal hemangioma. Vascular dilatation and hypersecretion, increased transudation of fluid through the thin-walled

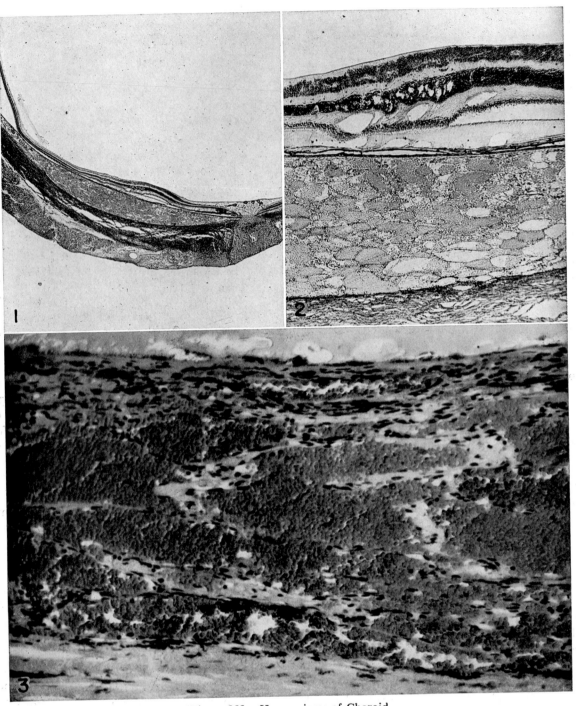

Figure 363. Hemangioma of Choroid

1. Hemangioma of choroid adjacent to optic disk. ×8. AFIP Acc. 171647.
2. Same tumor extending beneath macular region. ×45.
3. Large, engorged blood spaces lined by thin layer of endothelial cells and fibroblasts. ×240. AFIP Acc. 45225

vessels of the tumor, and variations in the size of the tumor are other possible causes of ocular hypertension in cases of uveal angiomatosis. In a histologic study of 36 cases of choroidal hemangioma, the associated glaucoma always seemed to be due to the chamber angle changes, either of a congenital type or secondary to the choroidal hemangioma.

The Sturge-Weber syndrome

Description. The Sturge-Weber syndrome, or encephalotrigeminal angiomatosis (Fig. 364), combines hemangioma of the skin, usually over the area of distribution of one or more branches of the fifth cranial nerve (nevus flammeus), glaucoma, and angiomatous changes in the vessels of the meninges of the brain. Nevus flammeus and glaucoma may be present without meningeal involvement. Glaucoma may be absent in nevus flammeus with meningeal involvement. Incomplete forms are more frequent than complete syndromes. When all features are present, they almost always occur on the same side.

Numerous instances of the association of glaucoma and facial hemangioma have been reported (Ballantyne, 1930; O'Brien and Porter, 1933; and Joy, 1950). Nevus flammeus usually is unilateral but may be bilateral, and, associated with glaucoma, involves the lids or conjunctiva. Glaucoma may be congenital, of the open angle type, or due to synechias.

Manifestations. The ocular manifestations associated with nevus flammeus include dilated conjunctival vessels, vascular nevus of the conjunctiva and the episclera, peripheral anterior synechias, heterochromia of the iris, a dense iris stroma with dilated, somewhat varicose vessels or a frank hemangioma, dilated, tortuous or varicose retinal or choroidal vessels, dark red fundus, changes in the pigment epithelium of the retina, retinal detachment, hemangioma of the choroid, and cavernous atrophy of the optic nerve. The most common intraocular vascular malformation is a hemangioma of the choroid.

Neurologic symptoms. The neurologic symptoms, which are due to intracranial pressure or hemorrhage from the abnormal vessels of a diffuse meningeal hemangioma, include generalized epileptiform seizures, hemiplegia, hemianopia, mental deficiency, contralateral homonymous hemianopia, and epilepsy.

Causes of glaucoma in Sturge-Weber syndrome. The glaucoma occurring in the Sturge-Weber syndrome usually is considered to be related to a choroidal hemangioma. The pathogenesis of glaucoma associated with choroidal hemangioma has already been discussed. Possibly, dilated conjunctival vessels or a hemangioma of the conjunctiva and episclera may impede the outflow of aqueous from the anterior ciliary veins. In some cases peripheral anterior synechias mechanically block the anterior chamber angle. They are congenital or occur secondarily due to anterior chamber angle closure by forward displacement of the iris-lens diaphragm by a detached retina. This causes apposition of the iris root to the trabeculas. At times there is organization of particulate matter, especially blood, in the anterior chamber angle. The hyperpigmentation and increased density of the stroma in the iris produce a darker color in the affected eye but do not influence the intraocular pressure. The hyperpigmentation is due to an increase in the number of melanocytes in the iris stroma, but no angioma is present.

Dilated and varicose vessels of the iris stroma may upset the interchange of water and electrolytes between the aqueous and the iris and block the anterior chamber angle mechanically. An iris or ciliary body hemangioma may infiltrate the angle and produce glaucoma.

The presence of tortuous retinal vessels and varicosities of the retinal veins in an otherwise normal fundus was noted clinically in a number of the reported cases of the Sturge-Weber syndrome in which a choroidal hemangioma was demonstrated later.

EPITHELIAL TUMORS

Epithelial tumors arise mainly in the ciliary body. They include pseudoadenomatous hyperplasia, benign epithelioma, carcinomas, and medulloepitheliomas. These may arise from pigmented as well as nonpigmented ciliary epithelium. Similar lesions occur in the iris and retina but they are rare.

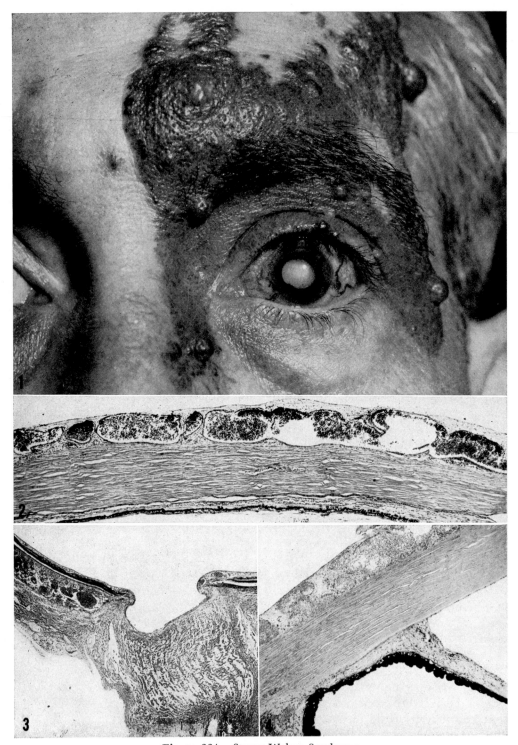

Figure 364. Sturge-Weber Syndrome

1. Facial hemangioma involving eyelid; huge anomalous episcleral vessels; absolute glaucoma; and mature cataract. AFIP Acc. 761707.

2. Cavernous hemangioma of episclera. ×47. Same case.

3. Cavernous hemangioma of choroid on temporal side (left); deep excavation of optic disk. ×14. Same case.

4. Cavernous hemangioma of limbus; broad peripheral anterior synechias. ×45. Same case.

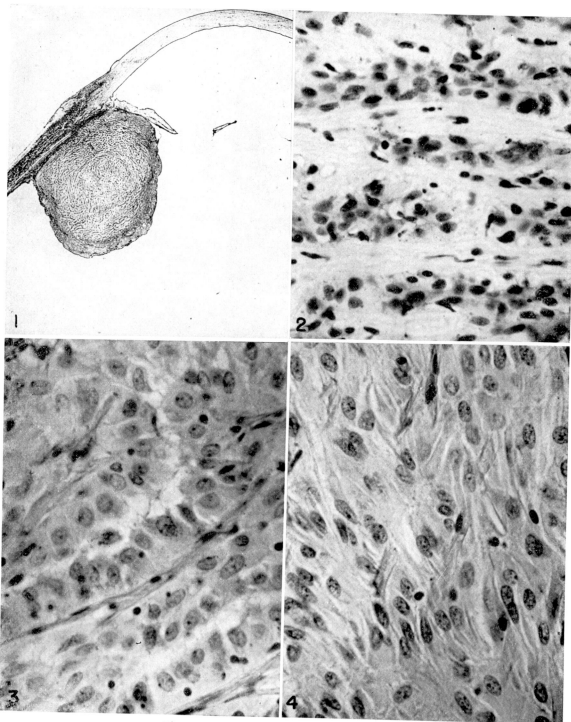

Figure 365. Hyperplasia, Ciliary Epithelium

1. Hyperplasia of pars ciliaris retinae, suggesting neoplasm. AFIP Acc. 169585.
2. Hyaline material between strands of hyperplastic cells. Same case. ×500.
3. Tubular proliferation of epithelial cells from pars ciliaris retinae. Same case. ×500.
4. Sheet-like proliferation of epithelial cells from pars ciliaris retinae. Same case. ×500.

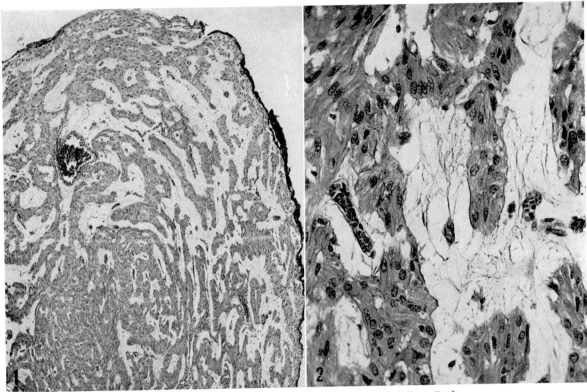

Figure 368. Benign Epithelioma or Adenoma of Ciliary Body

This tumor, excised from a 15 year old boy, was suspected clinically of being a malignant melanoma of the ciliary body. AFIP Acc. 821536. 1. ×50. 2. ×305.

rounded on its inner aspect by pigment epithelium (Fig. 368). This epithelium most often contains very little pigment. A similar tumor may arise from the pigment epithelium of the ciliary body and iris but is extremely rare.

Embryonal Type

Diktyoma. Badal and Lagrange first described the tumor of this group in 1892. Verhoeff, in 1904, was the first to emphasize the embryonal character of these tumors. The diktyoma (Figs. 369, 370) usually is observed at birth or becomes apparent in early childhood, is not preceded by trauma or inflammation, and generally is conceded to be choristomatous.

Usually the tumor is detected by the parents, who observe a peculiar pupillary reflex, but it may become obvious only after it results in glaucoma or atrophy with poor vision.

Diktyomas infiltrate the zone around the lens, and may spread forward into the angle,

iris and onto the cornea. They may push the iris forward, and obstruct the angle. Rare tumors extend through the scleral emissaria.

These tumors contain poorly differentiated neural tissue which in places resembles embryonic retina. They also contain columnar epithelial cells arranged in sheets, tubes or solid masses. Some areas resembling retinoblastoma may be seen. Ependyma-like spaces, cerebral tissue, and cartilage may be present (Fig. 370). There is little stromal tissue. The epithelium shows frequent mitosis in the marginal zone of the growth.

Medulloepithelioma (Carcinoma)

The adult type of medulloepithelioma (Figs. 371, 372) may or may not be pigmented. It is composed of cuboidal or columnar epithelial cells in a tubular arrangement. Sometimes the arrangement is rather regular and alveoli dominate the picture, but in other instances the alveoli are not as large or as apparent because of tremendous

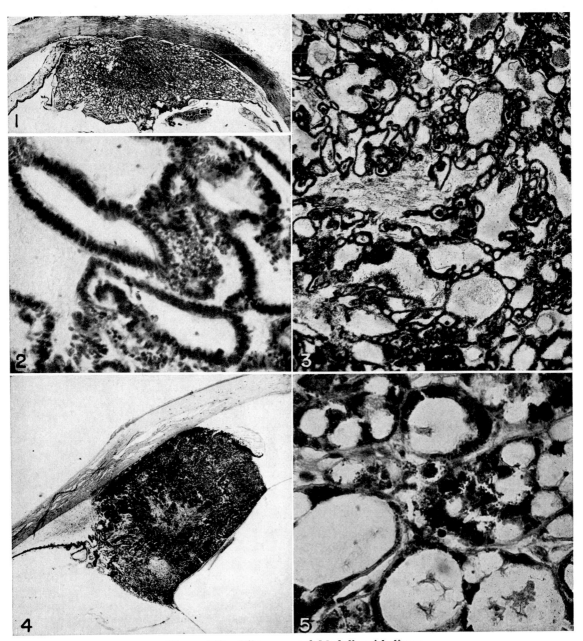

Figure 369. Diktyoma and Medulloepithelioma

1. Tumor arising from ciliary epithelium. ×22. AFIP Acc. 46745.
2. Glandlike proliferation of cells of pars ciliaris retinae. ×275. AFIP Acc. 311828.
3. Glandlike structure of tumor arising in pars ciliaris retinae. ×30. AFIP Acc. 311828.
4. Tumor arising in pigment epithelium of iris. ×20. AFIP Acc. 67470.
5. Glandlike structure of tumor arising in pigment epithelium of ciliary body. ×515. AFIP Acc. 46745.

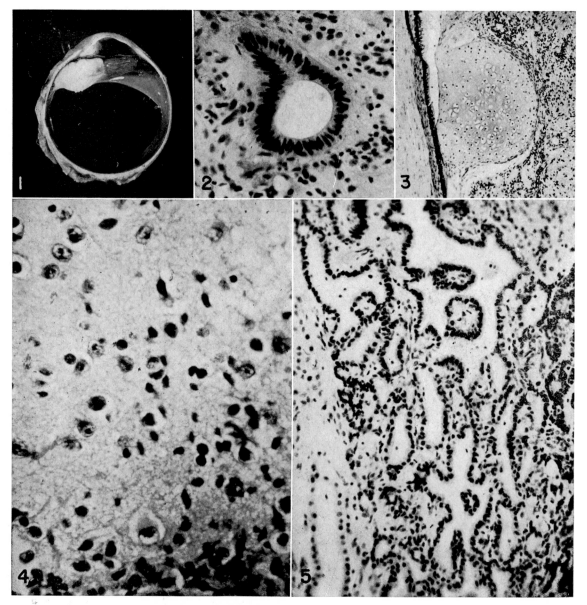

Figure 370. Diktyoma

1. Tumor in ciliary region. AFIP Acc. 196709.
2. Epithelium-lined space simulating ependymal cleft. Same case. ×500.
3. Cartilage at base of tumor. Same case. ×150.
4. Ganglion and glia cells in glioneuromatous portion of tumor, resembling cerebral cortex. Same case. ×485.
5. Papillary structure simulating choroid plexus. Same case. ×385. (Case reported by Fralick and Wilder, 1949.)

cellular proliferation. Both features may be present in the same tumor. A similar tumor may arise from the iris epithelium (Fig. 369–4).

Leiomyoma

Origin. Tumors of the dilator and sphincter muscles are cytogenetically retinal and topographically iridic. The muscles are differentiated from that portion of the retinal pigment epithelium which extends over the posterior surface of the iris, and are therefore neuroectodermal in origin. Nevertheless, these tumors appear to be true leiomyomas, indistinguishable histologically from smooth muscle tumors found elsewhere in the body. Among the cases which have been reported, all tumors have appeared benign and none has metastasized.

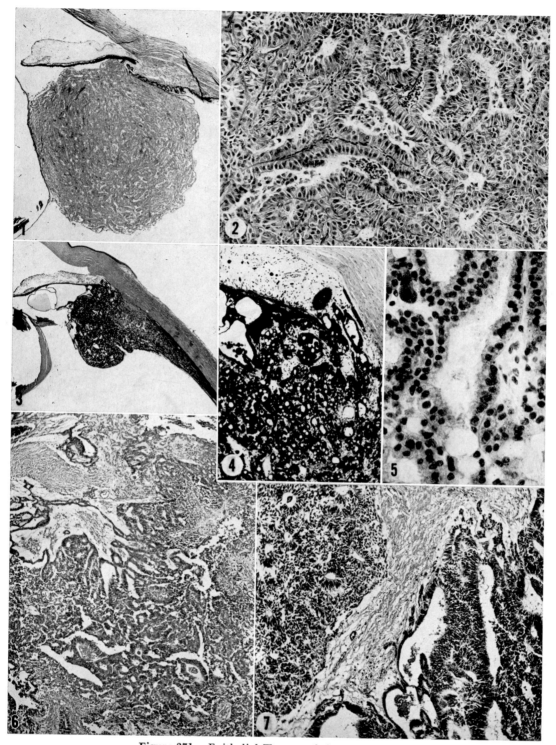

Figure 371. Epithelial Tumors of the Ciliary Body

1 and 2. Adenoma of nonpigmented ciliary epithelium. ×13 and ×115, respectively. AFIP Acc. 911701.

3 to 5. Well differentiated adenocarcinoma of pigmented ciliary epithelium with invasion of ciliary body. No. 5 is a bleached preparation. ×9, ×50, and ×305, respectively. AFIP Acc. 954743.

6 and 7. Poorly differentiated neuroepitheliomatous tumor invading orbit, believed to have arisen from the ciliary body in a 13 year old boy. The neoplasm extended through the frontal bone and into the brain. (Case reported by de Buen and González-Angulo, 1960.) ×50 and ×115, respectively. AFIP Acc. 846123.

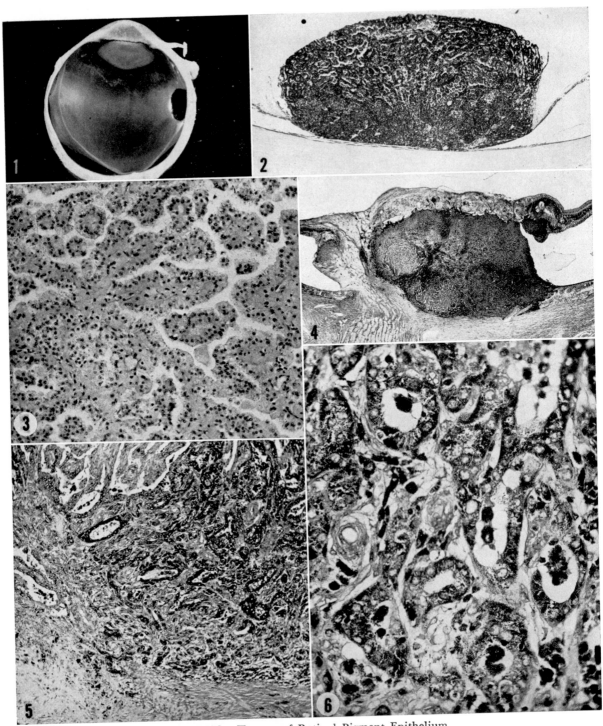

Figure 372. Tumors of Retinal Pigment Epithelium

1 to 3. Very highly differentiated adenocarcinoma with minimal invasion of choroid. No. 3 is a bleached preparation. ×2, ×13, and ×130, respectively. AFIP Acc. 848819.

4 to 6. Moderately well differentiated adenocarcinoma with broad area of invasion of choroid and optic disk. (Case reported by Fair, 1958.) ×12, ×70, and ×305. AFIP Acc. 503113.

Clinical and histologic appearance. It is impossible to differentiate these tumors from certain nevi and lightly pigmented malignant melanomas on the basis of clinical examination. In fact, even histologic studies fail to provide satisfactory criteria for a clear cut separation of these two seemingly different groups of tumors. When it is realized that the melanocytes of the iris may have similar neural crest derivation the similarity of nevi and leiomyomas becomes more comprehensible. Leiomyomas usually are observed as pinkish-brown nodules which more often involve the pupillary than the ciliary zone (Fig. 373). Histologically, they are amelanotic or lightly pigmented tumors composed of cells with long narrow nuclei which sometimes, but not always, have flat ends. Sometimes nucleoli are evident. The cytoplasm, instead of having an ill-defined spindle shape such as occurs in malignant melanomas of the spindle cell type, frays out into many fine fibrils. In the leiomyomas in the Registry of Ophthalmic Pathology, reticulin fibers were demonstrated with silver stains only around blood vessels and between cell bundles, not among the tumor cells. The cells have a parallel arrangement within bundles and are comparatively uniform in size and shape. Where the bundles are cut in cross section the cells appear round, as do those of spindle cell malignant melanoma, and the fibrillar processes are seen as dots. Gold impregnation or Mallory's phosphotungstic acid hematoxylin may be helpful in demonstrating the myofibrils. O'Day (1949) makes particular mention of the long fibrils which do not anastomose and in which there are many and prominent fusiform dilatations. Cystic degeneration, hemorrhage into the tumor, and hyphema may occur.

Leiomyoma of the ciliary body is extremely rare (Blodi, 1950). The tumor arises from the ciliary muscle.

Neurilemoma

Histologic appearance. Neurilemoma (Schwannoma, neurofibroma, neurinoma) is a benign encapsulated tumor arising from the Schwann cells sheathing peripheral nerves. Within the eye it is associated with the ciliary nerves as they pass through the scleral canals or enter the uveal tract. Intraocular tumors of this type are quite rare. Clinically most of them are misdiagnosed as malignant melanomas. The growth is nonpigmented and is composed of spindle-shaped cells with nuclei that, in general, appear longer and narrower than those of the spindle A type of malignant melanoma, but are sufficiently like them to present a problem in histologic diagnosis (Fig. 374). As in neurilemomas elsewhere, the nuclei show some degree of palisading, in this respect resembling somewhat the fascicular type of malignant melanoma, although they do not behave like them in regard to malignancy.

Neurofibromatosis

Another tumor which contains schwannian elements is a diffuse, benign congenital or developmental growth often associated with widespread neurofibromatosis (von Recklinghausen's disease). In many instances there exists an associated developmental anomaly of the filtration angle and in others peripheral anterior synechias result in glaucomatous enlargement of the globe and to enucleation. The association of glaucoma with the congenital type is, however, not invariable, and occasional small tumors of this type are to be found on routine postmortem examination of eyes in which no disease has been suspected clinically. Although the condition is in itself benign, it often is a component of the potentially malignant von Recklinghausen's disease (multiple neurofibromatosis) (Figs. 63, 64), and is regarded as one of the phakomatoses. Occasionally, large tumor masses may be found in the uveal tract of a patient who has von Recklinghausen's disease. In such cases the tumor may prove either to be a neurofibroma or a malignant melanoma and the two cannot be differentiated clinically.

Histologic appearance. In neurofibromatosis there often is a generalized thickening rather than a circumscribed mass (Figs. 63–2; 64–2). The process may involve the ciliary body and iris, as well as the choroid. The cellular character varies within certain limits. In addition to cells derived from the sheaths of Schwann of the ciliary nerves, ganglion

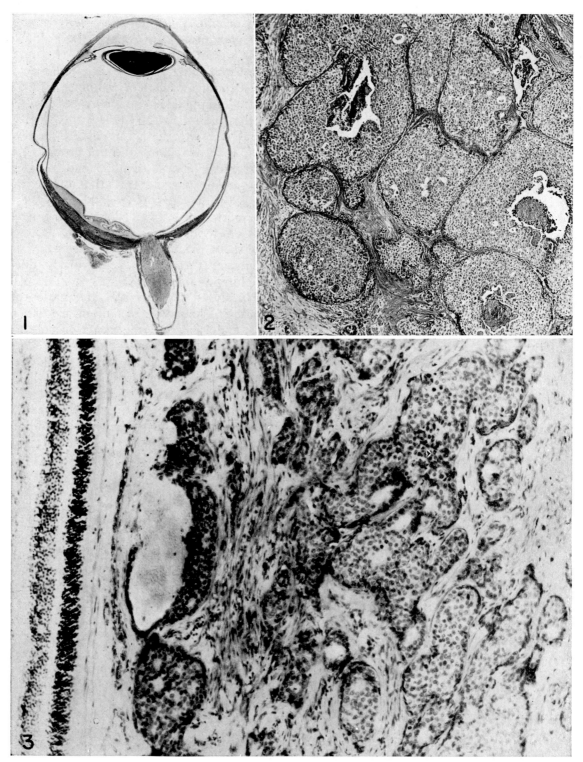

Figure 379.   Metastatic Carcinoma

1. Carcinoma in choroid, metastatic from breast. AFIP Acc. 37637.

2. Carcinoma in choroid, metastatic from breast, well defined stromal pattern. ×48. AFIP Acc. 309867.

3. Carcinoma in choroid, metastatic from breast, with fibrous proliferation around nests of tumor cells. ×375 AFIP Acc. 48880.

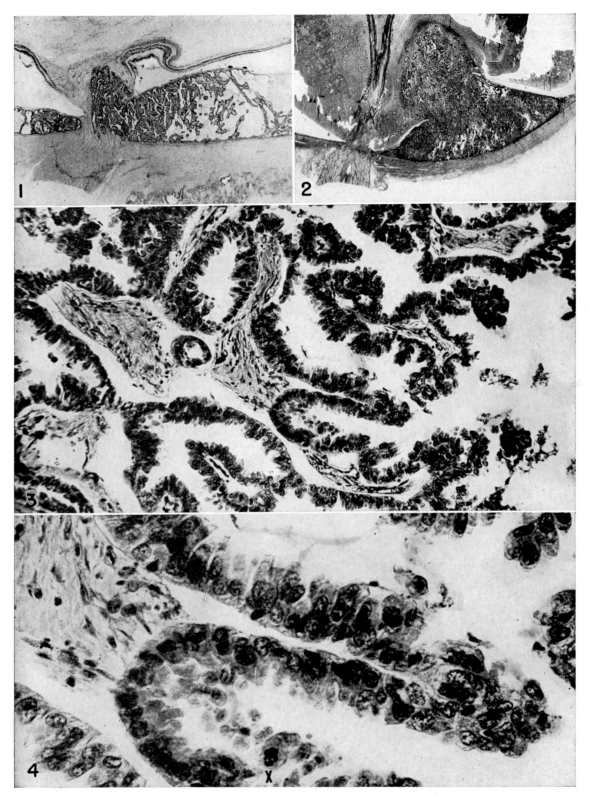

Figure 380. Metastatic Carcinoma

1. Carcinoma in choroid, metastatic from lung. Invasion of nerve head. AFIP Acc. 81665.

2. Mushroom-shaped carcinoma in choroid, simulating malignant melanoma, metastatic from lung. **AFIP Acc.** 86871.

3. Papillary adenocarcinoma in choroid, metastatic from lung. ×200. AFIP Acc. 153347.

4. **Columnar epithelium, with mitosis (X), lining alveolus. ×500. AFIP Acc. 153347.**

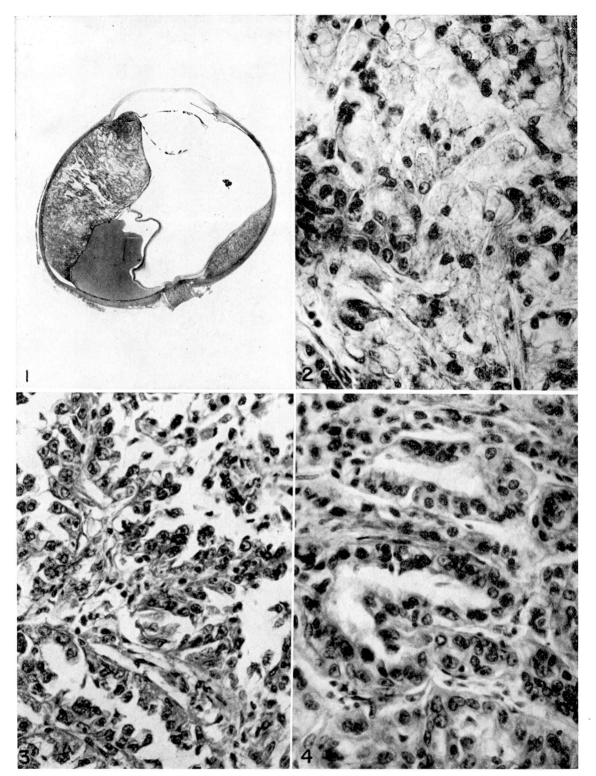

Figure 381. Metastatic Carcinoma

1. Two metastases to uveal tract from carcinoma of kidney. Serous detachment of retina. AFIP Acc. 140909.
2. Characteristic clear cells of hypernephroid tumor in uveal metastasis. Same case. ×360.
3. Papillomatous area, same tumor. ×360.
4. Adenomatous area simulating kidney tubules in which the tumor originated. Same tumor. ×680.

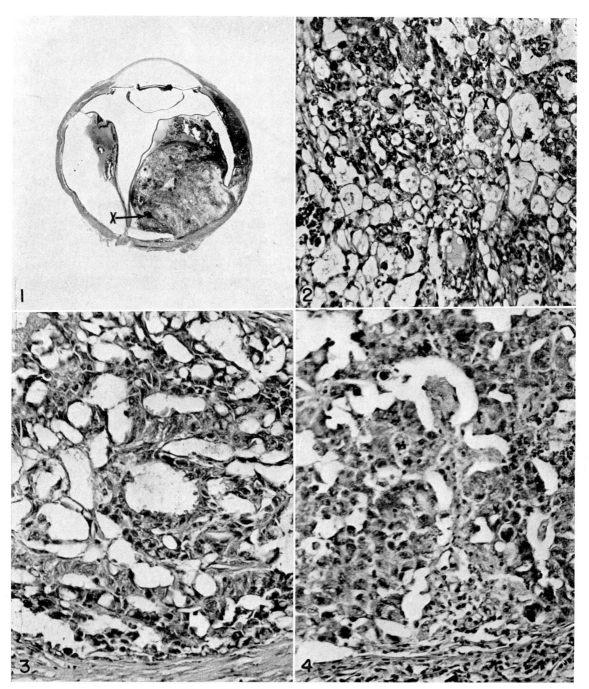

Figure 382. Metastatic Chorioepithelioma

1. Chorioepithelioma, metastatic in eye from testicle. X, hemorrhage. AFIP Acc. 213695.
2. Same tumor. Multinucleated syncytial cell (X). ×180.
3. Same tumor. Branching strands of syncytial cells. ×205.
4. Same tumor. Cytotrophoblasts. ×205.

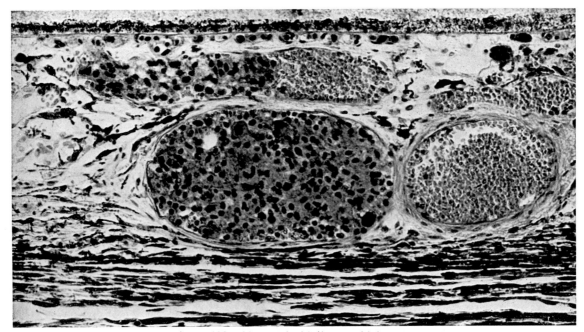

Figure 383.   Metastatic Malignant Melanoma

Tumor cells in choroidal veins and capillaries, metastatic from skin. ×250. AFIP 131550.

istics may be lost to a large extent through lack of differentiation, so that without clinical evidence it frequently is not possible to determine the site of the primary tumor by examination of the ocular metastasis. Few authenticated cases of intraocular metastasis from malignant melanoma of the skin have been recorded (Fig. 383).

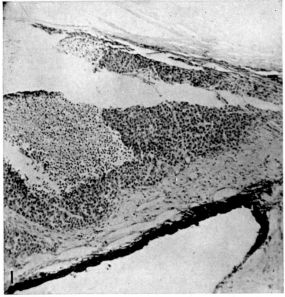

Figure 384.   Carcinoma in iris, metastatic from lung.
AFIP Acc. 82616.

Lymphomatous Tumors

Ocular involvement in tumors of the hematopoietic tissues is sometimes seen. Granulocytic (myelogenous) and lymphocytic leukemia, and malignant lymphomas have been observed in the eye (Figs. 385, 386). Usually the ocular involvement is part of a generalized disease. Primary malignant lymphoma of the uvea is of doubtful occurrence.

The most common tumors of this type to involve the eye are the granulocytic and lymphocytic leukemias. The acute leukemias of childhood are particularly apt to produce ocular lesions.

The posterior choroid most commonly is involved, although the anterior uvea and retina often are the sites of infiltration. Tumor cells may appear in the vitreous or in the anterior chamber. The typical ophthalmoscopic signs in leukemia are engorgement of the retinal vessels, scattered retinal hemorrhages, exudates and alteration in the red color of the fundus to a pale yellowish or greenish-yellow hue. The cause of the vascular dilatation is unknown. The retinal hemorrhages often are capped by yellowish exudates which on histologic examination are found to be composed of masses of leukemia cells. The altered fundus color is attributable to the diffuse

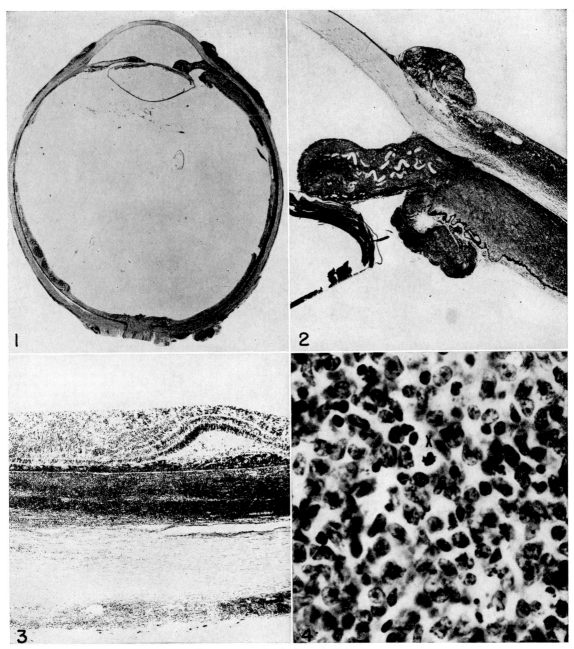

Figure 385. Reticulum Cell Sarcoma

1. Diffuse neoplastic thickening of uveal tract in patient with reticulum cell sarcoma. AFIP Acc. 205805.
2. Neoplastic invasion of iris and ciliary body. Same case. ×16.
3. Cells of the lymphatic series invading choroid and retinal pigment epithelium. Partial destruction of retina by hemorrhage. Same case. ×48.
4. Cells resembling those of germinal centers of lymph follicles. Mitosis (X). Same case. ×705.

leukemic infiltration of the choroid which is common and occasionally is massive. When the iris is involved in leukemic infiltration there may be a pale greenish hypopyon.

Occasional lymphomatoid tumors are seen in the eyes of patients who show no evidence of blood dyscrasia, palpable glands, or other systemic disease. Moreover the patients have remained without symptoms for years following enucleation. In many of these cases the multiplicity of cell types, and the presence of plasma cells in particular, suggest that the tumors are reactive inflammatory processes rather than neoplasms (Fig. 387).

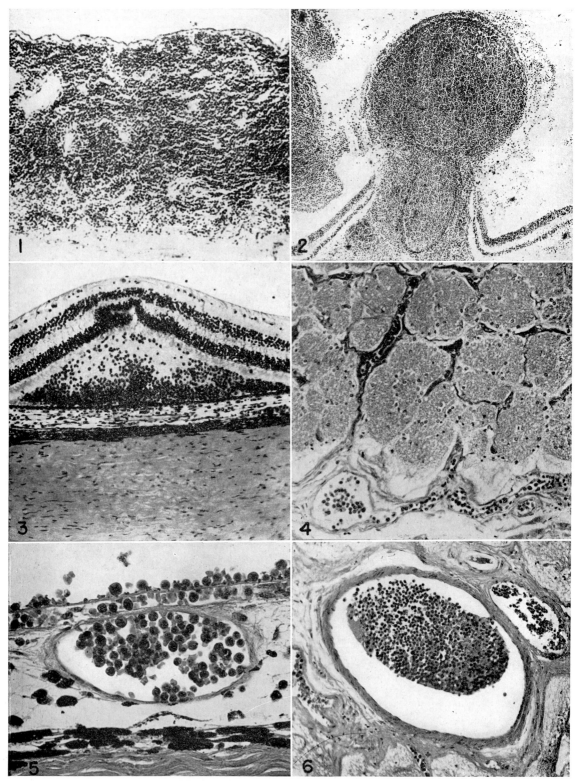

Figure 386. Lymphosarcoma and Leukemia

1. Lymphosarcoma, choroid. ×175. AFIP Acc. 28190.
2. Lymphatic leukemia. Lymphocytes forming tumefaction at site of retinal hemorrhage. ×91. AFIP Acc. 28163.
3. Lymphatic leukemia. Lymphocytes in subretinal hemorrhage. ×125. AFIP Acc. 81362.
4. Lymphatic leukemia. Lymphocytes in septal and meningeal vessels of optic nerve. ×145. AFIP Acc. 81362.
5. Myelogenous leukemia. Myeloid cells in choroidal vein and capillaries. ×400. AFIP Acc. 493367.
6. Myelogenous leukemia. Myelocytic cells in central vein of optic nerve. ×125. AFIP Acc. 493367.

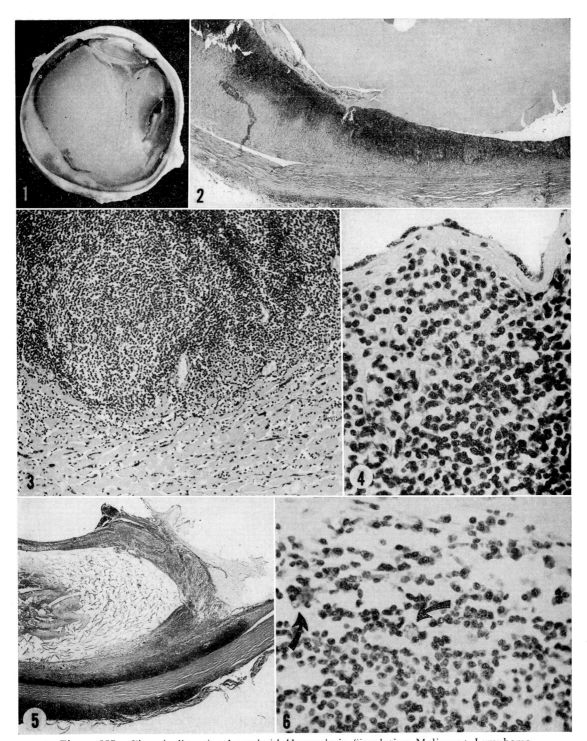

Figure 387. Chronic Reactive Lymphoid Hyperplasia Simulating Malignant Lymphoma

1 to 4. Massive diffuse thickening of the choroid by a sclerosing chronic inflammatory process of obscure etiology. Lymphocytes and plasma cells are the predominating cells. ×1½, ×10, ×115, and ×380, respectively. AFIP Acc. 788145.

5 and 6. Massive diffuse thickening of the choroid and episclera by chronic inflammatory cells. In addition to lymphocytes and plasma cells, Russell's bodies are present (arrows). ×9 and ×380. AFIP Acc. 890079.

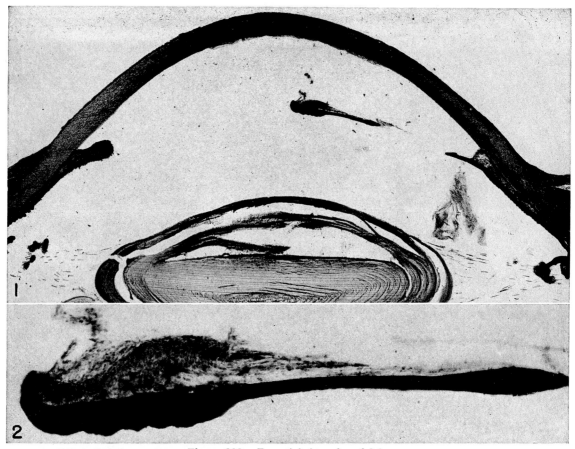

Figure 388. Essential Atrophy of Iris

1. Hole in iris, sparing pupillary zone (right). Peripheral anterior synechia. Ectropion uveae (left). AFIP Acc. 27355.

2. Same case. Atrophy of iris stroma. Sphincter muscle intact. ×110.

DEGENERATIVE CHANGES

Essential progressive atrophy of the iris. Essential progressive atrophy of the iris is a disease of unknown cause, characterized by an initial degeneration and disappearance of the iris stroma, followed by loss of the epithelium with hole formation, progressive displacement of the pupil, ectropion of the pupillary margin, and eventually glaucoma due to peripheral anterior synechias. It is unilateral, occurs almost exclusively in women and the onset is fairly early in life. The holes enlarge or coalesce; eventually large areas may disappear and the pupil is displaced toward the limbus.

Gonioscopic examinations performed before onset of glaucoma in a number of cases show a varying picture of partial to complete adhesion of the iris to the trabecular area. In some cases synechias are seen only on the side toward which the pupil is displaced, the remainder of the angle being open.

Microscopic examination in the advanced stages reveals much of the iris to have vanished and the tissues are not replaced by scar. Some iris tissue is drawn into the angle and there may be widespread adhesions of the iris root to the trabecular area and even onto the peripheral cornea. Opposite the coloboma the stroma may appear thickened and fibrotic, and an ectropion may be present (Fig. 388). A hyaline membrane, continuous with Descemet's membrane, may extend around the synechias onto the iris. The corneal endothelium is usually normal.

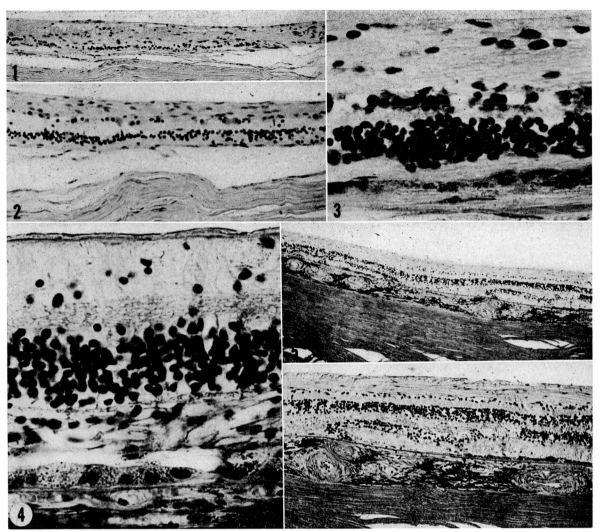

Figure 389. Choroideremia

1 and 2. Advanced stage of disease in 76 year old man. Case I reported by McCulloch, 1950 (Courtesy of Dr. A. B. Reese). ×115 and 145, respectively. AFIP Acc. 264106.

3 and 4 Advanced stage of disease in 78 year old man. Case II reported by McCulloch, 1950 (Courtesy of Dr. A. B. Reese). Persistence of part of the choriocapillaris in macular region is shown in 4. ×485. AFIP Acc. 931483.

5 and 6. Incomplete retinal degeneration in 84 year old female "carrier." ×50 and ×100, respectively. AFIP Acc. 858614.

Choroideremia. Choroideremia is a hereditary choroidal degeneration characterized by night blindness from very early childhood, but no cases have been reported in children younger than three years of age. McCulloch and McCulloch, from the study of 86 cases in two families, reported that it has different manifestations in the male and female, the former having a progressive course to blindness, the latter, a benign and nonprogressive course. Choroideremia in the families studied by these authors was transmitted in a recessive sex-linked manner. In such a large series the course of the disease may be traced from its earliest stages. The onset in males may be in early childhood but usually is in the second and third decades. The earliest symptom is night blindness, which becomes absolute in ten years when the visual field loss begins. Blindness usually occurs within 35 years after the onset. The earliest fundus changes are pigmentary, followed by progressive atrophy, especially in the midperiphery of the fundus, until the sclera is bared. Progressive atrophy

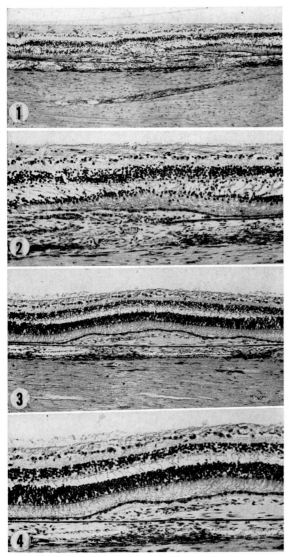

Figure 390. Angioid Streaks

Postmortem specimens obtained from a 53 year old man with bilateral angioid streaks who died of a cerebral hemorrhage. AFIP Acc. 273307. (Case reported by Klien, 1949.)

1 and 2. Bruch's membrane is interrupted; the pigment epithelium and sensory retina exhibit marked degeneration over an area where connective tissue has invaded the subretinal space from the choroid. ×40 and ×100, respectively.

3 and 4. In other areas Bruch's membrane exhibits irregular thickening and basophilia but is intact. In some such areas the pigment epithelium is lifted off Bruch's membrane by connective tissue plaques. ×80 and ×130, respectively.

then proceeds toward the periphery and the macula, leaving a small patch of normal-appearing retina and choroid in the macular area. The retinal vessels and optic disk show no changes until the very late stages, when atrophy of the disk becomes evident.

The female carriers do not have visual complaints, and their fundi show a combination of pigmentation and depigmentation, most marked in the midperiphery. The pigment granules have an irregular squared appearance and lie both in front of and behind the retinal vessels, singly or in groups. Toward the macula the granules are finer and more evenly distributed. Associated areas of depigmentation up to half a disk diameter in size are noted in the midperiphery of the fundus. The retinal vessels and disks are normal. There is no evidence that any progression occurs in the female.

Pathologic examination reveals thickening and hyalinization of the peripheral choroidal blood vessels. The posterior choroidal blood vessels are hyalinized and their lumina almost obliterated. The choroid is reduced to a thin fibrous strand (Fig. 389). Bruch's membrane is intact at the equator, but halfway between the equator and posterior pole the choroid and Bruch's membrane are absent. Degeneration of the retinal pigment epithelium and of the rods and cones and their nuclei is complete, but the bipolar and ganglion cells are unchanged. In the macular area some thin fibrous choroid may remain, along with a tiny bit of pigment epithelium, a few cone fibrils, some of the outer nuclear layer, remnants of Henle's layer, bipolar cells and inner retina. The ganglion cells seem normal. There are occasional clumps of pigment in the retina. The blood vessels of the remainder of the eye, including the posterior and long ciliary arteries and the central retinal artery, are normal (McCulloch).

Angioid streaks. The bilateral fundus changes which characterize this condition consist of dark reddish-brown bands of irregular contour which radiate outward from the region of the disk. Frequently they are associated with such other lesions as disciform degeneration, hemorrhages at the macular region, and colloid deposits. The bands are somewhat wider and more uneven in contour than a blood vessel. Some pigmentary disturbance may occur at the margins, and in the later stages the bands may be bounded by a whitish border that represents proliferation of fibrous tissue. The bands may remain stationary or may progress.

Angioid streaks may occur in Paget's disease and in pseudoxanthoma elasticum (Groenblad-Strandberg syndrome). In the latter the angioid streaks may precede the skin lesions. This heredofamilial syndrome is characterized by softening, wrinkling and relaxation of the skin around the neck and in the region of the joints, abdomen and axillas. Histologically, the elastica of the corium shows swelling, disruption and basophilic de-

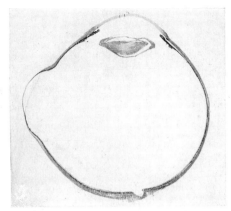

Figure 391. Severe atrophy of retina, choroid, and sclera in equatorial staphyloma due to secondary glaucoma. AFIP Acc. 107046.

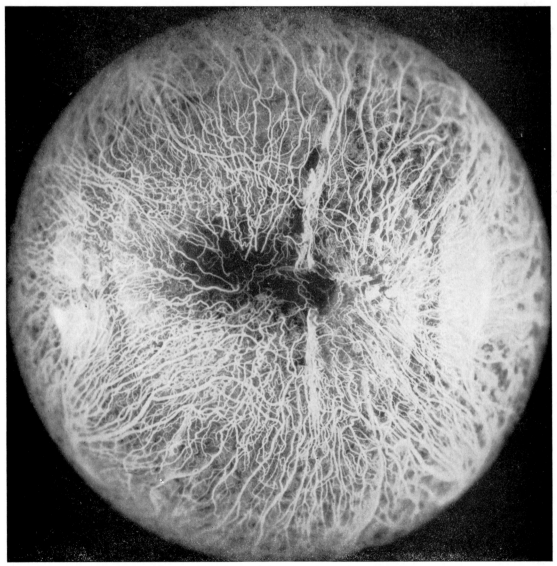

Figure 392. Central Areolar Choroidal Sclerosis
Neoprene cast of choroidal vessels of right eye reveals a well demarcated avascular zone extending from the submacular region to the disk. Elsewhere the choroidal vessels are not abnormal. (From Ashton, 1953.)

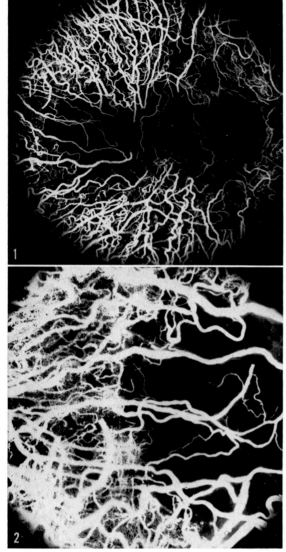

Figure 393. Central Areolar Choroidal Sclerosis

The affected portion of the choroid illustrated in Figure 392 is shown at greater magnification, revealing complete absence of the choriocapillaris and only a few remaining larger vessels. (From Ashton, 1953.)

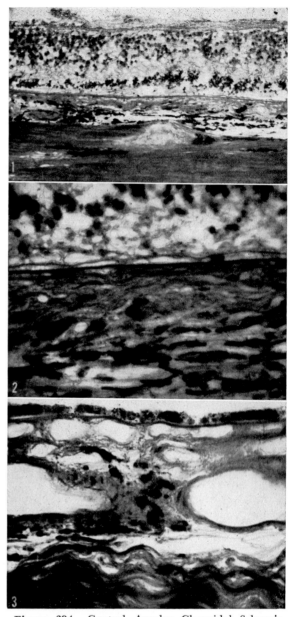

Figure 394. Central Areolar Choroidal Sclerosis

1 and 2. Section through macular region of left eye reveals advanced degeneration of retinal pigment epithelium and of all the outer layers of sensory retina. Bruch's membrane is intact. There is marked fibrosis of the choroid and disappearance of the choroidal vessels. Mallory's triple stain. ×140 and ×550, respectively.

3. In other areas the choroid is unaffected. Equatorial choroid. Mallory's triple stain. ×500. (From Ashton, 1953.)

generation, alterations reminiscent of those seen in pingueculas.

Pathologic studies (Böck; Hagedoorn; Klien) have shown that the histologic lesion responsible for angioid streaks involves Bruch's membrane which is interrupted at the sites of the streaks (Fig. 390). The lamina vitrea takes a basophilic stain, and shows a variation in thickness and staining properties. The defects and ruptures in this membrane are irregular, with jagged edges and varying breadth. Fibrovascular tissue from the cho-

roid can be seen to fill the defects and even to extend through them beneath the adjacent pigment epithelium (Fig. 390). The pigment epithelium over the breaks may be normal, elevated by scar, or partially degenerated.

The choriocapillaris beneath and adjacent to large defects may be replaced by collagenous connective tissue.

Senile choroidal atrophy. Senile choroidal atrophy occurs predominantly in three regions, the extreme periphery of the fundus, the peripapillary zone, and the posterior polar region. In the aged it is found quite regularly in the extreme periphery of the fundus and to a lesser extent in the peripapillary zone. The specific relation of these lesions to local occlusive or partially occlusive atherosclerotic manifestations has not been demonstrated.

Pressure atrophy. In the localized areas of sclerectasia (commonly called scleral staphylomas) observed in many cases of advanced glaucoma (Fig. 391), the choroid becomes so atrophic that it virtually disappears. The retinal pigment epithelium rests directly on the sclera and the retina exhibits advanced degeneration.

Central areolar choroidal sclerosis. Central areolar choroidal sclerosis (Sorsby and Crick) begins as a central exudative edematous reaction or a central pigmentary mottling, which is followed by exposure of the choroidal vessels centrally in an areolar fashion. This progresses to an obliteration of the exposed choroidal vessels and choriocapillaris. The condition occurs in males and females between the ages of 20 years and 50 years.

Ashton made a Neoprene cast of the choroidal vessels in one eye of a patient of Sorsby and Crick by injecting the ophthalmic artery (Figs. 392, 393). A well-demarcated avascular zone in the macular area extending over to the disk was found. Histologic examination of the other eye showed the avascular zone to be atrophic and fibrosed, and over it the outer retinal layers had disappeared, without glial replacement. Despite the extreme avascularity of the submacular choroid in these cases, Bruch's membrane appeared healthy (Fig. 394).

REFERENCES

Adler, F. H.: Physiology of the Eye. St. Louis, C. V Mosby, 1950.

Anderson, J. R.: Hydrophthalmia or Congenital Glaucoma. London, Cambridge University Press, 1939.

Ashton, N.: Central Areolar Choroidal Sclerosis: A Histopathological Study. Brit. J. Ophthal. 37:140–147, (March) 1953.

Ashton, N.: Observations on the Choroidal Circulation. Brit. J. Ophthal. 36:465–481, 1952.

Badal, and Lagrange, F.: Carcinome primitif des procès et du corps ciliare. Arch. d'opht. 12:143–148, 1892.

Ballantyne, A. J.: Buphthalmos with Facial Nevus and Allied Conditions. Brit. J. Ophthal. 14:481–495, (Oct.) 1930.

Barber, A. N.: Embryology of the Human Eye. St. Louis, C. V. Mosby, 1955.

Batson, O. V.: The Function of the Vertebral Veins and Their Role in the Spread of Metastases. Ann. Surg. 112:138–149, (July) 1940.

Behçet, H.: Some Observations on the Clinical Picture of So-called Triple Syndrome Complex. Dermatologica 81:73–83, 1940.

Berliner, M. L.: Biomicroscopy of the Eye. New York, Paul B. Hoeber, Inc., 1949.

Blank, H., Eglick, P. G., and Beerman, H.: Nevoxantho-Endothelioma with Ocular Involvement. Pediatrics 4:349–354, 1949.

Blodi, F. C.: Leiomyoma of the Ciliary Body. Amer. J. Ophthal. 33:939–942, (June) 1950.

Blodi, F. C.: Sympathetic Uveitis as an Allergic Phenomenon. With a Study of Its Association with Phaco-anaphylactic Uveitis and a Report on the Pathological Findings in Sympathizing Eyes. Trans Amer. Acad. Ophthal. Otolaryng. 63:642–649, 1959.

Blodi, F. C., and Sullivan, P. B.: Involvement of the Eyes in Periarteritis Nodosa. Trans. Amer. Acad. Ophthal. Otolaryng. 63:161–165, 1959.

Böck, J.: Zur Klinik und Anatomie der gefässähnlichen Streifen im Augenhintergrund. Ztschr. f. Augenh. 95:1–50, 1938.

Boeck, C.: Multiple Benign Sarcoid of the Skin. J. Cutan. and Genito-Urin. Dis. 17:543, 1899.

Boniuk, M., and Zimmerman, L. E.: Necrosis of the Iris, Ciliary Body, Lens, and Retina following Scleral Buckling Operations with Circling Polyethylene Tubes. Trans. Amer. Acad. Ophthal. Otolaryng. 65:671–693, 1961.

Braley, A. E.: A Case of Behçet's Disease. Tr. Amer. Acad. Ophthal. Otolaryng. 62:712–715, 1958.

Braley, A. E.: Unpublished data.

Brown, W. C., Kellenberger, R. E., and Hudson, K. E.: Granulomatous Uveitis Associated with Disseminated Coccidioidomycosis. Amer. J. Ophthal. 45:102–104, 1958.

Bruins Slot, W. J.: Besnier-Boeck's disease and Uveoparotid Fever (Heerfordt). Nederl. tijdschr. v. geneesk. 80:2859–2863, 1936.

de Buen, S., and González-Angulo, A.: Diktyoma (Embryonal Medullo-epithelioma): Review of the Literature and Report of a Case. Amer. J. Ophthal. 49:606–612, 1960.

de Buen, S., and Velázquez, T.: Histopathologia ocular en la hipertension arterial maligna. Sob. Rev. An. Soc. Mexicana Oftal. 33:1–17, 1960.

Callender, G. R.: Malignant Melanotic Tumors of the Eye: A Study of Histologic Types in 111 Cases. Trans. Amer. Acad. Ophthal. Otolaryng. 36:131–142, 1931.

Callender, G. R., and Thigpen, C. A.: Two Neurofibromas in One Eye. Amer. J. Ophthal. 13:121–124, 1930.

Callender, G R., Wilder, H. C., and Ash, J. E.: Five-Hundred Malignant Melanomas of the Choroid and Ciliary Body Followed Five Years or Longer. Amer. J. Ophthal. 25:962–967 (Aug.) 1942.

Chandler, P. A., and Braconier, H. E.: Spontaneous Intra-epithelial Cysts of Iris and Ciliary Body with Glaucoma. Amer. J. Ophthal. 45:64–74, (April) 1958.

Christensen, L., Swan, K. C., and Huggins, H. D.: The Histopathology of Iris Pigment Changes Induced by Miotics. A.M.A. Arch. Ophthal. 55:666–671, 1956.

Collins, R. C.: Experimental Studies on Sympathetic Ophthalmia. Amer. J. Ophthal. 32:1687–1699, 1949.

Daily, R. K.: Hemangioma of the Ciliary Body; Report of a Case. Amer. J. Ophthal. 14:653–654, (July) 1931.

Dalén, A.: Zur Kenntnis der sogenannten Chorioiditis sympathica. Mitt. a.d. Augenklin. d. Carolin, med-chir. Inst. zu Stockholm, Jena, 1904, Hft. VI, 1–21.

Derby, G. S., and Verhoeff, F. H.: Sarcoid of the Eyelid. A.M.A. Arch. Ophthal. 46:312–319, 1917.

Duke-Elder, W. S.: Text-book of Ophthalmology. Vol. I.: The Development, Form and Function of the Visual Apparatus. St. Louis, The C. V. Mosby Company, 1940.

Duke-Elder, W. S.: Text-book of Ophthalmology. Vol. 3: Diseases of the Inner Eye. St. Louis, C. V. Mosby Co., 1942, Chaps. 35–37, pp. 2097–3101.

Duke-Elder, W. S.: Text-book of Ophthalmology. St. Louis, C. V. Mosby Co., 1954, Vol. VI.

Elschnig, A.: Studien zur Sympathischen Ophthalmie. 2. Die Antigene Wirkung des Augenpigmentes. Arch. f. Ophth. 76:509–546, 1910.

Fair, J. R.: Tumors of the Retinal Pigment Epithelium. Amer. J. Ophthal. 45:495–505, 1958.

Fine, B. S., and Gilligan, J. H.: The Vogt-Koyanagi Syndrome. Amer. J. Ophthal. 43:433–440, 1957.

Flocks, M., Gerende, J. H., and Zimmerman, L. E.: The Size and Shape of Malignant Melanomas of the Choroid and Ciliary Body in Relation to Prognosis and Histologic Characteristics. A Statistical Study of 210 Tumors. Trans. Amer. Acad. Ophthal. Otolaryng. 59:740–758, 1955.

Flocks, M., Littwin, C. S., and Zimmerman, L. E.: Phacolytic Glaucoma: A Clinicopathologic Study of One-hundred Thirty-eight Cases of Glaucoma Associated with Hypermature Cataract. A.M.A. Arch. Ophthal. 54:37–45, 1955.

Flocks, M., and Zweng, H. C.: Studies on the Mode of Action of Pilocarpine on Aqueous Outflow. Amer. J. Ophthal. 44:380–387, (Nov.) 1957.

Fralick, F., and Wilder, H. C.: Intraocular Diktyoma and Glioneuroma. Trans. Amer. Ophthal. Soc. 47:317–324, 1949.

Francois, J.: Cystes des procés ciliaires, observés par la gonioscopie après enclavement de l'iris. Ophthalmologica, 116:313–316, 1948.

Friedenwald, J. S.: Melanoma of the Choroid and Allied Tumors. In Penfield, W.: Cytology and Cellular Pathology of the Nervous System. New York, Paul B. Hoeber, Inc., 1932, Vol. 3, pp. 1063–1082.

Friedenwald, J. S.: Retinal Arteriosclerosis. In Cowdry, E. V.: Arteriosclerosis. A Survey of the Problem. J. H. Macy, Jr. Foundation. New York, The MacMillan Co., 1933, pp. 363–395.

Friedenwald, J. S.: Notes on the Allergy Theory of Sympathetic Ophthalmia. Amer. J. Ophthal. 17:1008–1018, 1934.

Friedenwald, J. S.: The Formation of the Intraocular Fluid. Amer. J. Ophthal. 32:9–27, (June, Part II) 1949.

Friedenwald, J. S., and Rones, B.: Ocular Lesions in Septicemia. A.M.A. Arch. Ophthal. 5:175–188, 1931.

Friedenwald, J. S., and Stiehler, R. D.: Circulation of the Aqueous. VII. A Mechanism of Secretion of the Intraocular Fluid. A.M.A. Arch. Ophthal. 20:761–786, 1938.

Fuchs, E.: Über sympathisierende Entzündung (Nebst. Bermerkungen über seröse traumatische Iritis). Arch. f. Ophthal. 61:365–458, 1905.

Gartner, S.: Malignant Melanoma of the Choroid and von Recklinghausen's Disease. Amer. J. Ophthal. 23:73–78, (Jan.) 1940.

Gilbert, W.: Klinisches und Anatomisches zur Kenntniss der Herpetischen Augenerkrankung. Arch. f. Augenh. 89:23, 1921.

Godtfredsen, E.: On the Frequency of Secondary Carcinomas in the Choroid. Acta Ophthal. 22:394–400, 1944.

Godtfredsen, E.: Choroid Metastasis in Chorionepithelioma of the Testicle. Acta Ophthal. 22:300–310, 1944.

Goldsmith, J.: Periarteritis Nodosa with Involvement of the Choroidal and Retinal Arteries. Amer. J. Ophthal. 29:435–446, 1946.

Greear, J. N., Jr.: Metastatic Carcinoma of the Eye. Amer. J. Ophthal. 33:1015–1025, (July) 1950.

Greer, C. H.: Choroidal Carcinoma Metastatic from the Male Breast. Brit. J. Ophthal. 38:312–315, (May) 1954.

Greer, C. H.: Metastatic Carcinoma of the Iris. Brit. J. Ophthal. 38:699–701, 1954.

Greeves, R. A.: A Contribution to the Microscopical Anatomy of the Sympathizing Eye. Brit. J. Ophthal. 32:545–550, 1948.

Guyton, J. S., and Woods, A. C.: Etiology of Uveitis: A Clinical Study of Five-hundred and Sixty-two Cases. A.M.A. Arch. Ophthal. 26:983–1018, 1941.

Hagedoorn, A.: Angioid Streaks. A.M.A. Arch. Ophthal. 21:746–774; 935–965, 1939.

Harada, Y.: Beiträge zur klinischen Kenntris von nichteitriger choroiditis. Nipp. Gank. Zass. 30:356, 1926.

Heath, P.: Tumors of the Iris Muscle. Trans. Amer. Ophthal. Soc. 49:147–166, 1951.

Heath, P.: Essential Atrophy of the Iris: Histopathologic Study. Amer. J. Ophthal. 37:219–234, (Feb.) 1954.

Heerfordt, C. F.: Über eine Febris uveo-parotidea subchronica an der Glandula parotis und der Uvea des Auges lokalisiert und häufig mit Paresen cerebrospinaler Nerven kompliziert. Arch. f. Ophth., Leipz., LXX: 254–273, 1909.

Holmberg, A.: Studies of the Ultrastructure of the Non-pigmented Epithelium in the Ciliary Body. Acta Ophthal. 33:377–381, 1955.

Holmberg, A.: The Fine Structure of the Ciliary Epithelium and Its Relationship to Aqueous Secretion. In: Conference on Glaucoma, Transactions of the

Fourth Conference. F. W. Newell, Editor. Josiah Macy, Jr. Foundation, New York, 1960, pp. 179–202.

Holmberg, A.: Ultrastructure of the Ciliary Epithelium. Arch. Ophthal. 62:935–948, 1959.

Holmberg, A.: The Ultrastructure of the Capillaries in the Ciliary Body. Arch. Ophthal. 62:949–951, 1959.

Jacobs, L., Fair, J. R., and Bickerton, J. H.: Adult Ocular Toxoplasmosis. Report of a Parasitologically Proved Case. A.M.A. Arch. Ophthal. 52:63–71, 1954.

Joy, H. H.: Nevus Flammeus Associated with Glaucoma. Amer. J. Ophthal. 33:1401–1409, (Sept.) 1950.

Kirk, H. Q., and Petty, R. W.: Malignant Melanoma of the Choroid: a Correlation of Clinical and Histological Findings. A.M.A. Arch. Ophthal. 56:843–860, 1956.

Klien, B. A.: Diktyoma Retinae. A.M.A. Arch. Ophthal. 22:432–438, (Sept.) 1939.

Klien, B. A.: Clinical and Histopathologic Aspects of Angioid Streaks. Amer. J. Ophthal. 32:1134–1135, 1949.

Koyanagi, Y.: Dysakusis, Alopecia und Poliosis bei schwerer Uveitis micht traumatischen Ursprungs. Klin. Monatsbl. f. Augenh. 82:194–211, 1929.

Le Moignic, and Pinoy: Les vaccins en émulsion dans les corps gras ou "lipo-vaccins". Compt. rend. Soc. de biol. Paris 79:201–203, 1916.

Leopold, I. H.: Symposium: The Diagnosis and Management of Intraocular Melanomas. Trans. Amer. Acad. Ophthal. Otolaryng. 62:517–555, (July-Aug.) 1958.

Longcope, W. T.: Sarcoidosis, or Besnier-Boeck-Schaumann Disease; Frank Billings Memorial Lecture. J.A.M.A. 117:1321–1327, 1941.

Lucic, L. H., and Gifford, S. R.: The Etiology of Sympathetic Ophthalmia. Further Notes. A.M.A. Arch. Ophthal. 1:468–474, 1929.

McCulloch, J. C.: The Pathologic Findings in Two Cases of Choroideremia. Trans. Amer. Acad. Ophthal. Otolaryng. 54:565–572, (May-June) 1950.

McCulloch, C., and McCulloch, R. J. P.: A Hereditary and Clinical Study of Choroideremia. Trans. Amer. Acad. Ophthal. Otolaryng. 52:160–190, (Jan.-Feb.) 1948.

McGavic, J. S.: Lymphomatoid Disease Involving the Eye and Its Adnexa. A.M.A. Arch. Ophth. 30:179–193, (Aug.) 1943.

Machek, E.: Über Herpes Zoster der Regenbogenhaut im Verlaufe von Herpes Zoster frontalis. Arch. f. Augenh. XXXI:1–9, 1895.

MacLean, A. L., and Maumenee, A. E.: Hemangioma of the Choroid. Trans. Amer. Ophthal. Soc. 57:171–194, 1959.

Makley, T. A., and Teed, R. W.: Unsuspected Intraocular Malignant Melanomas. A.M.A. Arch. Ophthal. 60:475–478, 1958.

Malone, R. G. S.: Diktyoma. Brit. J. Ophthal. 39:429–436, (July) 1955.

Mann, I. C.: Developmental Abnormalities of the Eye. London, Cambridge University Press, 1937.

Mann, I. C.: The Development of the Human Eye. Second Ed. New York, Grune and Stratton, 1950.

Marchesani, O.: Weitere Beiträge zur Frage der Beziehungen der Herpesvirus zur Sympathischen Ophthalmie. Arch. f. Augenh. 97:575–590, 1926.

Masson, P.: Les naevi pigmentaires tumeurs nerveuses. Ann. d'anat. path. 3:417–453; 657–696, 1926.

Masson, P.: Pigment Cells in Man. In New York Academy of Sciences: Biology of Melanomas (Special Publications, Vol. IV.) New York, The Academy, 1948, pp. 15–51.

Mauthner, L.: Ein Fall von Choroideremia. Ber. d. naturw. Vereins in Innsbruck 2, Nos. 2 and 3, 1872 (cited from Nettleship).

Milares, T.: Structural Differences in Intraocular Tumors and Their Metastases. Ophthalmologica 98:271–284, 1940.

Müller, H.: Clinical and Pathological Findings in Recurrent Hypopyon Iritis with Obliterative Arterial Changes in the Retina. Klin. Monatsbl. Augenh. 129:289–300, 1956.

Nordman, J.: Les Tumeurs de la Retine Ciliare. Ophthalmologica 102:257–274, (Nov.) 1941.

O'Brien, C. S., and Porter, W. C.: Glaucoma and Nevus Flammeus. A.M.A. Arch. Ophthal. 9:715–728, (May) 1933.

O'Day, K.: Leiomyoma of the Iris: Report of a Case. Brit. J. Ophthal. 33:283–290, (May) 1949

Pappas, George D.: Ultrastructure of the Ciliary Epithelium and its Relationship to Aqueous Secretion. In: Conference on Glaucoma, Transactions of the Fourth Conference. F. W. Newell, Editor. New York, Josiah Macy, Jr. Foundation, 1960, pp. 141–178.

Puig Solanes, M., Heatley, J., Arenas, F., and Guerrero Ibarra, G.: Ocular Complications in Brucellosis. Amer. J. Ophthal. 36:675–689, 1953.

Reese, A. B.: The Occurrence of Ciliary Processes on the Iris. Amer. J. Ophthal. 18:6–9, 1935.

Reese, A. B.: Pigment Freckles of the Iris (Benign Melanomas): Their Significance in Relation to Malignant Melanoma of the Uvea. Amer. J. Ophthal. 27:217–226, (March) 1944.

Reese, A. B.: Pigmented Tumors (The de Schweinitz Lecture). Amer. J. Ophthal. 30:537–565, (May) 1947.

Reese, A. B.: Spontaneous cysts of the Ciliary Body Simulating Neoplasms. Amer. J. Ophthal. 33:1738–1746, 1950.

Reese, A. B.: Tumors of the Eye. New York, Paul B. Hoeber, Inc., 1951.

Reese, A. B.: Tumors of the Eye and Adnexa, Atlas of Tumor Pathology, Section X, Fascicle 38, Washington, D. C., Armed Forces Institute of Pathology, 1956.

Reese, A. B., and Blodi, F. C.: Hematopoiesis in and Around the Eye. Amer. J. Ophthal. 38:214–221, (June, Part II) 1954.

Rones, B.: A Mechanistic Element in Trabecular Function. Amer. J. Ophthal. 45:189–192, 1958.

Rones, B.: Unpublished Data.

Rones, B., and Linger, H. T.: Early Malignant Melanoma of the Choroid. Amer. J. Ophthal. 38:163–170, (Aug.) 1954.

Rones, B., and Zimmerman, L. E.: The Production of Heterochromia and Glaucoma by Diffuse Malignant Melanoma of the Iris. Trans. Amer. Acad. Ophthal. Otolaryng. 61:447–463, (July-Aug.) 1957.

Sanders, T. E.: Intraocular Juvenile Xanthogranuloma (Nevoxanthogranuloma): A Survey of 20 Cases. Trans. Amer. Ophthal. Soc. 58:59–74, 1960.

Schepens, C. L.: Clinical Aspects of Pathologic Changes in the Vitreous Body. Amer. J. Ophthal. 38:8–21, (July, Part II) 1954.

Schreck, E.: Uber Wesen und Migrations weg der sympathischen Ophthalmie. Arch. f. Ophth. 148:361–419, 1948.

Schreck, E.: Weitere Beiträge zur Frage der Klinik, Microbiologie und pathologischen Anatomie der sympathischen Ophthalmie. Arch. f. Ophth. 149:656–678, 1949.

Schreck, E.: The Micro-organisms Causing Sympathetic Ophthalmia. A.M.A. Arch. Ophthal. 46:489–500, 1951.

Sezar, F. N.: Isolation of a Virus as a Cause of Behcet's Disease. Amer. J. Ophthal. 36:301–315, 1953.

Sinskey, R. M., and Anderson, W. B.: Miliary Blastomycosis with Metastatic Spread to Posterior Uvea of Both Eyes. A.M.A. Arch. Ophthal. 54:602–604, 1955.

Sorsby, A., and Crick, R. P.: Central Areolar Choroidal Sclerosis. Brit. J. Ophthal. 37:129–139, (March) 1953.

Stokes, J. J.: The Ocular Manifestations of the Sturge-Weber Syndrome. Southern Med. J. 50:82–89, 1957.

Stokes, J. J.: Unpublished data, personal communication.

Szily, A. von: Ergebnisse der Infectionsüberleitung von Bulbus zu Bulbus mit Herpesvirus (experimentelle sympathische Ophthalmie beim Kaninchen), unter besonderer Berücksichtigung des Impfmodus, der Übertrittswege und der Spätstadien. Klin. Monatsbl. f. Augenh. (Beilageheft) 78:11–32, 1927.

Theobald, G. D.: Neurogenic Origin of Choroidal Sarcoma. A.M.A. Arch. Ophth. 18:971–997, (Dec.) 1937.

Tousimis, A. J., and Fine, B. S.: Ultrastructure of the Iris: an Electron Microscopic Study. Amer. J. Ophthal. 48:397–417, (Part II) 1959.

Tousimis, A. J., and Fine, B. S.: Ultrastructure of the Iris: the Intercellular Stromal Components. A.M.A. Arch. Ophthal. 62:974–976 and 1077–1087, 1959.

Tousimis, A. J., and Fine, B. S.: Electron Microscopy of the Pigment Epithelium of the Iris. In Smelser. G. K.: Structure of the Eye, Academic Press, 1961.

Usher, C. H.: Cases of Metastatic Carcinoma of the Choroid and Iris. Brit. J. Ophthal. 7:10–54, (Jan.) 1923.

Vail, D., Merz, E. H.: Embryonic Intra-epithelial Cyst of the Ciliary Processes. Trans. Amer. Ophthal. Soc. 49:167–183, 1951.

Verhoeff, F. H.: Sarcoma of the Choroid with Destructive Hemorrhage. A.M.A. Arch. Ophthal. 32:241–251, 1904.

Verhoeff, F. H.: A Rare Tumor Arising from the Pars Ciliaris Retinae (Terato-neuroma), of a Nature Hitherto Unrecognized, and its Relation to the So-called Glioma Retinae. Trans. Amer. Ophthal. Soc. 10:351–377, 1904.

Verhoeff, F. H.: The Experimental Product of Sclerokeratitis and Chronic Intraocular Tuberculosis. A.M.A. Arch. Ophthal. 42:471–485, 1913.

Verhoeff, F. H.: Mycosis of the Choroid Following Cataract Extraction, and Metastatic Choroiditis of the Other Eye, Producing the Clinical Picture of Sympathetic Uveitis. A.M.A. Arch. Ophthal. 53:517–530, 1924.

Vogt, A.: Frühzeitiges Ergrauen der Zilien und Bemerkungen über den sogenannten plötzlichen Eintritt dieser Veranderung. Klin. Monatsbl. f. Augenh. Stuttg. XLV:228–242, 1906.

Wadsworth, J. A. C.: Epithelial Tumors of the Ciliary Body. Amer. J. Ophthal. 32:1487–1501, (Nov.) 1949.

Walsh, F. B., Hogan, M. J., and Sabin, A. B.: Symposium. Toxoplasmosis. Trans. Amer. Acad. Ophthal. Otolaryng. 54:177–206, 1950.

Wilder, H. C.: Intraocular Tumors in Soldiers, World War II. Mil. Surgeon 99:459–490, (Nov.) 1946.

Wilder, H. C.: Relationship of Pigment Cell Clusters in the Iris to Malignant Melanoma of the Uveal Tract, in New York Academy of Sciences; Biology of Melanoma. (Special Publications, Vol. IV) New York, The Academy, 1948, pp. 137–143.

Wilder, H.: Toxoplasma Chorioretinitis in Adults. A.M.A. Arch. Ophthal. 48:127–136, 1952.

Wilder, H.: Unpublished data.

Wilder, H. C., and Callender, G. R.: Malignant Melanoma of the Choroid: Further Studies on Prognosis by Histologic Type and Fiber Content. Amer. J. Ophthal. 22:851–855, (Aug.) 1939.

Wilder, H. C., and Paul, E. V.: Malignant Melanoma of the Choroid and Ciliary Body: A Study of 2535 Cases. Mil. Surgeon 109:370–378, (Oct.) 1951.

Wolff, E.: The Anatomy of the Eye and Orbit. 3rd Ed., Philadelphia, The Blakiston Co., 1948.

Woods, A. C.: Allergy in its Relation to Sympathetic Ophthalmia. New York J. Med. 36:67–85, 1936.

Woods, A. C.: Sympathetic Ophthalmia. Amer. J. Ophthal. 19:9–15; 100–109, 1936.

Woods, A. C.: Endogenous Uveitis, Baltimore, Williams and Wilkins, 1956.

Woods, A. C.: An Adventure in Ophthalmic Literature: Manuel Straub and the Tradition of Toxicity in Lens Protein. Amer. J. Ophthal. 48:463–472, 1959.

Wright, C. J. E.: Prognosis in Cutaneous and Ocular Malignant Melanomas; A Study of 222 Cases. J. Path. Bact. 61:507–525, (Oct.) 1949.

Wybar, K. C.: Vascular Anatomy of the Choroid in Relation to Selective Localization of Ocular Disease. Brit. J. Ophthal. 38:513–527, 1954.

Wybar, K. C.: Anastomoses between the Uveal and Retinal Circulation and Their Significance in Vascular Occlusion. Acta XVII Conc. Ophth. 1954, Canada-U.S.A., 1955, pp. 294–302.

Zimmerman, L. E., Paul, E. V., and Parnell, B. L.: Evaluation of Prognostic Factors in Intraocular Melanoma. Cited in Symposium: The Diagnosis and Management of Intraocular Melanoma. Trans. Amer. Acad. Ophthal. Otolaryng. 62:517–555, (July-Aug.) 1958.

Chapter VIII

Retina

ANATOMY AND HISTOLOGY

The retina is composed of the tissues arising from the optic vesicle, and consists of a pigment layer derived from the outer wall of the cup and a complex sensory layer derived from the inner wall.

The *pigment epithelium* consists of a single layer of hexagonal cells of uniform size (16 microns in diameter) and regular arrangement (Fig. 395). The cells have a round nucleus which is situated near the base, and rod-shaped and elliptical melanin granules which concentrate in the inner portion of the cell. Each cell has a large number of fine processes on its inner surface which extend inward between the rods and the cones. The cells are bound to each other by a neuro-keratin cement substance, which also covers the base of the cell and binds it to the cuticular layer of the lamina vitrea (Bruch's membrane of the choroid). The only variations in the regular arrangement of these cells are in the region of the fovea, where they are higher, narrower, and of a darker color, and at the ora serrata, where there often are larger and multinucleated cells.

The *sensory retina* is a delicate transparent layer. It is firmly attached only at two points: posteriorly at the optic disk, and anteriorly at the ora serrata. Elsewhere the attachment to the underlying pigment epithelium is weak.

It is not easy to picture the complex microscopic anatomy of the retina because the delicacy and perishability of the tissue allows early postmortem changes and artifacts, and because ordinary histologic technique and staining methods do not reveal its structural details. Special stains, employing silver and

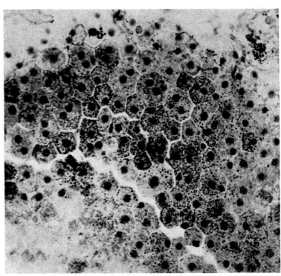

Figure 395. Pigment Epithelium of Retina

Transverse section reveals cells to have pentagonal or hexagonal contours. Plane of section passes through basal part of cells which contains the nucleus but very few pigment granules. ×380. AFIP Acc. 38095.

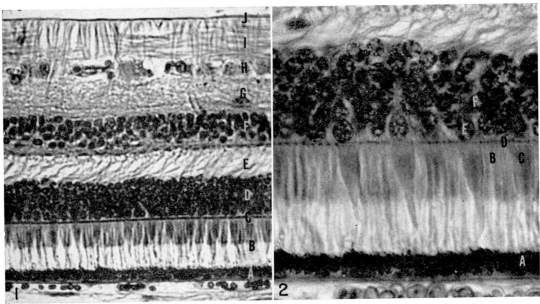

Figure 396. Normal Retina

1. A, retinal pigment epithelium. B, rods and cones. C, external limiting membrane. D, outer nuclear layer. E, outer plexiform layer. F, inner nuclear layer. G, inner plexiform layer. H, ganglion cell layer. I, nerve fiber layer: nerve fibers are horizontal, Müller fibers vertical. J, internal limiting membrane. ×425. AFIP Acc. 47846.

2. A, pigment epithelium. B, rods. C, cone. D, external limiting membrane. E, cone nucleus. F, rod nucleus. ×1000. AFIP Acc. 47846.

gold, are necessary to show the glia and neurons. The sensory retina is considered to be made up of nine layers; from without inward these are (Fig. 396):

1. Layer of rods and cones
2. External limiting membrane
3. Outer nuclear layer
4. Outer plexiform layer
5. Inner nuclear layer
    a. Horizontal cells
    b. Bipolar cells
    c. Amacrine cells
    d. Müller cells
6. Inner plexiform layer
7. Ganglion cell layer
8. Nerve fiber layer
9. Internal limiting membrane

These layers are interconnected by broad contacts between axons and dendrites in each layer, and by a system of special supporting fibers.

The *layer of rods and cones* has a palisaded arrangement of its constituent elements (Fig. 396). The rods are slender and cylindrical; their length corresponds to the thickness of the entire layer. Each rod is made up of a somewhat longer, more slender, highly re-

fractile outer segment containing the photosensitive visual purple, and a shorter, thicker and finely granular inner segment. The cones are flask-shaped and about half the length of the rods, but, like the latter, are composed of an outer and an inner segment. The cones are said to contain no visual purple. Different areas of the retina contain different proportions of rods and cones. At the fovea only cones are found, and these are long and slender, resembling rods. The cones become relatively scarcer toward the periphery.

Recent investigations have demonstrated the presence of a mucoid interstitial substance coating the rods and cones, particularly their outer segments. Because it is unstained by dyes which are ordinarily used in ophthalmic pathology, this hyaluronidase-resistant mucoid material escaped recognition until the introduction of newer special staining methods for the demonstration of mucopolysaccharides (Zimmerman; Sidman; Zimmerman and Eastham).

The *external limiting membrane* is a delicate membrane with perforations which serve as exits for the fibers from the rods and cones. This membrane belongs to the supporting tissue of the retina. It is believed by some to be formed by the union of the outer ends of Müller's fibers, although Verhoeff advanced the theory that it is elaborated by the rod and cone cells.

The *outer nuclear layer* is composed of eight or nine layers of cells with densely staining nuclei. Two kinds of cells can be discerned because of the nuclear morphology. The smaller, more densely stained nuclei belong to the rods, and the larger, more weakly stained nuclei, which tend to lie just within the external limiting membrane, belong to the cones. Dendrites extend from both types of cells into the outer plexiform layer. Occasionally cone nuclei are found to be displaced into the rod and cone layer as a normal variation (Fig. 397).

The *outer plexiform layer* consists of fibers which are loosely arranged and is composed of the axons of the rod and cone fibers and the dendrites of the bipolar and horizontal cells. In the macular region these fibers are greatly elongated and radiate outward from the fovea, forming the fiber layer of Henle.

The *inner nuclear layer* is a closely packed mass of cells, resembling the outer nuclear layer, but much thinner. The extremely complicated structure of this layer is revealed by electron microscopy and when the methods of Golgi and Cajal are utilized. Three types of neurons are present in this layer. The *bipolar cells* have dendrites which are in contact with the axons of the rod and cone cells. Their axons end in the inner plexiform layer, forming synapses with dendrites of the ganglion cells. The *horizontal cells* have complex arborizing processes in the outer plexiform layer which synapse with the rod and cone processes, as well as adjacent bipolar fibers. Occasional processes extend from the cell into the inner plexiform layer. The *amacrine cells* are pear-shaped and have processes which extend into the inner plexiform layer, where they synapse widely with the dendrites of the ganglion cells. The nuclei of Müller's fibers also are found in the inner nuclear layer. These fibers extend internally to form the inner limiting membrane, and externally to form a great part of the external limiting membrane.

The *inner plexiform layer* consists of a fine reticulum of fibers; several sublayers may be recognized. This layer is formed by the syn-

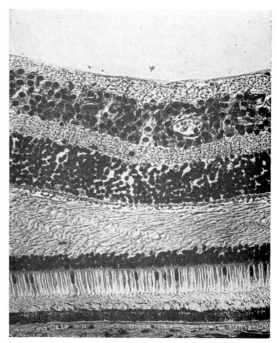

Figure 397.   Normal Macula (Perifoveal Tissue)

Ganglion cell layer is thicker than elsewhere; nerve fibers of Henle's layer radiate obliquely away from the fovea, and some cone nuclei appear external to the outer limiting membrane (a normal variation observed most often in the macula). ×275. AFIP Acc. 321406.

apses of the bipolar cells, the stratified amacrine cells, and by the ganglion cells.

The *ganglion cell layer* consists of a row of ganglion cells separated from each other by Müller's fibers and neuroglia. The ganglion cells are multipolar with large nuclei and prominent Nissl granules. Their numerous dendrites arise in the inner plexiform layer, and their long axons constitute the nerve fiber layer and form the optic nerve pathway. In the macular region the ganglion cells are much more numerous, forming a layer five to eight cells deep.

The *nerve fiber layer* is composed almost entirely of the axons of the ganglion cells, which extend via the optic nerve to the brain. This layer also contains some neuroglia. Because the fibers radiate toward the optic nerve, it follows that this layer is thickest near the disk because of the piling up of fibers from the retina as they converge on the disk.

The *internal limiting membrane* in the normal eye of a young person is a very delicate basement membrane structure applied

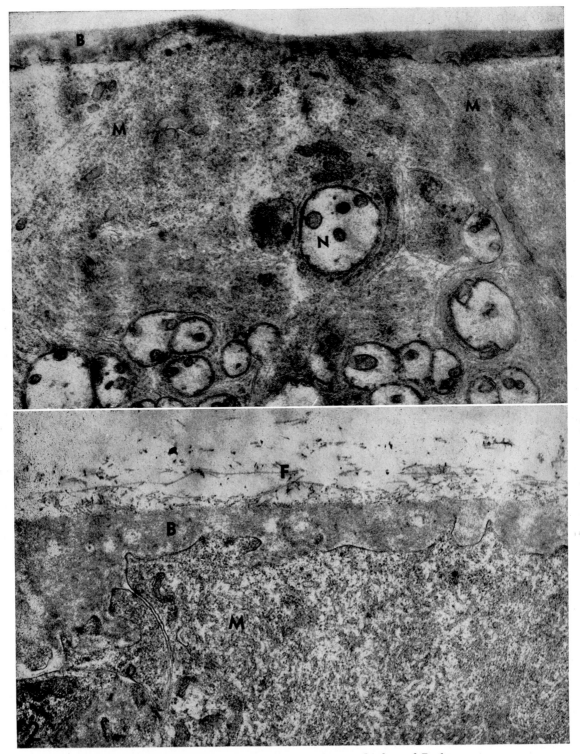

Figure 398. Electron Micrographs of Inner Surface of Retina

1. The inner surface of the retina is formed by the expanded ends of Müller's cells (M) which are covered by a basement membrane (B). A group of nerve fibers (N) sectioned transversely is observed along the bottom of the field. Adult human. ×14,200. (From Dr. B. S. Fine, unpublished work.)

2. The filamentous component (F) of the vitreous is inserted into the basement membrane (B) of the retina. The inner end of Müller's cells (M) contains much filamentous material, tubules of smooth surfaced endoplasmic reticulum and a few mitochondria. Adult human. ×22,140. (Courtesy Dr. B. S. Fine.)

to the broad flat expansions of Müller's fibers. The fine fibrillar insertions of the vitreous body are attached to its inner surface (Fig. 398). Occasional broad flat cells containing round or reniform nuclei are present along the inner surface of the internal limiting membrane (Fig. 399), but these probably are identical with the macrophagic cells of the cortical vitreous as described by Szirmai and Balazs.

Special staining techniques have been shown by Wolter to reveal several types of glial tissue in the retina:

1. Müller's fibers form a skeleton to support the nerve cells. The inner processes of Müller's fibers form a mosaic-like pattern known as the internal limiting membrane. The outer processes form the outer limiting membrane through which the rods and cones send their processes to the outer nuclear layers. Kuwabara et al. have found Müller's fibers to reduce tetrazolium, indicating the presence of dehydrogenase and suggesting a further function of these scaffolding cells.

2. In the nerve fiber layer numerous bipolar cells with elongated nuclei and long straight processes accompany the axons (Fig. 55-1). These cells run in a plane at right angles to Müller's fibers and have no connection with them; they appear to be identical with the cells of Remak or lemmocytes. Recent studies suggest that these are astroglia.

3. In the ganglion cell and inner plexiform layers, there are well differentiated astrocytes (Fig. 54). They are star-shaped with

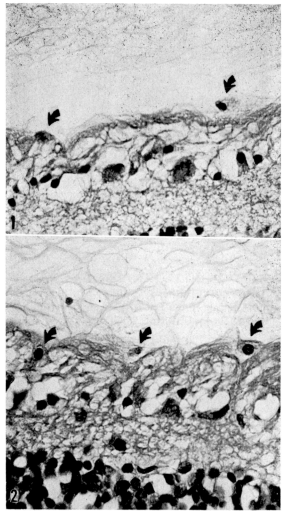

Figure 399. Cells in cortical vitreous along vitreo retinal interface (internal limiting membrane of retina), probably histiocytic in type.
1. ×450. AFIP Acc. 822982.
2. ×525. AFIP Acc. 822982.

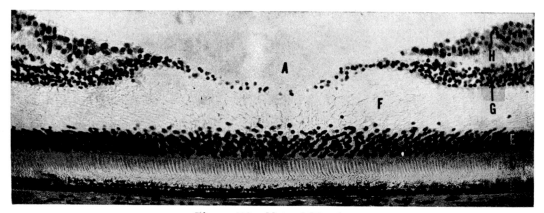

Figure 400. Normal Macula

A, fovea; B, retinal pigment epithelium; C, modified cones; D, external limiting membrane; E, outer nuclear layer; F, Henle layer; G, inner nuclear layer; H, inner plexiform layer; I, ganglion cell layer; ganglion cells piled up around fovea, absent in fovea. ×210. AFIP Acc. 84236.

ized in the full term infant. The temporal periphery is farther from the optic disk; therefore, incomplete vascularization more frequently is observed on the temporal side. These developmental considerations are of importance in relation to the pathogenesis of retrolental fibroplasia (p. 511).

With aging the melanin granules in the pigment epithelium tend to lose their oval or rod-like contour and become rounded. The cuticular basement membrane thickens and focal irregular mound-like excrescences known as drusen form in this part of Bruch's membrane (Fig. 313–2). They are called drusen because of their glistening crystalline ophthalmoscopic appearance. Accumulations of acid mucopolysaccharide and dystrophic calcification are observed in these drusen. Bruch's membrane in older persons may contain large amounts of lipid and finely dispersed calcareous granules.

In the sensory retina Müller's fibers and the limiting membranes become thicker with age. Atrophic changes are seen at the periphery and there is diminution of the neuronal elements with proliferation of glia. Pigment cells from the epithelial layer may wander into the retina in this region. Near the ora serrata, particularly on the temporal side, and extending posteriorly in varying degrees to the equator, vacuoles appear in the retina. At first these are seen most prominently in the inner nuclear and outer plexiform layers, but they enlarge and coalesce to form the so-called peripheral cystoid degeneration between the limiting membranes (Blessig-Iwanoff cysts) (Fig. 403–1). These spaces in reality are not cystoid, but are formed by an interlacing pattern of tunnels which can be demonstrated in flat sections of the retina. Recently these seemingly empty spaces have been shown by Zimmerman to contain a mucoid material which is sensitive to hyaluronidase. This is a continuous change with advancing years and it also may be seen in young persons in the presence of local disease. Less often a similar cystoid degeneration occurs in the maculas of older persons (Fig. 403–2). Retinoschisis is believed to be an exaggerated example of the same mucoid degeneration that is responsible for peripheral cystoid degeneration (see p. 553).

There are other atrophic and degenerative retinal changes which can be explained on the basis of a gradual and progressive decrease in the vascular supply to the area due to profound arteriolosclerosis. There is a loss of retinal sensory cells and a coincident increase in the neuroglial elements.

The peripheral retina is nourished by the distal arterioles of the retinal vascular tree; therefore, any decrease in the flow of blood through the large vessels produces its greatest effect on the tissue of the peripheral retina. The foveal area is dependent on its nutrition from the choriocapillaris. In general, senile degeneration of the retina is most apt to involve the periphery and macula, leaving the remainder of the fundus relatively free of gross evidence of degeneration.

CONGENITAL ABNORMALITIES

Congenital abnormalities of the retina itself are rather uncommon. Most often other structures are seriously affected.

Coloboma. Typical colobomas of the retina are localized defects which contain defective retinal tissue. Usually they are found in the lower nasal area, and are associated with abnormal closure of the fetal fissure (see Chapter VII). Atypical colobomas histologically resemble typical colobomas and are found in areas other than the lower nasal, usually associated with partial or complete coloboma of the choroid, ciliary body, iris, lens, and optic nerve. The pigment epithelium may be entirely absent in the area of the coloboma or merely represented by scattered cells. The retina may be represented by a membrane containing scattered retinal elements. Rosettes, glial tissue, and scattered rods and cones may be present (Fig. 319).

Medullated nerve fibers. Normal medullation of the optic nerve fibers is a centrifugal process which stops at the lamina cribrosa at birth. Occasionally myelinated fibers may be observed in the retina near the disk or elsewhere. The presence of such a sheath usually does not interfere with the function of the affected fibers, but does diminish the

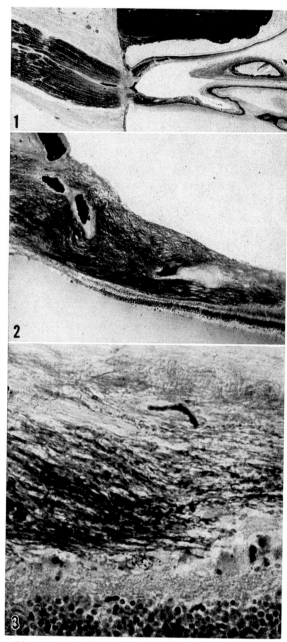

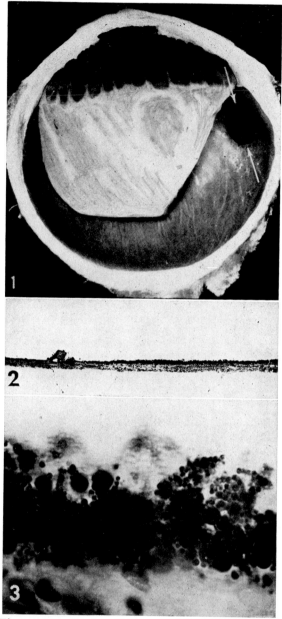

Figure 404. Myelinated Nerve Fibers in Retina

1. Most of the nerve head is not myelinated (pale zone) but myelinated fibers extend into the retina. Myelin sheath stain. ×7. AFIP Neg. 58–14517.

2. Lower half of retina shown in 1. ×50. AFIP Neg. 58–14518.

3. Lower right corner of retina shown in 2. ×305. AFIP Neg. 58–14516.

Figure 405. Benign Melanoma (Nevus) of Pigment
Epithelium.

1. Sharply circumscribed deeply pigmented lesion (arrows) near ora serrata. AFIP Acc. 901684.

2 and 3. The lesion consists of a great enlargement of the cells in the retinal pigment epithelium. The pigment granules contained in these cells are larger and more irregularly spheroidal than normal. ×50 and ×990, respectively.

transparency of the affected retina, producing a scotoma (Fig. 404). Ophthalmoscopically, medullated fibers present an unchanging picture.

Grouped pigmentation. Grouped pigmentation of the retina is a congenital condi-

tion which is characterized by varying-sized areas of failure of development of the rods and cones, and by proliferation of the cells of the pigment epithelium to form plaque-like lesions. Some of these clumps of cells are surrounded by acellular eosinophilic material resembling that forming the hyaline por-

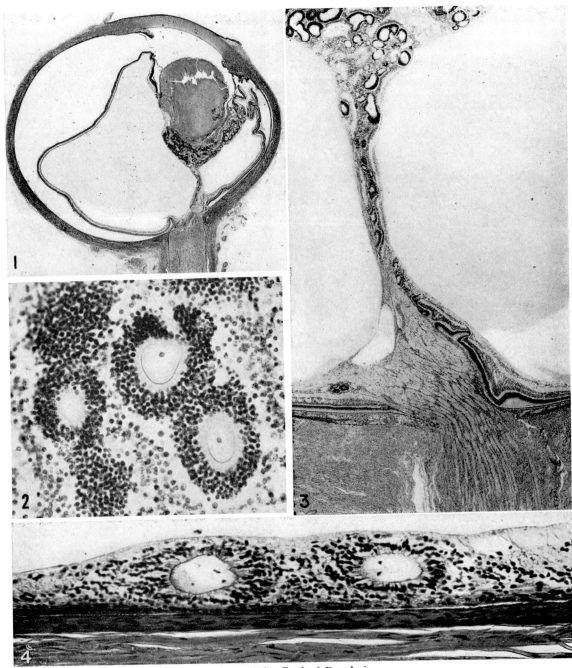

Figure 406. Retinal Dysplasia

1. ×5. AFIP Acc. 38159.   2. ×300. AFIP Acc. 45389.   3. ×25. AFIP Acc. 53033.   4. ×250. AFIP Acc. 43952.

tion of Bruch's membrane. Ophthalmoscopically, this process gives rise to the peculiar picture in which smaller pigmented plaques affect one sector of retina near the disk and other plaques are formed which become larger as they approach the periphery (bear-track pigmentation).

Another type of congenital pigmentation of the retina is characterized by the presence of a solitary, elevated, usually nonprogressive pigmented tumor. Microscopically, these tu-

mors are caused by a proliferation of the pigment epithelium associated with an increased pigment content in the subjacent choroid (Fig. 405) (Reese, 1958; Duke and Maumenee, 1959).

Abnormalities of the macula. Complete absence of the macula has been described in albinotic eyes. Such a condition often is associated with other gross abnormalities of the eye. Hypoplasia of the macula may be found in extreme hyperopia or microphthalmus.

Temporal displacement of the macula may be associated with an abnormal position of the optic disk. Vascular abnormalities often accompany heterotopia of the macula.

Oguchi's disease. Oguchi's disease is a congenital and stationary condition in which the most prominent symptom is a retardation of dark adaptation. Microscopically, an abnormal number of cones are present, especially in the temporal retina; rods are almost absent. A nondescript amorphous tissue containing pigment granules lies between the cones and the pigment epithelium. The pigment granules in the pigment epithelium are crowded to the inner aspect of the cells while the basal parts of the cells are rich in lipoid.

Retinal dysplasia. Retinal dysplasia is a developmental aberration which is present at birth. It is characterized by bilateral abnormalities of the eyes, systemic changes, and a familial tendency. There is no relationship to prematurity.

Grossly, the affected eyes are smaller than normal although the degree of microphthalmus may vary. Cataractous changes may be present, but the lens often is sufficiently clear to visualize the white vascularized retrolental tissue. Large ciliary processes may be seen to insert into the periphery of a retrolental mass composed of fibrous tissue and retinal elements. In some cases the membrane covers only part of the lens, permitting visualization of the persistent primary vitreous and retinal folds. Secondary glaucoma may develop as the result of malformation of the anterior chamber angle (Fig. 406).

The common feature of the ocular abnormality is a developmental defect involving the inner layer of the optic cup (Figs. 406, 407). It seems to result from a proliferation and infolding of the outer layers of the retinal stroma. Microscopically, a series of straight branching tubes is formed, composed of abortive elements of the rod and cone layer, external limiting membrane, and outer nuclear layer. Serial sections reveal a communication between the lumen of these tubes and the subretinal space. The late stages are characterized by an obliteration of the tubes with formation of rosettes similar to those seen in retinoblastoma. Neoplastic rosettes, however, usually are small spherical clusters, whereas elliptical rosettes and tubes are characteristic of dysplasia. A dysgenesis of the entire retina, including the ganglion cells, may account for the reduced vision, even in the nondetached areas. Gliosis of the retina may be extensive. Persistence of the primary vitreous and a failure in the formation of the secondary vitreous may accompany the retinal

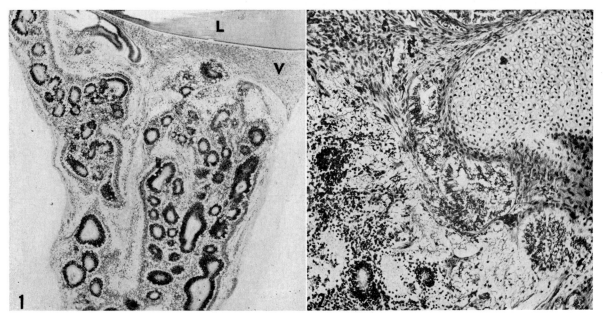

Figure 407. Retinal Dysplasia

1. Mass behind lens (L) is composed of dysplastic retina and hyperplastic primary vitreous (V). ×35. AFIP Acc. 45389. (From Reese and Straatsma, 1958.)

2. Focus of metaplastic cartilage (upper right corner) in hyperplastic primary vitreous in a case of retinal dysplasia. ×115. AFIP Acc. 523225. (From Reese and Straatsma, 1958.)

dysplasia (Fig. 407). Other anomalies such as microphthalmus, fetal filtration angle, with congenital glaucoma, and coloboma of uveal tract and optic nerve may accompany retinal dysplasia. The central nervous system, respiratory, gastrointestinal, cardiovascular, and genitourinary systems may be severely affected. The condition may be familial, suggesting that retinal dysplasia is due to an environmental disturbance or a genetic defect. Minor changes may be found in the retina in otherwise healthy individuals which greatly resemble retinal dysplasia. These isolated changes, however, rarely permit the diagnosis of retinal dysplasia to be made.

INFLAMMATION

Inflammations of the retina may arise as a primary disease during the course of a systemic infection, or they may be secondary to extension of disease from other parts of the eye or orbit. Those originating in the retina may remain localized to this tissue as a small

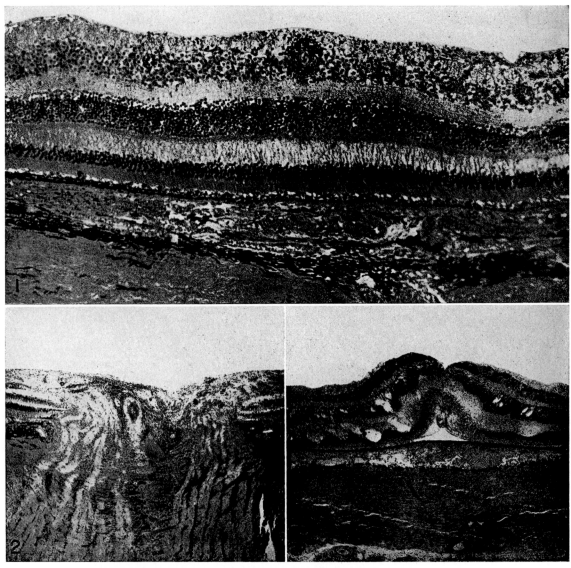

Figure 408. Retinitis and Papillitis Secondary to Chronic Iridocyclitis

1. Lymphocytic periphlebitis in retina. ×130. AFIP Acc. 86403.
2. Lymphocytic periphlebitis in nerve head. ×60. AFIP Acc. 86403.
3. Edema of macula with serous exudates in inner nuclear and outer plexiform layers. ×40. AFIP Acc. 182157.

focus which eventually heals, or may spread to involve the vitreous, optic nerve, and uveal tract. The general effect in such cases is to produce an endophthalmitis or panophthalmitis. Often the inflammation localizes in the posterior eye to form a vitreous abscess (metastatic ophthalmia). The etiology and the general course of these more widespread inflammations have been discussed in some detail in Chapter II.

The general pathology of retinal inflammation is characterized by the *vascular response* which is similar to that observed in other inflamed tissues (see Chapter I). The dilated ves-

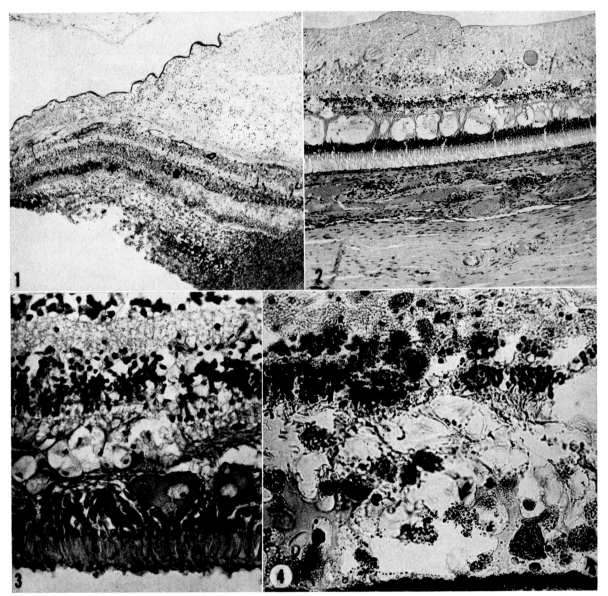

Figure 409. Retinal Exudates

1. Fibrinopurulent exudate in septic retinitis. The exudate has ruptured the internal limiting membrane (upper right corner) and has extended into the subretinal space (lower right). ×50. AFIP Acc. 213298.

2. Serosanguineous exudates in hemorrhagic infarction of retina, secondary to cavernous sinus thrombosis. ×80. AFIP Acc. 61137.

3. Lipoidal histiocytes (microglia) and hyaline exudates in area of retinal degeneration. ×300. AFIP Acc. 30034.

4. Fat stains on frozen sections reveal the cytoplasm of lipoidal histiocytes to contain myriad lipoidal granules (arrows). ×300. AFIP Acc. 867773.

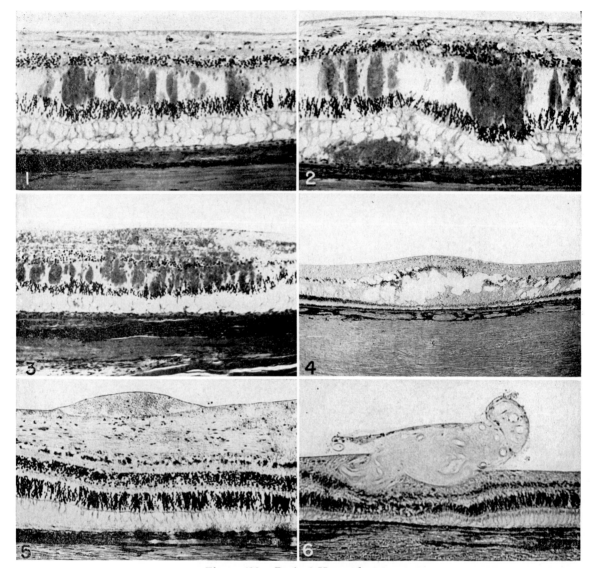

Figure 410. Retinal Hemorrhages

1. Hemorrhages in outer plexiform layer of retina. ×125. AFIP Acc. 186516.
2. Hemorrhages in outer plexiform layer of retina. Small subretinal hemorrhage. ×125. AFIP Acc. 186516.
3. Hemorrhages in nerve fiber, outer plexiform and intervening retinal layers. ×125. AFIP Acc. 186516.
4. Cystoid degeneration of retina resulting from hemorrhages which have been absorbed. ×45. AFIP Acc. 117032.
5. Hemorrhage between nerve fiber layer and internal limiting membrane. ×98. AFIP Acc. 161187.
6. Vascular membrane extending into vitreous from retinal vessel. ×83. AFIP Acc. 177901.

sels in the inner retinal layers show margination and migration of leukocytes into the tissues and accumulation of cells in the perivascular spaces (Fig. 408). *Edema* soon follows, with localization of a protein-rich fluid in the tissues around the blood vessels. The fluid gradually diffuses into adjacent nonvascular areas, where it accumulates in large pools (Fig. 408–3). The products of the inflammatory process and pressure exerted by the fluid soon lead to degeneration of the retinal elements, forming larger areas containing fibrin, cellular debris, inflammatory cells and lipoids. Macrophages from the tissues and blood

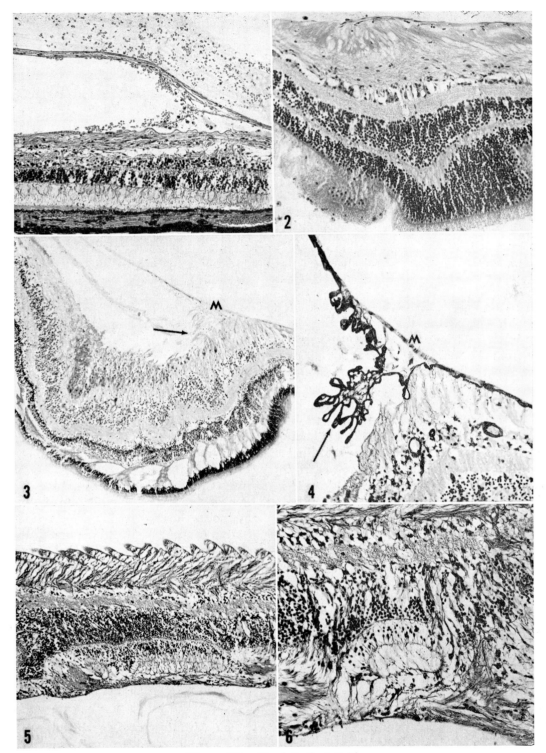

Figure 411. Fixed Retinal Folds

1. Vitreous hemorrhage; fibrous tissue anchored to retina has produced wrinkles in the internal limiting membrane. ×115. AFIP Acc. 730699.

2. Preretinal membrane has puckered the inner retinal surface. ×115. AFIP Acc. 694444.

3 and 4. Pronounced retinal fold and detachment produced by preretinal membrane (M) which has also torn off much of the inner limiting membrane (arrow) from the retina. 3. H and E, ×50. 4. Periodic acid-Schiff reaction. ×130. AFIP Acc. 905244.

5 and 6. Many retinal folds produced by marked gliosis along posterior surface of retina. ×70 and ×140, respectively. AFIP Acc. 980758.

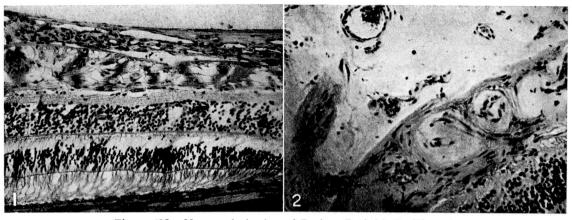

Figure 412. Neovascularization of Retina (Retinitis Proliferans)

1. Newly formed vessels on inner surface of retina. ×125. AFIP Acc. 210125.

2. Newly formed vessel in nerve fiber layer of retina with a budding capillary extending into vascular membrane on inner retinal surface. ×165. AFIP Acc. 69605.

stream accumulate in the cavities and become filled with debris and lipoid from the degenerating retinal cells (Fig. 409). These soon depart from the foci via the blood stream or disintegrate in situ. Chemical changes in this fluid later lead to formation of a uniform, eosinophilic staining material which is called hyalin (Fig. 409). *Hemorrhage* may occur in the vessel layers. Most often small linear hemorrhages lie in the nerve fiber or inner retinal layers. Larger, round hemorrhages extend into the outer retinal layers, or break through the inner limiting membrane (Fig. 410). Persistence or recurrence of such hemorrhages leads to additional necrosis and inflammation followed by repair, scarring, and deformity.

Alterations may occur in the *pigment epithelium*. If the inflammation is severe the epithelium is destroyed, and the pigment granules are phagocytized by adjacent cells or macrophages, which tend to migrate into the retina and localize around blood vessels. Adjacent cells most often proliferate to form clumps of pigment which are commonly seen ophthalmoscopically and microscopically around chorioretinal scars (Figs. 321, 328, 333, 339). The proliferation of these cells, and alteration of their shape to a spindle form, may produce a large, heavily pigmented tumor-like mass between retina and choroid (Fig. 366).

Healing occurs by removal of the fluid by the vessels, and cells and debris by the macrophages; subsequent proliferation of connective tissue elements occurs from the region of the blood vessels, and glia from the inner retinal layers, these and the new blood vessels produce a fibroglial scar. Organization of the scar leads to distortion and folding of the retina (Fig. 411).

Damage and loss of the inner limiting membrane adjacent to the focus of inflammation leads to accumulation of cells and fluid on the inner retina and in the nearby vitreous. New capillaries bud from the retinal vessels and invade this exudate (Fig. 410–6). Eventually a dense thin vascular scar may line the retina and extend into the vitreous, producing the changes known as *retinitis proliferans* (Fig. 412). Most inflammations which affect the retina or choroid involve both structures simultaneously (Figs. 25, 72) and the healing process eventually leads to fusion of the outer limiting membrane of the retina to the lamina vitrea of the choroid. The retinal epithelium often is missing in the region of such chorioretinal scars. If the lamina vitrea has been destroyed a dense scar unites the choroidal stroma to the retina.

Old chorioretinal scars, therefore, show moderate to severe damage in the retinal stroma with loss of neural and supporting cells. The choroidal stroma shows a loss of the lamina vitrea and inner vessel layers, and a dense connective tissue scar containing more or less pigment unites these two structures (Figs. 321, 328, 333, 339). Hyaline and calcareous degeneration is common, especially around vessels.

Purulent retinitis. Endogenous purulent

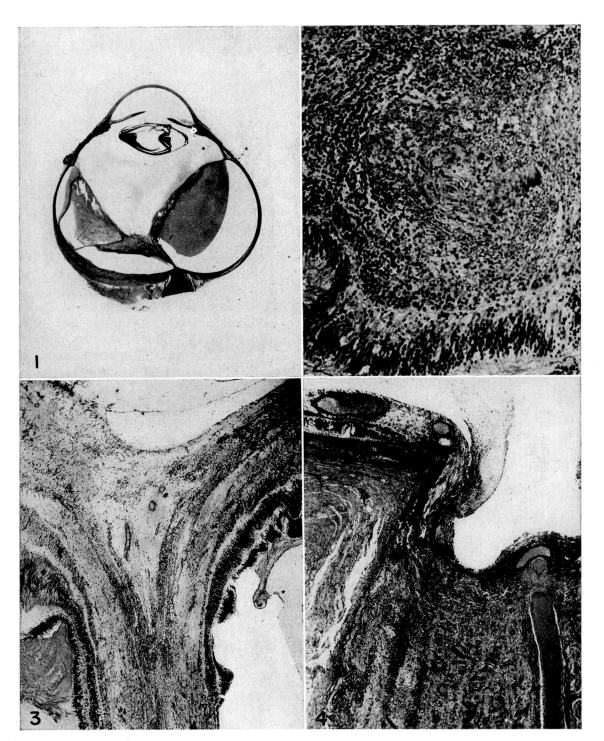

Figure 413. Syphilis

1. Chorioretinitis in patient with positive Wassermann reaction; retinitis proliferans, serous separation of retina. AFIP Acc. 79699.

2. Small gummatous lesion with ill-formed giant cell in retina of same eye. ×190.

3. Retinitis proliferans (vascular membrane extending into vitreous from retina), same eye. ×48.

4. Optic neuritis in patient with positive Wassermann reaction. Inflammatory and hemorrhagic membrane arising from excavated optic disk in eye with secondary glaucoma. ×48. AFIP Acc. 68481.

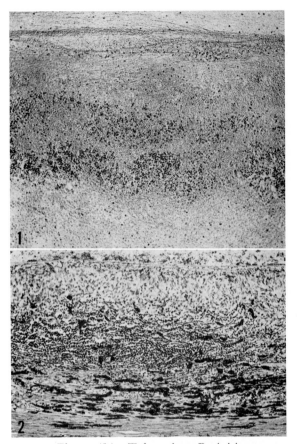

Figure 414. Tuberculous Retinitis

1. Extensive necrosis of retina. ×100. AFIP Acc. 693164.

2. Granulomatous chronic inflammatory reaction in choroid adjacent to necrotic retina. ×100. (Case reported by Theobald, 1958.)

retinitis may develop during the course of any systemic infection such as puerperal sepsis, meningococcemia, and gonococcal and streptococcal infections. Antibiotic therapy has lowered the incidence of such complications. The inflammation may be localized or it can spread rapidly and lead to severe necrosis of the retina and its blood vessels, with secondary hemorrhage. In the early stages the retina is edematous, the vessels are congested, there is intense perivasculitis, and a seropurulent exudate forms in the tissue and beneath the rods and cones to produce retinal separation. The optic nerve and vitreous rapidly become infiltrated with purulent exudate. Organisms often can be demonstrated. The eventual outcome of such infections has been discussed in Chapter II.

Embolic retinitis. Septic retinitis is a toxic or embolic affection of the retinal blood vessels occurring in septicemia due to various causes. White opaque spots, often with hemorrhage, are seen in the retina and represent an area of infarction of the nerve fiber layer with resulting retinal edema and necrosis. The causative organism may be found in the lesion. Microscopically, the picture of a cotton-wool exudate is seen, with swelling and degeneration of the nerve fibers. Most often the lesion heals without spread to other areas.

Subacute and chronic endogenous retinitis. Subacute and chronic endogenous retinitis occurs when a less virulent organism reaches the retina or when the virulence of a pyogenic organism is attenuated by therapy. Clinically the disease may be of relatively sudden onset and great severity; however, the predominant cell in the exudate most often is the lymphocyte. It has been pointed out in Chapter I that many acute intraocular inflammations are characterized by exudation of lymphocytes and plasma cells. The inflammation may remain active for one to two months during which time there is marked vitreous exudation. Healing is characterized by gliosis, fibrosis, and new-vessel formation. In long-standing chronic disease, the retina may be detached by the shrinkage of vitreous membranes and show degenerative changes.

Granulomatous. The retina may be the primary site of a granulomatous inflammation of acute or chronic type in which there is development of an exudate containing lymphocytes, epithelioid, and giant cells. The uveal tract frequently shows a secondary inflammation, but the retina is the primary site of the affection. A discussion of the basic disease processes in many of these entities is included in Chapter I.

Syphilis. The retina may participate in early or late syphilitic infections. Congenital syphilis may lead to widespread disease in the posterior eye (Fig. 339).

In syphilis of the adult, the initial pathology is one of lymphocytic perivascular infiltration, with extensive edema and secondary destruction of the retinal elements. Exudative and edematous changes involve the inner retinal layers, and the disk often is affected (Fig. 413). The inflammation usually is granulomatous although it may have a nonspecific character. Organisms may be identified in the acute lesions. The vitreous is heavily infiltrated with exudate and cells. The rods and

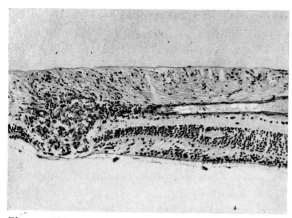

Figure 415. Granulomatous periphlebitis, possibly tuberculous, retina. ×75. AFIP Acc. 28137.

cones often degenerate and the retina and choroid become adherent to each other. The pigment from the degenerating pigment epithelial layer is scattered into adjacent tissues and the inflammatory exudate. If the disease is severe and chronic, the choroid becomes involved and the late picture resembles retinitis pigmentosa. A differentiating feature is the marked formation of chorioretinal adhesions with involvement of the lamina vitrea in postinflammatory pigmentary degeneration, in contrast to the absence of such destruction in primary pigmentary degeneration. In postinflammatory pigmentary degeneration the retinal vessel walls are thickened and their lumens are obliterated. Pigment accumulates about the vascular tree just as in the primary disease. The optic nerve becomes atrophic. Gummatous lesions of the retina are rare.

Tuberculosis. Tuberculosis of the retina often is secondary to involvement of the uvea. Acute necrotizing inflammations of the retina due to tubercle bacilli do occur, however, and in such cases there often is an associated granulomatous reaction in the choroid (Fig. 414). A severe endophthalmitis may result (Fig. 23). Tubercle bacilli frequently cannot be demonstrated with special stains (Fig. 415).

Eales' disease. Although a variety of retinal hemorrhages occur in association with generalized vascular disease, one form, primary retinal hemorrhage in young males, involves only the eye and was first described by Eales. Although this disease essentially is of unknown origin it frequently has been found in association with pulmonary tuberculosis

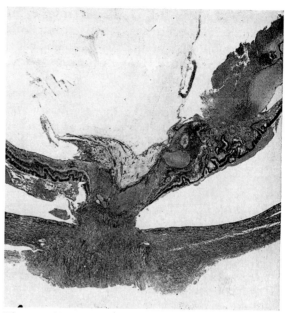

Figure 416. "Eales' disease." Retinal hemorrhages. Retinitis proliferans. ×10. AFIP Acc. 108045.

and in several instances the tubercle bacillus has been demonstrated in histologic preparations. Clinically, the retinal vessels are obscured by the vasculitis and show sheathing and telangiectasia. Pathologically, they are inflamed or occluded and often are surrounded by lymphocytes. Hemorrhages initially occur within the retina, but recurrences lead to damage to the inner limiting membrane and bleeding into the vitreous, finally being complicated by retinitis proliferans and retinal detachment (Fig. 416). As the hemorrhages organize and absorb, wandering cells, fibro-

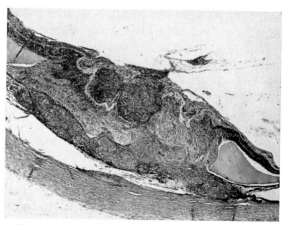

Figure 417. Granulomatous chorioretinitis in a patient who later died of sarcoidosis. ×20. AFIP Acc. 733320.

blasts, and sprouting capillaries invade the vitreous from the retina and tend to contribute further to the vitreous hemorrhage. The usual outcome is extensive retinal detachment with secondary glaucoma.

Occasionally, while the lesion is in the posterior pole, there may be more anterior foci of chorioretinitis which were not apparent clinically. At times foci of choroiditis affect the retina in such a fashion that the vessels are damaged and recurrent hemorrhages occur (secondary retinal vasculitis).

Sarcoidosis. The retina may be affected in sarcoidosis and single (Fig. 22) or multiple lesions may be present. Usually the retinal lesions are minute, but large granulomatous nodules producing detachment may occur. The hard tubercles have the features of sarcoidosis elsewhere and are associated with pulmonary and other changes (Figs. 18, 417).

Toxoplasmosis. Toxoplasmosis has a world-wide distribution in humans, and nearly all domestic and wild animals may become affected. The exact method of transmission of the disease is not known, but it is thought that it may be by ingestion of food, by insect vectors, or by direct contact.

Toxoplasma is a protozoan parasite, which produces either congenital or acquired chorioretinitis. In fixed tissue the extracellular organism is crescentic in shape, but intracellular organisms are somewhat more rounded. Cyst formation occurs very frequently as a result of parasitization of cells. The cysts contain many Toxoplasmas but they are surrounded by a tough membrane rather than a true capsule.

Infants may be born with acute toxoplasmosis, or it may not become apparent until within a short time after birth. The clinical findings include encephalomyelitis, visceral inflammation, and chorioretinitis. These lead to the classic findings of congenital toxoplasmosis: convulsions, fever, paralyses of various types, chorioretinitis, cerebral calcification, and hydrocephalus. The diagnosis most often can be made with the methylene blue dye and complement fixation tests, which become strongly positive within three to four weeks after onset of the infection. Such infections result in the fetus by transmission from the mother during pregnancy. A maternal history of an acute infection rarely is obtained in these cases. Therefore, it is believed the mother has a chronic latent infection which in some manner is passed to the infant. Remmington and coworkers have isolated Toxoplasma from uterine muscle, and this suggests that the uterus contains Toxoplasma cysts which are capable of transmitting the disease to the fetus. The unlikely chance that a placenta might be implanted in the region of a cyst helps explain why mothers who give birth to one toxoplasmic infant do not transmit the disease to subsequent offspring.

In some toxoplasmic infants the disease is so mild it may be unrecognized for months or even years. A subsequent relapse calls attention to the probable congenital origin of the disease. Infections transmitted from a mother with considerable immunity may explain milder or less apparent infections in the infant. Also, organisms of lesser virulence may produce less severe infections.

The *Sabin-Feldman syndrome* is characterized by chorioretinitis and cerebral calcifications. The microscopic findings are similar to those seen in toxoplasmosis, but the methylene blue dye test is negative.

Cytomegalic inclusion disease may produce choroiditis and encephalitis with calcifications. Microscopic examination of a chorioretinal inflammation in such cases has not been possible. The virus can be isolated from the mouth, urine, and liver biopsies in these cases.

Acute chorioretinitis occurs at birth or shortly thereafter and is one of the most constant clinical findings in congenital toxoplasmosis. The infection usually is bilateral. *Subacute chorioretinitis* may occur and not be recognized until later when mild generalized signs of infection develop. By this time the chorioretinal lesion may be either active or healed. Late relapses often occur by the apparent reactivation of dormant organisms near an old healed scar.

The acute chorioretinitis begins in the retina with severe inflammation and necrosis and exudation into the vitreous (Fig. 25). Single or multiple foci occur. Secondary involvement of the choroid always is present. The acute or primary stage may last for several months, depending on the severity of the infection. Organisms almost always are found in cysts or are free in the region of the

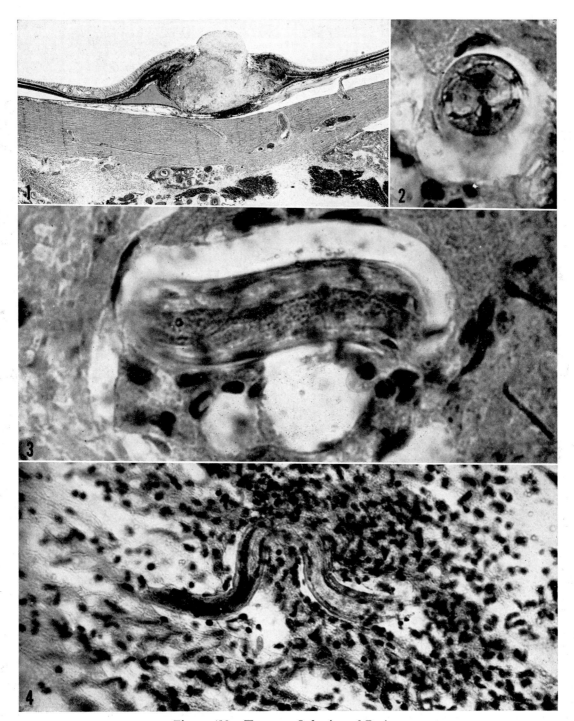

Figure 418. Toxocara Infection of Retina

1. A mound of sclerosing chronic inflammatory tissue projecting from the choroid replaces part of the macula The subjacent choroid is infiltrated by lymphocytes, plasma cells, and eosinophils. (Case 1 reported by Ashton 1960.) ×13. AFIP Acc. 220297.

2. Transverse section through fragment of Toxocara larva found in lesion shown in 1. ×880.

3. Longitudinal section through same larva shown in 2. ×960.

4. Toxocara larva. (Case 4 reported by Ashton, 1960.) ×350.

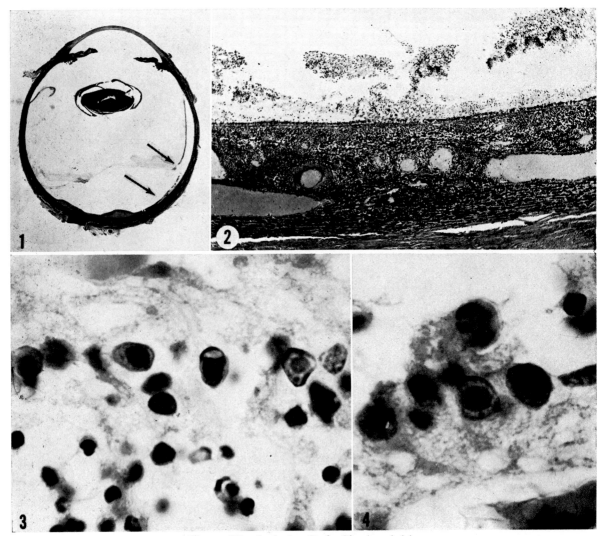

Figure 419. Inclusion Body Chorioretinitis

1. Localized area of necrosis of retina (arrows) and serous detachment about optic disk. ×2. AFIP Acc. 62192.

2. Same area indicated by arrows in 1. The necrotic retina is extremely friable and there is a diffuse chronic choroiditis.

3 and 4. Intranuclear inclusion bodies resembling those of cytomegalic inclusion body disease, found in necrotic portion of retina. ×1280 and ×1620, respectively. (Case reported by Foerster, 1959.)

acute lesions. Eventually the inflammation subsides, leaving a pale atrophic scar surrounded by pigmented margins. The cysts may be found in the tissue adjacent to these scars. They contain viable, resting organisms surrounded by a zone which is argyrophilic and often PAS positive. Rupture of these cysts may lead to reactivation of the disease.

Some cases of adult chorioretinitis are known to be due to Toxoplasma, but the establishment of an exact diagnosis is difficult. In the adult the infection produces a necrotizing retinitis with heavy vitreous ex-

udation. Organisms often can be demonstrated in these lesions, in either the free or intracellular form. Animal inoculation of tissue from such lesions may result in acute toxoplasmosis. The adjacent choroid shows a typical granulomatous inflammation, and, at times, the sclera may be thickened and inflamed (Figs. 25, 31, 32). Upon healing the retina shows severe destruction in the area of the infection and chorioretinal adhesions are present. Recurrences are common. Toxoplasma cysts are found in the retina near the scar. The recovery of the Toxoplasma gondii by animal inoculation from the infected ocular tissue provides the final proof of the nature of the infection.

Nematode retinitis and chorioretinitis. Discrete tumor-like retinal and chorioretinal masses may be seen as isolated manifestations of visceral larva migrans. Wilder, in 1950, first showed that ectopic migration of nematode larvae into the eye produced a disease which was often mistaken for retinoblastoma. This entity, in fact, proved to be one of the most important etiologic categories in her study of pseudoglioma, and justified the conclusion that nematodiasis was undoubtedly a much more important cause of blindness in children than had previously been realized. In almost all of her cases the wandering larvae had produced an endophthalmitis (Fig. 27) which led to massive retinal detachment and formation of a retrolental mass. Within the chronically inflamed and contracted vitreous there were abscesses or granulomas in which the nematode larvae were found (see Chapter X). Subsequently, Nichols identified four of the better preserved larvae as those of Toxocara canis, the cosmopolitan intestinal parasite of the dog intestine.

Ashton, in 1960, reported four cases of larval granulomatosis of the retina due to Toxocara. These cases had so much in common, yet were sufficiently different from those in Wilder's study, that Ashton concluded they formed a new clinicopathologic entity. The patients were children aged 4, 6, 8 and 16 years. Each presented a solitary retinal tumor involving the macula or situated between the disk and the macula. The vitreous was not involved except in the immediate vicinity of the retinal lesion. Microscopically,

the retina was elevated, distorted, and partially replaced by an inflammatory mass containing an abundance of dense scar tissue (Fig. 418). The immediately adjacent choroid was infiltrated by chronic inflammatory cells and eosinophils. The nematode larvae were buried within the retinal mass, but, judging from the breaks in Bruch's membrane and in the pigment epithelium, the Toxocara may well have invaded the retina from the choroid.

Viral chorioretinitis. Sabin and Feldman presented the findings in a condition similar to toxoplasmosis, but in which the methylene blue dye test was negative, and organisms were not found in the tissues.

Theobald described a chorioretinitis, associated with encephalomyelitis, and widespread visceral inflammation in a newborn infant in which cytoplasmic and intranuclear inclusions were observed in the tissues. The observations in this condition resemble closely those of toxoplasmosis.

Cytomegalic inclusion disease of the newborn may produce a clinicopathologic syndrome similar to that of congenital toxoplasmosis, though the retinal lesions in the one proved case that has been reported (Guyton, et al. 1957; Burns, 1959) were smaller, more discrete, and more peripheral than those of toxoplasmosis. In one adult whose eye was enucleated after 2 years of recurrent unilateral uveitis, Foerster found extensive retinal necrosis and a granulomatous reaction in the choroid. Intranuclear inclusion bodies, similar to those of cytomegalic inclusion disease, were found within the necrotic retina (Fig. 419).

INJURIES

Contusions. Contusion of the eye as a result of a blow through the closed eyelids or a concussion by a bomb or underwater blast produces profound disturbances not only in the cells of the retina, but in the capillaries and arterioles. The blow or force so distorts the globe and alters pressure relationships in the tissues that changes occur in the retinal cells and walls of the retinal vessels. Vasoparalysis leads to alteration of vascular pressure, slowing of the blood stream, and

leakage of fluid into the tissues. A contrecoup type of injury produce a characteristic retinal lesion which is known as Berlin's edema. Ophthalmoscopically, there is swelling and haziness of the retina surrounding the fovea. After three to four weeks the edema gradually subsides, and the macular area appears somewhat atrophic and pigmented. Most often there is partial permanent central visual loss. Microscopically, the edema is most marked in the outer plexiform layer, which is broad and

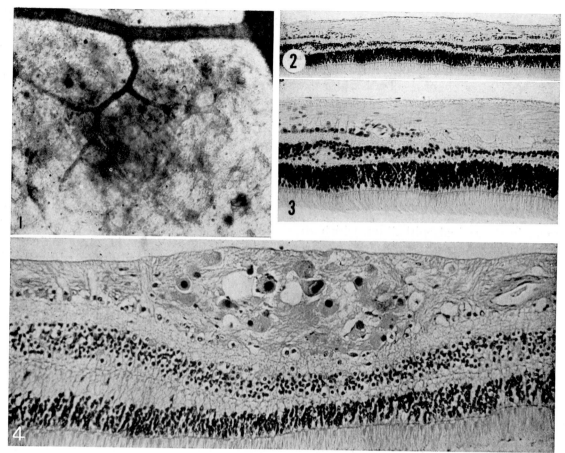

Figure 423. Microinfarcts of Retina

1. Relationship to a terminal arteriole demonstrated in flat preparation stained by the periodic acid-Schiff reaction. AFIP Acc. 219548. (From Friedenwald, 1949.)

2 and 3. Within the microinfarct ganglion cells have disappeared, the inner nuclear layer is much reduced in thickness, and the nerve fiber layer is very edematous. ×75 and ×160, respectively. AFIP Acc. 625745.

4. Cytoid bodies in swollen nerve fiber layer within microinfarct. The alterations in the ganglion cell and inner nuclear layers are less advanced than those shown in 2 and 3. ×210. AFIP Acc. 62937.

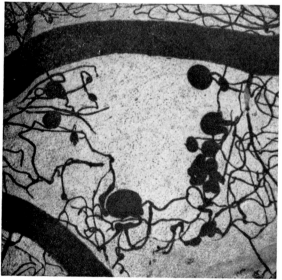

Figure 424. Capillary microaneurysms about the margins of a cotton-wool spot. (From Ashton, 1959.) The retinal capillaries have been injected with India ink revealing the cotton-wool spot to be an area in which the capillaries are obliterated. ×88.

in the tissue supplied by a single terminal arteriole and correspond to the pattern of damage which might be expected from occlusion of such an arteriole (Fig. 423). Examination revealed in his cases, however, that the afferent vessel to the affected region usually is patent. He attributed the lesion, therefore, to arteriolar spasm.

Small hemorrhages and varicose, dilated capillaries often are found at the margins of these lesions. Ashton (1959) injected the retinal vessels with India ink in several cases of malignant hypertension and frequently found microaneurysms situated at the junction of normal and avascular tissue (Fig. 424). During healing, new-formed capillaries grow into the area from the venous side. These new capillaries usually are wide, their contours are irregular and angular, and their persistence serves to establish the location of healed lesions.

On section these cotton-wool spots are seen to be disk-shaped areas of thickening of the retinal nerve fiber layer. They contain great numbers of globular bodies, ten to twenty microns in diameter, each usually containing a central structure resembling a cell nucleus in size and shape, but eosinophilic in its staining reactions.

During the 100 years cytoid bodies have been known, there has been much debate concerning their composition and histogenesis; and even today little agreement exists. Christensen recently has reviewed the literature dealing with the nature of the cytoid body and he has shown that the dark central zone

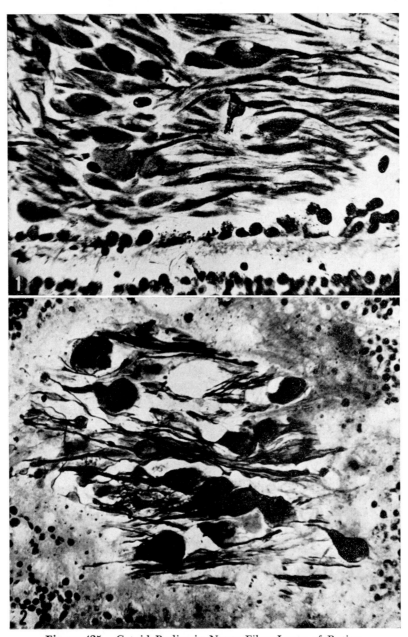

Figure 425. Cytoid Bodies in Nerve Fiber Layer of Retina

1 and 2. Special techniques of silver impregnation demonstrate the globoid structures to be varicose swellings in the damaged axis cylinders. Since the tapered ends of these cytoid bodies are continuous with those parts of the axons connected with the respective ganglion cells, the blunt ends are directed towards the optic nerve (which is to the left in 1 and to the right in 2). (Courtesy of Dr. J. R. Wolter.)

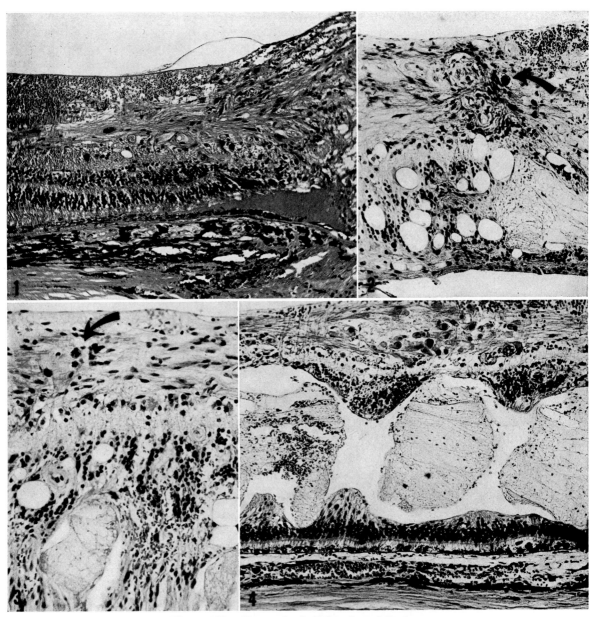

Figure 426.   Hemorrhagic Infarction of Retina

1. Absorbing hemorrhages and marked gliosis in nerve fiber and ganglion cell layers. ×130. AFIP Acc. 779256.

2 and 3. Absorbing hemorrhage, hemosiderin deposits (arrows), edema, gliosis, and architectural disarray involving all layers. ×140 and ×190, respectively. AFIP Acc. 640467.

4. Collection of cytoid bodies in nerve fiber layer and fibrinous exudate within an area of retinoschisis. ×130. AFIP Acc. 640467.

(Compare with Figure 50.)

has staining reactions characteristic of fibrin while the outer zone probably consists of precipitated mucopolysaccharide ground substance. The old idea that the cytoid bodies in cotton-wool exudates represent degenerative changes in the nerve fibers has been given support by the recent neuropathologic studies of Wolter who showed that they were terminal nerve fiber swelling of Cajal (see Chapter I). The fact that these structures develop in the nerve fiber layer of the retina and in the optic nerve, and that their free blunt extremities are directed towards the optic disk (away from the ganglion cells) is in keeping with this hypothesis (Figs. 52, 425). The lack of detectable functional change is explained by the fact that the lesions are minute and only a few of the nerve fibers passing

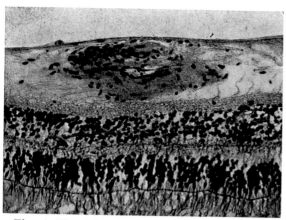

Figure 427. Sclerosis of retinal artery, endothelial proliferation and occlusion of adjacent retinal vein. ×165. AFIP Acc. 210125.

through the microinfarcts seem to be affected.

Cotton-wool exudates have no specific diagnostic implications but they are especially common in hypertensive retinopathy, lupus erythematosus, dermatomyositis, occlusion of the central retinal vein, and papilledema. They do have a prognostic importance in hypertensive retinopathy, however, in that they signify a serious disease.

Retinal venous occlusions. The events that follow *retinal venous occlusions* are more complex. The retinal capillaries become markedly congested. There is marked edema of the affected tissues, and hemorrhages occur in great numbers (Fig. 410). Superficial retinal hemorrhages are most common. These follow the plane of nerve fibers and form linear streaks and flame-shaped configurations. Deeper hemorrhages often are delimited by Müller's fibers and tend to be rounded. Larger hemorrhages involve the full thickness of the retina and erupt through the internal limiting membrane to form preretinal hemorrhages, or dissect posteriorly, separating the sensory retina from the pigment epithelium. Focal necroses appear in scattered areas, leading to the invasion of the tissue by microglia (macrophages). Sometimes edema fluid accumulates in large irregular cystic areas and it may escape subretinally to produce a localized flat detachment of the retina. In the organization of the hemorrhages and in the formation of new collateral vascular channels, a net of new-formed vessels develops on the inner retinal surface, sometimes extending into the vitreous (Fig. 410–

6). The occluded vein tends to become recanalized. These new channels are of capillary dimensions, and sections through the original vessel may reveal several such capillary channels within its lumen. Eventually the hemorrhages and exudates become absorbed, though this may take a very long time. Hemosiderin-laden macrophages usually persist (Fig. 426). These, together with the great disorganization of retinal architecture and the marked gliosis, help differentiate the final histopathologic picture from that seen after central retinal artery occlusion (Fig. 426).

Occlusions that involve only a branch of the retinal vein (Fig. 427) generally heal with some recovery of the affected area. In cases of occlusion of the central retinal vein the damage not only is more extensive but also is more thoroughly destructive. In about half the cases secondary glaucoma occurs, especially in eyes which already have an impaired facility of outflow. Usually this is a late complication occurring about three months after the venous occlusion. It is associated with vascularization of the anterior surface of the iris (Fig. 428), and formation of a delicate endothelial membrane in the anterior chamber angle and over the inner surface of the trabecula (see Chapter XII). Anterior synechias soon close the chamber angle, but there is clinical and pathologic evidence that the glaucoma begins before this complication. Glaucoma of the open angle type in an eye with central retinal vein sclerosis may precipitate a vein occlusion, and following such an occlusion it suddenly may become more severe. In such a case the fellow eye most often has open angle glaucoma.

These are the retinal vascular changes seen as complications of atherosclerosis. There now follows a discussion of changes in the retina which are related to those systemic diseases which involve the function and structure of smaller retinal blood vessels.

Hypertensive retinopathy. Purely hypertensive changes in the retina must be distinguished from those which are both hypertensive and arteriosclerotic. Essential hypertension may exist as a chronic or intermittent disease for many years without observable changes in the fundus. Also, it may develop rapidly and produce sudden retinal alterations such as gen-

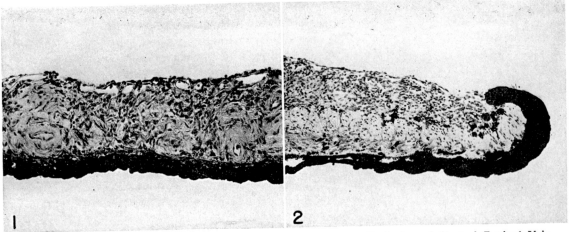

Figure 428.   Rubeosis Iridis in Hemorrhagic Glaucoma Due to Occlusion of Central Retinal Vein

1. Vascularization of anterior surface of iris. ×145. AFIP Acc. 130053.
2. Vascularization of anterior surface of iris with ectropion uveae. ×95. AFIP Acc. 88720.

eralized and localized narrowings of the arterioles, hemorrhages, edema residues, and cotton-wool patches. A more fulminating course may be followed, as in malignant hypertension, in which the findings include the ones just mentioned, as well as those of papilledema (hypertensive neuroretinopathy).

Chronic hypertension with a persistent variable pressure eventually produces arteriolar vascular damage, followed by the sequelae of arteriolosclerosis and phlebosclerosis, such as vascular occlusions with retinal edema and hemorrhages. Arteriolar changes of this type probably do not occur in the absence of hypertension. Atherosclerotic plaques may form in the arterioles in the absence of hypertension, but they rarely produce significant retinal changes. However, because they are less capable of reacting, vessels with changes of this type do not behave as do healthy ones if hypertension develops late. Correlation of the ophthalmoscopic and microscopic findings in hypertensive retinopathy is essential for an understanding of the pathogenesis of many of the changes. The following classification is useful, but it should be understood that disease processes are variable, and the findings may change rapidly.

I. Chronic hypertensive retinopathy
   A. Early
      1. Generalized narrowing of the arterioles
   B. Late
      1. Sclerosis
         a. Changes in the light reflex
         b. Copper-wire arterioles
         c. Crossing changes
            (1) Interruption of the veins
            (2) Deflection of the veins
         d. Silver-wire arterioles
         e. Sheathing
         f. Occlusive changes
            (1) Venous—central and tributary
            (2) Arteriolar—central and branch
      2. Retinal changes
         a. Atrophy
         b. Edema and hemorrhage
II. Angiospastic hypertensive retinopathy
   A. Vascular changes
      1. Generalized narrowing
      2. Localized narrowings
         a. Active
         b. Quiescent
      3. Increased tortuosity
      4. Arteriolosclerosis
   B. Retinal changes
      1. Edema
      2. Hemorrhages
      3. Cotton-wool patches
III. Malignant hypertension
   The changes are the same as those observed in angiospastic hypertensive retinopathy with the additional finding of hypertensive neuroretinopathy.

IV. Eclampsia

The changes are similar to those of malignant hypertension.

This clinical classification of the ocular manifestations of hypertensive states is presented simply to serve as a stepping stone for correlation with the microscopic findings. It should be understood that all changes are not detectable in microscopic sections and that a certain amount of interpretation is necessary, based on observations made of the changes in other tissues. Furthermore, the type of hypertension itself may change, and alter the clinical and histologic findings.

Chronic hypertension. Changes rarely are detectable in early and moderate hypertension, but sclerosis invariably occurs in persistent moderate or severe hypertension.

The earliest ophthalmoscopic sign of sclerosis is a *change in the arteriolar light reflex.* The normal retina and its blood vessel walls are not visible with the ophthalmoscope but the blood column is. The normal light reflex of the ophthalmoscope forms a bright stripe along the center of the blood column. This is produced by a reflection of light from the interface between the column of blood and the vessel wall. Arteriolosclerosis alters the density of the vessel wall, therefore the reflection of light, so that the central reflex is less bright and more diffused.

The next early change is the development of a *copper wire arteriole* in which the central light reflex becomes even more diffused, and the arteriolar color changes to a reddish-brown color. Microscopically this is brought about by an increasing sclerosis of the wall of the arteriole, so that the reflection of light from the blood column is altered. The arterioles show thickening of their walls, with hyalinization of the media (Figs. 43, 427). The preceding changes may exist for years before other lesions appear, or the hypertension suddenly may become severe and progressive, producing rapid vascular and retinal changes.

In the former case advanced sclerosis gradually becomes evident with *crossing changes.* One of the earliest of these is *nicking.* Normally at arteriovenous crossings the adventitia forms a common sheath for the arteriole and vein, and the walls of these two vessels are intimately united, the arteriole usually crossing internal to the vein. Arteriolosclerosis, therefore, also is associated with phlebosclerosis at the crossings (Fig. 427). Normally at the crossing the artery can be seen to cross the vein, and the blood column in both vessels is seen quite distinctly. Increasing sclerosis interferes with visualization of the vein at the crossing. If the sclerotic process extends out into the wall of the vein beyond the crossing it interferes with visualization of the blood column here also. In addition the vein is compressed and its lumen is narrowed. As a result of this reduction in calibre the vein becomes dilated distal to the crossing, then tapers and seems to lose its blood column at some distance before it crosses under the arteriole. After passing under the arteriole it does not reappear for a short distance, and when it does, it again is tapered and reduced in calibre. All of this change, then, is produced by extension of the sclerotic process from the arteriole into the wall of vein and from here beyond the crossing. A certain amount of deep displacement of the vein by the arteriole may assist in production of the phenomenon. Constant twisting movements of these vessels, caused by their normal pulsation, may lead to stress on the walls and predispose to such crossing changes in hypertension.

A second important sclerotic crossing change is *deflection of the veins.* This may be produced much in the same fashion as the tortuosity of the radial arteries in Mönckeberg's sclerosis. Ordinarily the radial arteries become tortuous because they elongate as they become sclerotic. The retinal arterioles either may elongate or shorten with sclerosis. The common sheath at arteriovenous crossings causes the vein to be deflected from its course by the change in length of the artery. Normally the vein passes under the arteriole at a rather acute angle. If it is deflected it crosses more at an obtuse angle. A combination of nicking and deflection of the veins is important for the diagnosis of sclerosis.

Longstanding hypertension leads to severe arteriosclerosis with marked thickening and hyalinization of the arterioles, and reduction in calibre of the lumen. This change may completely interfere with visualization of the blood column, the vessels appearing as *silver wires.*

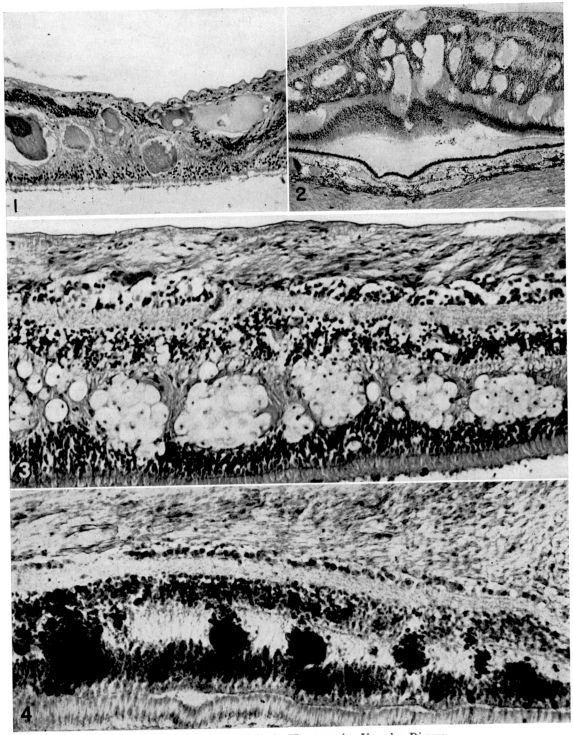

Figure 429. Retinopathy in Hypertensive Vascular Disease

1. Serous exudates in outer plexiform layer of posterior portion of retina. ×100. AFIP Acc. 55972.

2. Serous exudates resulting in cystoid degeneration of retina in macular region. ×60. AFIP Acc. 105307.

3. Lipoidal histiocytes ingesting exudates in outer plexiform layer of retina near macula. ×170. AFIP Acc. 30034.

4. Lipoidal histiocytes in outer plexiform layer of retina. Fat stain. ×170. AFIP Acc. 30034.

Occlusive changes in the main or tributary arteriolar and venous channels are extremely frequent in longstanding hypertension. *Tributary venous occlusions* are most common and occur at crossings because of the sclerotic process, compression, and deflection of the veins. The upper temporal vein most often is affected possibly because it has more arterial crossings. Central venous occlusions are not uncommon. Branch arteriolar and central artery occlusions are much less common, probably because of the stronger construction of these vessels, lack of compression by other vessels, and their more direct course.

Longstanding hypertension with retinal vascular sclerosis can lead to gradual *atrophy* of the retina with reduction in the number and size of the cells, as well as in their function.

Edema and hemorrhages are not characteristic of this type of retinopathy, except in the case of a vascular accident.

Acute or angiospastic hypertension. Vascular changes in the early stages are the most prominent finding, the severity depending on the degree of hypertension. The hypertension may be severe for three to six months, then gradually change to a more chronic form, or a chronic hypertension suddenly may become severe, with rapid changes in the retinal vascular tree. Such variability in the hypertension modifies the ophthalmoscopic picture.

Generalized narrowing of the arterioles can be detected ophthalmoscopically without difficulty, but cannot be demonstrated microscopically in the early stage. Persistence of the hypertensive state leads to arteriolosclerosis and the vessels become fixed in a narrowed position. In such a case the wall is thickened and hyalinized, and the lumen is narrowed.

Localized (angiospastic) *narrowings* are easy to detect clinically. During the active phase they appear, then disappear, so they cannot be demonstrated microscopically. If they become fixed, localized arteriosclerotic changes occur, frequently with adventitial proliferation due to previous edema. In such case the narrowing shows a gray sheathing. As shown by Friedenwald some localized narrowings are produced by atherosclerosis, but these characteristically affect one side of the wall of the vessel only.

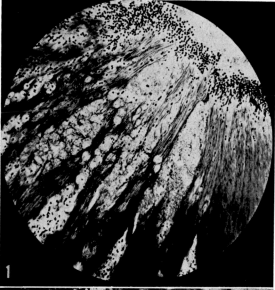
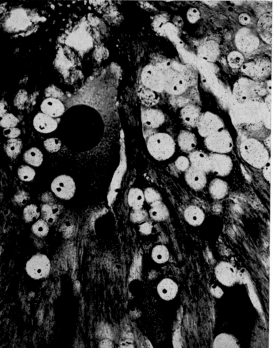

Figure 430. Star-Figure of Macula

1. Flat section passing through Henle's layer reveals great numbers of lipid-laden macrophages, many of which are necrotic. Hortega method, ×100.

2. Similar preparation of opposite eye reveals free lipids and hyaline bodies in addition to the many macrophages between the compressed nerve fibers in Henle's layer. Hortega method, ×400.

(Courtesy of Dr. J. R. Wolter.)

The smaller arterioles in the macular area may show an *increased tortuosity* due to production of a change in their length by the arteriolosclerotic process. This does not occur in chronic hypertension and therefore may

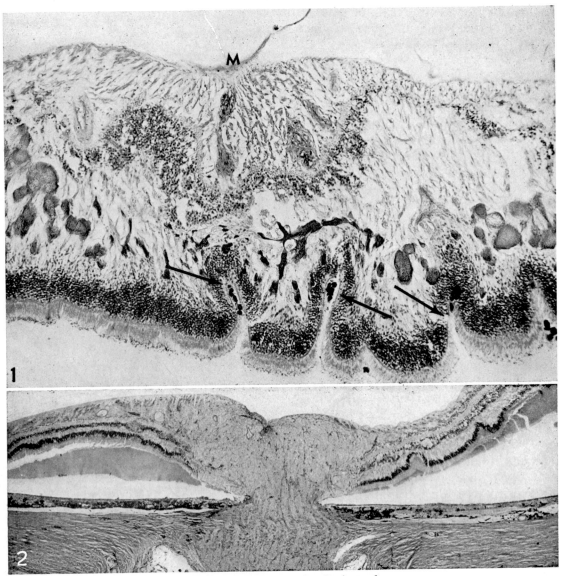

Figure 431. Hypertensive Retinopathy

1. Serofibrinous exudates and marked edema of outer plexiform layer; preretinal membrane (M) and fixed fold; partial detachment with degeneration of rods and cones within retinal folds (arrows). ×90. AFIP Acc. 46391.

2. Papilledema and serous detachment of peripapillary retina. ×26. AFIP Acc. 64722.

be a reflection of the severity of the disease.

Sudden onset of this type of hypertension usually results in local tissue changes usually classified as a *retinopathy*. *Hemorrhages* of the *flame-shape type* (nerve fiber layer) or *round type* (deeper layers) are striking and result from diapedesis, or actual necrosis of the capillary wall.

Edema invariably is found, and may be present for a considerable period before it is seen ophthalmoscopically because the edema fluid has the same index of refraction as the retina. The fluid diffuses through all layers

and even produces slight separation of the retina, especially near the disk. It soon collects in pools in the fiber layers and inner nuclear layer and produces degeneration of the retinal cells. As a result the fluid changes in character, containing lipoids, proteins, fibrin, and debris. At this stage it becomes visible as an edema *exudate* or *residue*. Microscopically, it is localized in the nuclear and fiber layers of the retina, is rather sharply localized, and is eosinophilic (Fig. 429). The retina quite often shows numerous areas which are filled with macrophages, as a result of degeneration of the tissue. These exudates usually form in the posterior fundus, around the disk and macula, and extend out to the equator. They last two to four weeks before being absorbed. If they occupy the macular region they form the *macular star* figure, in which case the exudates are found in the long fibers of the external plexiform layer (Henle's layer) microscopically (Figs. 57, 429).

Pathologically, these spoke-like lesions are composed of hyaline material and phagocytes (microglia) (Fig. 430). The surrounding fibers of Henle's layer usually show severe damage by compression. In the late stage the phagocytes disintegrate, freeing the lipid which later becomes hyalinized.

In the full-blown cases there is a profuse outpouring of serous fluid in the retina. The tissue may be swollen to twice its normal thickness. The edema is most marked in the posterior pole and, in malignant hypertension, includes the optic disk in its distribution. This neuroretinal edema generally is much more diffuse than that found in papilledema resulting from increased intracranial pressure. Cerebral edema and increased cerebrospinal fluid pressure may also be present in patients with malignant hypertension, so that true papilledema may exist independent of retinopathy or superimposed upon retinopathy (Fig. 431). Though the distribution of fluid is diffuse, especially prominent accumulations occur where retinal tissue structure is loosest and most easily spread apart. Irregular cyst-like spaces develop, particularly in Henle's fiber layer near the disk. Some fluid generally leaks out of the retina into the subretinal region, causing a flat detachment of the retina. The detachment is usually slight and not recognizable on ophthalmoscopic examination, but rarely is absent in postmortem specimens. On the other hand, the detachment may be voluminous in eclampsia. In the experimental form of the disease produced in dogs, retinal detachment generally is massive.

Cotton-wool patches also form in the posterior retina around the macula and disk (Figs. 424, 425, 432). They constitute a grave sign when found in any type of hypertension. Ophthalmoscopically, they always lie in the nerve fiber layer near the main arteriolar vessels or their branches. They have a soft, gray-

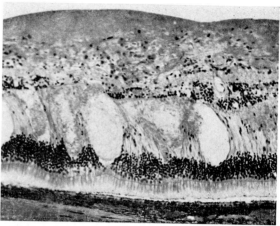

Figure 432. Microinfarct of retina in malignant hypertension; cytoid bodies in nerve fiber layer and marked edema of outer plexiform layer. ×100. AFIP Acc. 103975.

white, cottony appearance, with frayed edges, as if they had been pulled from a roll of cotton. They appear suddenly, and last four to six weeks, but always disappear without leaving an ophthalmoscopically visible scar, although, as has been discussed, the damage they produce can be detected microscopically.

Finally, persistence of this type of hypertension leads to severe sclerosis, and all the changes described in chronic hypertension.

The changes produced in the retina by *malignant hypertension* are identical with those of acute angiospastic hypertension except that in the former the disease process develops more rapidly, the retinal changes are more severe, and there is a neuroretinopathy.

Choroidal vascular changes also are found in malignant hypertension (Fig. 348). At times there is severe sclerosis with thrombosis. In more acute cases a necrotizing vasculitis occurs.

The changes in the retina in the hypertension associated with eclampsia are very similar to those seen in malignant hypertension. Extensive serous separation of the retina is more common. After control of the hypertension or delivery of the child permanent sclerotic changes often are seen in the retinal vessels.

Periarteritis nodosa. In periarteritis nodosa there often is renal damage and hypertension which produces generalized arteriolar sclerosis or is associated with angiospasm which gives rise to a full-blown hypertensive

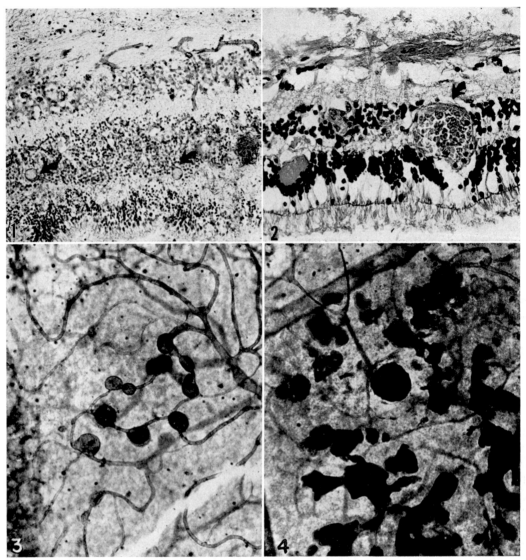

Figure 433. Retinal Microaneurysms in Diabetes

   1. Capillary aneurysms (arrows) in outer nuclear and outer plexiform layers. Periodic acid-Schiff reaction. ×145. AFIP Acc. 213298.
   2. Huge capillary aneurysm involving outer plexiform and both nuclear layers. ×240. AFIP Acc. 721735.
   3. Capillary aneurysms, flat preparation of retina with Hotchkiss stain. AFIP Acc. 219548 (Friedenwald, 1949).
   4. Exudates around capillary aneurysm in flat preparation of retina. AFIP Acc. 219548 (Friedenwald, 1949).

retinopathy. The retinal and uveal blood vessels rarely exhibit the typical inflammatory lesions which characterize the pathologic anatomy of this disease in other organs (Fig. 46), but the small choroidal arterioles may show typical inflammatory infiltrates (Fig. 349). The nodular periarterial lesions may reach such a size that they can be recognized on ophthalmoscopic examination.

Disseminated lupus erythematosus. In disseminated lupus erythematosus the retinal blood vessels are affected in the same manner

as they are elsewhere in the body. Cotton-wool patches are the most common finding in the retina, and microscopically these are identical with those occurring in hypertension.

Diabetic retinopathy. Sclerosis of larger arteries in diabetics does not differ from that of nondiabetics except for its earlier appearance, greater severity and higher incidence. On the other hand, lesions of the capillaries and venules, particularly as they are seen in the retina and kidney, are so characteristic that they are virtually diagnostic of the diabetic state (Ashton). It is a well-recognized fact that modern therapy has greatly decreased the mortality in diabetes and that this increased survival and longer life span have led to a corresponding increase in degenerative vascular diseases. Retinopathy is the most frequent and it may be the earliest demonstrable evidence of these complicating conditions. A number of observers have reported a threefold increase in the incidence of diabetic retinopathy during the past two decades. This is partly the result of wider recognition of the early lesions, but mostly it is due to the longer survival of juvenile diabetics. The incidence is higher in females. The most significant factor appears to be the duration of the disease, and after 15 to 25 years the eyes of a majority of patients are affected. Most writers report that retinopathy occurs equally in mild and severe diabetes but there is much conflicting evidence concerning a possible relationship between the severity of diabetes and the severity of retinopathy.

Diabetic retinopathy almost always is bilateral. The earliest ophthalmoscopic observation is the presence of minute, sharply defined "dot hemorrhages," now known to be capillary aneurysms, situated mostly in the posterior fundus. Frequently, they are preceded by venous engorgement but often the fundus appears otherwise normal. This is especially true of juvenile diabetic retinopathy. They are so characteristic as to suggest the diabetic state, even in the absence of other clinical signs or symptoms. Subsequently, in the same areas that contain the microaneurysms, irregular "blot" hemorrhages and multiple, small, glistening yellow-white exudates appear. The retinal veins become increasingly engorged, sclerotic, and distorted. Delicate fronds of new vessels grow into the vitreous (rete mirabile), particularly at sites where blood flow is obstructed. This often leads to vitreous hemorrhage and fibro-

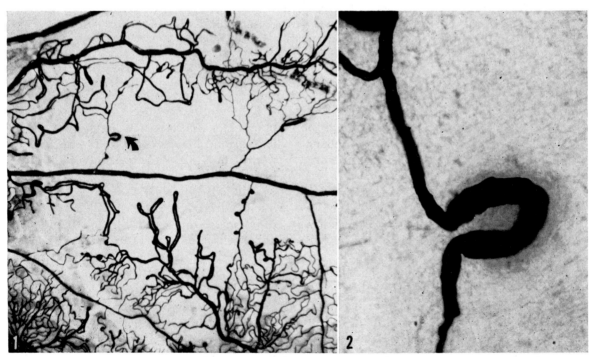

Figure 434. Diabetic Microangiopathy

1. Artery coursing horizontally across the field. The arterial side of the circulation is undergoing obliteration; numerous new channels project towards the artery from the venous side. Arrow indicates early stage of microaneurysm-formation. Periodic acid-Schiff reaction. ×52.

2. The capillary has a dilated (varicose) lumen and has formed a conspicuous loop. Some exudate has escaped from the capillary into the adjacent tissue. ×430.

(From Ashton, 1958.)

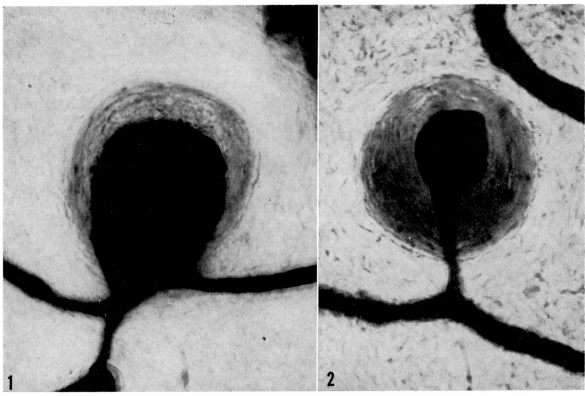

Figure 435. Diabetic Microangiopathy

1. A more advanced stage of capillary aneurysm development than that shown in Fig. 434–2. The opposing walls of the capillary loop have fused and the escaped exudate has formed a laminated cap over the convex surface of the loop. ×500.

2. Fully developed microaneurysm of retinal capillary with thick laminated cap of inspissated exudate. ×800.

(From Ashton, 1953 and 1958.)

vascular proliferation (retinitis proliferans) followed by retinal detachment. Secondary glaucoma, uveitis, and cataract formation are often associated.

The pathologic anatomy of the retina and kidney in diabetes has been studied most thoroughly by Ashton (1958) who recently prepared an excellent review of the entire subject of diabetic microangiopathy. It is a remarkable fact that although the clinical aspects of diabetic retinopathy have been controversial for over a century, virtually no effort was made to study the problem histologically until very recent years. According to Ashton, up to 1943 histopathologic descriptions of only 12 diabetic eyes had been published and most of these were valueless. At this time the virtually pathognomonic capillary aneurysms, originally described and illustrated in 1877, were rediscovered and their identity with the "dot hemorrhages" seen

ophthalmoscopically was recognized. To Ballantyne and his associates we owe the foundation of our present knowledge of the pathologic histology of diabetic retinopathy. Friedenwald (1949) and Ashton (1949) subsequently introduced new methods and special staining techniques to demonstrate the aneurysms more dramatically.

Diabetic retinopathy is considered to be a distinct morphologic entity. The process commences on the venous side of the capillary circulation at a time when the arterial side is still normal. The veins are engorged and there may be widespread or localized beading, looping, kinking, or coil-formation. New capillary channels form and these may extend into the vitreous (rete mirabile). The microaneurysms develop on the venous side of the capillary network, mainly in the inner nuclear layer, on the course of the capillaries which link the deep and superficial capillary

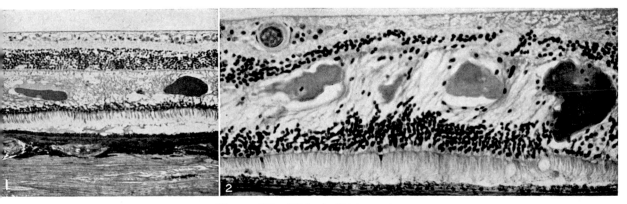

Figure 436. Diabetic Retinopathy

1. Discrete intensely eosinophilic exudates in edematous outer plexiform layer of macula. ×100. AFIP Acc. 40413.

2. Exudates in outer plexiform layer of retina posteriorly. Retinal ganglion cells have disappeared as result of secondary glaucoma. ×205. AFIP Acc. 100161.

plexuses. Typically, they measure 20 to 30 microns in diameter but may reach 70 to 100 microns (Fig. 433). The diabetic microaneurysm develops in a unique fashion. A small focal segment of the capillary undergoes degenerative changes leading to varicose dilatation, and forms a U-shaped kink (Fig. 434). Exudate oozes through the capillary walls and the two limbs of the kink become adherent and fuse. This gives rise to a saccular configuration which appears to represent a focal aneurysmal dilatation of one side of the capillary wall (Fig. 435). In view of the characteristic way that these "aneurysms" develop and the fact that they show no particular tendency to occur at bifurcations, there is no valid reason for believing them to be related

pathogenetically to embolic or miliary aneurysms of the cerebral arteries. Retinal microaneurysms are found in other conditions besides diabetes (e.g., retinal venous occlusions, Eales' disease, malignant hypertension, posttraumatic uveitis), but it is their frequent occurrence, great numbers, and mode of development which makes them so much more characteristic of diabetic retinopathy.

The exudate which leaks out of the microaneurysms and forms discrete retinal lesions is rich in lipids and mucopolysaccharides (Fig. 433). It becomes incorporated in the vessel walls and accumulates both inside and outside the capillary. This produces a thick

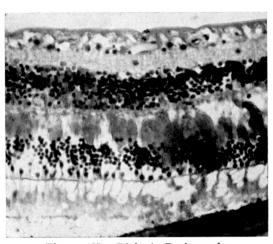

Figure 437. Diabetic Retinopathy

Hemorrhages in outer plexiform layer of retina. ×230. AFIP Acc. 40413.

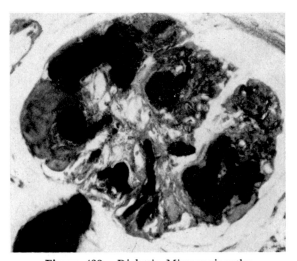

Figure 438. Diabetic Microangiopathy

Glomerulus in diabetic glomerulosclerosis. Aneurysmal dilatations in the capillary tuft are revealed by injected India ink in relation to the hyaline nodules. ×320. (From Ashton, 1958.)

laminated or homogeneous hyaline nodule which may completely replace the lumen. Some of the escaping exudate seeps out to the external plexiform layer, where it accumulates to form the discrete waxy refractile hyaline exudates which are particularly characteristic of advanced diabetic retinopathy (Fig. 436). Hemorrhages also are most likely to occur at the site of microaneurysms, but, like the exudates, they may develop wherever the capillary walls have degenerated (Fig. 437).

It is well known that all types of arteriosclerosis occur earlier and in a more extensive fashion in diabetics than in nondiabetics, and the retina is no exception. Hyalinization of the terminal arterioles and precapillary retinal vessels leads to their gradual occlusion and consequent atrophy of the arterial side of the capillary bed. On the venous side of the capillary bed there is irregular dilatation and neovascularization.

Diabetic retinopathy is frequently associated with the Kimmelstiel-Wilson syndrome (nephrotic edema, massive proteinuria, and hypertension in longstanding diabetes mellitus). The incidence of retinopathy coincides poorly with that of glomerulosclerosis, for example, in Ashton's postmortem study the incidence of the latter was only 36 per cent while retinopathy was present in 68 per cent. When the two lesions coexist there seems to be no correlation in their degree of severity. Although not completely identical, the two lesions of retina and glomerulus probably are closely related histogenetically. Ashton showed that histopathologic lesions exactly comparable to retinal micro-aneurysms (except that they are arterial) are present in the diabetic glomerulus (Fig. 438). In both sites there is localized capillary dilatation and degeneration with exudation of a PAS-positive hyaline material and deposition of lipid. In fact, glomerulosclerosis has been described as a retinopathy in miniature.

The fundamental disturbance responsible for these vascular, retinal, and renal lesions, be it an abnormality in serum mucopolysaccharides, lipids, or lipoproteins, disturbed adrenal cortical function, a miscellany of mechanical factors, or a combination of these, remains to be determined. The literature pertaining to these etiologic considerations is reviewed in the admirable monographs of Ashton (1958), and Larson (1960).

Circinate retinopathy. A circinate pattern of large and small, yellowish, sharply defined intraretinal exudates may form around the macula in patients who have no systemic disease. Presumably, circinate retinopathy is due to hereditary factors and it is most common in middle age, especially in women. It is an uncommon disease, and should not be confused with the circinate pattern of exudates which occur in the same area in diabetes and disciform degeneration of the macula. Microscopically, the exudates are lipoidal (Fig. 429), either within phagocytes or forming solid masses between the retinal fibers, especially in Henle's fiber layer and the inner nuclear layer. According to Klien, these exudates develop primarily as a result of disease of the small arterioles which supply the macula.

Leukemia. Infiltrates frequently are seen in the retina of patients with all types of leukemia. In the advanced stages of the disease some retinal infiltrates are almost constantly found. Histologically, there is a leukemic infiltration which concentrates in the perivascular areas. Such a process may cause destruction of the vessel wall. Hemorrhages and exudates also are seen throughout the retina (Fig. 386-2, 3). The latter changes may be explained on the basis of the usually severe associated anemia.

Anemia. Ischemia of the retina may follow the acute loss of blood or more commonly may occur after repeated small hemorrhages. Histologically, the changes are similar to those seen in central artery occlusion.

Some chronic anemias, such as pernicious anemia, may be associated with retinal hemorrhages of the round or linear types, and transient edema exudates.

INTOXICATIONS

Retrolental fibroplasia. The most important retinal disease which may be classified as an intoxication is retrolental fibroplasia, the oxygen-induced retinopathy of premature in-

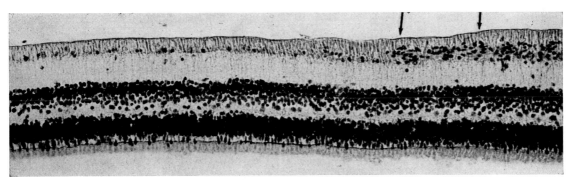

Figure 439. Early Retrolental Fibroplasia

In the premature infant, the peripheral retina (left half of field) is incompletely vascularized. The growing tips of the retinal vessels (arrows) are most responsive to the toxic effects of oxygen. ×195. AFIP Acc. 488849.

fants. The incompletely vascularized peripheral retina of premature infants (Fig. 439) and newborn animals is sensitive to variations in oxygen concentration of the circulating blood. According to Campbell, a lowered oxygen tension reduces the capillary-free zone around the arteries and Ashton and co-workers have shown that increased oxygenation widens the zone. Experimentally, oxygen in high concentrations has been shown to obliterate the terminal arterioles and the arterial side of the capillary bed. The effect spreads to involve the whole capillary bed and finally the entire vasculature (arterial, capillary, and venous) closes down. This phenomenon is peculiar to the incompletely vascularized retina. Once the retinal vessels have reached the periphery they no longer are susceptible. Were it not for the diffusion of oxygen from the choriocapillaris, the reaction would be self-limited, and Ashton (1957) has shown that it is for this reason that it is not observed when the retina is detached from the choroid.

The immediate vaso-obliteration induced by oxygen is transient and after about ten minutes the retinal vessels dilate again. In spite of continuous hyperoxygenation they remain dilated for about six hours. Then a delayed vaso-obliteration occurs which at first is reversible after normalization of oxygen tension. Gradually the process becomes irreversible. At this stage the vessel walls have become adherent to each other or show degeneration. By this time, whether oxygen tension is normalized or not, vasoproliferative changes occur from those vessels immediately adjacent to the obliterated areas (Figs. 440, 441). Glomeruloid capillary tufts appear. The

newly formed capillaries invade the retina, penetrate the internal limiting membrane, and proliferate into the vitreous (Figs. 442, 443).

Leakage of plasma, hemorrhages, and reactive gliosis complicate the picture. Organization of hemorrhages and exudates in the vitreous and formation of preretinal membranes may lead to partial or complete retinal detachment (Fig. 444). In severe cases, the completely detached retina and the organized vitreous may form an opaque retrolental mass which produces a white pupil (leukokoria) and a cat's eye type of reflex when the pupil is illuminated in the dark. For this reason, and because both conditions are often bilateral, retrolental fibroplasia and retinoblastoma may be very difficult to differentiate clinically. Ultimately in the most advanced cases, the eye becomes somewhat phthisical and sinks into the orbit (enophthalmos). Transient secondary glaucoma may be observed, but buphthalmos is unusual. Histopathologic diagnosis is exceedingly difficult in these advanced cases because secondary changes tend to obscure the essential vaso-obliterative and vasoproliferative process. If the examination of the peripheral retina reveals an absence of capillaries, this provides important circumstantial evidence of prematurity and therefore susceptibility to oxygen toxicity.

In the less severe cases only a part of the retina may be involved. Reese and Stepanik showed the retina to be affected on the temporal side in 90 per cent of such cases. This is believed to reflect the longer period required for vascularization of the retina to occur on

(Continued on p. 516.)

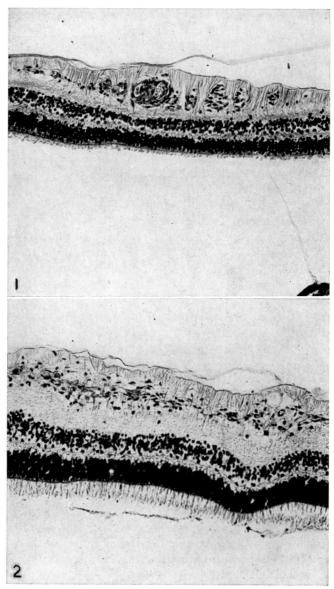

Figure 440.   Retrolental Fibroplasia

1. Proliferated endothelium and surrounding glial cells which have formed whorls **resembling glomerular** tufts. Müller's fibers pushed aside with no evidence of destruction of normal retinal cells.

2. Retina just behind ora serrata showing numerous proliferating capillaries surrounded **by glial cells in nerve** fiber layer.

(From Friedenwald et al., 1951.)

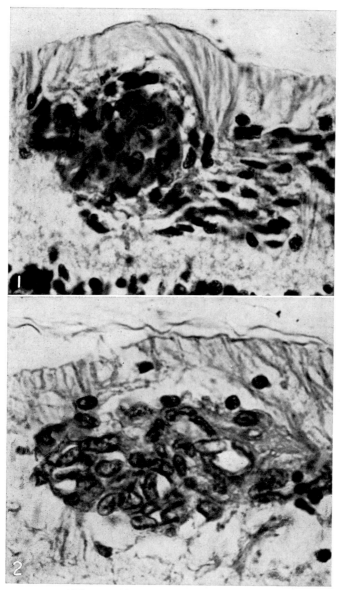

Figure 441. Retrolental Fibroplasia

1. Nerve fiber layer showing the whorl-like endothelial proliferation with surrounding glial cells.
2. Proliferated capillary endothelium in whorl resembling a glomerulus.
(From Friedenwald et al., 1951.)

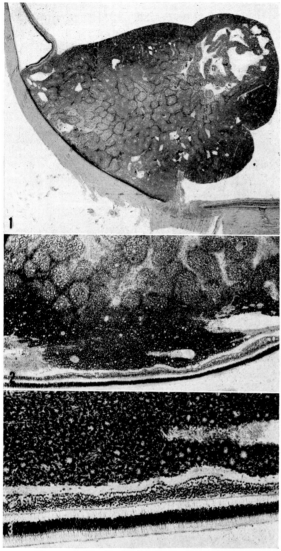

Figure 446. Endophytic Retinoblastoma

1. The tumor projects from the inner surface of the retina into the vitreous, overlapping the optic disk. AFIP Acc. 747443.

2 and 3. In the plane of section this endophytic tumor appears to have arisen from the inner retinal layers, but there are many characteristic rosettes. ×35 and ×106, respectively. AFIP Acc. 205156.

tumors, calling them gliomas in the belief that they arose from glial cells of the retina. In 1891 Flexner, in reporting a single case, first described the rosettes which are sometimes present, and in 1897 Wintersteiner described them in a large series. Both authors advanced the opinion that the rosettes represented an attempt to form rods and cones. Flexner designated his tumor "neuroepithelioma" and Wintersteiner adopted this term as a substitute for "glioma," whether or not the tumor contained rosettes. Later, Verhoeff suggested "retinoblastoma" as the designation for the entire group, to indicate that these tumors are composed of embryonic retinal cells. This term was officially adopted by the American Ophthalmological Society in 1926. Since that time some authors have adopted the classification of Grinker. According to him, the tumors without rosettes arise from hypothetical pluripotential undifferentiated cells produced by primitive retinal epithelium and capable of differentiating either to the neuroblastic series, forming neurons, or to the spongioblastic series, forming glia. He, like Flexner, Wintersteiner and others, looked upon the rosettes as evidence of rod and cone origin, and for tumors with rosettes he retained the name neuroepithelioma. Parkhill and Benedict reverted to the original term glioma, subdividing the group into a retinoblastoma type and a neuroepithelioma type. They, like Virchow, considered all of these tumors to be of glial origin, arising most frequently from the inner nuclear layer where glial cells are most abundant, and rarely, if ever, from the outer layers where glial cells seldom have been demonstrated. They postulated a derivation from normal glial cells, either astrocytes (spider cells) or the cells of Müller fibers which have undergone dedif-

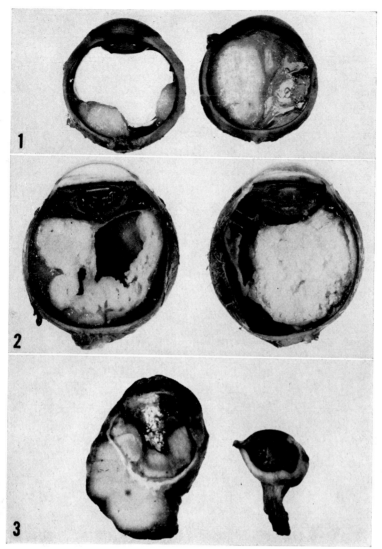

Figure 447. Bilateral Retinoblastoma

1. The tumor mass in the right eye is much larger than in the left, though the latter contains two separate neoplasms. AFIP Acc. 687292.

2. In each eye the tumor has reached massive proportions and has largely replaced the vitreous. AFIP Acc. 635460.

3. An extremely unusual case in which spontaneous tumor necrosis led to phthisis bulbi in one eye while extraocular spread was taking place in the other. AFIP Acc. 570989.

ferentiation, rather than from embryonic rests or primitive epithelium. In their opinion rosette formation is an attempt to reproduce the primitive epithelium of the neural tube rather than the more highly specialized rods and cones. They called attention to the resemblance of the retinoblastoma type to the medulloblastoma of the central nervous system, and of the rosette cells of the neuroepithelioma type to primitive spongioblasts. The American Registry of Pathology has, with the American Ophthalmological Society, adhered to Verhoeff's terminology, and until the histogenesis of these tumors is clarified they will be referred to as retinoblastomas with rosettes and retinoblastomas without rosettes.

Retinoblastoma is the most common intraocular tumor of childhood and it is second only to malignant melanoma of the uvea among all intraocular tumors. Falls and Neel have estimated its frequency as 1 for each 20,288 live births. According to Reese, the neoplasm always is congenital even though

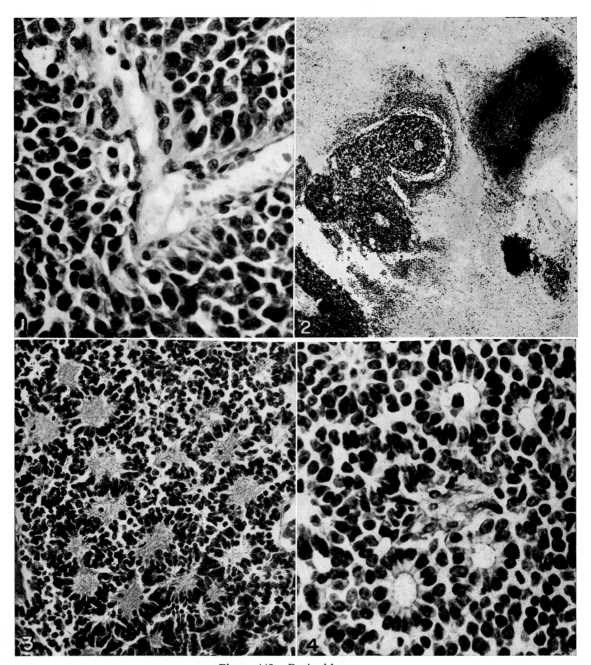

Figure 448. Retinoblastoma

1. Poorly differentiated tumor without rosettes. ×400. AFIP Acc. 190088.

2. Viable tumor cells form a collar about prominent vessels; elsewhere there is necrosis with foci of calcification. ×180. AFIP Acc. 39579.

3. Incomplete rosette formation. ×275. AFIP Acc. 481110.

4. Well-formed rosettes. ×605. AFIP Acc. 293627.

in bilateral cases the tumor in the second eye may not be detectable clinically for a considerable interval. Ordinarily the tumor is clinically apparent by the time the child is two years old although many cases are not recognized for two to five years. After the fifth year the incidence falls off sharply and only a few rare cases have been diagnosed in adults. There is no significant sex or race distribution. Although most cases of retinoblastoma are sporadic, no other members of the family being affected, according to Weller, and Benedict and Parkhill, there nevertheless is a strong hereditary tendency in that the offspring of survivors are likely to be affected. Reese (1954) reported that in his series of 30 children whose mother or father had confirmed retinoblastoma, 23, or 77 per cent, also had the tumor.

It is postulated that the development of a retinoblastoma is dependent upon the presence of a single dominant gene. The number of such genes in the population is constantly increasing as a result of mutations, and also is diminishing because of deaths of affected persons. Falls and Neel have calculated this rate of mutation to be 2.3×10^{-5} per generation. Without therapy most retinoblastoma genes would be eliminated because the affected persons would not live long enough to transmit their mutant genes. With the increasing survival rate obtained during recent years, the pool of retinoblastoma genes in the population is increasing. For reasons not now understood, all persons who possess this particular gene do not develop a retinoblastoma. This "failure of penetrance" probably accounts for those unusual kindreds exhibiting "horizontal" rather than "vertical" constellations (i.e., several affected siblings whose parents are normal). One explanation for failure of penetrance is that a cellular alteration to malignant change is required and that in certain cases such changes do not occur. This concept would also account for the occurrence of unilateral cases and explain the multicentric origin that commonly is observed.

Bilaterality is observed in about one fourth of the cases (Fig. 447). This does not represent spread from one eye to the other, for de Buen has shown that such an occurrence is distinctly rare. It is a reflection of the

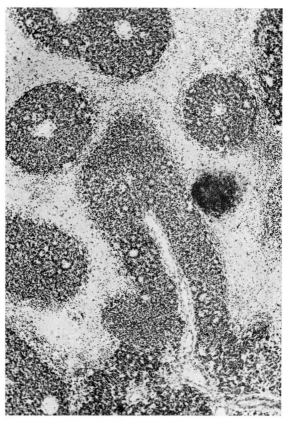

Figure 449. Retinoblastoma

Living tumor cells around blood vessels with necrosis in areas remote from vascular supply. One deeply stained focus of calcification is present in a necrotic area. ×80. AFIP Acc. 147292.

tendency for the neoplasm to have multicentric foci of origin in one or both retinas. Ordinarily one eye is much more extensively involved than the other.

Microscopically, the tumor usually presents a characteristic appearance. It is composed principally of undifferentiated neuroblastic cells ("retinoblasts") which exhibit large hyperchromatic nuclei and a very scanty cytoplasm (Fig. 448). Mitotic figures usually are numerous but may be scarce. Varying degrees of differentiation are observed and in many retinoblastomas a few neuroepithelial rosettes are seen. A well differentiated Flexner-Wintersteiner rosette is formed by cells which appear more mature and less anaplastic than those which constitute the bulk of the tumor. Generally they appear as uniform cuboidal or short columnar cells arranged in an orderly fashion about a small round lumen (Fig. 448–4). The nuclei are contained at the base

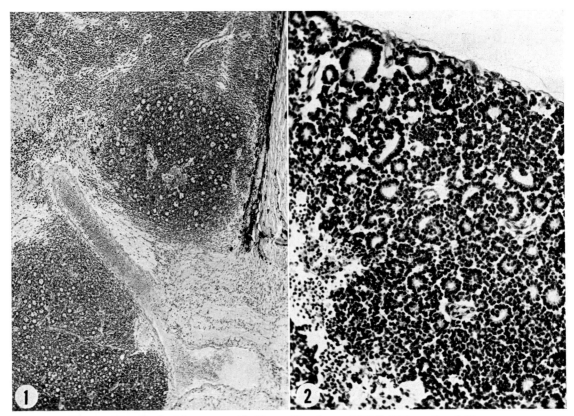

Figure 450. Retinoblastomas with Large Numbers of Well Differentiated Rosettes

1. ×50. AFIP Acc. 753671.
2. ×200. AFIP Acc. 747443.

of the cell away from the lumen and occasionally a fine filamentous process extends into the lumen. Condensations of the cell border about the lumen may closely resemble the external limiting membrane of the normal retina. Many observers have been impressed by the close resemblance of these well differentiated rosettes of retinoblastomas to those seen in retinal dysplasia and to a stage in the embryologic differentiation of rods and cones from the outer nuclear layer. Recently it has been shown that a mucoid material, resistant to hyaluronidase and similar to that which normally coats the surface of rods and cones, may be found in the lumen of the rosettes in retinoblastomas and in retinal dysplasia. In many tumors an attempt to form rosettes is observed (Fig. 448–3), but there are no well differentiated structures. Many retinoblastomas contain minute focal areas of necrosis which to the uninitiated may be misinterpreted as rosettes. These meaningless configurations as well as the collars of tumor

cells about nutrient blood vessels (Fig. 449) have often been called "pseudorosettes" but this term has also been used to describe poorly differentiated rosettes. Hence it has been robbed of any potential usefulness. For this reason and because it is really unnecessary, the term should be dropped.

There are two reasons for paying so much attention to the occurrence of rosettes. One concerns histogenesis, the other prognosis. At one time it was suspected that the presence of rosettes in exophytic tumors signified an origin from the outer nuclear layer, but it has been impossible to establish this point. In fact, the general belief today is that rosettes may be found in any type of retinoblastoma and that their presence provides no clue as to histogenesis. Furthermore, there are two main schools of thought concerning the nature of the rosettes: one (Willis) championing the view that they represent abortive visual cells, the other (Parkhill and Benedict; Reese) maintaining that, in the same manner as rosette-containing neuroepitheliomatous tumors of other locations, they are differentiating as cells lining the primitive neural tube. On the other hand, there is general agreement that those tumors containing an abundance of well formed rosettes (Fig. 450) represent more highly differentiated, less anaplastic, and therefore less malignant neoplasms.

In most tumors a large percentage of the cells exhibit severe degenerative changes and large areas of necrosis are present. Very little stroma is present, but a system of nutrient vessels ramifies through the tumor. A mantle of viable cells usually surrounds these vessels while those areas farther removed become necrotic. Accumulations of mucoid ground substance and dystrophic calcification are observed in many of the necrotic areas (Fig. 448–2). These calcific deposits sometimes can be visualized ophthalmoscopically in the case of endophytic tumors and they can also be demonstrated roentgenographically.

Because of the lack of cohesion of the cells and the necrosis, retinoblastomas are often friable, and they seed into the vitreous (mainly in endophytic tumors) or subretinal fluid (in exophytic tumors) (Fig. 451). Occasionally, with widespread invasion and seeding, tumor cells get into the aqueous and accumulate in the anterior chamber, simulating hypopyon (Fig. 452). Necrotic retinoblastomas are not nearly so irritating as necrotic melanomas; hence, uveitis, endophthalmitis, and panophthalmitis rarely are observed as presenting manifestations, but hypopyon in a small child should always arouse suspicion of retinoblastoma.

As the retinoblastoma grows it forms an opaque mass in the vitreous. In the case of endophytic growths ophthalmoscopic examination reveals the tumor in front of the retina, while in the case of exophytic neoplasms the retina with its vessels is detached and lifted up by the tumor mass. In either case when the mass becomes sufficiently large it produces a "cat's eye" reflex when light is thrown onto the eye. Many other pathologic processes may create similar manifestations in a child's eye and therefore may be misinterpreted as retinoblastoma. Some of the more important are retrolental fibroplasia, persistent hyperplastic primary vitreous, retinal dysplasia, Coats' disease, nematode en-

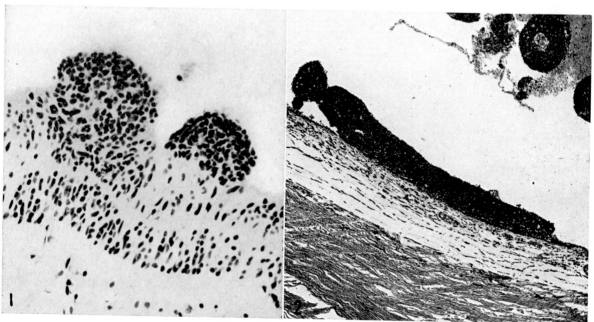

Figure 451. Retinoblastoma

1. Implantation (seeding) of tumor cells on inner surface of retina from primary tumor in same eye. ×610. AFIP Acc. 28130.

2. Implantation growth on inner surface of retinal pigment epithelium with early invasion of choroid. ×50. AFIP Neg. 57–351.

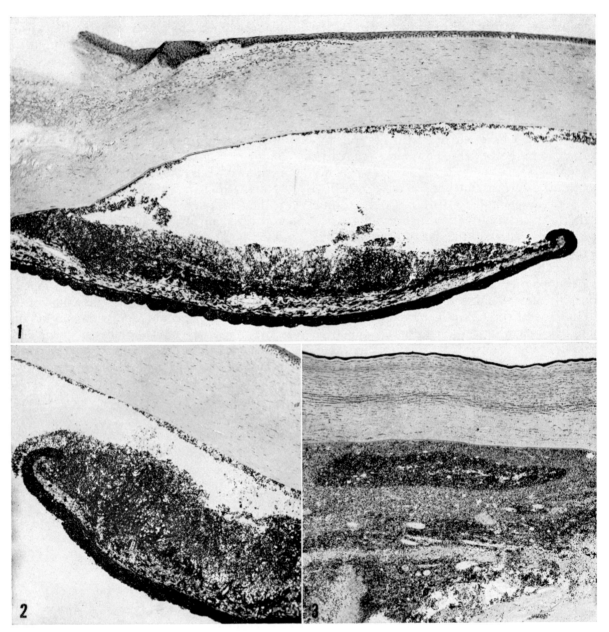

Figure 452. Retinoblastoma in Anterior Chamber Simulating Hypopyon

1 and 2. Most of the retinoblastoma cells in the anterior chamber of this case are viable. ×75 and ×80, respectively. AFIP Acc. 297415.

3. In this case the tumor cells are largely necrotic and there is an associated acute keratitis. ×50. AFIP Acc. 150880.

dophthalmitis, and organization of the vitreous following unsuspected penetrating wounds. These are described elsewhere.

In exceptional cases where relatively small tumors are located in the macula, strabismus may be an early sign (Fig. 453). For this reason the occurrence of strabismus in an infant or small child should always arouse a suspicion of retinoblastoma. At the other extreme, neglected cases may be observed only after massive growth produces secondary glaucoma and buphthalmos (Fig. 454). In some cases there may be broad peripheral anterior synechias, advanced neovascularization of the iris, and ectropion of the pupil. Proptosis produced by massive orbital extension of the neoplasm is another late manifestation (Figs. 447, 454–4).

In the ordinary small or medium-sized tumor a variety of growth patterns may be seen. Because of the tendency for seeding to occur, implantation growths, as well as independent foci of neoplasia often are present in the retina. These implants are observed both on the inner and on the outer surfaces of the retina. Implants on the pigment epithelium may erode through the lamina vitrea to invade the choroid.

A most important characteristic of retinoblastoma is its tendency to invade the optic disk and nerve (Fig. 454–1, 2). Over the years, this feature has become so generally recognized that ophthalmic surgeons make efforts to ascertain that 15 mm. or more of optic nerve is attached to the globe when an eye is enucleated because of a suspected retinoblastoma. This therapy, together with earlier diagnosis, has been responsible for great progress in obtaining five-year cures. The retinoblastoma, as it invades the nerve, spreads by direct infiltration along the nerve fibers and also along the central vessels. Tumor cells continue along the sheath of these vessels as they leave the nerve to traverse the meningeal space. There they gain access to the circulating subarachnoid fluid and may be carried by it to the brain. Reese indicates that about one half of fatal cases at autopsy are found to have brain and meningeal involvement. Thus, it is of prognostic importance for the pathologist to determine not only whether the nerve is involved, but to what extent it is invaded. Herm and Heath have

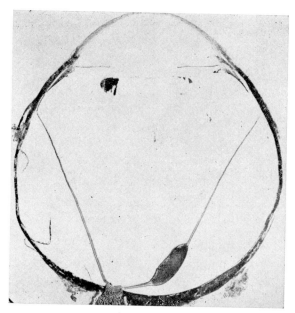

Figure 453. Retinoblastoma

This small tumor located in the macula produced a convergent strabismus first noted when the child was 12 months old. The patient's twin also had a retinoblastoma. ×4. AFIP Acc. 260992.

shown that choroidal invasion also is believed to carry an unfavorable prognosis and presumably this invasion is responsible for the widespread hematogenous metastases that may be found in about half the fatal cases.

Rarely the tumor may undergo complete spontaneous necrosis and lead to phthisis bulbi (Fig. 455). This may happen in one eye while extraocular extension develops in the other (Fig. 447). Similar necrosis and calcification may be observed after the lesion is treated with x-rays (Fig. 456).

Astrocytoma. Astrocytes normally are present in the retina. Therefore, it is to be expected that an occasional astrocytoma would be discovered. Such tumors do occur but are extremely rare, except in patients with tuberous sclerosis. They usually are discovered in childhood, and produce damage only by local extension (Fig. 457). These tumors are thought to be hamartomatous (Figs 458, 459). In association with Bourneville's syndrome or von Recklinghausen's disease, they are often multicentric; otherwise they are solitary masses.

Histologically the tumors are composed of elongated fibrous astrocytes containing small oval nuclei. Their cytoplasmic processes in-

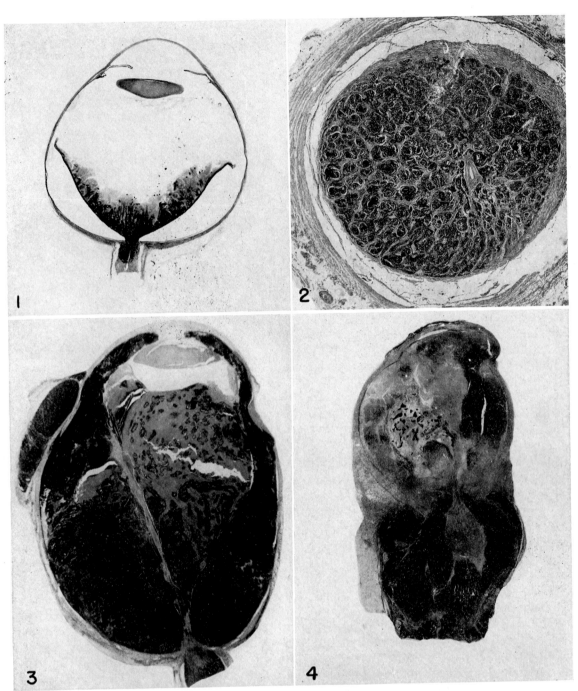

Figure 454. Retinoblastoma

1. Retinoblastoma invading optic nerve beyond lamina cribrosa, but not to line of excision. AFIP Acc. 211405.

2. Invasion of optic nerve by retinoblastoma. ×16. AFIP Acc. 39376.

3. Detachment and destruction of retina by tumor. Invasion of uveal tract. Extension through sclera to form an epibulbar nodule. Extension into optic nerve beyond line of excision. Lobulated appearance of tumor where living cells are grouped around blood vessels with necrotic areas intervening. AFIP Acc. 34764.

4. Retinoblastoma filling and destroying globe and extending into orbit posteriorly. Note calcium deposits (X) in area of necrosis. AFIP Acc. 40642.

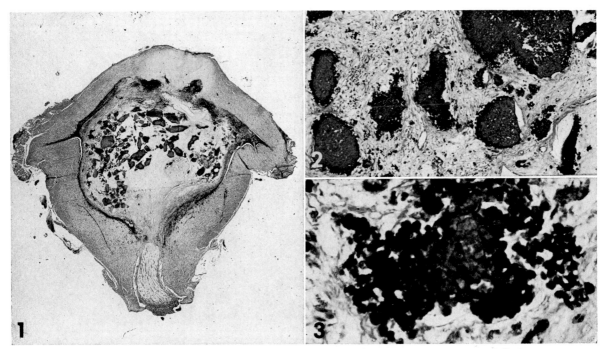

Figure 455. Phthisis Bulbi Secondary to Spontaneous Retrogression of Retinoblastoma

1. Retrogressed retinoblastoma with calcium deposits. Phthisis bulbi. ×6. AFIP Acc. 193695.

2. Calcium deposits in fibrous tissue matrix in retrogressed retinoblastoma. No living tumor cells seen. ×75. AFIP Acc. 235121.

3. Calcium deposits in tumor cells. Same case. ×400. AFIP Acc. 235121.

terlace to form a fine feltwork. The tumor is purely retinal and does not destroy the internal limiting membrane or infiltrate other structures. When very small, as in certain cases of tuberous sclerosis, they may be confined to the nerve fiber layer.

Glioneuroma. Tumors of the retina which combine both neuronal and glial elements are very rare. Since they are congenital, they are properly classified as choristomas. They have not been observed to metastasize, and therefore are considered to be benign. Both glial and ganglion cells may be identified in these tumors, and glial and nerve fibers can be demonstrable by special staining.

Kuhlenbeck and Haymaker reported one glioneuroma without other neural tumors in association with a coloboma of the iris and ciliary body. It contained ependymal elements and, in some areas, resembled normal cerebral cortex. It was believed to be a neoplasm of the edge of the primitive optic cup, preventing the formation of iris and retina at this point. In Fralick's case of glioneuroma in the eye of an otherwise normal infant,

some areas resembled brain cortex, but the tumor was associated with a diktyoma which had invaded the iris (Fig. 370). Cartilage and cellular arrangements resembling ependymal cleft and choroid plexus also were present.

Angiomatosis retinae. Angiomatous tumors of the retina are rare, but there are two important diseases to be considered here: von Hippel-Lindau's and Coats'. The former, angiomatosis retinae, is a congenital, often bilateral, frequently familial angioblastic retinal tumor with associated lesions in the

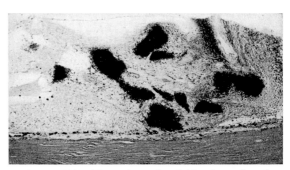

Figure 456. Necrosis and calcification of retinoblastoma following radiation therapy. ×40. AFIP Acc. 185791.

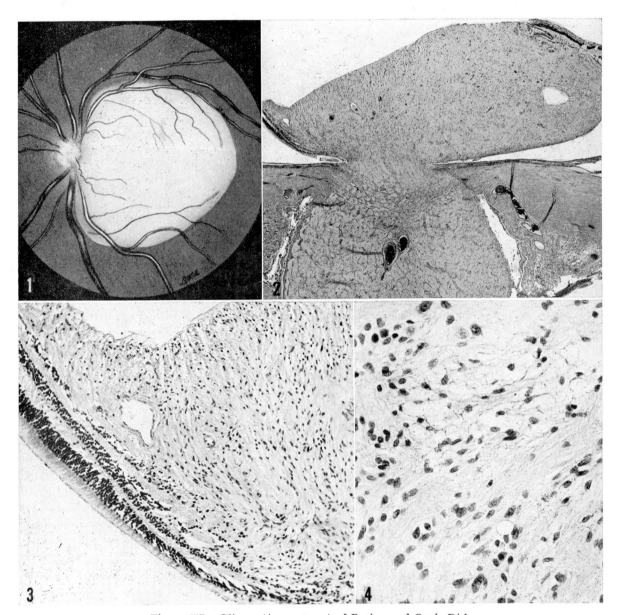

Figure 457. Glioma (Astrocytoma) of Retina and Optic Disk

1. Painting of fundus of 6 year old girl who presented no evidence of tuberous sclerosis or neurofibromatosis. (Case reported by Boles et al., 1957.)

2 to 4. Microscopic appearance of well differentiated tumor arising in nerve fiber layer of retina and in optic disk. Same case shown in 1. (Courtesy Dr. J. H. Allen.) ×25, ×115 and ×305, respectively. AFIP Acc. 862102.

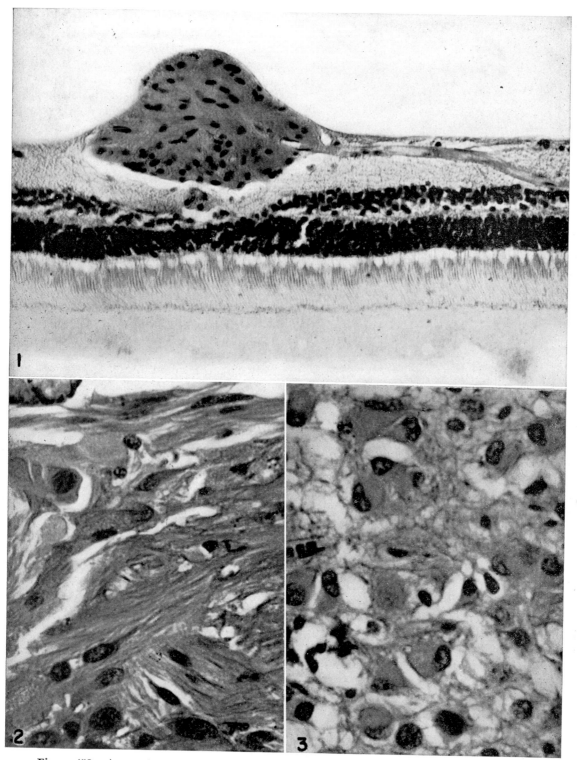

Figure 458. Astrocytic Hamartoma of Retina in Tuberous Sclerosis (Bourneville's Syndrome)

1. Small circumscribed tumor involving nerve fiber and ganglion cell layers of retina. This was one of multiple lesions. ×322. AFIP Acc. 68196.

2. Glial cells in retinal tumor. Same case. ×855.

3. Glial cells in brain tumor. Same case. ×855.

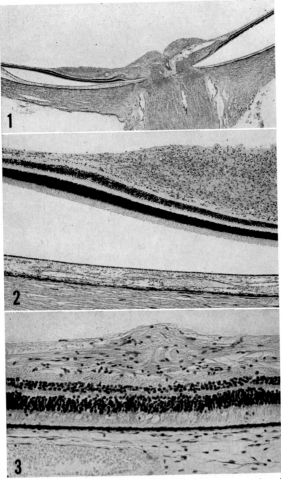

Figure 459. Gliomas (Astrocytic Hamartomas) of Retina and Optic Disk

Two year old child whose father and sister had von Recklinghausen's neurofibromatosis. ×8, ×45 and ×155, respectively. AFIP Acc. 219976.

viscera and brain. Clinically, the course of the disease follows a typical pattern: (1) angiomatous dilatation and tumor formation; (2) hemorrhages and exudates; (3) massive detachment; and (4) glaucoma. Ophthalmoscopically, there is a yellow retinal tumor of moderate size which is supplied by a large artery and vein. The tumor may be located in any part of the fundus, and in some patients there are multiple tumors. The artery and vein are tortuous and convoluted. The tumor is composed of vascular channels which may be small due to capillary hyperplasia (Fig. 460). Other areas of angioblastic cells are present, which exhibit growth tendencies. Among the capillaries are large foamy macrophages containing lipoid. These cells

probably are present because of degeneration of the retinal cells. Gliosis is common.

The usual pathologic specimens demonstrate only the advanced stages of the disease. Added to the primary vascular overgrowth of capillary or larger vessels is the marked glial reaction, which is analogous to the connective tissue proliferation which occurs in response to some primarily epithelial tumors. As the nutrition of retinal cells is compromised, cystoid spaces develop and lipoid (some cholesterol) accumulations are found. Hemorrhage, reactive fibrosis, and gliosis obscure the basic lesion. Studies of enucleated eyes occasionally have revealed the presence of angiomatous tissue in an eye with massive fibrosis of the retina resulting from repeated hemorrhages. By the time enucleation is performed, secondary changes leading to phthisis bulbi (Fig. 461) may obscure the fundamental lesion, and the correct histopathologic diagnosis may not be made. The disease probably is more common than previously suspected.

Coats' disease. Telangiectasis of the retina (Leber's miliary aneurysms or capillary hemangioma) is a vascular malformation which may remain static or progress to complete retinal detachment (Coats' disease), or, according to Reese (1956), may give rise to hemorrhage from time to time with no serious secondary changes. The term "Coats' disease" has been subjected to great variations in usage and there are certain authorities, including Duke-Elder, who do not regard it as a clinical entity, but include under this designation a number of conditions characterized by massive exudation between the retina and choroid. Reese and many others, however, believe the term should be restricted exclusively to the characteristic and rather constant clinical picture of the dark, perhaps greenish colored, bullous detachment of the retina of young children, the angiomatous nature of which can often be appreciated at some site where the retina still is more or less in situ.

The characteristic retinal lesion of telangiectasis is a circumscribed slightly elevated area over which there are numerous, small, sharply outlined red globules resembling hemorrhages or capillary aneurysms (Fig.

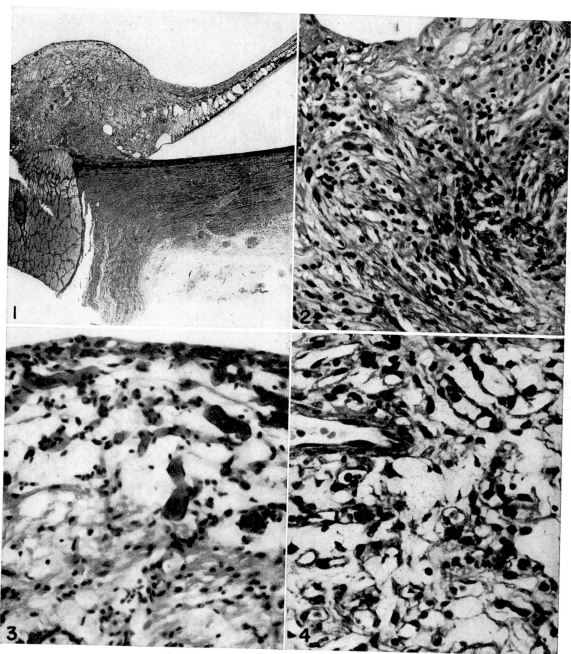

Figure 460. Von Hippel's Hemangiomatosis

1. Vascular and glial mass involving nerve head and adjacent retina. Cystoid degeneration of retina near tumor. ×14. AFIP Acc. 154481.

2. Glial proliferation in tumor. ×250. AFIP Acc. 154481.

3. Numerous capillaries in superficial portion of tumor. ×250. AFIP Acc. 154481.

4. Thin-walled blood channels, some containing red blood cells, in deep portion of tumor. ×500. AFIP Acc. 154481.

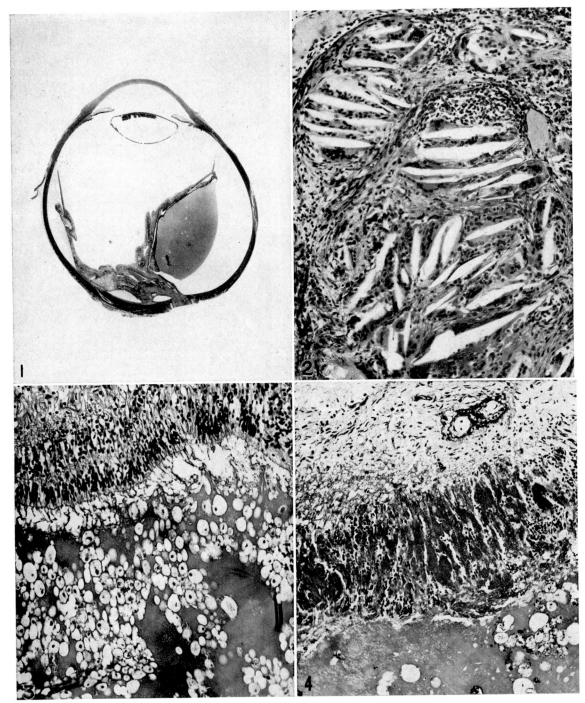

Figure 463.   Coats' Disease

1. Posterior chorioretinal adhesions. Subretinal serous exudate. Retinal separation. ×2. AFIP Acc. 203583.

2. Cholesterol slits surrounded by foreign body giant cells in organized hemorrhagic subretinal exudate. ×125. AFIP Acc. 105527.

3. Foamy cells (bladder cells) in subretinal serous exudate. ×125. AFIP Acc. 206444.

4. Eosinophilic PAS-positive exudate engorges the outer retinal layers. ×95. AFIP Acc. 889042.

DEGENERATIONS

Senile macular degeneration. Senile macular degeneration comprises a group of conditions, usually described as separate entities, which are characterized in some eyes by a gradual reduction of nutrition to the retinal layers which results in cystic degeneration of the retina, and in other eyes by the occasional development of a subretinal hemorrhage with formation of a disk-like area (disciform degeneration). These lesions result from vascular disease in the afferent macular vessels and in the choriocapillaris of the choroid, which may show severe sclerosis. In some cases there is basophilia of the lamina vitrea, or a variable thickening of the cuticular portion of this layer, accompanied by fissuring or cracking, which may lead into the region of the capillary layer. This retinal condition may occur as a presenile form in the 40 to 50 year age groups, at times with a family history of macular degeneration. Most often, however, a family history is lacking, in which case the disease is considered to be a macular dystrophy.

The various changes which occur in senile macular degeneration appear in the older age groups, most often are bilateral, and are independent of any systemic disease, such as hypertension and arteriosclerosis. They are characterized by macular degeneration either of a very slow, intermittent type, or by rapid progression to hole or cyst formation. Some cases may show an early degenerative macular change in one eye, and a typical disciform degeneration in the other. Others may show a typical senile macular degeneration in one eye, and a degeneration with a circinate retinopathy in the other. At any time during the course of a macular degeneration a hemorrhage may occur, producing the picture of a disciform degeneration.

The typical senile macular degeneration commences with visual disturbance and faint depigmentation and clumping of pigment in the macular region. Over a period of months or years progressive depigmentation occurs, accompanied by alterations in the retina itself, characterized by cystoid degeneration. At first small cysts appear, which sooner or later coalesce to form larger ones; at times a large macular cyst results from this process, and rupture of the inner wall may produce the picture of macular retinoschisis. These cysts may persist for years. In other instances the walls of the cyst may disappear, resulting in hole formation.

Microscopic examination rarely has been done in early cases, but those which have been examined show choriocapillary sclerosis in the macular choroid, with some obliteration or even disappearance of vessels (Fig. 464). The lamina vitrea may show basophilia or the cuticular portion is considerably thickened (Fig. 313). Fine fissures may be present in the cuticular layer, through which these sheets of fibroblasts proliferate, and extend out under the pigment epithelium. The most pronounced changes occur in the pigment epithelium, which shows degenerative changes. Some cells simply lose their pigment, while others are completely degenerated (Fig. 464). Adjacent epithelial cells proliferate moderately and appear rounded. Macrophages may appear and become heavily filled with pigment; they lie outside the rods and cones. The rods and cones in the foveal and macular area show degenerative changes, and the outer limiting membrane of the retina almost may be in contact with the lamina vitrea. Henle's fiber layer, and the outer nuclear and inner plexiform layers may show small areas of cystoid degeneration (Fig. 403–2). More advanced cases show larger cysts, often completely surrounding the fovea. If the cystic degeneration extends into the fovea a large macular cyst results (Fig. 465), the innermost wall being composed of the inner limiting membrane, and a small amount of inner retinal tissue and the outermost wall being the remainder of the retinal tissue and the external limiting membrane. Rarely the walls of the cyst disappear, leaving a macular hole which has smooth rounded edges (Fig. 465). The retina almost never detaches as a result of such hole formation because the degenerative changes in the pigment epithelium and outer retina adjacent to the macula lead to more or less firm adhesions. Also there is no traction on the margins of the retina surrounding the hole by vitreous bands. Occasionally extensive areas of retinoschisis are observed in the macula (Fig. 466).

Another type of macular degeneration, possibly a precursor of typical senile macular degeneration, has been described by Klien

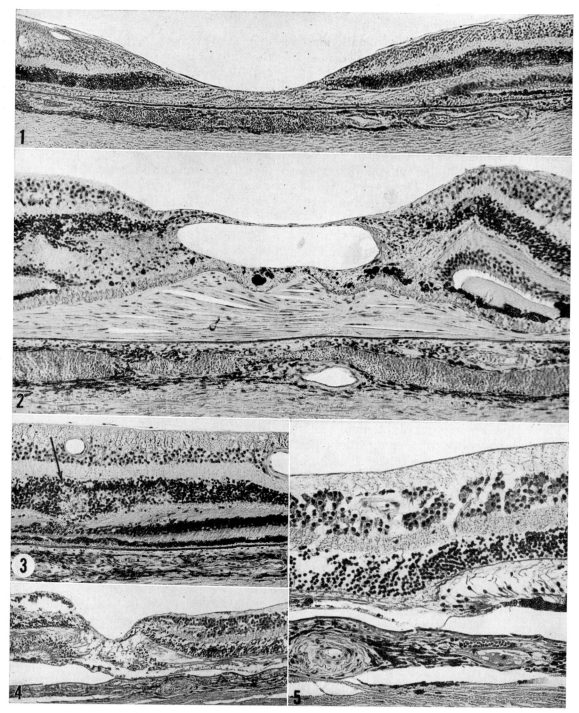

Figure 464. Senile Macular Degeneration

1. Extensive degeneration of retinal pigment epithelium and outer retinal layers of macula believed to be secondary to severe choroidal sclerosis (left eye). (Case 1 reported by Klien, 1951.)

2. Much more advanced stage of disease in macula of right eye, same case. ×130. AFIP Neg. 60–2791.

3. Periphery of macular lesion in right eye. The nest of lipoidal histiocytes (arrow) corresponds to white flecks of circinate retinopathy which had been observed clinically. (Courtesy of Dr. B. A. Klien.) ×115. AFIP Neg. 60–2648.

4 and 5. Severe degeneration of retinal pigment epithelium and outer layers of retina due to advanced sclerosis of choroidal vessels. ×80 and 180, respectively. **AFIP Acc. 911086.**

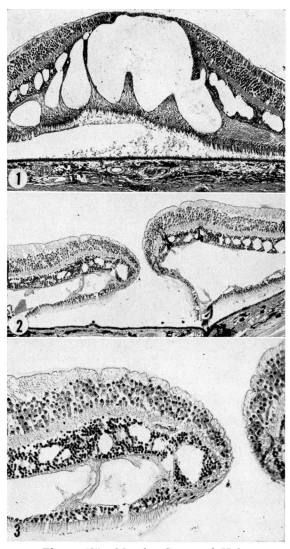

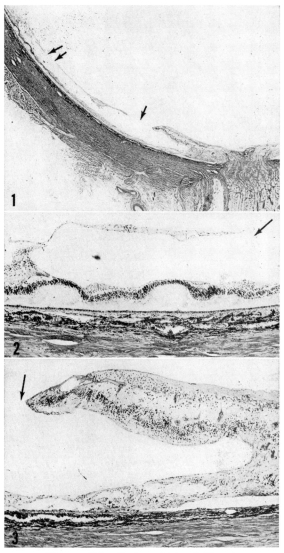

Figure 465. Macular Cysts and Holes

1. Cystic degeneration of macula. ×55. AFIP Acc. 952752.

2 and 3. Cystic degeneration of macula with hole in fovea. ×80 and ×165, respectively. AFIP Acc. 747444.

Figure 466. Retinoschisis of Macula

1. There is a broad area of confluent cystic degeneration involving the macula. The outer layers of the degenerated retina are adherent to the pigment epithelium. Several holes (arrows) are present in the very attenuated inner wall of the split retina. ×9. AFIP Acc. 937290.

2. Peripheral margin of field shown in 1. Arrow indicates a small hole in the inner wall of the split retina. ×50.

3. Central margin of same lesion. Hole indicated by arrow corresponds to position of the fovea. ×50.

and is characterized by depigmentation of the retinal epithelium in situ and degeneration of the rods and cones in a circumscribed zone in or near the fovea. The choriocapillaris may be absent in the affected area, or show extreme sclerosis.

Senile disciform degeneration. Senile disciform degeneration of the macula usually affects persons over the age of 60, and in approximately 50 per cent of cases becomes bilateral. It may appear suddenly without antecedent senile changes, and, according to Keeney and Jain, may follow senile macular degeneration in 4 per cent of cases. The sexes

are affected equally. The etiology appears to be the same as for senile macular degeneration, the choroidal vessels often showing advanced sclerosis. The choriocapillaris frequently is atrophic, with reduction in the caliber and number of vessels.

This condition commences with subretinal macular hemorrhage which may be large or

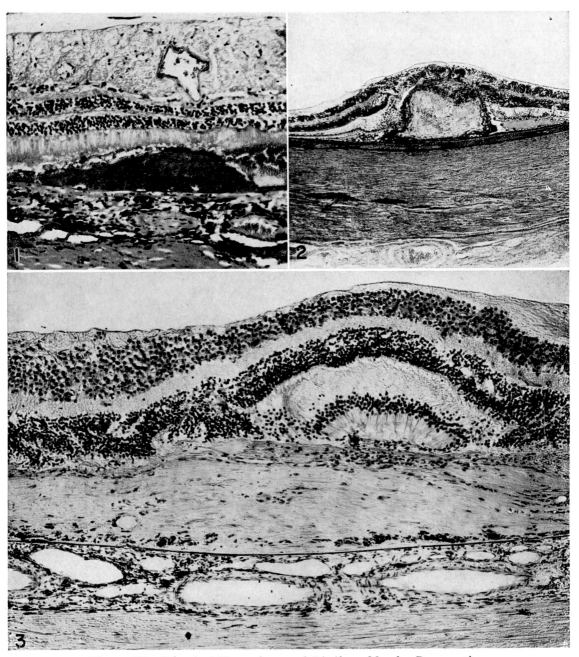

Figure 467. Subretinal Hemorrhage and Disciform Macular Degeneration

1. Hemorrhage from choriocapillaris beneath retinal pigment epithelium. ×125. AFIP Acc. 299242.
2. Organized submacular hemorrhage. ×48. AFIP Acc. 283077.
3. Submacular fibrous plaque, probably organized hemorrhage. Small breaks in Bruch's membrane. ×130 AFIP Acc. 120292.

small (Fig. 467). Larger hemorrhages penetrate the pigment epithelium and separate the retina. Even more brisk hemorrhages infiltrate the retina or even break through into the preretinal area. Subsequent events are determined by efforts of the adjacent tissues to heal the lesions and remove the blood. Eventually a large or small, elevated, pale or pigmented, macular scar is formed, leading to severe loss of macular vision.

Microscopically, there is sclerosis or obliteration of the choroidal capillaries, basophilia or marked thickening of the lamina vitrea, especially the cuticular portion, and small dehiscences in this layer. A considerable number of examinations of eyes has been

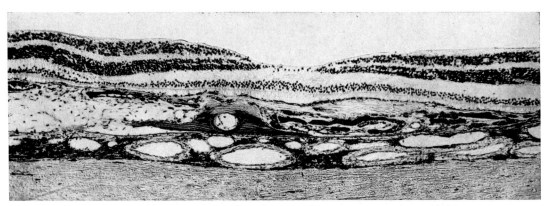

Figure 468. Disciform macular degeneration. ×55. AFIP Acc. 183551.

made in the early stages, because these eyes are suspected to have neoplasms and are enucleated. Early, there is an infiltration of fresh blood beneath the pigment epithelium, through the pigment epithelium, and into the subretinal area, with elevation of the retinal layers. Usually the blood infiltrates a considerable distance toward the disk, and a short distance around the macula. Organization of this clot occurs by proliferation of connective tissue from the choroid, mobilization of macrophages from the retina and choroid, and proliferation and alteration of the pigment epithelial cells to become macrophages (Fig. 467). A good portion of the blood cells undergo spontaneous lysis, liberating hemoglobin and its products into the coagulated plasma beneath the retina. Moderate numbers of lymphocytes are found in the clot, but inflammation is minimal throughout the process. Eventually a young scar is formed. Fibroblastic proliferation occurs from the region of the choriocapillaris through the breaks in the lamina vitrea and extends laterally along the inner surface of the cuticular layer, lifting up the epithelium (Figs. 467, 468). The epithelium may show extensive loss in the area of the lesion, and marked proliferation near its periphery. The retina is elevated by a dense layer of connective tissue which is relatively avascular, and contains large or small amounts of pigment in cells, derived either from the previous hemorrhage, or from the proliferating pigment epithelium. Metaplastic bone may also be observed in the subretinal scar (Fig. 468). The outer retinal elements are completely degenerated, and the scar is firmly fixed to the outer limiting membrane. The inner retinal ele-

ments show marked atrophy and folding. The scar may be extensive and flat, extending from the region of the disk to beyond the macula, or quite elevated and more circumscribed.

Juvenile disciform macular degeneration. The nature of this condition has not been settled. It was first described by Junius as an example of juvenile exudative macular retinitis. Two apparent forms now are considered in this category, and they may or may not be related, but often produce similar symptoms and findings. Since the one form must be differentiated from central serous retinopathy, the latter condition also is considered in this section. One type always is associated with hemorrhage from the inner choroidal vessels under the epithelium and with spread from this area to cause detachment of the retina. Vision is reduced immediately, and on ophthalmoscopic examination the vitreous is clear, and the retina is elevated by a varying-sized macular hemorrhage. Recurrences of small hemorrhages are the rule, and in about 50 per cent of cases the condition becomes bilateral. Often the lesion is displaced eccentrically from the macula and gradually extends into this area. The subsequent course is for the hemorrhage to become organized much in the same manner as has been discussed in senile disciform degeneration. Microscopic examinations have been made on quite a number of advanced lesions of this type, and the changes resemble those of the senile type. The choroid, however, shows no inflammation or evidence of vascular disease which might produce the hemorrhage. Early examinations have been done in a few cases, notably by Maumenee

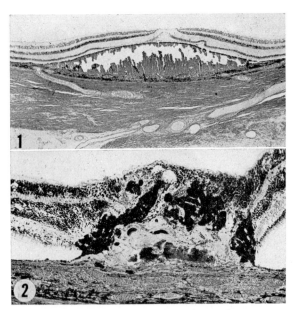

Figure 469. Submacular Hemorrhage

1. Hematoma separating pigment epithelium from Bruch's membrane and choriocapillaris. Enucleation performed because of suspected malignant melanoma of choroid. ×22. AFIP Acc. 595574.

2. Scar tissue separating proliferated pigment epithelium from choroid, possibly the end result of hematoma similar to that shown in 1. Enucleation performed because of suspected malignant melanoma of choroid. ×80. AFIP Acc. 797119.

with the observation of a hemorrhage under the pigment epithelium (Fig. 469), or one which has broken through this layer and spread beneath the retina. Those cases in which the hemorrhage remains beneath the epithelium have a better prognosis, often clearing completely. A prolonged or delayed period of healing may be associated with cystic degeneration of the macula. The prognosis in most cases for recovery of central vision is poor.

Central serous detachment. Another group of cases is characterized by a serous detachment of the macula in an area of one and one-half to two disk diameters, which persists for two to three months, and gradually subsides, leaving normal vision in more than 50 per cent of cases. It may be associated with or followed by hemorrhage. If the serous detachment persists for a long period (over six months) secondary macular degeneration often occurs. This condition most often is unilateral and affects males four times more frequently than females. Microscopically there is an accumulation of serous fluid between the choroid and the retinal pigment epithelium. The choroid itself appears normal, and there is no inflammation. Except in prolonged cases the retinal receptors are normal, and the retina itself shows no evidence of edema or degeneration. The cause of this serous outpouring of fluid is not known.

Central serous retinopathy. The condition known as central serous retinopathy, central serous chorioretinopathy, and central angiospastic retinopathy also probably comprises a number of entities, and at least three clinical types are recognized: (1) A retinal form in which vision becomes reduced in one eye, and examination shows macular edema of a type which produces a cyst-like appearance. The area of edema usually is larger than the disk, is sharply circumscribed, is elevated 1 to 2 diopters, and shows a loss of the foveal reflex. Examination with a contact lens and slit lamp microscope shows diffuse retinal edema and the inner limiting membrane is separated from the retina. Microscopic examination in one case (Klien) showed a detachment of the inner limiting membrane from the retina, retinal edema, and, possibly, separation of the pigment epithelium by serous fluid (Fig. 470). (2) A retinal form in which the patient develops hazy vision in one eye. Ophthalmoscopic examination shows a circumscribed area of retinal edema similar to that described in type (1). Contact lens and slit lamp microscope examination shows the accumulation of fluid to lie mainly in the area between the rods and cones and the pigment epithelium (Fig. 471–1). Microscopic examination shows a separation of the retina by a serous fluid. A variable amount of fluid also may lie under the pigment epithelium. The choroid shows no alteration. The prognosis in this form of the disease, as in the first type, is good if the edema does not persist too long. In most of the reported cases the vision has returned to normal or near normal. Recurrences are common and may lead to permanent damage (Fig. 471–2). (3) A type which is subretinal is similar to that described already in juvenile central serous detachment of the macula. This form was described by Walsh as idiopathic flat detachment of the macula. Early there is blurring of vision in one eye, and ophthalmoscopically a sharply localized elevated area, the size of about 2 disk diameters, is seen in the macular area. Refraction shows the eye to have become more hyperopic, and vision

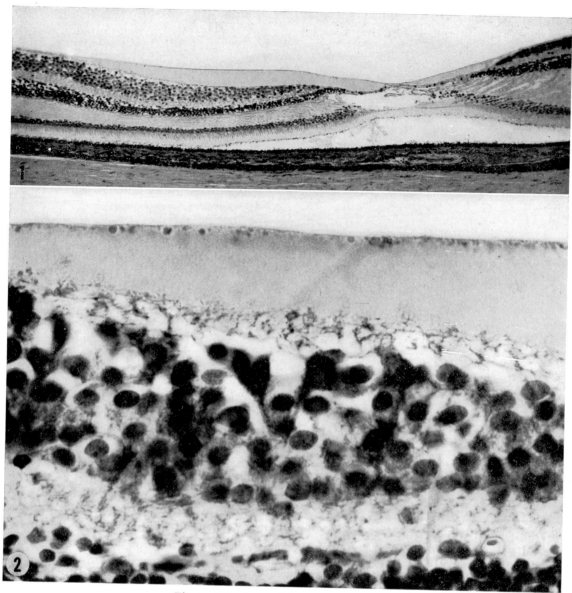

Figure 470. Central Serous Retinopathy

Intraretinal edema with serous separation of internal limiting membrane of retina from nerve fiber layer, and degeneration of foveal tissue. ×100 and ×900. (Case reported by Klien, 1956 and 1958.)

rarely corrects better than 20/40. After one to two months the lesion subsides, leaving normal vision. Recurrences are common. Microscopic examination of some cases by Maumenee and Klien shows that the choroid is normal, and the retina and its epithelium are detached by an eosinophilic serous fluid (Fig. 472). The epithelium and retinal receptors are normal.

The etiology of all these conditions is unknown, and their relationship to each other is obscure. They probably are closely related, and serous and hemorrhagic forms of the retinopathy have been seen in the same patient on different occasions. Also a patient may have the retinal type of disease at one time and the subretinal type on another.

Primary degenerations. Primary degenerations of the retina may be diffuse (retinitis pigmentosa with and without pigment, retinitis punctata albescens), or localized (macular degenerations, Doyne's choroiditis). Those which are secondary to choroidal diseases have been discussed in Chapter VII. Most are considered to be heredofamilial and genetically determined; however, many spo-

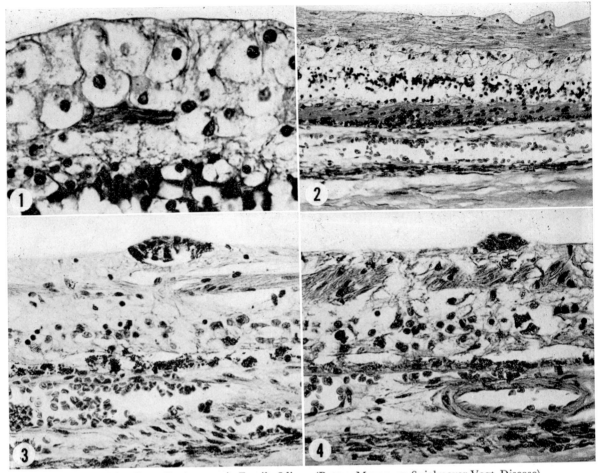

Figure 477. Juvenile Amaurotic Family Idiocy (Batten-Mayou or Spielmeyer-Vogt Disease)

1. Swollen ganglion cells in macula, similar to those observed in infantile type (see Fig. 476). ×600. AFIP Acc. 920375.

2. Other layers of macula reveal severe degenerative changes that are not observed in Tay-Sachs disease. ×195. Same case.

3 and 4. Peripheral retina reveals complete degeneration of outer retinal layers and alterations in pigment epithelium simulating those of retinitis pigmentosa. ×380. Same case.

spread damage in the brain and spinal cord, whereas in the juvenile form there is less damage to the cortex and thalamus and the spinal cord changes are milder. In general, it may be said that the earlier these diseases commence, the more severe are the nervous system and eye changes.

Spielmeyer-Vogt form. Amaurotic family idiocy of the juvenile form may occur at puberty or in late teen ages. It differs from the infantile form in that the rapidly progressive degeneration of ganglion cells does not occur; therefore, a cherry-red spot is rarely seen. The changes seen in the macula greatly resemble those previously described under heredomacular degenerations and nonfamilial macular degenerations. These cases differ from the

latter, however, in that there is development of cerebral lesions. In addition to the macular degeneration there may be peripheral pigmentation of the retina, or a diffuse fine pigmentary disturbance. The optic nerve eventually becomes pale and atrophic, and the retinal vessels much reduced in caliber. Microscopically, a most interesting feature is the primary degeneration of the retinal receptors and pigment epithelium (Fig. 477). The rods and cones partially or completely disappear, and the macula always is most affected. They are replaced by proliferating neuroglia. The retinal epithelium shows degeneration, and the liberated pigment is phagocytized. Other cells show proliferation and migration into the retina. The pattern of migration never resembles that seen in retinitis pigmentosa, however. Coincident with these retinitis-pigmentosa-like changes is a simultaneous degeneration of a lipoidal type in the retinal ganglion cells and their axons and dendrites.

Niemann-Pick type. In Niemann-Pick disease (essential lipoid histiocytosis), the eye and central nervous system develop changes which are similar to those seen in Tay-Sachs disease. In addition, there is an extensive lipoidal infiltration of the cells of all the other body organs, especially the liver and spleen. At times the central nervous system and eye show little involvement. The fundi show changes similar to those seen in infantile amaurotic family idiocy. Coincident changes may occur in the outer retina and pigment epithelium, producing a diffuse pigmentary disturbance. Microscopically there are changes in the retina characterized by an infiltration of lipoidal material into the ganglion cells, and the cells of the inner and outer nuclear layers. The glial cells of the optic nerve and nerve fiber layer also are affected, as are the cells in the choroid and episclera. The nature of the defect in metabolism which produces this condition is not known.

RETINAL DETACHMENT

From the optic disk to the ora serrata there normally are only weak attachments between the rod and cone layer and the pigment epithelium of the retina. A potential space exists here, the vestige of the central cavity of the optic vesicle in the early embryo. Accumulation of fluid within this potential space constitutes a separation of the retina. Strictly speaking, a detachment of the retina would be a detachment of the pigment epithelium from the lamina vitrea of the choroid. Usage, however, allows us to speak of a separation of the rods and cones from the pigment epithelium of the retina as a detachment of the retina. There are three major mechanisms by which such detachment can be brought about.

1. The accumulation of subretinal fluid may result from an extravasation in the retina or choroid. In retinal inflammation the accumulation of fluid beneath the retina is common. In panophthalmitis seropurulent subretinal exudation is the rule and may be massive. In less severe and more localized retinal inflammation the subretinal fluid tends to form only small pools. In choroiditis the retina over the choroidal lesion usually is necrotic and adherent to the choroid, but minor and sometimes major accumulations of subretinal fluid may surround the focal lesion.

Disturbances of the retinal and choroidal circulation commonly lead to retinal detachment. In retinal venous occlusion and in hypertensive retinopathy flat detachment of the retina is often present. Occasionally in the retinopathy of pregnancy the detachment may be extensive and bullous. In papilledema slight peripapillary detachment of the retina is often present.

Serous detachment of the choroid in cases of fistulizing wounds of the eye and in delayed healing of ocular surgical wounds usually is associated with moderate flat detachment of the retina. Massive subretinal extravasations occur in the growth of choroidal tumors. Retinal detachments occurring in the course of retinal angiomatosis (von Hippel's disease) are in part attributable to a similar mechanism.

2. The retina may be pulled away from its normal position by fibrous bands in the vitreous. Such bands arise in the organization of inflammatory exudates and of hemorrhages in the vitreous. In severe endophthalmitis the organization of exudate over the ciliary body and in the anterior vitreous leads to the formation of a cyclitic membrane. Posteriorly this membrane generally attaches to the retina near the ora serrata and its contraction commonly leads to detachment of the retina. The process can and usually does continue until the vitreous cavity has completely disappeared, the retina being completely detached, its anterior portions firmly bound onto the retrolental cyclitic membrane and its posterior portions forming a stalk extending back to the optic disk.

Organization of vitreous hemorrhages may produce much the same result. Neovascularization from the retina may lead to the formation of vascular strands extending out into the vitreous from the nerve head or elsewhere in the fundus. Contraction of these strands causes retinal detachment, which may be partial or complete. It should not be concluded that the retina is entirely inelastic and that traction invariably leads to detachment. Some stretching of the tissue can take place, and under rare conditions extensive folds may form without accumulation of subretinal fluid.

3. The third mechanism for accumulation of subretinal fluid is the escape of fluid from the vitreous into the subretinal space through a hole or tear (break) in the retina. The possible causes of retinal holes or tears are numerous. Direct contusion of the eye can be responsible although it accounts for less than 10 per cent of the cases of retinal detachment. It is an occupational hazard among prize fighters. Indirect injury, a blow on the head or a sudden jolt, often is reported in the history as a prelude to retinal detachment. The significance of such injuries is difficult to evaluate.

Spontaneous detachments and those occurring after trivial injuries are more frequent in myopic than in hyperopic eyes, also more frequent in old than in young people. In many of these cases tears and holes in the retina are readily discovered. Factors favoring the formation of tears and holes are atrophy and cystoid degeneration of the peripheral retina with adhesions between retina and vitreous. If the retina is sufficiently friable, sudden rotation of the eye may put a sufficient tug on the vitreous adhesion to cause a tear.

Retinal detachments, therefore, may be classified as follows:

1. Secondary to disease of the retina and vitreous
   a. Degeneration with hole formation
      (1) Peripheral retinal degeneration
      (2) Lattice degeneration
      (3) Peripheral cystoid degeneration
      (4) Retinoschisis
   b. Exudative
      (1) Inflammation
   c. Traumatic
   d. Circulatory
      (1) Eales' disease
      (2) Vasculitis
      (3) Hypertension

2. Secondary to disease of the choroid
   a. Exudative
      (1) Inflammations
      (2) Tumors
   b. Traumatic
   c. Circulatory
3. Secondary to general disease of the eye
   a. Hypotony
   b. Myopia

The pathogenesis of retinal detachment now is sufficiently understood that such terms as idiopathic, spontaneous, and primary can be eliminated. All detachments are secondary to some local ocular condition; the latter, in turn, may be the result of a systemic disease (e.g., diabetes, hypertension, eclampsia, etc.). If trauma, inflammation, hemorrhage, and systemic diseases are eliminated there remain a large number of detachments which are due to some obscure retinal or vitreoretinal degeneration. These detachments are more common in males (60 to 70 per cent), usually develop in the age group between 45 and 65, frequently are bilateral (20 to 30 per cent, depending on the series), and are more common in myopic than in hyperopic eyes.

Detachments due to degenerative disease occur after the development of asymptomatic retinal, chorioretinal, and chorioretinovitreal lesions. The final stage in the evolution of these lesions is the retinal hole. The exact reason for development of these presenile degenerative lesions in the retina is not known, but because of their frequency and because they principally affect certain portions of the retina, it can be concluded that some defect in nutrition or blood supply plays a part.

Peripheral cystoid degeneration. Posterior retinal degenerations already have been considered in this section. It now remains to consider those which affect the area from the equator forward. The one which is best known is *peripheral cystoid degeneration* (Blessig's cysts; Iwanoff's cysts) (Fig. 403–1). This condition probably should be considered as physiologic, even though there is variation in the findings in different eyes. Peripheral retinal cystoid degeneration has been observed in the eyes of some children, but generally it is found after the age of 20 years. The microcysts increase in number

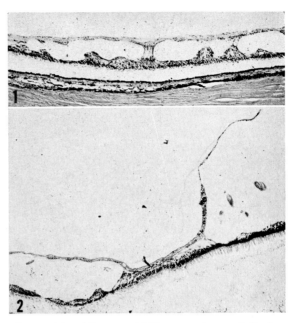

Figure 479.   Microcystoid Degeneration and Retinoschisis

1. Confluent microcystoid degeneration or early
retinoschisis. ×50. AFIP Acc. 905244.
2. More advanced stage of retinoschisis. ×50. AFIP
Acc. 858415.

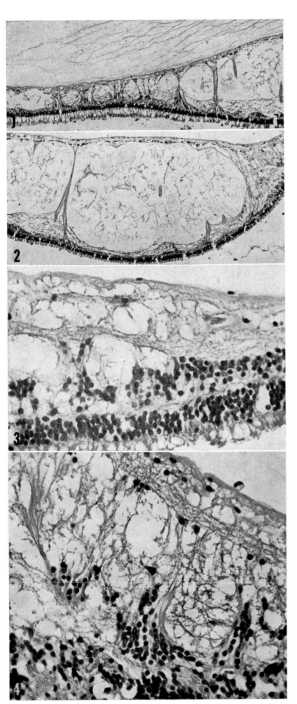

Figure 478.   Microcystoid Degeneration of Peripheral
Retina

1 and 2. Mucoid material sensitive to hyaluronidase fills the intraretinal microcysts. Alcian blue stain
for acid mucopolysaccharides. ×50. AFIP Acc.
908999.

3 and 4. Advancing edge of involved area reveals
mucoid degeneration of retinal tissue. Alcian blue.
×305.

and size, extending backward into the retina
from the ora serrata often as far as 7 mm.
They first appear immediately behind the
dentate processes of the retina at the ora
serrata as small isolated cystoid areas. They
increase in size, both by accumulation of
mucoid material (Fig. 478), and by coalescence with adjacent cysts. These cysts arise
first in the external plexiform layer, usually
encroaching upon the nuclear layers. Coalescence produces stretching of Müller's fibers,
both longitudinally as well as laterally. Eventually the cysts extend almost to the inner
and outer limiting membranes, and their
walls are formed of compressed glial fibers.
When these walls give way, the retina becomes split into two layers (Fig. 479), hence
the term, *retinoschisis*. Such cystoid degeneration is most prominent on the temporal side
of the eye, which presumably undergoes the
most stretching during development. Viewed
macroscopically in enucleated eyes, the cysts
appear as small rounded slightly translucent
areas, or as lobulated irregularly branching
tortuous channels in the peripheral retina

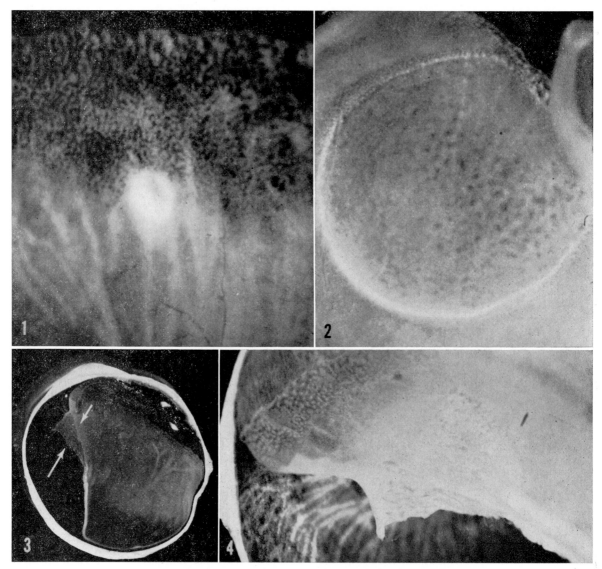

Figure 480.   Microcystoid Degeneration and Retinoschisis

1. Microcystoid degeneration has produced a series of tunnels within the peripheral retina (upper half of field); a patch of chorioretinal degeneration is present in the center of the field. (From Okun, 1960.)

2. Microcystoid degeneration and retinoschisis have led to the formation of a large hemispherical cyst in the peripheral retina; ora serrata and edge of lens are present in upper right corner. AFIP Acc. 777702.

3 and 4. Microcystoid degeneration is present along the ora serrata and on one side, indicated by arrows, there is retinoschisis. AFIP Acc. 905244.

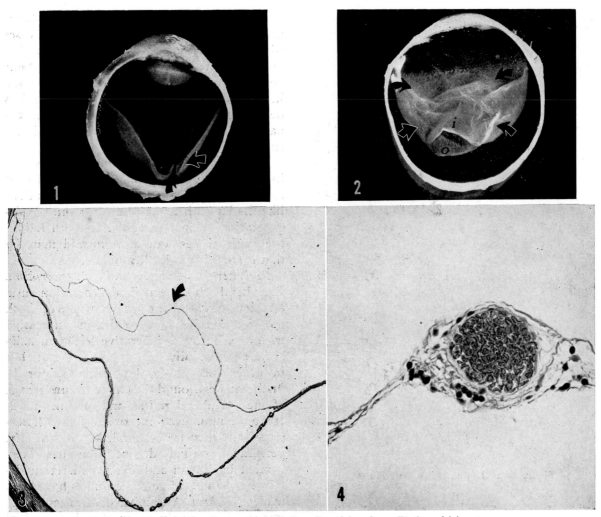

Figure 481. Large Retinal Cyst Resulting from Retinoschisis

This eye was enucleated because the macrocyst was thought to be a choroidal tumor. AFIP Acc. 858415. (Case reported by Zimmerman and Spencer, 1960.)

1. Most of the eye appeared grossly normal: arrows indicate posterior margin of area of retinoschisis.

2. The area of retinoschisis (outlined by arrows) was located in the upper temporal quadrant: i, inner layer; o, outer layer.

3 and 4. There is marked attenuation of the anterior (inner) wall of the retinal cyst through which pass the retinal blood vessels. Position of vessels shown in 4 is indicated by arrow in 3. ×7 and ×390, respectively.

(Fig. 480). They most commonly extend from the region of the dentate processes backward, and tend to be concentric with the ora, temporally.

Senile retinoschisis. Microcystoid degeneration which is observed so frequently in the peripheral retina occasionally may lead to extensive splitting of the retina, particularly on the temporal side in older persons. According to Shea et al., this senile retinoschisis frequently is bilaterally symmetrical. When the condition is unilateral or when the process is considerably more advanced on one side than on the other, Zimmerman and Spencer have found it to be confused with retinal detachment or a uveal tumor (Fig. 481). Retinoschisis may be seen in any part of the retina; however, it characteristically is found in the lower temporal periphery. It often is slowly progressive, spreading circumferentially to a much greater extent than posteriorly. Rarely is the macula involved as a result of progression from the periphery, but a similar pathologic process does occur in the macula as a rare complication of senile macular degeneration (Fig. 466).

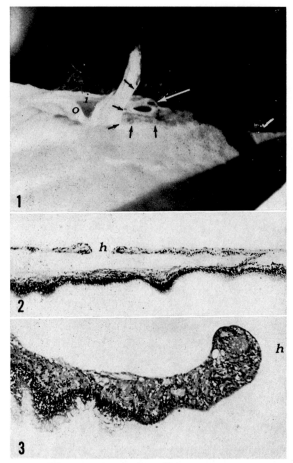

Figure 482. Retinoschisis with Holes

This eye was enucleated because the retinoschisis led to retinal detachment which simulated an intraocular tumor. AFIP Acc. 905244. (Case reported by Zimmerman and Spencer, 1960.)

1. Area of retinoschisis: i, inner layer of split retina; o, outer layer. Large white arrow indicates two of several small holes in the inner layer while the five small black arrows outline part of the single large hole in the outer layer.

2. One of the small holes (h) in the inner layer. ×50.

3. Edge of the large hole (h) in the outer layer. ×80.

PATHOLOGIC ANATOMY. Typically there is observed a broad dome-shaped sessile cyst within the retina (Fig. 481). The retinal blood vessels course through the inner layer of the split retina, and these may show severe sclerosis. Often this inner wall consists only of a very delicate glial membrane containing few nuclei, and it may have multiple small round holes (Fig. 482). The posterior layer tends to remain intact and the rods and cones are relatively well-preserved and in apposition

with the pigment epithelium. Rarely, holes may develop in this layer also. In such cases where holes form in both layers, retinoschisis may lead to retinal detachment. Even without detachment, retinoschisis produces an absolute scotoma with sharply outlined borders because the neural pathway between the visual cells and the ganglion cell layer is interrupted.

Retinoschisis is of unknown etiology but its relation to Blessig-Iwanoff cystoid degeneration of the peripheral retina suggests that, like the latter, it is the result of a mucoid degeneration related to aging. In both lesions the cystic spaces contain a mucoid material that is sensitive to hyaluronidase.

Peripheral chorioretinal degeneration. Peripheral chorioretinal degeneration usually develops after the age of forty, with both the size and incidence of lesions increasing with age. These degenerative lesions usually are seen inferiorly near the ora serrata, but in older individuals they often appear in small patches around the entire circumference of the peripheral retina, and at times reach 10 to 12 mm. from the ora serrata. Characteristically they are bilateral. Microscopically, peripheral retinal degeneration has been studied by Katzin and Teng, and recent detailed gross and microscopic studies have been made by Okun. A number of changes occur; some areas greatly resemble chorioretinal scars and others show a type of pigment degeneration at times with hole formation in the retina. The lesions resembling chorioretinal scars actually are not inflammatory foci, but appear to be due to localized areas of chorioretinal degeneration.

Macroscopically, these lesions vary from a single minute round or oval spot of complete depigmentation to large patches with irregularly scalloped edges (Fig. 483). The larger lesions usually contain some residual pigment within their centers or increased amounts of pigment about their edges.

Microscopically, the involved retina reveals sharply defined areas of degeneration often involving all layers. Characteristically there is an abrupt disappearance of the pigment epithelium, sensory cells, and the outer nuclear layer (Fig. 484). Lesser degrees of degeneration and disorganization are observed in the other layers. Usually the retinal vessels are

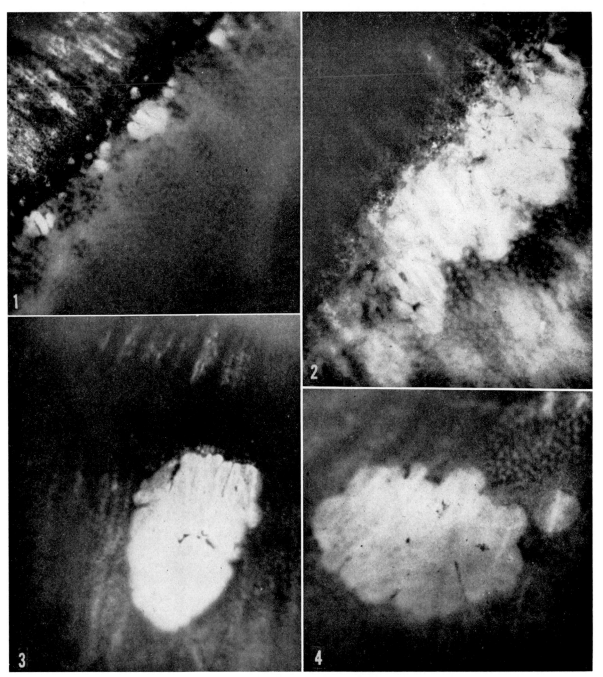

Figure 483. Peripheral Chorioretinal Degeneration

1. Small discrete spots of depigmentation just posterior to the ora serrata within an area of microcystoid degeneration.

2. Confluence of similar lesions produces a large area of depigmentation with scalloped margins.

3. Small foci containing residual pigment are present within the center of this large patch.

4. In places the scalloped margin of the large lesion reveals hyperpigmentation; the small round spot would probably have coalesced with the large patch as it grew in diameter.

(From Okun, 1960.)

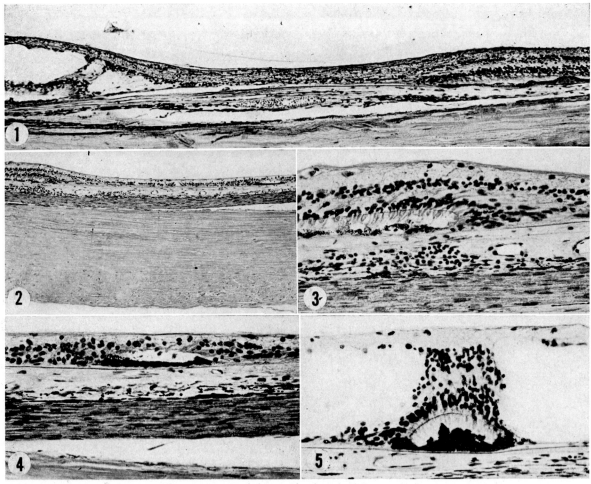

Figure 484. Peripheral Chorioretinal Degeneration

1. Microscopic appearance of discrete ovoid patch of depigmentation adjacent to larger area of peripheral microcystoid degeneration shown in Fig. 480–1. ×120. AFIP Neg. 61–07.

2. Part of lesion shown in Fig. 483–4: abrupt termination of retinal pigment epithelium and disappearance of retinal architecture. ×35. AFIP Neg. 61–11.

3. Edge of lesion shown in 2. ×220. AFIP Neg. 61–08.

4. Island of residual pigment epithelium shown in upper right corner of 2. ×220. AFIP Neg. 61–09.

5. Section through linear pigmented area in center of lesion shown in Fig. 483–3 reveals island of residual retina and pigment epithelium. Elastic stain. ×220. AFIP Neg. 60–12.

(From Okun, 1960.)

not significantly altered. The choroidal vessels, however, are extremely attenuated and often replaced by fibrous connective tissue. The choriocapillaris is generally absent throughout the lesion, and there is marked hyalinization of the choroidal stroma. Okun (1960) found these lesions to be related to aging and generalized atherosclerosis.

When there are similar alterations in the retinal vessels, the combination leads to severe chorioretinal degeneration with extreme degrees of retinal thinning (Figs. 485, 486) and hole-formation.

The vitreous usually adheres to or is firmly bound to the degenerated zone, and the inner limiting membrane is thickened (Fig. 487). Traction on these very thin, degenerated areas by the retinovitreous adhesions during movements of the eye may lead to partial or complete hole formation (Fig. 488). If one of the retinal vessels (Fig. 489) which crosses the area is torn during this process a vitreous hemorrhage may occur. The retinochoroidal adhesions may be so firm posterior to the hole that they prevent development of a detachment, but often the tear extends beyond the adhesion and a detachment develops later. This type of tear of the retina

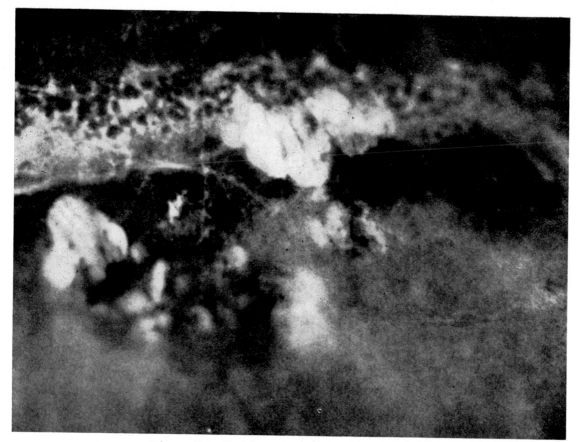

Figure 485. Peripheral Chorioretinal Degeneration

The depigmented areas are similar to those shown in Fig. 483. In the dark area (upper right) the pigment epithelium is not destroyed but the sensory retina is reduced to an extremely thin layer of cells (see Fig. 486) (From Okun, 1961.)

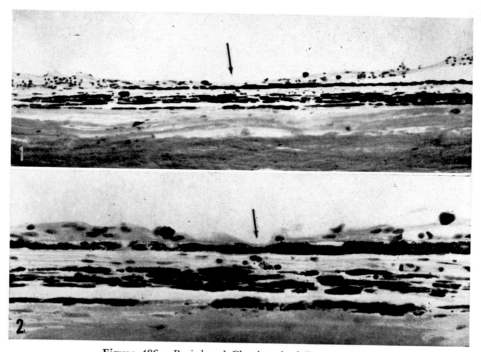

Figure 486. Peripheral Chorioretinal Degeneration

1 and 2. Microscopic examination of dark area in upper right corner of Fig. 485 reveals extreme attenuation of retina with virtual hole-formation in minute foci (arrows). ×110 and 320, respectively. (From Okun, 1961.)

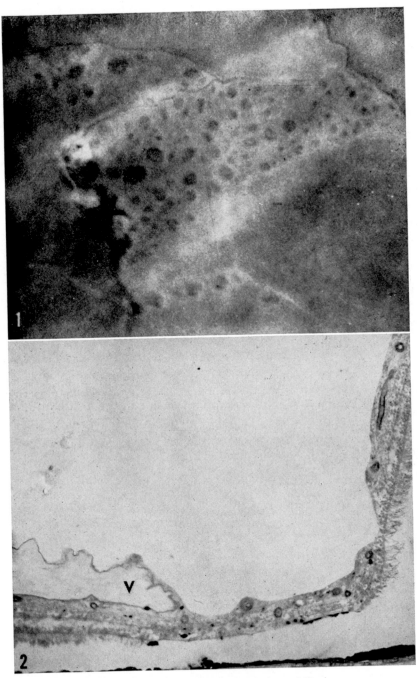

Figure 487. Peripheral Degeneration of Retina

1. The "moth-eaten" appearance of the retina is the result of marked attenuation, focally, but with incomplete hole-formation.

2. Partial hole-formation is observed on the right. In this area the thickened internal limiting membrane and portions of the degenerated inner retinal layers have been peeled off by the partially detached vitreous (V). (From Okun, 1961.)

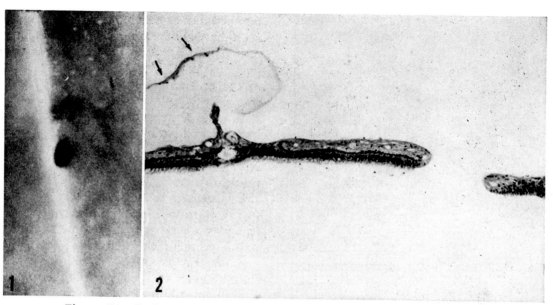

Figure 488. Retinal Degeneration, Vitreous Detachment, and Hole Formation

1. Small round hole in peripheral retina found at autopsy; no detachment. Photographed with Noyori slit beam.

2. Microscopic examination of same hole reveals detachment of vitreous over the hole; small amount of retinal tissue peeled off with vitreous is indicated by arrows.

(From Okun, 1961.)

leads to arrowhead or horseshoe types of tear, with the convexity of the horseshoe toward the disk, and the operculum (the retina in the concavity of the tear) pulled inward by a vitreous traction band on the distal (ora serrata) concave side (Figs. 489, 490). Most of these tears occur in the upper retina (90 per cent), especially temporally. At times a combination of traction forward by a vitreous band and traction backward by retinal degeneration and the retinal vessels leads to stellate, round (Fig. 491), or other type holes. The horseshoe tear is one of the most common types of retinal hole, and is a frequent cause of retinal detachment. This particular type of presenile or senile retinovitreal degeneration, therefore, probably is the cause of most retinal detachments. It is not certain why this type of degeneration should affect the peripheral retina, choroid, and vitreous, but a combination of abnormal attachment of the base of the vitreous to the inner limiting membrane, thinning and loss of the nerve fiber layer in the peripheral retina, general attenuation of the neural and supporting cells, poor vascular supply, and greater movement of the upper vitreous during downward movements of the eye may lead to the changes described. The thickening of the cuticular portion of the lamina vitrea and adhesions between the retina and choroid probably result from all these factors.

Lattice degenerations. Lattice degeneration of the retina is characterized by patches of fine gray lines which intersect each other at irregular intervals in the peripheral retina (Fig. 492). These areas of degeneration may be localized or gradually form moderately broad bands in the retina, concentric with the ora serrata. Within the affected area there may be associated changes in pigmentation, and the retina appears atrophic. Microscopically, the retina and vitreous are extremely degenerated, and the vessels which pass through the area have thickened hyalinized walls and lumina which are obliterated (Fig. 492).

Dialysis. Disinsertion or dialysis of the retina from its attachment to the ora serrata may occur spontaneously as a consequence of atrophy of the peripheral retina and cystoid

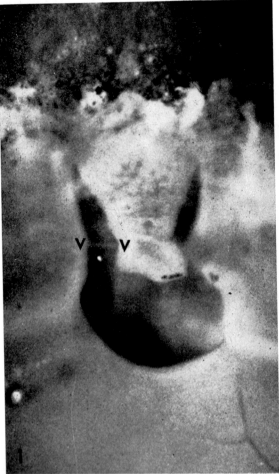

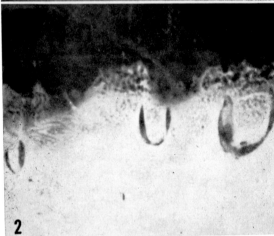

Figure 489. Horseshoe-Shaped Tears (Flap Tears) in Peripheral Retina

1. The base of the flap is close to the ora serrata while the convexity of the horseshoe is directed posteriorly. A vessel (V-V) bridges the tear on one side (see Fig. 490–1). There is evidence of microcystoid degeneration in the flap and some proliferated pigment epithelium remains attached to the free end of the flap (see Fig. 490–2). (From Okun, 1961.)

2. Three flap tears of peripheral retina. AFIP Acc. 957714.

degeneration or develop as a result of trauma. Most dialyses develop in the inferior temporal retina, the thinnest and least developed portion, but disinsertion related to contusion of the eye may occur in the superior nasal sector.

Vitreous degeneration plays a part in retinal detachment. Vitreous degeneration and detachment are discussed in detail in Chapter X. Vitreo-retinal adhesions, which occur as a result of peripheral retinal degeneration, lattice degeneration, and small unrecognized foci of chorioretinitis in childhood and adult life, play a great part in development of retinal detachment. Small foci of healed chorioretinitis and peripheral retinal degeneration may be associated with defects in the inner limiting membrane, and thin strands of fibroblasts can be seen to extend from the retinal stroma into the bands. These are particularly visible in microscopic sections through holes, where the operculum can be seen to be adherent to the strand by a delicate fibrous band.

Once hole formation has been accomplished the development of detachment depends on passage of fluid from the vitreous through the hole, where it accumulates under the retina. Movements of the eye, the inertia of the vitreous and subretinal fluid, and continued movement of fluid through the hole produces more and more detachment. A detachment may become localized when there is sufficient friction or irritation to produce a proliferation of the pigment epithelium. Metaplasia of these cells produces a fibrous adhesion to the retina, and may prevent further detachment. The momentum of the eye or continued vitreous traction may loosen the adhesion, allowing more retina to become detached. Succeeding friction lines may produce a series of concentric lines as the retina pulls away. It is of interest that the retina overlying these friction lines is atrophic and most of the neural and supporting cells have disappeared. New holes may form at a friction line because of this atrophy. Complete detachment almost always occurs if treatment is not instituted.

The changes which occur in detached retinas are of importance and have a profound influence on the success of corrective surgery. The retina has a high rate of metabolism, which is supported by the central artery and

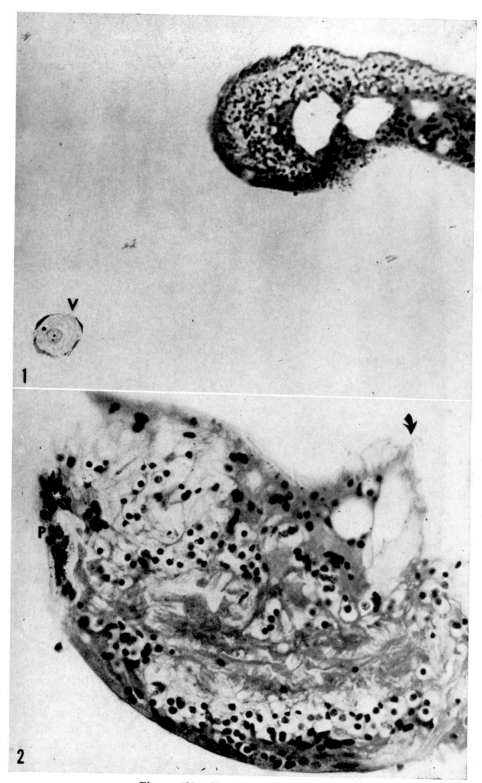

Figure 490. Horseshoe-Shaped Tear

1. Section through lateral edge of flap and vessel (V) bridging hole (same lesion shown in Fig. 489–1). ×200.

2. Section through posterior tip of flap in area containing pigmented line (see Fig. 489–1). Free edge is at upper left where proliferated pigment epithelium (P) is present. Tenting of inner surface of flap (arrow) is produced by traction of adherent vitreous. ×350.

(From Okun, 1961.)

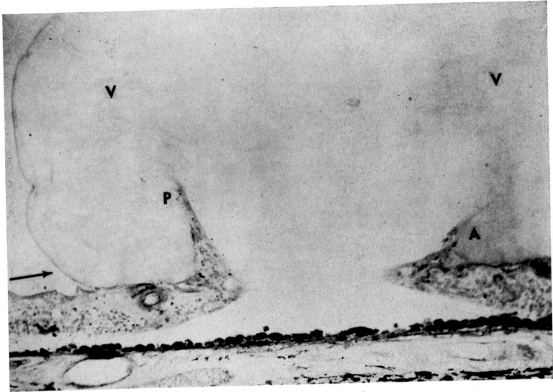

Figure 491. Round Hole Near Ora Serrata

Incidental observation at autopsy; no detachment of retina. The vitreous (V) is firmly adherent to both the anterior (A) and posterior (P) edges of the hole in the peripheral retina but is detached posteriorly (arrow). ×130. (From Okun, 1961.)

choriocapillaris of the choroid. Detachment separates the outer layers from the region of choriocapillaris, hence from their immediate source of nourishment. The subretinal fluid contains some nutriments, but as time passes secondary changes occur in the subretinal fluid and choroid, and the outer retina suffers. The macula appears to be most susceptible, undergoing cystic changes and degeneration of the rods and cones if it is separated from the choroid for more than four to six weeks. The retina elsewhere also tends to become edematous and atrophic, particularly in the outer layers, after two to three months detachment. Microcystoid degeneration first occurs, followed by coalescence of the cystoid spaces to form larger and larger cysts (Fig. 493). These cysts produce the orange peel effect seen clinically in a detachment of longstanding. A certain amount of glial and connective tissue proliferation also occurs in detached retinas, and this results in shortening of the retina so that instead of having a bullous appearance it becomes more

flattened and tightly stretched between the ora serrata and disk. At other times the deep folds between bullae become adherent to each other, leading to fixation of the retina in this position. Microscopic examination shows minute interruptions of the internal limiting membrane in such cases with proliferation of thin layers of fibroblasts from the retina along the inner surface to unite two folds. All this tends to create further shortening of the retina.

The choroid often shows rather marked degenerative changes in longstanding detachments. Proliferative and degenerative changes in the pigment epithelium, thickening of the lamina vitrea, and formation of drusen (Fig. 494) are generally observed. The walls of the vessels in the choriocapillaris become hyalinized.

When the retina has been detached for some time marked degenerative changes occur, and the shortening and folding produces a complete funnel-shaped detachment. Often the folding and proliferation of glia obliter-

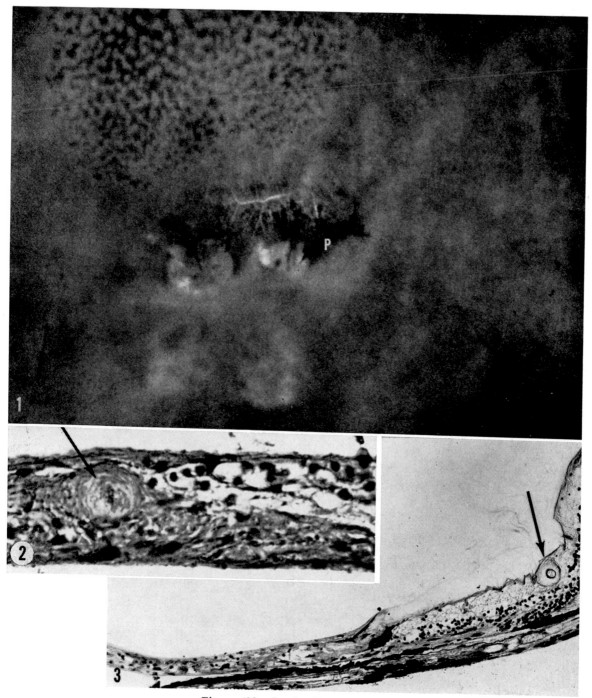

Figure 492. Lattice Degeneration

1. Lattice degeneration is the result of severe sclerosis of retinal vessels. The small white vessels in center of field can be traced to the large patent vessel in the lower right corner. Perivascular pigmentation (P) and white areas of retinal degeneration are also observed in the center of the field while at the far periphery (upper half of field) there is marked cystoid degeneration.

2 and 3. Sections from same lesion reveal severe chorioretinal degeneration with extensive sclerosis and obliteration of retinal blood vessels (arrows). ×500 and ×185, respectively.

(From Okun. 1961.)

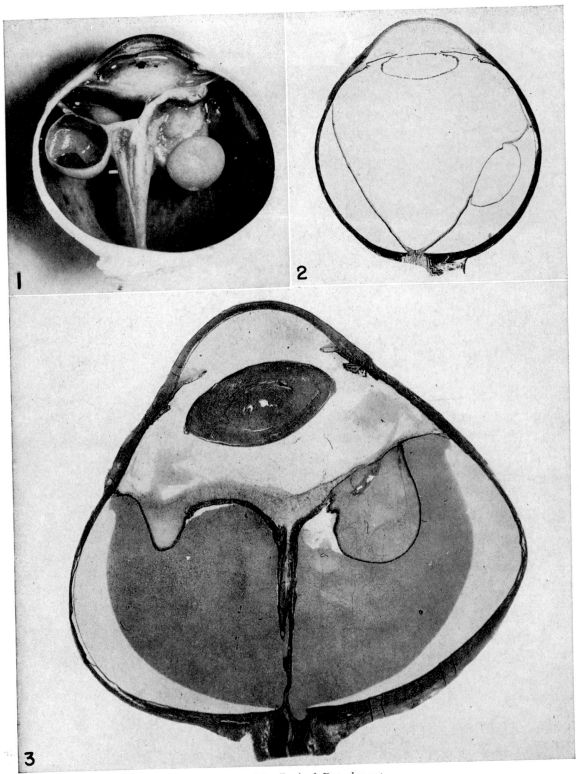

Figure 493.   Retinal Detachment

1. Macrocystoid degeneration of detached retina. AFIP Acc. 309727.
2. Macrocystoid degeneration of detached retina. AFIP Acc. 200201.
3. Serous detachment and macrocystoid degeneration of retina in a glaucomatous eye. AFIP Acc. 41828.

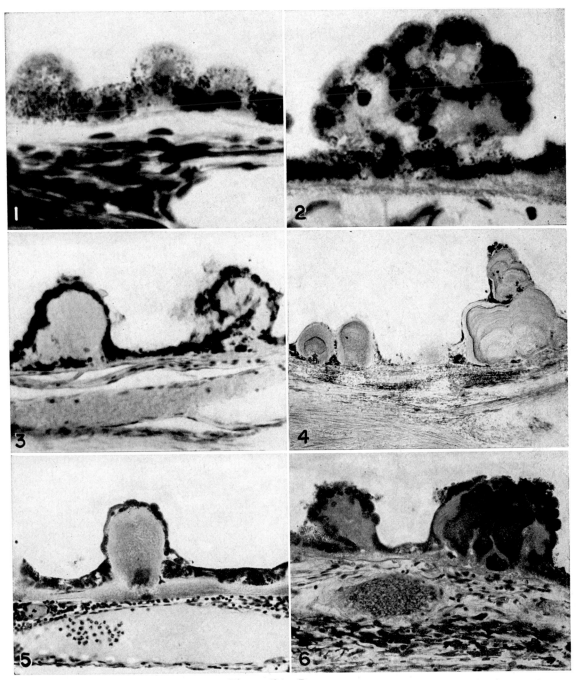

Figure 494. Drusen

1. Early swelling of retinal pigment epithelial cells. ×1050. AFIP Acc. 50725.

2. Proliferation of retinal pigment epithelial cells. ×800. AFIP Acc. 50725.

3. Accumulation of colloid material secreted by pigment epithelial cells, forming excrescences (drusen) on Bruch's membrane. ×420. AFIP Acc. 51052.

4. Old laminated excrescences containing calcium deposits. Epithelial cells have disappeared. ×40. AFIP Acc. 23440.

5. Excrescence with calcium at base. Atrophy of overlying epithelium. ×500. AFIP Acc. 52733.

6. Calcified drusen on Bruch's membrane. ×250. AFIP Neg. 67233.

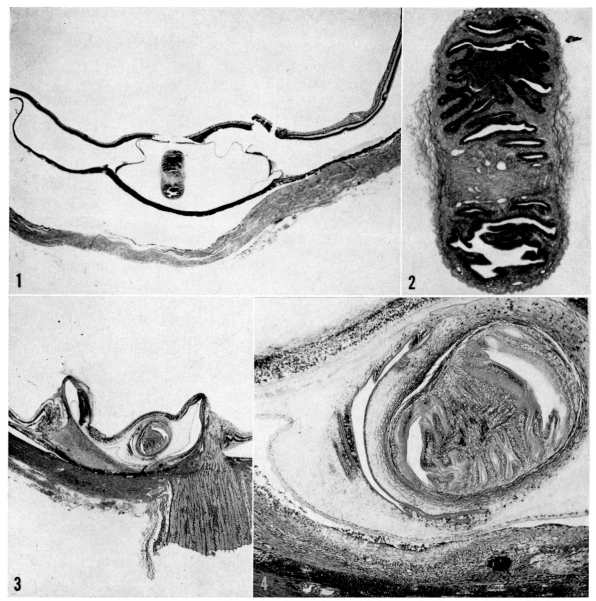

Figure 495. Subretinal Cysticercus

1 and 2. The parasite appears viable and there is minimal inflammatory reaction. (From Kirk and Petty, 1956.)
3 and 4. The parasite in this case has incited a marked inflammatory reaction in the retina and choroid. ×8 and ×50, respectively. AFIP Acc. 229753.

ate the holes and the subretinal fluid is trapped. In this case the choroid also has developed degenerative changes and is incapable of removing the fluid. Macrophages, proliferating pigment cells, cholesterol crystals from small hemorrhages, and toxic products accumulate in the fluid, act as irritants, and produce secondary uveitis. Secondary glaucoma may develop as a result of this uveitis and lead to enucleation. Hemorrhages are common from the degenerating retina and choroid, further leading to inflammation.

Retinal detachment due to trauma may have a varied pathogenesis. At times a contusion produces a macular hole and detachment. Inferior temporal dialyses of the retina at the ora serrata often are due to trauma. Localized areas of chorioretinitis may be produced by trauma, and have vitreous adhesions which later produce holes by traction. Foreign bodies may lodge in the retina, produce scars, and later detachment by the same mechanism. Vitreous hemorrhage may result in membrane formation, traction

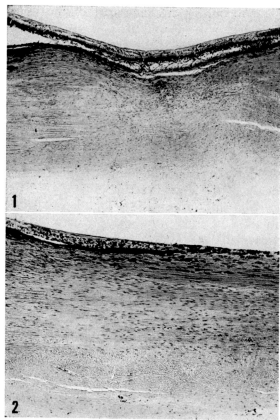

Figure 496. Chorioretinal and Scleral Scarring following Perforating Diathermy

1. ×50. AFIP Acc. 743282.
2. ×115. AFIP Acc. 743282.

bands, and tent-like detachments. Hemorrhagic detachments may be due to the trauma of surgery of an eye already predisposed to retinal hole formation. At other times spontaneous choroidal hemorrhages occur following surgery, leading to serous detachment of the retina. Hypotony following glaucoma and cataract surgery may be followed by choroidal and retinal detachment of a serous type. Loss of vitreous during surgery leads to detachment by formation of traction bands (see Chapter X). Discissions of congenital cataracts are particularly apt to lead to subsequent detachment.

Most detachments follow injuries of a minor type, such as a sudden jar, a bump on the head, an unusual strain, or a sudden movement, and probably produce the detachment by the mechanisms described previously. Most often it is difficult to correlate the injury with the detachment, but those detachments which follow minor injuries or a sudden strain often are accompanied by a

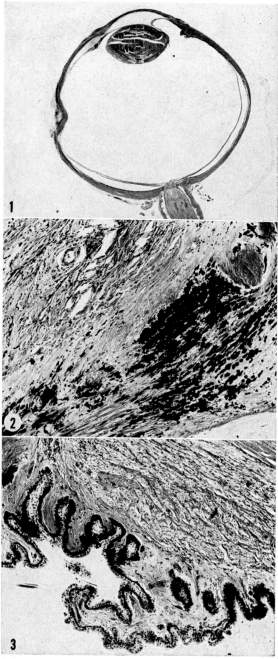

Figure 497. Reattachment of Retina by Perforating Diathermy

1. Necrosis and postnecrotic scarring in episclera, sclera, choroid, and retina in equatorial region. The anterior uvea on the same side shows severe necrosis. ×3. AFIP Acc. 634398.
2. Necrosis of ciliary body on treated side. ×80.
3. Viable ciliary body on opposite side. ×80.
(Case reported by Wilson and Irvine, 1955.)

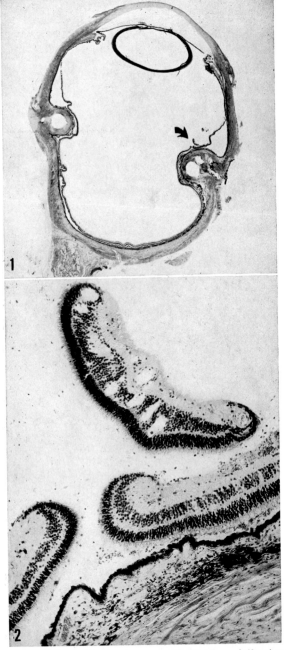

Figure 498. Reattachment of Retina following Scleral Buckling with Circling Polyethylene Tube

1. Postmortem specimen obtained 5 days after operation: arrow indicates retinal hole and operculum. ×4.

2. Same area indicated by arrow in 1. ×100. AFIP Acc. 958422.

(From Boniuk and Zimmerman, 1961; courtesy of Dr. H. Q. Kirk.)

sudden flashing in some part of the visual field when the tear forms.

Inflammations of the eye produce detachments either of a serous type (choroiditis of the Harada form), or by formation of vitreous bands (cyclitic membrane) which produce traction on the peripheral retina. The detachment due to minor foci of chorioretinitis already has been discussed. Infections with parasites such as Cysticercus may produce detachment of an exudative type following death of the organism (Fig. 495).

Following surgery for retinal detachment a number of interesting changes occur in the treated tissues (Figs. 346, 496 to 498). Those cases treated with nonperforating diathermy show localized areas of scleral necrosis early, followed by infiltration with inflammatory cells and scarring. Often it is difficult to find the scar in late cases. The choroid shows similar changes, with localized necrosis of the stromal cells and melanocytes, edema and infiltration by lymphocytes and plasma cells, and subsequent fibroblastic repair. The pigment epithelium degenerates in the affected area and proliferates in adjacent areas. The choroiditis is transmitted to the adjacent retina which becomes fastened to the choroid by adhesions. The cells forming the adhesion most often are derived by metaplasia from the pigment epithelium.

REFERENCES

Ashton, N.: Vascular Changes in Diabetes with Particular Reference to Retinal Vessels. Brit. J. Ophthal. *33*:407–420, 1949.

Ashton, N.: Arteriolar Involvement in Diabetic Retinopathy. Brit. J. Ophthal. *37*:282–292, 1953.

Ashton, N.: Retinal Vascularization in Health and Disease. Amer. J. Ophthal. *44*:7–17, 1957.

Ashton, N.: Diabetic Micro-Angiopathy. Adv. Ophthal. *8*:1–84, 1958.

Ashton, N.: Diabetic Retinopathy; a New Approach. Lancet *2*:625–630, 1959.

Ashton, N.: Larval Granulomatosis of the Retina Due to Toxocara. Brit. J. Ophthal. *44*:129–148, 1960.

Ashton, N., Ward, B., and Serpell, G.: Effect of Oxygen on Developing Retinal Vessels with Particular Reference to the Problem of Retrolental Fibroplasia. Brit. J. Ophthal. *38*:397–432, 1954.

Ballantyne, A. J., and Loewenstein, A.: The Pathology of Diabetic Retinopathy. Trans. Ophthal. Soc. U. K. *63*:95–115. 1943.

Ballantyne, A. J., and Loewenstein, A.: Retinal Microaneurysms and Punctate Haemorrhages. Brit. J. Ophthal. *28*:593–598, 1944.

Ballantyne, A. J., and Michaelson, I. C.: Some Aspects of Disease Affecting the Retinal Veins. Trans. Ophthal. Soc. U. K. 67:59–81, 1947.

Benedict, W. L., and Parkhill, E. M.: Glioma of Retina in Successive Generations. Amer. J. Ophthal. 26:511–521, 1943.

Boles, W. M., Naugle, T. C., and Samson, C. L. M.: Glioma of the Optic Nerve; Report of a Case Arising from the Optic Disc. A.M.A. Arch. Ophthal. 59:229–231, 1958.

Boniuk, M., and Zimmerman, L. E.: Necrosis of the Iris, Ciliary Body, Lens, and Retina following Scleral Buckling Operations with Circling Polyethylene Tubes. Trans. Amer. Acad. Ophthal. Otolaryng. 65:671–693, 1961.

Boniuk, M., and Zimmerman, L. E.: Necrosis of Uvea, Sclera, and Retina Following Operations for Retinal Detachment. A.M.A. Arch. Ophthal., 66:318–326, 1961.

Burns, R.: Cytomegalic Inclusion Disease Uveitis. A.M.A. Arch. Ophthal. 61:376–387, 1959.

Callahan, A., and Klien, B. A.: Thermal Detachment of the Anterior Lamella of the Anterior Lens Capsule; a Clinical and Histopathologic Study. A.M.A. Arch. Ophthal. 59:73–80, 1958.

Campbell, F. W.: The Influence of a Low Atmospheric Pressure on the Development of the Retinal Vessels on the Rat. Trans. Ophthal. Soc. U. K. 71:287–300, 1951.

Christensen, L.: The Nature of the Cytoid Body. Trans. Amer. Ophthal. Soc. 56:451–473, 1958.

de Buen, S.: Retinoblastoma; with Spread by Direct Continuity to the Contralateral Optic Nerve: Report of a Case. Amer. J. Ophthal. 49:815–819, 1960.

Duke, J. R., and Maumenee, A. E.: An Unusual Tumor of the Retinal Pigment Epithelium. Amer. J. Ophthal. 47:311–317, 1959.

Duke-Elder, W. S.: Text-book of Ophthalmology. Vol. III, St. Louis, C. V. Mosby Co., 1941, pp. 2610–2612.

Fair, J. R.: Tumors of the Retinal Pigment Epithelium. Amer. J. Ophthal. 45:495–505, 1958.

Falls, H. F., and Neel, J. V.: Genetics of Retinoblastoma. A.M.A. Arch. Ophthal. 46:367–389, 1951.

Fine, B. S.: Limiting Membranes of the Sensory Retina and Pigment Epithelium: An Electron Microscopic Study. To be published.

Fine, B. S., and Tousimis, A. J.: The Structure of the Vitreous Body and the Suspensory Ligaments of the Lens. A.M.A. Arch. Ophthal. 65:95–110, 1961.

Flexner, S.: A Peculiar Glioma (Neuroepithelioma?) of the Retina. Bull. Johns Hopkins Hosp. 2:115–119, 1891.

Foerster, H. C.: In Maumenee, A. E.: Uveitis Symposium, Survey Ophthal. 4:296–299, No. 3 (Pt. II), 1959.

Fralick, F. B., and Wilder, H. C.: Intraocular Diktyoma and Glioneuroma. Trans. Amer. Ophthal. Soc. 47:317–324, 1949.

Friedenwald, J. S.: Ocular Lesions in Fetal Syphilis. Bull. Johns Hopkins Hosp. 46:185–202, 1930.

Friedenwald, J. S.: A New Approach to some Problems of Retinal Vascular Disease. The Jackson Memorial Lecture. Amer. J. Ophthal. 32:487–498, 1949.

Grinker, R. R.: Gliomas of the Retina; Including the Results of Studies with Silver Impregnations. A.M.A. Arch. Ophthal. 5:920–935, 1931.

Guyton, T. B., et al.: New Observations in Generalized Cytomegalic Inclusion Disease of the Newborn. New England J. Med. 257:803–807, 1957.

Herm, R. J., and Heath, P.: A Study of Retinoblastoma. Amer. J. Ophthal. 41:22–30, 1956.

Hoeve, J. van der: Phakomatoses. In Ridley, F., and Sorsby, A.: Modern Trends in Ophthalmology, Vol. 1, New York, Paul B. Hoeber, Inc., 1940, pp. 124–131.

Junius, P.: Erscheinungsformen und Ablauf der Juvenilen Retinitis exsudativa macularis. Ztschr. f. Augenh. 70:129–148, 1930.

Keeney, A. H., and Jain, M.: Macular Disease of Involutional Type: Classification and Therapeutic Approaches. Trans. Amer. Ophthal. Soc. 56:247–262, 1958.

Kirk, H. Q., and Petty, R. W.: Malignant Melanoma of the Choroid; a Correlation of Clinical and Histological Findings. A.M.A. Arch. Ophthal. 56:843–860, 1956.

Klien, B.: The Heredodegeneration of the Macula Lutea. Amer. J. Ophthal. 33:371–379, 1950.

Klien, B.: Macular Lesions of Vascular Origin. Amer. J. Ophthal. 34:1279–1289, 1951.

Klien, B.: Macular Lesions of Various Origin. Part II. Functional Vascular Conditions Leading to Damage of the Macula Lutea. Amer. J. Ophthal. 36:1–13, 1953.

Klien, B.: Retinal Lesions Associated with Uveal Disease: Part I. Amer. J. Ophthal. 42:831–847, 1956.

Klien, B.: Diseases of the Macula. A.M.A. Arch. Ophthal. 60:175–186, 1958.

Kuhlenbeck, H., and Haymaker, W.: Neuroectodermal Tumors Containing Neoplastic Neuronal Elements: Ganglioneuroma, Spongioneuroblastoma, and Glioneuroma. Mil. Surgeon 99:273–304, 1946.

Kuwabara, T., Cogan, D. G., Futterman, S., Kinoshita, J. H.: Dehydrogenases in the Retina and Müller's Fibers. J. Histochem. Cytochem. 7:67–68, 1959.

Larsen, H. W.: Diabetic Retinopathy, Acta Ophthal. 38, Suppl. 60. 1960.

McFarland, C. B.: Heredodegeneration of the Macula Lutea. A Study of the Clinical and Pathologic Aspects. A.M.A. Arch. Ophthal. 53:224–228, 1955.

Maumenee, A. E.: Serous and Hemorrhagic Disciform Detachment of the Macula. Trans. Pacif. Coast. Oto-ophthal. Soc. 40:139–160, 1959.

Meyer-Schwickerath, G.: Light Coagulation. Transl. by S. M. Drance. St. Louis, C. V. Mosby, 1960.

Nichols, R. L.: The Etiology of Visceral Larva Migrans. I. Diagnostic Morphology of Infective Second-stage Toxocara Larvae. J. Parasit. 42:349–362, 1956.

Okun, E.: Gross and Microscopic Pathology in Autopsy Eyes. Part I. Introduction and Long Posterior Ciliary Nerves. Amer. J. Ophthal. 50:424–429, 1960. Part II. Peripheral Chorioretinal Atrophy. Amer. J. Ophthal. 50:574–583, 1960. Part III. Retinal Breaks without Detachment. Amer. J. Ophthal. 51:369–391, 1961.

Parkhill, E. M., and Benedict, W. L.: Gliomas of the

Retina. A Histopathologic Study. Amer. J. Ophthal. 24:1354–1373, 1941.

Patz, A.: Oxygen Studies in Retrolental Fibroplasia. IV. Clinical and Experimental Observations. Amer. J. Ophthal. 38:291–308, 1954.

Reese, A. B.: Frequency of Retinoblastoma in the Progeny of Parents Who Have Survived the Disease. A.M.A. Arch. Ophthal. 52:815–818, 1954.

Reese, A. B.: Telangiectasia of the Retina and Coats' Disease. Amer. J. Ophthal. 42:1–8, 1956.

Reese, A. B.: Atlas of Tumor Pathology, Section X, Fascicle 38, Washington, D. C., Armed Forces Institute of Pathology, 1956.

Reese, A. B., and Jones, I. S.: Benign Melanoma of the Retinal Pigment Epithelium. Amer. J. Ophthal. 42: 207–212, 1956.

Reese, A. B., and Stepanik, J.: Cicatricial Stage of Retrolental Fibroplasia. Amer. J. Ophthal. 38:308–316, 1954.

Reese, A. B., and Straatsma, B. R.: Retinal Dysplasia. Amer. J. Ophthal. 45:199–211, 1958.

Remington, J. S., Jacobs, L., and Kaufman, H. E.: Studies on Chronic Toxoplasmosis. The Relation of Infective Dose to Residual Infection and to the Possibility of Congenital Transmission. Amer. J. Ophthal. 46:261–268, 1958.

Sabin, A. B., and Feldman, H. A.: Chorioretinopathy Associated with Other Evidence of Cerebral Damage in Childhood. A Syndrome of Unknown Etiology Separable from Congenital Toxoplasmosis. J. Pediat. 35:296–309, 1949.

Shea, M., Schepens, C. L., and von Pirquet, S. R.: Retinoschisis. I. Senile Type: A Clinical Report of One Hundred Seven Cases. A.M.A. Arch. Ophthal. 63:1–9, 1960.

Sidman, R. L.: Histochemical Studies on Photoreceptor Cells. Trans. N. Y. Acad. Sci. 74:182–195, 1958.

Szirmai, J. A., and Balazs, E. A.: Studies on the Structure of the Vitreous Body. III. Cells in the Cortical Layer. A.M.A. Arch. Ophthal. 59:34–48, 1958.

Teng, C. C., and Katzin, H. M.: An Anatomic Study of the Periphery of the Retina. Part I. Nonpigmented Epithelial Cell Proliferation and Hole Formation. Amer. J. Ophthal. 34:1237–1248, 1951.

Teng, C. C., and Katzin, H. M.: An Anatomic Study of the Peripheral Retina. II. Peripheral Cystoid Degeneration of the Retina; Formation of Cysts and Holes. Amer. J. Ophthal. 36:29–39, 1953.

Teng, C. C., and Katzin, H. M.: An Anatomic Study of the Peripheral Retina. III. Congenital Retinal Rosettes. Amer. J. Ophthal. 36:169–185, 1953.

Theobald, G. D.: Cytomegalic Inclusion Disease: Report of a Case. Amer. J. Ophthal. 47:52–56, 1959.

Theobald, G. D.: Acute Tuberculous Endophthalmitis: Report of a Case. Amer. J. Ophthal. 45:403–407, 1958.

Verhoeff, F. H., and Jackson, E.: Minutes of the Pro-

ceedings, Sixty-Second Annual Meeting. Trans. Amer. Ophthal. Soc. 24:33–34, 38–43, 1926.

Virchow, R.: Die Krankhaften Geschwülste. Vol. 2. Berlin, Hirschwald, 1864–65, p. 151.

Walsh, F. B., and Sloan, L. L.: Idiopathic Flat Detachment of the Macula. Amer. J. Ophthal. 19:195–208, 1936.

Weller, C. V.: The Inheritance of Retinoblastoma and Its Relationship to Practical Eugenics. Cancer Research 1:517–535, 1941.

Wilder, H. C.: Nematode Endophthalmitis. Trans. Amer. Acad. Ophthal. Otolaryng. 54:99–109, 1950.

Willis, R. A.: Pathology of Tumours. St. Louis, C. V. Mosby, 1948.

Wilson, W. A., and Irvine, S. R.: Pathologic Changes following Disruption of Blood Supply to Iris and Ciliary Body. Trans. Amer. Acad. Ophthal. Otolaryng. 59:501–502, 1955.

Wintersteiner, H.: Das Neuroepithelioma Retinae. Eine Anatomische und Klinische Studie. Leipzig, F. Deuticke, 1897.

Wolter, J. R.: The Human Optic Papilla: A Demonstration of New Anatomic and Pathologic Findings. Amer. J. Ophthal. 44:(Part II) 48–65, 1957.

Wolter, J. R.: Perivascular Glia of the Blood Vessels of the Human Retina. Amer. J. Ophthal. 44:766–773, 1957.

Wolter, J. R.: Pathology of a Cotton-wool Spot. Amer. J. Ophthal. 48:473–485, 1959.

Wolter, J. R., and Liss, L.: The Evolution of Hyaline Corpuscles (Cytoid Bodies) in the Human Optic Nerve. Amer. J. Ophthal. 43:885–892, 1957.

Wolter, J. R., Goldsmith, R. I., and Phillips, R. L.: Histopathology of the Star-Figure of the Macular Area in Diabetic and Angiospastic Retinopathy. A.M.A. Arch. Ophthal. 57:376–385, 1957.

Wolter, J. R., Phillips, R. L., and Butler, R. G.: The Star Figure of the Macular Area; Histopathologic Study of a Case of Angiospastic (Hypertensive) Retinopathy. A.M.A. Arch. Ophthal. 60:49–59, 1958.

Zimmerman, L. E.: Demonstration of Hyaluronidase-Sensitive Acid Mucopolysaccharide in Trabecula and Iris in Routine Paraffin Sections of Adult Human Eyes. Amer. J. Ophthal. 44:1–4, 1957.

Zimmerman, L. E.: Application of Histochemical Methods for the Demonstration of Acid Mucopolysaccharides to Ophthalmic Pathology. Trans. Amer. Acad. Ophthal. Otolaryng. 62:697–703, 1958.

Zimmerman, L. E., and Eastham, A. B.: Acid Mucopolysaccharide in the Retinal Pigment Epithelium and Visual Cell Layer of the Developing Mouse Eye. Amer. J. Ophthal. 47:488–499 (Part II), 1959.

Zimmerman, L. E., and Spencer, W. H.: The Pathologic Anatomy of Retinoschisis, with a Report of Two Cases Diagnosed Clinically as Malignant Melanoma. A.M.A. Arch. Ophthal. 63:10–19, 1960.

Chapter IX

Optic Nerve

ANATOMY AND HISTOLOGY

Topography. The optic nerve provides a nervous connection between the retina and the brain. It is not a true peripheral nerve but rather is a white fiber tract of the central nervous system. Its total length from the eye to the chiasm averages about 50 mm. (Fig. 499). This includes a very short intraocular segment of 0.7 mm., a long, somewhat redundant intraorbital part measuring about 33 mm., a firmly anchored intracanalicular section about 6 mm. in length, and the intracranial portion which varies in length with the position of the chiasm, but averages 10 mm. The diameter of the orbital portion of the nerve with its meningeal sheaths is 3 to 4 mm. The nerve tapers to 1.5 mm. in the scleral canal where the meninges terminate and the fibers lose their myelin sheaths.

The nerve emerges from the eye just above and somewhat nasal to the posterior pole. The intraorbital segment courses in an upward and inward direction, entering the optic foramen at the apex of the orbit. Since this portion of the nerve is considerably longer than the actual distance from the back of the globe to the apex of the orbit, an ample excess of nerve is provided for normal eye movements. This excess also allows for con-

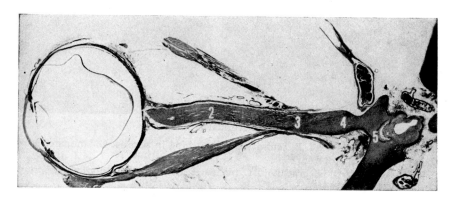

Figure 499. Normal Optic Nerve

The 4 topographical segments of the nerve and the chiasm are shown: 1, intrascleral; 2, intraorbital; 3, intracanalicular; 4, intracranial; and 5, optic chiasm. AFIP Acc. 315737.

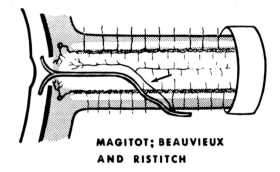

MAGITOT; BEAUVIEUX
AND RISTITCH

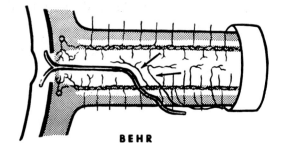

BEHR

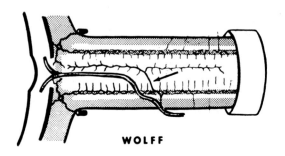

WOLFF

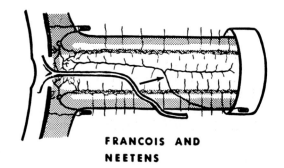

FRANCOIS AND
NEETENS

ARTERIAL SUPPLY OF OPTIC NERVE

Figure 501. Variations in arterial supply of optic nerve reported by different investigators. (Courtesy of Dr. J. W Henderson, redrawn from François and Neetens.) Arrows indicate central artery of optic nerve.

the axial and periaxial pial systems is uncertain, but it does seem reasonable to infer that involvement or sparing of the papillomacular fibers in various diseases may be related to the separate blood supply to the central and peripheral portions of the nerve. The apparently much more limited contribution to the supply of the macular fibers would seem to be especially important.

In the region of the lamina cribrosa and optic nerve head there is an extensive capillary network derived from the arterial circle of Zinn-Haller. The latter is formed by the short posterior ciliary arteries. According to François and Neetens, there are abundant anastomoses between the terminal branches of the central artery of the optic nerve and those derived from the Zinn-Haller arterial circle, but no contributions from the central retinal artery which supplies the retina exclusively. Wybar (1955), on the other hand, reported that in each of 44 human eyes studied by injection of Neoprene through

the central retinal artery, branches arose anteriorly from the central retinal artery. These not only supplied the optic papilla, but formed anastomoses with the circle of Zinn-Haller and with the pial vessels at the anterior end of the nerve.

The mode and site of passage of the central retinal vessels across the sheaths to enter the optic nerve may have important clinical implications. It has been shown that the central retinal artery passes directly through the subarachnoid space to enter the nerve, but that the vein has a variable course (Fry, 1930). In less than half the cases it crosses directly, and in the remainder the meningeal course is more irregular (Fig. 502). This exposes the relatively compressible vein to the effects of increased cerebrospinal fluid pressure, and is thought to be a major factor in the production of papilledema associated with increased intracranial pressure.

The site of a lesion in relationship to the point of entrance of the central retinal vessels into the optic nerve probably determines whether or not early visible swelling will occur in the optic disk. Lesions anterior to this level are likely to produce swelling in the optic nerve head, while those situated further back produce little or no swelling in their acute phase.

Histology. The essential histologic components of the optic nerve consist of (1) the partially myelinated nerve fibers; (2) the interstitial cells which include (a) oligodendrocytes, (b) astrocytes, and (c) microglia; and (3) the fibrovascular septums of pia mater.

There are approximately the same number of nerve fibers in the optic nerve as there are ganglion cells in the retina (Arey and Gore, 1942). This 1:1 ratio is in contrast with the 1000:1 ratio of visual cells to ganglion cells. Thus most of the nerve fibers in the optic nerve represent the axons of retinal ganglion cells, carrying afferent visual and pupillomotor impulses. Normally in the human eyes these axons are nonmyelinated until they have passed through the lamina cribrosa. Behind the lamina they acquire a myelin sheath, probably derived from oligodendrocytes. In addition there are comparatively small numbers of fine efferent fibers which probably are vasomotor in function. As seen in cross section, the principal myelinated optic nerve fibers appear as small, faintly stained, eosinophilic dots (the axons) surrounded by relatively clear halos (the myelin sheaths) (Figs. 500, 503). Thus the normal nerve has a rather pale, somewhat spongy microscopic appearance, and since the normal glia are neither large nor numerous, the tissue appears hypocellular. Disease often produces a loss of the myelin sheaths and an increase in the collagenous fibrils which invest the pial capillaries within the septums of the nerve. This results in a less spongy, more compact, more acidophilic tissue which also contains an increased number of glial and mesenchymal cell nuclei.

Papillomacular bundle. About one-third

RELATIONSHIP OF CENTRAL RETINAL VESSELS TO SUBARACHNOID SPACE (AFTER FRY)

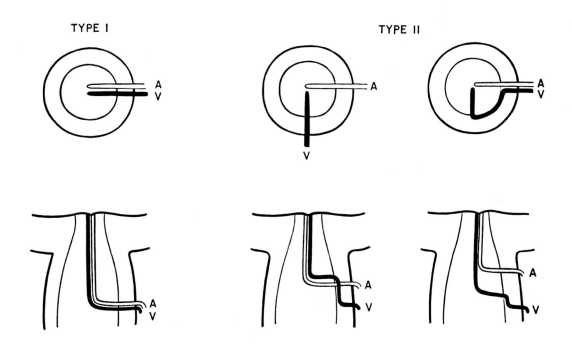

TYPE I

TYPE II

42% OF CASES (15 NERVES)   58% OF CASES (21 NERVES)

Figure 502. Anatomical variations in the course of the central retinal vein. (Courtesy of Dr. J. W. Henderson, redrawn from Fry.)

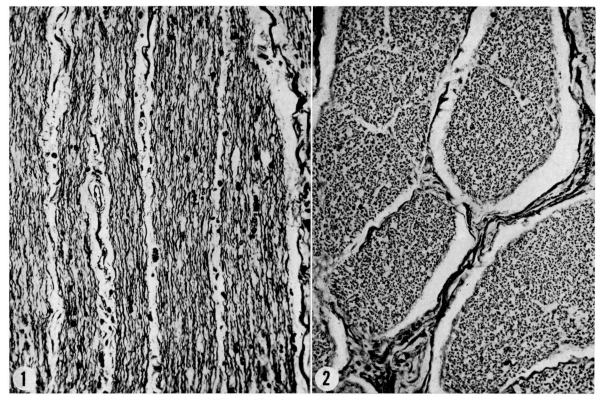

Figure 503. Normal Optic Nerve

1. Five bundles of nerve fibers sectioned longitudinally. Black filamentous structures are the axis cylinders stained by Bodian's method. ×265. AFIP Acc. 114419.

2. Another portion of same nerve sectioned transversely. Black dot-like structures are the axis cylinders. Clear space about each dot is the unstained myelin sheath. ×265.

of the afferent nerve fibers of the optic nerve are the fibers from the macular portion of the retina. These fibers are known as the papillomacular fibers. At the disk the bundle of these fibers is spread over an area which is triangular in section and occupies the temporal disk margin with its apex in the center of the nerve. The fibers from other parts of the retina are found in the remaining upper, nasal, and lower parts of the optic nerve head. Posteriorly the macular fibers become more and more centrally located while those from other retinal areas are grouped about the periphery.

Glial elements. The supporting glial cells of the optic nerve, like those of the brain, include two basic types which are derived from the neuroectoderm (the astroglia and the oligodendroglia) plus the mesenchymal microglia which are the central nervous system's principal phagocytes (Figs. 53, 54, 57).

Astrocytes. Astrocytes are large cells which contain long, coarse, branching fibers which

give the cell a star-like appearance. With routine histologic staining methods the cell processes are not demonstrable and the cell nuclei appear naked. Special methods of fixation, sectioning, and staining, such as those devised by Cajal, Hortega, and their followers, are required to reveal the various glial processes both in normal and pathologic tissues (Figs. 53 to 56). Some of the astrocytic processes have foot-like endings (suckers) which ensheath the capillaries and unite with similar processes from other astrocytes to form limiting membranes about the periphery of the optic nerve fiber bundles. Thus the ramifying extensions of pia which subdivide the optic nerve into compartments are separated from the nerve fibers by a very delicate astroglial membrane. The astroglial processes also form extensive criss-crossing networks throughout the nerve, much like the iron rods laid in reinforced concrete. Some astroglial processes are believed to furnish nutritional as well as mechanical support to the nerve fibers by transporting metabolites between the capillaries and the inner parts of the avascular nerve bundles. Behind the lamina cribrosa astrocytes are outnumbered by the oligodendrocytes, but within the lamina and in the nervehead the astroglia becomes much more highly developed.

Oligodendrocytes. Oligodendrocytes are arranged about the nerve fibers and correspond to the Schwann cells of peripheral nerves. They are believed to be concerned with the elaboration and metabolism of myelin. They are numerous posterior to the lamina cribrosa where the nerve fibers are myelinated, but are absent in the nerve head and retina, except where anomalous myelinated nerve fibers are present. Contrariwise, when there is a congenital incompleteness of myelination posterior to the lamina cribrosa, oligodendrocytes are absent in the foci where there are no myelin sheaths (Fig. 53–1, 2). Oligodendrocytes do not have the regenerative capacity of Schwann cells. Injuries and other pathologic processes which destroy these cells and myelin sheaths cause irreparable nerve damage.

Microglia. Microglia cells are the phagocytes (macrophages) of the central nervous system (Fig. 57). These mesodermal cells ordinarily are present in very small numbers and are difficult to demonstrate in the normal optic nerve. With special staining methods they appear as dendritic cells with short branching processes. In pathologic states they may be mobilized rapidly. They phagocytize a variety of materials, especially lipids, and become markedly swollen (gitter cells).

Glia of disk. In the nerve head there are astrocytes with especially long branching processes known as "spider cells" (Wolter). Anterior to the lamina cribrosa the optic nerve framework is formed by these spider cells together with a meshwork of capillaries (Fig. 55–3). The sieve-like lamina cribrosa includes an anterior network of spider cells, and the more rigid posterior collagenous framework derived from the sclera. In addition to the spider cells, other specialized arrangements of astroglia are found lining the inner surface of the physiologic cup (the "central connective tissue meniscus of Elschnig") (Fig. 53–3) and along the boundary of the optic nerve head where it comes into contact with the choroid and sclera (border tissue of Jacoby and intermediate tissue of Kuhnt).

GROWTH AND AGING

During infancy and early childhood, the optic nerves and their meninges, like many other tissues at this early age, appear somewhat more cellular and contain a paucity of connective tissue fibrils. The optic nerve is said to be one of the last tissues to complete its myelination and this process still may be active at birth. With growth and aging, the connective tissue fibers of the optic nerve and its meninges become more abundant and the cell nuclei become more widely separated. This accumulation of interstitial material may become significant physiologically. It should be recalled that normally in the pial septums there is a minimum of connective tissue surrounding the capillaries, and the astrocytic foot plates come into intimate relationship with these capillaries. In the optic nerves of elderly subjects there may be a considerable deposition of coarse collagenous fibers about these capillaries, forming a thick mantle which separates them from the nerve tissue (Fig. 504). It seems reasonable to assume that such accumulations might interfere with the efficient exchange of nutrients and other metabolites between the capillaries and the nerve fibers.

Arachnoidal cell nests. Several types of cellular and acellular deposits are recognized. These are classified either as products of growth and aging or as degenerative processes. Discrete concentrically whorled masses of meningothelial cells often are observed in the arachnoid (Fig. 505). They are more conspicuous in the optic nerves of young children, and are of practical significance when optic nerves are examined for possible evidence of posterior extension of a retinoblastoma. Occasionally these arachnoidal cell nests are mistaken for retinoblastoma infiltrates and the patient is given an unduly bad prognosis—and possibly radiation ther-

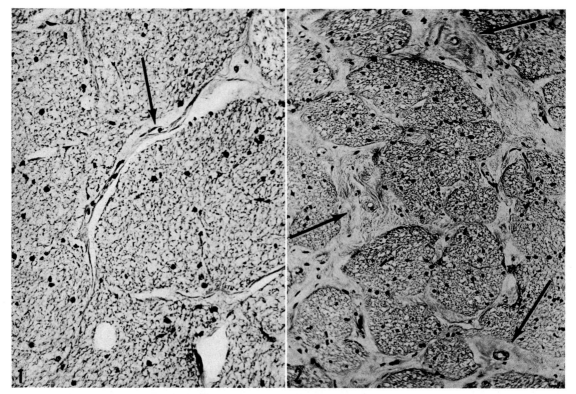

Figure 504. Aging of Optic Nerve

1. Normal optic nerve of a young man. There is a virtual absence of connective tissue about the septal capillaries (arrow). ×265. AFIP Acc. 114419.

2. Optic nerve of a 78-year old man. A thick mantle of collagenous fibers surrounds the septal vessels (arrows). ×160. AFIP Acc. 618132.

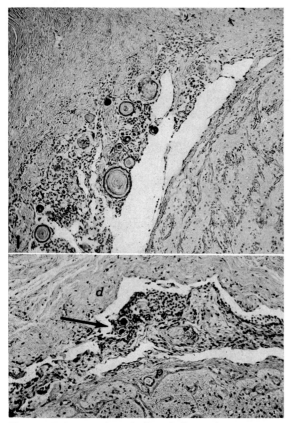

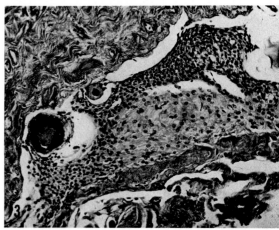

Figure 505. Meningothelial Cells and Psammoma Bodies in Arachnoid

1. Insertion of dura of optic nerve into sclera is observed at top and top left; arachnoid containing many psammoma bodies is present in center and at bottom left; optic nerve is present on right. ×90. AFIP Acc. 94594.

2. Dura (d) is relatively acellular, avascular collagenous tunic; arachnoid (a) is the most cellular layer of the meninges, especially in youth, and in it develop the psammoma bodies (arrow); pia (p), containing the blood vessels supplying the periaxial bundles of the optic nerve, forms a tight investment for the nerve. ×100. AFIP Acc. 684100.

3. Meningothelial cells of arachnoid, the cells which give rise to most meningiomas. ×135. AFIP Acc. 960514.

apy! These arachnoidal cells also are of interest in relation to neoplasms of the optic nerve. They are the specific cells believed to give rise to meningiomas. In the case of gliomas which have invaded the meninges, these cells frequently proliferate in an exuberant manner (see section on neoplasms, p. 613).

Psammoma bodies. Psammoma bodies, also called corpora arenacea, are formed in the arachnoid (Fig. 505). Whorls of meningothelial cells, often surrounding a minute capillary, lay down concentric masses of connective tissue. Eventually both the meningothelial cells and the capillary disappear and are replaced by an acellular laminated hya-

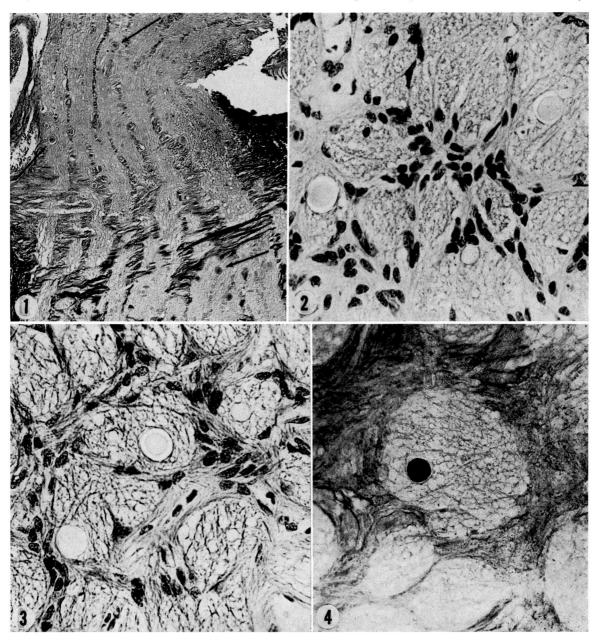

Figure 506. Corpora Amylacea

1. There are many spheroidal bodies (only a few of which are indicated by arrows) located within the nerve fiber bundles of the optic nerve and retina. ×110. AFIP Acc. 744396.

2. Corpora amylacea are only faintly stained with ordinary dyes and appear homogeneous or finely granulated. H and E. ×380. AFIP Acc. 674861.

3. Same case as 2. Masson trichrome stain. ×380.

4. Same case as 2 and 3. The bodies give a strongly positive reaction with the periodic acid-Schiff procedure. ×380.

line material which frequently becomes calcified. Typically these spheroidal psammoma bodies are located in the outer layers of the arachnoid near the dura and they become more numerous with advancing age. Certain meningiomas contain these bodies in abundance. Similar structures may be observed in other neoplasms, particularly papillary carcinomas of the thyroid and ovary.

Corpora amylacea. Corpora amylacea should not be confused with corpora arenacea (as they often are) for they are entirely different structures, morphologically and histogenetically. They are smaller, often completely homogeneous but sometimes concentrically laminated, noncalcified spheroidal bodies which are confined to the nerve fiber tissue of the optic nerve and retina (Fig. 506). They are not found in meninges. They appear to represent mucoid accumulations within the ground substance of nerve tissue, for they are typically acellular, apparently structureless, and brilliantly revealed by the Alcian blue stain, the Hale procedure, and the periodic acid-Schiff reaction. In ordinary hematoxylin and eosin stained sections they are pale blue.

Drusen. Drusen of the optic disk differ from corpora amylacea and also are unrelated to the drusen which develop in Bruch's membrane. A distinction should also be made between the relatively rare giant drusen which typically are associated with tuberous sclerosis (described in the section on tumors) and those which are considered here. The latter are laminated, acellular basophilic concretions of varying sizes and shapes contained within the substance of the optic disk. These bodies almost invariably are basophilic calcareous deposits and it is obvious that the term "drusen" is more appropriate for them than that of "hyaline bodies" which is preferred by many writers. They are always located anterior to the lamina cribrosa, but rarely reach the surface of the nerve head. If they are of large size and well covered by bundles of nerve fibers they may mimic papilledema ophthalmoscopically (Fig. 507). Varying degrees of nerve fiber degeneration and field defects may result from drusen (Rucker, 1944; Walsh, 1957). Their pathogenesis has not been established, but there would seem to be little support for the suggestion (Reese, 1940) that they represent minor manifestations (formes frustes) of tuberous sclerosis.

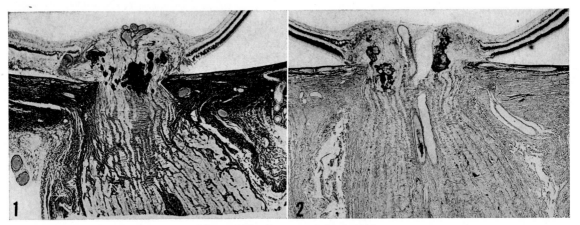

Figure 507. Drusen of Optic Disk

Discrete and conglomerate laminated calcareous deposits are present anterior to the lamina cribrosa. The nerve head is swollen and the peripapillary retina is displaced away from the margins of the disk.
1. ×18. AFIP Acc. 85674.
2. ×23. AFIP Acc. 185846.

ANATOMIC VARIATIONS AND CONGENITAL ANOMALIES

Fibroglial membranes. Failure in regression of the hyaloid system (Fig. 508) and Bergmeister's papilla (Fig. 509) may lead to persistence of twisted and convoluted vessels and also to fine membranes and perivascular sheaths on the surface of the disk. Occasionally these membranes may project into the vitreous.

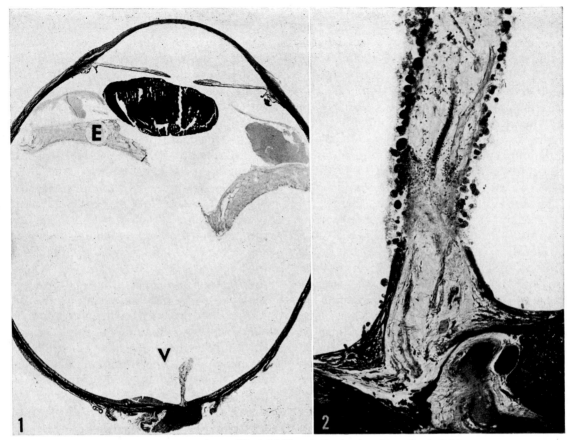

Figure 508. Persistent Hyaloid Vessels Projecting from Optic Disk

1. The serosanguineous exudate (E) located anteriorly probably was derived from the anomalous vessels (V) on the disk. The patient, a 46 year old man, had had recurrent intraocular hemorrhages for 5 years. ×4. Doheny Lab. No. 239–54.

2. Higher magnification of vascular stalk projecting from optic disk.

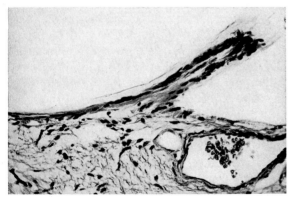

Figure 509. Tongue of Glial Tissue Projecting from Disk

Probably a remnant of Bergmeister's papilla. ×305. AFIP Acc. 772617.

Papillary vessels. The appearance and branching of the central artery and vein on the disk depend on (1) the size and depth of the cup and (2) the position in the nerve at which branchings occur. If the artery and vein form their first and second branches behind the lamina cribrosa, the branches to the retinal quadrants are apparent ophthalmoscopically at the lamina cribrosa. If branching first occurs after the lamina has been crossed, all the primary and secondary branchings can be seen in the disk and retina.

Optic disk. Many anatomic variations are observed in the configuration of the optic nerve, particularly at the disk and in the scleral canal. Normally the retinal receptor cells, the retinal pigment epithelium, Bruch's membrane, and the choroid terminate rather abruptly at the margins of the optic disk (Fig. 70). Variation from this pattern is common, and some layers may not reach the disk margin. If the pigment epithelium and choroid fall short the peripapillary retina is in contact with bare sclera. This produces the ophthalmoscopic appearance of a scleral crescent or conus adjacent to the disk. If the choroid is present in its normal position, and the pigment epithelium fails to reach the disk margin, the ophthalmoscopic picture of a choroidal ring or crescent is present (Figs. 69, 70). The opposite of these situations may also be observed. Pigment epithelium, Bruch's membrane, and choroidal tissue may extend over the scleral foramen forming an overhanging lip or ledge. This gives rise to the ophthalmoscopic appearance of a pigmented ring or crescent. At other times the pigment crescent is formed by a folding or duplication of pigment epithelium at the disk edge.

The scleral canal also may have numerous variations in form and direction. If the canal is wide the physiologic cup appears broad and flat, and if it is narrower the cup may be deep and funnel shaped or even may be absent. In such cases the ophthalmoscopic appearance may simulate papilledema. The canal may have a cylindrical or truncated shape and its course may be at right angles or oblique with respect to the sclera. In myopia the canal is extremely oblique, with the obliquity directed temporally. This obliquity together with the prominent overhanging nasal shelf often obscures the entering central vessels at the disk, and the vessels and nerve bundles on the nasal side are acutely angulated as they pass from the nasal retina into the nerve. On the temporal side, however, the nerve fibers and vessels most often pass directly into the nerve with almost no angulation.

Owing to the obliquity, the inner scleral wall of the optic nerve canal on the temporal side becomes more visible with the ophthalmoscope, making it difficult to determine the exact position of the disk edge.

The congenital absence of myelinated nerve fibers behind the lamina cribrosa and the converse occurrence of myelination in the retina already have been mentioned (Fig. 53).

Myopia. The general eye findings in myopia have been discussed in Chapter II. The disk and optic nerve have a characteristic ophthalmoscopic and histologic appearance in high myopia (Figs. 68, 70). On the temporal side of the disk, the pigment epithelium, Bruch's membrane, and the choroid each terminate at varying distances from the disk margin. Frequently there is a white crescent of sclera (scleral conus) immediately adjacent to the disk as the result of an absence of all these tissues. Temporal to this conus there may be a crescent of choroidal tissue, followed by a pigmented crescent of proliferated retinal epithelium. On the nasal side, the typical myopic disk shows a prominent shelf, consisting of pigment epithelium, Bruch's membrane and choroidal tissue which overhangs the scleral foramen, sometimes covering as much as half the normal circular opening (Figs. 69, 70). Since these abnormalities occur on the temporal and nasal sides of the disk, and obscure the real disk margin, the nerve head has an ovoid appearance with its long axis vertical.

Inferior conus. A similar malformation of the optic nerve head occurring in the vertical rather than the horizontal plane gives rise to the relatively common inferior conus. In this case the choroid, Bruch's membrane, and pigment epithelium terminate at varying distances below the optic disk and the retina over a crescentic area below the disk lies in direct contact with the sclera. The optic canal passes obliquely downward through the sclera, and the superior branches of the central retinal artery become sharply angulated as they turn upward from the nerve head. The reverse of these alterations giving rise to a superior conus is very unusual.

Minor anomalies. Occasionally, especially in persons having deep pigmentation, uveal melanocytes may be incorporated in the nerve head, most often in the region of the lamina cribrosa (Fig. 510), but also in the meninges. Marked pigmentation of the nerve head is observed in many animal species (Fig. 512). Tumors arising from these pigmented cells are described later in this chapter. (p. 608).

Aplasia and hypoplasia. Aplasia of the optic nerve is an exceedingly rare anomaly (Fig. 511). Virtually all cases reported as aplasias are in reality examples of hypoplasia. In true aplasia the optic nerve fails to develop and ophthalmoscopic examination reveals an absence of the optic disk and retinal blood vessels. There is a failure of the disk to form during closure of the fetal fissure.

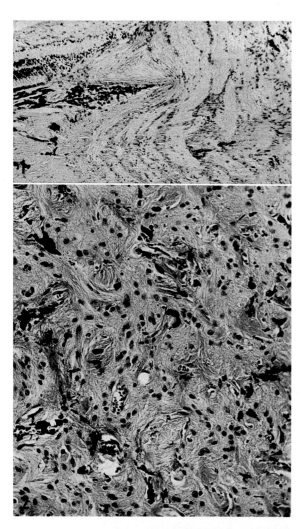

Figure 510. Melanocytes in Human Nerve Head

1. Heavily pigmented melanocytes are present in the papilla, lamina cribrosa, and sclera. ×70. AFIP Acc. 749631.

2. Many heavily pigmented melanocytes in a transverse section through posterior part of lamina cribrosa. ×180. AFIP Acc. 706594.

In hypoplasia (Fig. 513–1) the disk area does form and the central vessels gain access to the retina. It is not known whether ganglion cells fail to develop or if their axons degenerate to produce this condition. The optic nerve contains a markedly reduced number of anatomically and physiologically normal nerve fibers. The degree of hypoplasia may be extreme and both the clinician and the pathologist may experience great difficulty in identifying the nerve head. Light perception may be greatly reduced or completely absent and the central vessels may appear extremely small.

Dysplasia. Dysplasia of the optic nerve (Figs. 513, 514) is more frequently observed than either aplasia or hypoplasia. A great number of anatomical variations, such as the occurrence of retinal cells or pigment epithelium within the nerve, defective development of the meninges with neural tissue outside of the nerve proper, and colobomas and "pits" of the disk, are included here. More often

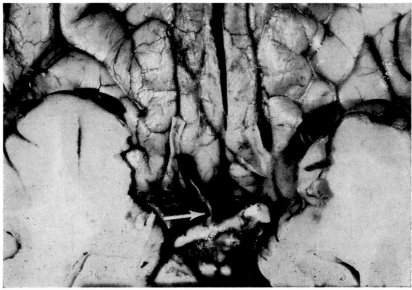

Figure 511. Aplasia of Optic Nerve

The right optic nerve (arrow) anterior to the chiasm is a thread-like structure. No optic nerve tissue was found in the ipsilateral orbit and the eye had no disk or retinal vessels. AFIP Acc. 630935.

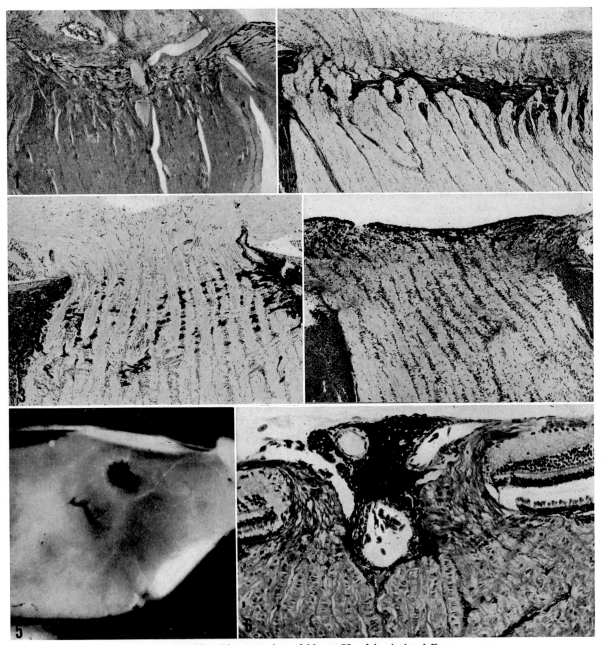

Figure 512. Pigmentation of Nerve Head in Animal Eyes

1. Melanocytes in lamina cribrosa of a camel's eye. ×15. AFIP Acc. 63753.
2. Melanocytes in lamina cribrosa of a German shepherd dog's eye. ×50. AFIP Acc. 65831.
3. Melanocytes in lamina cribrosa of a Kodiak bear's eye. ×50. AFIP Acc. 70597.
4. Melanocytes on surface of optic disk of a crocodile's eye. ×42. AFIP Acc. 67905.
5. Macroscopic appearance of pigmented optic disk of a snake's (C. horidus) eye. AFIP Neg. 59–6000.
6. Microscopic appearance of snake eye shown in 5. ×165. AFIP Neg. 59–6169.

than not these anomalies are associated with gross malformation of the entire eye. They are considered in other chapters.

Pit. Congenital pit or hole deserves special consideration for it is likely to be found in an otherwise normal eye. It is an atypical coloboma usually located on the temporal edge of the disk (Fig. 515). Irregular defects in the juxtapapillary choroid and pigment epithelium are seen. Macular fibers passing through this area often are affected and corresponding changes in the retinal ganglion cell layer and in the visual fields occur (Greear, 1942).

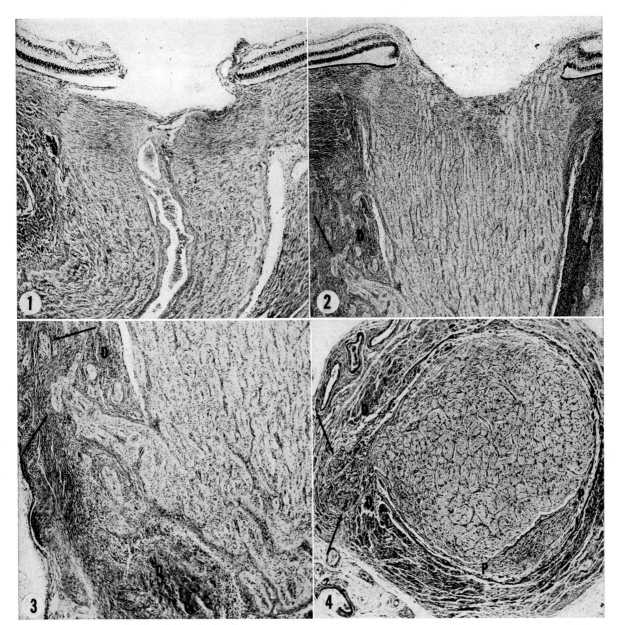

Figure 513. Hypoplasia and Dysplasia of Optic Nerve

1. Severe hypoplasia. The ganglion cells and nerve fiber layer of the retina have either failed to differentiate or to survive during intrauterine development. The nerve head consists only of the bare lamina cribrosa. ×40. AFIP Acc. 952335.

2 to 4. Dysplasia of optic nerve. Aberrant bundles of nerve and glial fibers (arrows) pass into the dura (D) and into the pia (P). ×34, ×50 and ×50, respectively. AFIP Acc. 704071.

Figure 514. Dysplasia of Optic Disk

The malformed nerve head is larger than normal, partly because the scleral aperture is abnormally large and partly because there is marked disorganization and gliosis of the nerve fibers and peripapillary retina. The retinal pigment epithelium along the disk margins is hyperplastic. ×22. AFIP Acc. 211587.

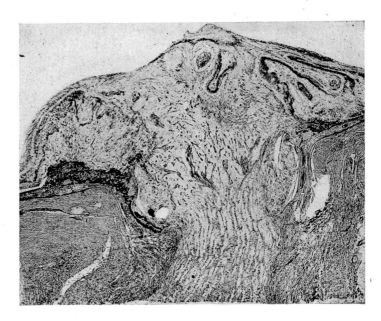

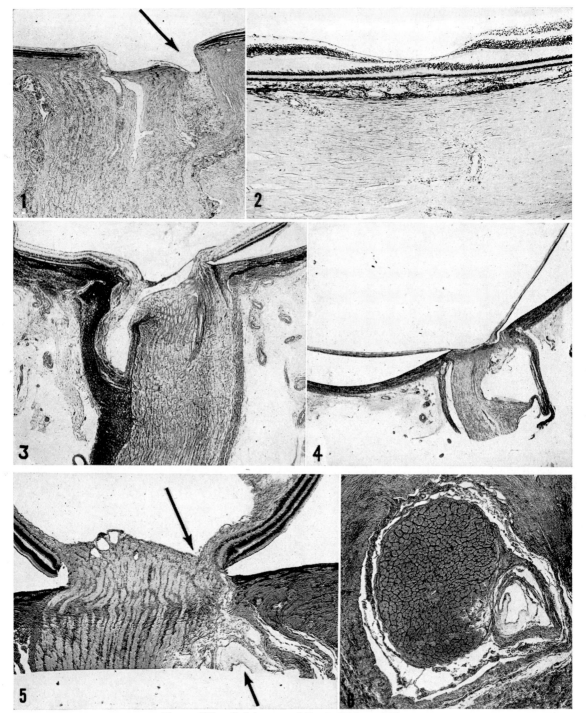

Figure 515. Colobomas of Optic Disk and Nerve

1. Congenital pit (atypical coloboma) involving temporal side of disk margin (arrow). Case reported by Greear (1942). ×29. AFIP Acc. 78995.

2. Macula of same case. The patient had a centrocecal scotoma extending almost to the point of fixation. Ganglion cells are virtually absent between the disk and the fovea while on the temporal side of the fovea (right side of photograph) ganglion cells appear to be present in normal numbers. ×48.

3. Coloboma of optic disk. ×16. AFIP Acc. 38159.

4. Coloboma of optic nerve. ×5. AFIP Acc. 43952.

5 and 6. Leptomeningeal cyst following closure of coloboma of optic disk. Arrows in 5 indicate glial scar along path of closed coloboma between lumen of meningeal cyst (lower arrow) and vitreous chamber (upper arrow). ×32 and ×20, respectively. AFIP Acc. 650243.

PAPILLEDEMA

Pathogenetic factors. Normally the tissues anterior to the lamina cribrosa are subject to the intraocular pressure which exceeds the intraorbital and intracranial pressures. There is, consequently, a sharp drop in tissue pressure across this narrow zone, and there is a small but appreciable flow of tissue fluid in an anterior-posterior direction through the optic nerve head. Any condition which tends to alter this pressure gradient and outward flow of tissue fluids may lead to papilledema. Space-occupying intracranial lesions, increased venous pressure, meningitis, orbital tumors and cellulitis all tend to increase the tissue pressure posterior to the lamina; penetrating wounds of the eye and uveitis may produce papilledema by lowering the intraocular pressure.

Alterations in intravascular pressure relationships also play a role in the pathogenesis of papilledema. It has been observed that whenever the ratio of arterial to venous pressure in the central retinal vessels of the nerve head changes from a normal of about 2:1 towards 2:1.4, the disk tends to swell (Lauber and Sobanski cited by Walsh, 1957). Elevation of intracranial venous pressure may be accompanied by elevated retinal venous pressure. Retinal venous pressure also may be increased if the central retinal vein becomes compressed by blood, tumor cells, exudate, or simply by an increased subarachnoid fluid pressure at its exit from the nerve (about 10 mm. posterior to the lamina cribrosa). Traumatic arteriovenous communications between the carotid artery and the cavernous sinus represent another major cause of elevated venous pressure with papilledema.

Although hypotony is a much more common cause of papilledema than is glaucoma, an *acute rise* in intraocular pressure also may be associated with swelling of the nerve head. Presumably in such cases there is a sudden interference with the venous return through the lamina cribrosa which lowers the arterial-venous pressure ratio.

Other factors besides the flow of tissue fluids across the lamina cribrosa and the ratio of arterial to venous pressure in the central retinal vessels would seem to play a role in papilledema. It appears, for example, that the nerve head tends to swell much more readily than does the nerve fiber layer of the retina. Duke-Elder has suggested that certain, as yet undefined, physiochemical factors peculiar to the nerve head may account for its special tendency to swell. The bunching together of nerve fibers as they enter the nerve head and the lack of the restraining effect of Müller's fibers (which are not present at the disk) account for some of this apparent difference in ability to swell.

Histopathologic characteristics. Regardless of the specific cause and pathogenesis of papilledema, the histopathologic alterations are similar. The vessels of the papilla are engorged and the bundles of nerve fibers appear unusually pale-staining because of their accumulation of watery interstitial fluid. The outermost fibers of the disk show the earliest and most accentuated changes (Fig. 516). As the nerve fibers take up fluid, they become swollen and tortuous. Clinically they may be observed as glistening striations radiating into the retina from the disk. The inner fibers are affected later and the anterior glial lamellas of the lamina cribrosa develop a forward bow in contrast to the more rigid scleral lamellas (Fig. 517). Swelling of the inner fibers leads to a reduction in size of the physiologic cup. When papilledema develops very *acutely* there are hemorrhages and exudates in the nerve head which are not often seen in the more chronic forms.

The most reliable microscopic changes indicative of papilledema are observed about the disk margins. The swollen nerve head not only protrudes forward against the vitreous but it bulges laterally, displacing sensory elements of the peripapillary retina away from the disk margins (Fig. 516). This frequently causes the retina to buckle inward, disturbing the intimate relationship of the visual cells with the pigment epithelium and the choriocapillaris. Often there also is a slight accumulation of proteinaceous exudate between the sensory retina and the pigment epithelium about the disk margins. These alterations in the peripapillary retina account for the enlarged blind spot which characterizes the visual field changes in papilledema.

Sequelae. In the early stages no perma-

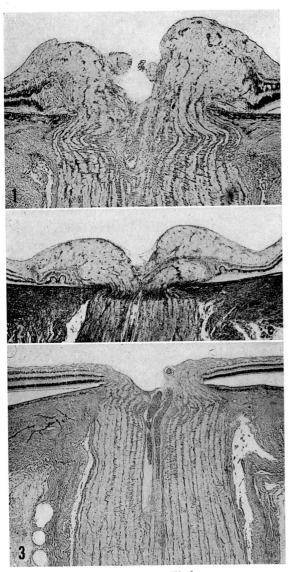

Figure 516. Papilledema

1 and 2. Papilledema due to metastatic tumors of brain. The greatly swollen nerve fibers protrude forward, narrow the physiologic cup, and displace the retina laterally away from the normal disk margins. In 2 the retina has buckled in several places and serous exudate is present beneath the retina about the nerve head. 1. ×28. AFIP Acc. 283414. 2. ×15. AFIP Acc. 210154.

3. Normal optic nerve head for comparison. ×23. AFIP Acc. 140999.

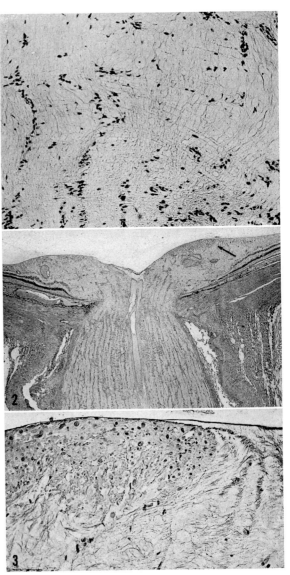

Figure 517. Papilledema

1. Marked forward bowing of glial fibers of lamina cribrosa. ×140. AFIP Acc. 283414.

2. Collection of cytoid bodies (arrow) in edematous nerve fiber layer at edge of disk. ×20. AFIP Acc. 682589.

3. Same lesion marked by arrow in 2. ×170.

nent alterations are observed and there is a conspicuous absence of inflammatory cells. Subsequently profound degenerative changes may be seen. Irregular varicosities and cytoid bodies identical with those of "cotton wool exudates" in the retina (see pp. 495 to 499) are observed in many cases (Figs. 517, 518). Longstanding papilledema is characterized by a readily recognized proliferation of glial cells. Their shrinkage may play a role in drawing the displaced retina back into position after subsidence of the swelling. Even so the blind spot may remain enlarged because of permanent damage to the peripapillary retinal receptors (Fig. 518–2). In such advanced cases visual acuity is reduced and other changes may be observed in the visual field examination.

Pseudopapilledema. Pseudopapilledema is of considerable importance because its ophthalmoscopic appearance may lead to the erroneous suspicion of a brain tumor. There are two definite anatomic changes which often simulate papilledema. One is a congenital noninflammatory enlargement of the papilla which persists through life, is stationary, and is accompanied by no visual defects. It is produced, not by any increased amount of glia or connective tissue, but by an unusually narrow canal and a coarse structure of the cribriform plate. Characteristically it is associated with small hypermetropic eyes and is usually bilateral (Guist). The other enlargement of the nerve head which often is mistaken for papilledema is that produced by drusen or hyaline bodies; these have already been described.

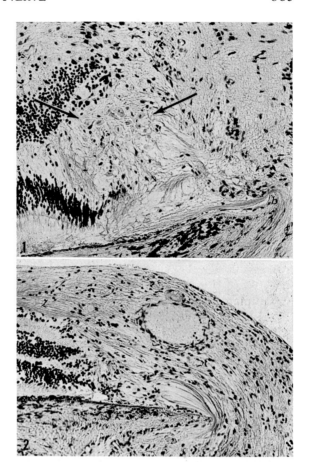

Figure 518. Sequelae of Chronic Papilledema

1. Degeneration of axons and formation of cytoid bodies (arrows). Note the extremely tortuous course of the peripheral bundles of nerve fibers as they pass from the retina into the nerve head around the end of Bruch's membrane (b). Same section shown in Fig. 516–1. ×160.

2. The papilledema has partially subsided but there is marked gliosis of the nerve head and the sensory cells at the disk margin reveal irreversible degenerative changes. ×150. AFIP Acc. 219949.

INFLAMMATIONS

Optic neuritis. The terms optic neuritis, papillitis, and neuroretinitis as they are generally employed in the ophthalmic literature are defined by clinical rather than histologic criteria. In fact, there is a dearth of material available for histopathologic study in the case of the more common clinical forms of optic neuritis. These lesions rarely require biopsy or enucleation and with few exceptions optic neuritis is not part of a fatal disease. Consequently much remains to be learned about the pathologic anatomy and pathogenesis of these conditions. Grouped together under "optic neuritis" are many pathologic processes which are basically non-inflammatory so that it is necessary to keep in mind the fact that the suffix "itis" often is inappropriate.

Retrobulbar neuritis, papillitis, neuroretinitis. The term "optic neuritis" implies involvement of any part of the optic nerve by a disease process, whether inflammatory, vascular, or degenerative, which impairs nerve conductivity as indicated by loss of visual acuity and by visual field changes. When the retrobulbar portion of the nerve is affected, ophthalmoscopic examination reveals no significant alterations and the disease is called "retrobulbar neuritis," but when the nerve head appears to be involved as determined by ophthalmoscopy, the term "papillitis" is appropriate. The ophthalmoscopic appearance of the nerve head in papillitis and in papilledema may be similar but the two conditions most often are distinguished by significant visual loss in the early phases of papillitis. Also there may be a faint vitreous haze and some opacification of the inner surface of the disk in papillitis. When there are associated alterations in the retina, the process is called "neuroretinitis." Since the essential criteria for use of these terms are based on ophthalmoscopy and visual field studies rather than on the character of the underlying pathologic process, there is bound to be much discrepancy between the diagnostic terminology applied by the clinician and that of the pathologist.

Topographical classification. Topographically and pathogenetically optic neuritis also may be subdivided into "perineuritis,"
"periaxial neuritis," "axial neuritis," and "transverse neuritis." Perineuritis is essentially a leptomeningitis of the optic nerve. This may represent an extension of a primary leptomeningitis of the brain along the meningeal coverings of the optic nerves and in such cases the process may be acute suppurative (e.g., meningococcal and pneumococcal meningitis), or granulomatous (e.g., tuberculous and coccidioidal meningitis) (Fig. 519). Optic perineuritis also may develop as a consequence of the direct extension of a localized inflammatory process in the paranasal sinuses, bony canal, orbit, or eye. When the meningeal inflammation extends along the pial septums into the parenchyma of the optic nerve, the term "periaxial optic neuritis" is used (e.g., tabetic optic neuritis) (Fig. 519).

While most of the inflammatory processes that affect the optic nerve by direct extension from contiguous structures damage the peripheral nerve bundles, degenerative processes due to malnutrition, toxic factors, such diseases as multiple sclerosis or unknown causes are more likely to selectively involve the inner portions of the nerve, including the macular fibers (axial neuritis) (Fig. 520). Both axial and periaxial optic neuritis may progress to a transverse neuritis. Such total devastation of the optic nerve is particularly characteristic of Devic's disease (neuromyelitis optica) (Fig. 521). Hematogenous infections may also produce a devastating transverse optic neuritis (Fig. 522). In addition to the foregoing, patchy foci without specific topographical orientation may be observed anywhere along the course of the nerve, particularly in multiple sclerosis. Some small lesions which spare the macular fibers remain asymptomatic.

Papillitis secondary to intraocular disease. The type of optic neuritis observed most frequently by the ophthalmic pathologist is the consequence of a primary intraocular process which has led to enucleation. Papillitis is an almost constant feature of suppurative endophthalmitis and panophthalmitis. Also, it is seen frequently in association with anterior uveitis, toxoplasmic chorioretinitis, phacoanaphylaxis, brawny scleritis, necrotic neoplasms, vitreous hemorrhage, and many other

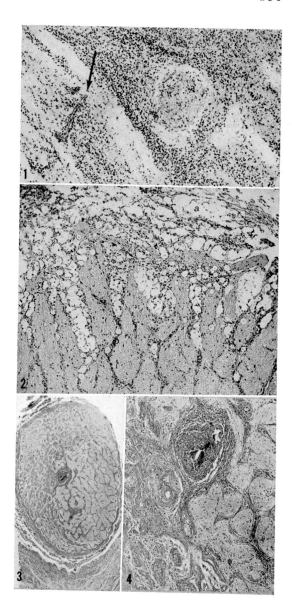

Figure 519. Infectious Perineuritis and Optic Neuritis

1. Mucormycosis of orbit. The fungi (arrow) have invaded the optic nerve. ×50. AFIP Acc. 219945.

2. Cryptococcus meningoencephalitis. The yeast cells in the arachnoid (a) have extended into the peripheral nerve bundles via the pial septums (p). ×75. AFIP Acc. 176358.

3. Partial optic atrophy following optic neuritis due to maxillary sinusitis and orbital cellulitis. Only the nerve bundles in the lower right sector remain relatively intact. ×18. AFIP Acc. 899385.

4. Center of field shown in 3, along junction of markedly atrophic part (on left) and the intact bundles (on right). The central retinal vessels are intensely infiltrated by inflammatory cells and their lumens are obliterated. ×60.

unrelated disease processes (Figs. 73, 328, 408, 413). The common denominator in all these is the diffusion into the nerve head of the irritating products of damaged tissues. The character of the tissue response in the nerve head varies considerably. Often there is merely hyperemia, edema, perivascular cuffing by lymphocytes, and proliferation of astrocytes. A flat serous separation of the peripapillary retina may occur.

Persistence of the edema and inflammation leads to secondary degenerative changes in

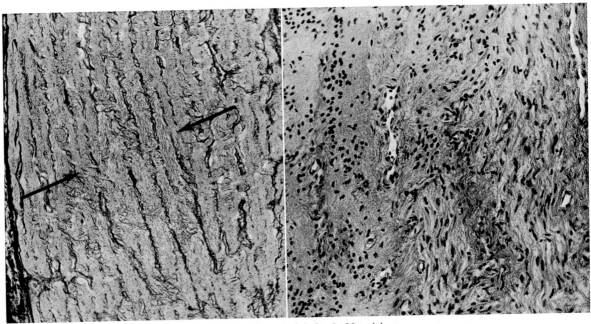

Figure 520.   Axial Optic Neuritis

1. There is selective degeneration and gliosis of the axial nerve bundles (arrows) of obscure etiology. ×45.
AFIP Acc. 505279.
of field. ×155.   2. Same case. Marked gliosis of degenerated nerve bundles is observed in the right half

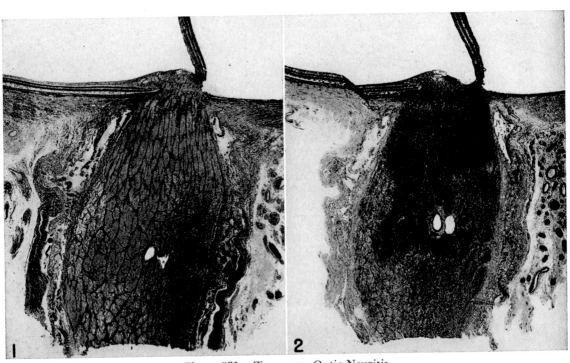

Figure 521.   Transverse Optic Neuritis

1. Neuromyelitis optica (Devic's disease). The degree of destruction of the optic nerve is not so evident in this hematoxylin and eosin-stained section.

2. This stain for myelin reveals destruction of myelin sheaths (pale areas) at bottom of field while close to the globe there appears to be no demyelination. Both ×15. AFIP Acc. 300459.

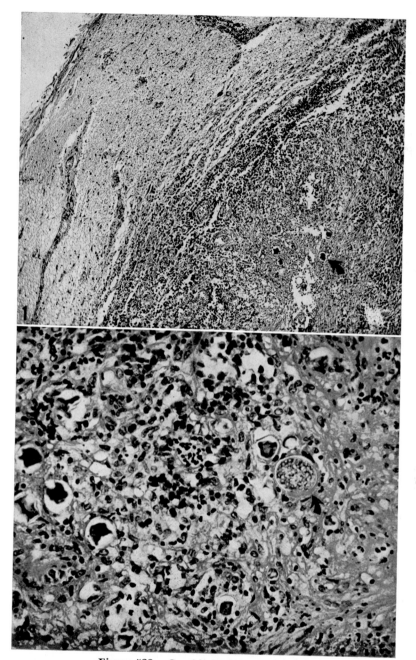

Figure 522. Coccidioidal Optic Neuritis

1 and 2. Massive destruction of optic nerve in a fatal case of coccidioidomycosis. Spherules (arrows) filled with endospores are present in great numbers. ×70 and ×300, respectively. AFIP Acc. 114120.

nerve fibers, with gliosis and fibrosis. New-formed connective tissue membranes appear on the inner surface of the disk and extend out over the inner surface of the retina particularly along branches of the central vessels. Thin bands of connective tissue spread out into the vitreous. The eventual picture is one of a slightly elevated scarred disk, with peripapillary fibrosis, and absence of the physio-logic cup. In other cases, particularly with fulminating infectious processes, the nerve head may become diffusely infiltrated by polymorphonuclear leukocytes. Suppurative or hemorrhagic necrosis also may be observed.

Demyelinating diseases. Optic neuritis frequently occurs in the demyelinating diseases. Multiple sclerosis, neuromyelitis optica,

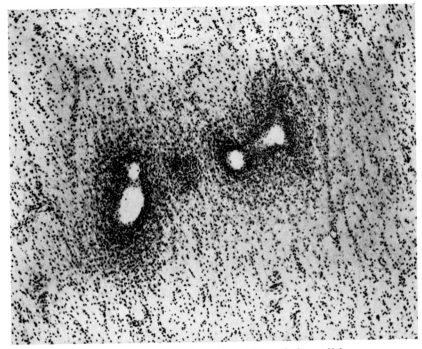

Figure 527. Acute Disseminated Encephalomyelitis

Intense perivascular infiltration by lymphocytes and plasma cells is especially characteristic of the postexanthematous encephalomyelitides. From a case that followed smallpox; Scholz collection, Registry of Neuropathology, **AFIP.**

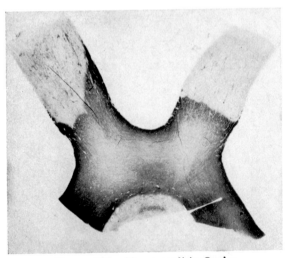

Figure 528. Neuromyelitis Optica

Massive demyelination (pale-staining areas) has occurred in almost the entirety of both optic nerves anterior to the chiasm. Myelin sheath stain. ×6. (Courtesy Dr. L. L. Calkins, from case reported by Dennis and Calkins, 1949.)

in great numbers. Later there is an astrocytic response leading to the characteristic glial sclerosis (Fig. 523). In addition to the demyelinating process, two other morphologic alterations are common to these diseases: perivenous distribution of lesions and perivascular exudation of inflammatory cells. Because of these pathologic similarities, it might seem reasonable to expect a similar pathogenesis. The alterations in these disorders are unlike those of known infectious and metabolic diseases of the central nervous system but are similar to those of experimental allergic encephalomyelitis. Hypersensitivity to some antigens, either of external origin or of the "auto-antigen" type, therefore, seems to explain best the genesis of the demyelinating diseases (Adams and Kubik, 1952).

Multiple sclerosis. Widely scattered, irregular plaques of varying ages and measuring from 1 mm. to 5 cm. or more in diameter occur characteristically throughout the white matter of the brain, spinal cord, and optic nerves (Figs. 524, 525). The disparity between the destruction of myelin sheaths and preservation of axis cylinders is greater in

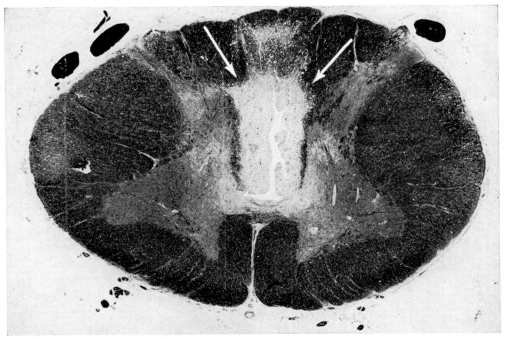

Figure 529. Neuromyelitis Optica

A large rectangular area of massive necrosis and total demyelination (arrows) is present just posterior to the gray commissure in the lower cervical spinal cord. At other levels there was almost total transverse myelitis. ×11. AFIP Acc. 300459.

multiple sclerosis than in the other demyelinating disorders.

Postinfectious and postvaccinal encephalomyelitis. In acute disseminated encephalomyelitis, the lesions are even more widespread throughout the central nervous system and involve the gray as well as the white matter (Figs. 526, 527). They are smaller, being not more than a few millimeters in diameter and show the most striking perivenous distribution. There is an especially intense inflammatory response with exudation of lymphocytes and plasma cells. The case for autosensitization is most suggestive in this disease since it typically occurs during recovery from an acute exanthematous disease or after vaccination.

Neuromyelitis optica. Devic's disease, considered by some to be a form of acute multiple sclerosis, is characterized by more massive lesions which often involve all of one or both optic nerves (Figs. 521, 523, 528) and extend completely across a section of the spinal cord, destroying gray as well as white matter (Fig. 529). The extent of the lesions, greater microglial response, involvement of gray matter, and greater destruction of axis cylinders serve to distinguish the pathologic

anatomy of Devic's disease from that of multiple sclerosis.

Diffuse sclerosis. Diffuse sclerosis, best exemplified by Schilder's disease, also is characterized by more massive lesions, but these involve predominantly or exclusively the hemispherical white matter (Fig. 530). The optic nerves often are affected. Destruction of axons is relatively great.

Sequelae. The changes that take place in the optic nerve and retina after the subsidence of the acute phases of optic neuritis depend upon the cause of the optic neuritis, the extent of the initial damage, and the position of the lesion within the nerve. Generally the reactive proliferation of mesenchymal and glial elements during the active and reparative phases is proportional to the extent of tissue damage. When the optic nerve is affected close to the papilla, the degree of vascular and connective tissue proliferation can be evaluated by ophthalmoscopic examination. When the lesions are more remotely situated the opthalmoscopic picture may be merely that of simple optic atrophy. The types of optic atrophy are considered later in this chapter (see p 621).

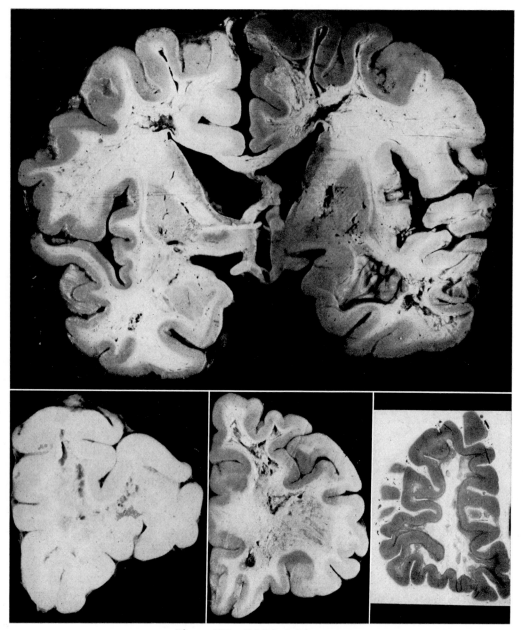

Figure 530. Schilder's Disease

There is diffuse softening of the hemispherical white matter bilaterally. The optic radiations are included in the extensive lesions involving the occipital lobes where the process characteristically begins. AFIP Acc. 631436.

INJURIES

Mechanical trauma to the optic nerve may be produced, not only by external physical violence applied directly or indirectly, but also by encroachment upon the nerve by tumors, hematomas, displaced tissues, foreign bodies, etc.

Pressure, distortion, and stretching. The intracranial portion of the nerve may be compressed by a neoplasm, granuloma, plastic exudate, a swollen or hydrocephalic brain, a pulsating sclerotic internal carotid artery, etc. If unrelieved such compression may lead to optic atrophy. In the case of space-occupying lesions within the pituitary fossa the damage produced by encroachment upon the chiasm may not be the result of compression but rather is due to stretching of the chiasmal fibers over the expanding mass. The intracranial segment of the nerve also may be damaged by sharp angulation against the inner aperture of the optic canal. Narrowing of the bony canal by hyperostosis, inflammatory or neoplastic cells, blood, or fluid injected during performance of a retrobulbar block may compress the nerve sufficiently to cause permanent damage. The intraorbital segment of the nerve is somewhat redundant and can be displaced considerably by neoplasms or other masses without being damaged. On occasion, however, meningiomas, inflammatory pseudotumors, or other lesions may completely encase and strangulate the retrobulbar segment of the optic nerve.

Avulsion. External violence may damage the nerve in several ways. Avulsion is usually the result of forceful separation of the nerve from the eyeball by a blunt instrument. This may either jerk the nerve backward or tear the globe from the orbit. Force applied to the lateral aspect of the orbit by a blunt fixed object may have a similar gouging effect, producing an avulsion of the nerve without visible evidence of an object having been applied to the orbit. Avulsion may be complete or incomplete. The extent of intraocular and intraorbital hemorrhage, tissue damage and reparative reaction varies greatly.

Division. The optic nerve may also be divided completely or incompletely by lacerations, stab wounds, missiles and fractured bones. With complete transection there is immediate loss of vision and the ophthalmoscopic picture resembles that resulting from thrombosis of the central retinal artery. Ophthalmoscopic evidence of optic atrophy usually appears about three weeks after such an injury. When visual loss is delayed following an injury, this is taken as proof that the nerve has not been severed and that the loss of function is the result of tissue swelling, pressure of a bone fragment, foreign body, hemorrhage, or interference with blood supply.

Hemorrhage into meninges. Subarachnoid hemorrhage about the optic nerve (Fig. 531) may be the result of extension from an intracranial bleeding point or there may be a primary bleeding point within the optic nerve

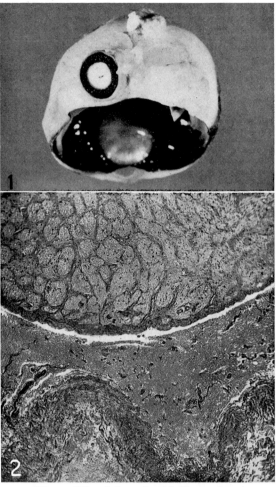

Figure 531. Subarachnoid Hemorrhage

1. The subarachnoid space is filled with blood from a ruptured aneurysm of the circle of Willis. AFIP Acc. 733102.

2. Massive subarachnoid hemorrhage associated with Eales' disease. ×75. AFIP Acc. 90537.

sheaths. In the case of subdural hemorrhages (Fig. 532), however, it is generally agreed that intracranial hemorrhages do not extend into the orbit via the subdural space. Independent bleeding points may be observed on the inner surface of the retina and disk, in the optic nerve sheaths and in the intracranial cavity following trauma, especially in infants.

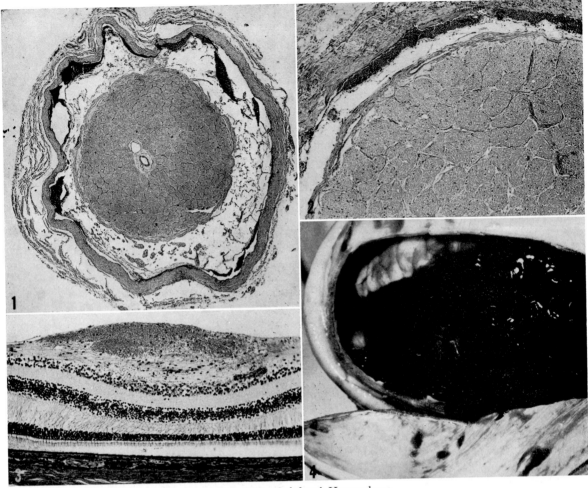

Figure 532. Subdural Hemorrhage

1 and 2. Multiple foci of subdural hemorrhage are present but the arachnoid is free of blood. ×22 and ×50 respectively. AFIP Acc. 219951.

3. Superficial macular hemorrhage in a 9 month old infant who had a massive subdural hemorrhage (see 4). ×90.

4. The entire left cerebral hemisphere is covered by clotted blood. AFIP Acc. 581133.

CIRCULATORY DISTURBANCES

The most common vascular lesions encountered in the optic nerve are occlusions of the central retinal artery and vein but, since the effects of these are upon the retina rather than in the nerve, they are considered in the chapter on the retina (see pp. 495, 499). Hypertensive vascular disease also is considered there.

Atherosclerosis of internal carotid artery. Partial or complete thrombosis of the internal carotid artery secondary to atherosclerosis (Fig. 42) is being diagnosed and treated with increasing frequency (Spalter, 1959; Hollenhorst, 1959). A history of transient obscurations of visions in one eye and episodes of contralateral hemiparesis and hemianesthesia should arouse suspicion. Ophthalmodynamometry may demonstrate a lowered pressure in the ophthalmic artery on the affected side. The pathologic anatomy of the affected optic nerve in such cases is yet to be described, but there should be varying degrees of ischemic necrosis (Fig. 533).

Occlusion of major arterial branches to the peripheral or axial portions of the optic nerve as a result of atherosclerosis leads to visual field loss corresponding to the portion of the nerve which is affected. Often the findings are identical with those encountered in retrobulbar optic neuritis, and the process may occur bilaterally.

Takayasu's disease. Pulseless disease is a

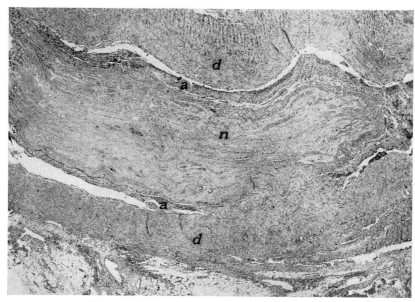

Figure 533. Ischemic Necrosis of Optic Nerve

Late stage with extensive post-necrotic scarring of optic nerve, most marked on left side of the field; d. dura; a., arachnoid; n., nerve. ×22. AFIP Acc. 628725.

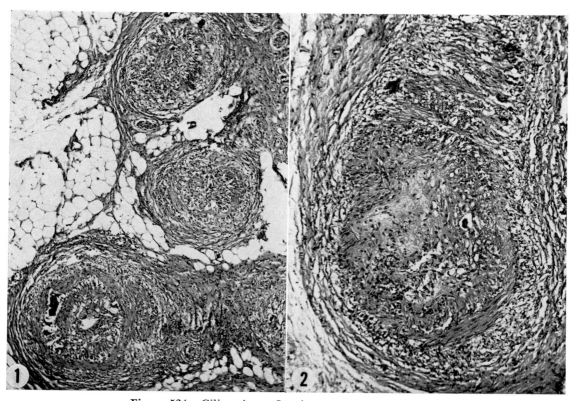

Figure 534. Ciliary Artery Involvement in Cranial Arteritis

1 and 2. Many arteries located in the orbital fat just behind the globe on one side are occluded by a chronic granulomatous inflammatory process. ×50 and ×90, respectively. AFIP Acc. 947299. Case reported by Spencer and Hoyt.

recently described syndrome which is being recognized with increasing frequency. It is due to gradual closure of the major arteries (Fig. 47) at their point of departure from the aortic arch (Ross and McKusick, 1953;

Pinkham, 1955; Caccamise and Okuda, 1954; Tour and Hoyt, 1959). Syphilitic arteritis is one cause but there is a large idiopathic group involving young women in particular. Characteristic symptoms include diminution

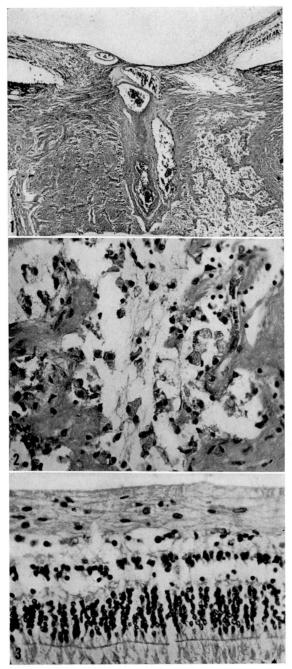

Figure 535. Ocular Involvement in Cranial Arteritis

1. There is an ischemic infarct which involves only the temporal half of the nerve and disk. ×30. From same case as Fig. 534.

2. Liquefaction necrosis and phagocytosis of debris by microglia. Same lesion shown in 1. ×305.

3. Ischemic infarction of retina. The ganglion cells and neurons of the inner nuclear layer have largely disappeared. Same case as Fig. 534. ×305.

or loss of pulsation in the major blood vessels, absence of measurable blood pressure in the arms, syncopal attacks, convulsions, and visual changes ranging from photopsia and blurring to blindness. Ophthalmologic examination has revealed arteriovenous anastomoses, retinal microaneurysms, neovascularization and atrophy of the iris, and cataracts.

Cranial arteritis. Cranial arteritis (also called temporal arteritis) is a disease of elderly persons characterized by a chronic granulomatous inflammatory reaction in the walls of large arteries, especially those of the head (Figs. 46, 534). Clinical features include anorexia, weight loss, headache, leukocytosis, fever, and a high sedimentation rate. In nearly half the cases, the arteries supplying the anterior portion of the optic nerve are involved and permanent visual loss ensues. If one eye is affected, the other also becomes involved within a few weeks in about half the cases. Ophthalmoscopic examination may reveal pallor and swelling of the optic disk which are characteristic of ischemic optic neuritis; subsequently the nerve head becomes atrophic. The temporal arteries may be painful, tender and swollen. Biopsy of these vessels establishes the diagnosis by revealing the characteristic granulomatous inflammatory reaction in the wall with thrombosis. Few cases have come to autopsy, but examination of the optic nerves in a few cases has revealed a massive ischemic necrosis (Fig. 535).

Buerger's disease. An inflammation of both arteries and veins occurs in thromboangiitis obliterans (Fig. 45). Thrombosis of the internal carotid artery may occur. Ophthalmologic complications include transient blindness due to vasospasm, partial or total obliteration of the vascular supply to the optic nerve and other ocular tissues, and recurrent vitreous hemorrhages.

Vasculitis of uncertain cause and apparently unrelated to any systemic or local ocular disease occasionally is observed in the optic nerve (Fig. 536).

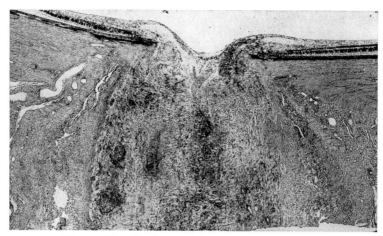

Figure 536.   Optic Neuritis, Cause Undetermined

The inflammatory reaction is centered about many of the blood vessels in the optic nerve but there was no known systemic vasculitis. ×22. AFIP Acc. 184267.

INTOXICATIONS

Much has been written on the clinical aspects of optic nerve damage produced by drugs and other poisons and the reader is referred to the comprehensive reviews of Carroll (1956) and Walsh (1957). There is, on the other hand, relatively little knowledge concerning the pathogenesis and pathologic anatonly of these toxic optic neuropathies. In many instances (e.g., methyl alcohol intoxication and plumbism) the optic nerve damage is merely part of a generalized central nervous system affection. In others there appears to be a selective involvement of the optic nerve. Judging from the frequency with which bilateral central and centrocecal scotomas are described it would appear that the papillomacular bundle is particularly vulnerable. This is not always the case, however, for in the case of certain poisons (e.g., tryparsamide) the usual field defect is a concentric contraction with preservation of central visual acuity.

Other pathogenetic factors. Even in some of the more extensively studied examples of "toxic amblyopia," the role of alleged toxins has been questioned. In the so-called tobacco-

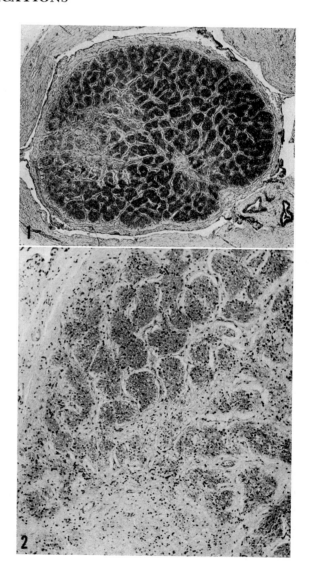

Figure 537.   Tobacco-Alcohol Toxic Amblyopia

1. There is severe atrophy of the papillomacular bundle. Myelin sheath stain. ×28. AFIP Acc. 683402.

2. Edge of same lesion. Normally myelinated nerve bundles are present in upper part of field while those in lower half are markedly degenerated. ×50.

alcohol amblyopia, for example, recovery may be complete if the patient takes large doses of vitamin B complex even though he continues his usual intake of alcohol or continues smoking (Carroll, 1956). The characteristic contraction of the peripheral field observed in tryparsamide amblyopia is believed by some to represent a form of Herxheimer reaction (Lees, cited by Walsh, 1957). Lillie's observations at autopsy in one case suggested that syphilitic periaxial neuritis, rather than a toxic amblyopia, was responsible for the contracted visual field (Walsh, 1957).

Many difficulties beset the investigator who wishes to study the pathology and pathogenesis of toxic optic neuropathy. In clinical situations, particularly in the more common forms such as "tobacco-alcohol" amblyopia, there is a complexity of potential pathogenetic factors and pathologic material is rarely obtainable (Fig. 537). In the more serious, often fatal intoxications, there still is a dearth of pathologic material because the eyes rarely are obtained at autopsy. Even when available, they usually show advanced postmortem alterations which make interpretations hazardous. This has been one of the great difficulties in evaluation of specimens obtained from patients who have died of methyl alcohol poisoning. The experimenter also has problems because of the great variations of susceptibility of different animals to the same poison, and by the lack of tests for minor damage to acuity and fields in experimental animals.

NUTRITIONAL DISEASES

Amblyopia was common among the World War II prisoners-of-war maintained on deficient diets by the Japanese. It also was observed among the American soldiers taken prisoner during the Korean conflict. It has probably occurred in all parts of the world as a result of serious malnutrition. Any age group may be affected. Typically the visual impairment develops gradually along with other signs of vitamin deficiency. Although the early changes are reversible, maintenance on a deficient diet may result in permanent amblyopia. Visual acuity may be reduced to 20/70 or less, and the fields show central or centrocecal scotomas. Fundus examination shows temporal pallor of the optic disks. Autopsies on 11 former prisoners-of-war revealed degeneration of the papillomacular bundles in four and demyelination of the posterior columns of the spinal cord in seven (Fisher, 1955) (Fig. 538).

Lesser degrees of nutritional amblyopia probably are more common than many ophthalmologists realize and there is good reason for believing that the so-called tobacco-alcohol amblyopia is really a form of nutritional amblyopia (Carroll, 1956). Prolonged postoperative vomiting, pernicious vomiting of pregnancy, and severe acute infectious diseases have been reported as probable causes.

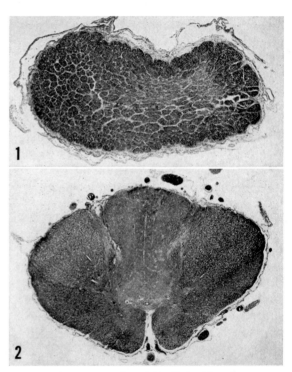

Figure 538. Nutritional Amblyopia

1. Demyelination of axial bundles of optic nerve in a Canadian prisoner-of-war of the Japanese during World War II. Case 1 reported by Fisher, 1955. Myelin stain; ×22. AFIP Acc. 714830.

2. Demyelination of posterior columns of thoracic spinal cord. Same case. Myelin stain; ×12.5.

NEOPLASMS AND OTHER TUMORS

Clinically and pathologically it is convenient to consider separately those space-occupying masses which involve the optic disk and those which arise in the orbital segment of the nerve. Optic nerve tumors confined to the intracranial part of the nerve fall within the domain of the neurosurgeon and neuropathologist, and they will therefore not be considered here.

Disk tumors. Tumors of the optic disk may be grouped into three categories: (a) primary neoplasms (including hamartomas), (b) secondary neoplasms (including metastases from distant primaries), (c) non-neoplastic tumor masses. Primary tumors of the optic nerve head are exceedingly rare and the majority are nonmalignant hamartomatous growths of glial, vascular, or melanocytic derivation.

Gliomas. Gliomas of the nerve head usually also arise in the adjacent retina, and they therefore should be considered both as disk and retinal tumors (Figs. 457, 459, 539). Typically they are very slow growing proliferations of spindle shaped astrocytic cells containing elongated, moderately chromatic nuclei. They seemingly are derived from those astrocytic cells located in the disk and nerve fiber layer of the peripapillary retina. These tumors have been observed primarily in children and young adults, most of whom have presented manifestations of tuberous sclerosis or von Reckinghausen's disease (Fig. 539). These gliomas, unlike those arising in the orbital segment of the optic nerve, show no tendency to invade adjacent structures. They may appear as flat discoid masses or bulge forward prominently into the vitreous. Cystic degeneration and calcification may be observed, but necrosis and hemorrhage are not characteristic.

Giant drusen. Lesions closely related to glioma are the giant drusen which occur almost exclusively in patients who have tuberous sclerosis. These are not to be confused with the much more common small calcareous deposits which have already been described on page 580. Ophthalmoscopically, the giant drusen appear as large protuberant masses resembling conglomerations of frog eggs or tapioca. Frequently the tumors are situated eccentrically and involve the adjacent retina. Though they may be composed almost entirely of acellular laminated calcific concretions, there may be cellular areas, composed of large glial cells and resembling other astrocytic hamartomas of the retina and nerve head (Fig. 540). It is for this reason that the

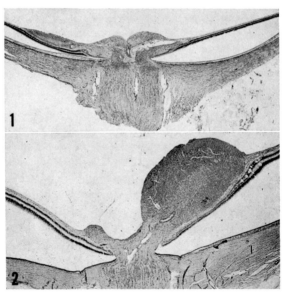

Figure 539. Gliomas of Optic Disk and Retina

1. Astrocytic hamartoma in a child whose father and sister had neurofibromatosis. ×8. AFIP Acc. 219976.

2. Astrocytic hamartoma in an infant who subsequently showed other evidence of tuberous sclerosis. ×14. AFIP Acc. 219942. (Case reported by McLean, 1956.)

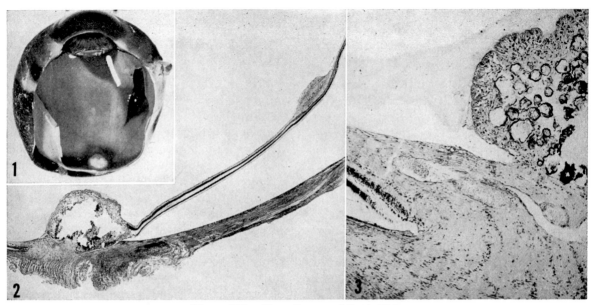

Figure 540. Giant Drusen of Optic Disk

1. The eye was enucleated because the 17 year old patient was thought to have a growing tumor of the optic disk; incomplete form of Bourneville's syndrome. (Case reported by Zimmerman and Walsh, 1956.) AFIP Acc. 511046.

2. Same case. In addition to the largely calcified astrocytic hamartoma of the disk and adjacent retina, there is another, smaller, glial hamartoma in the nerve fiber layer of the peripheral retina. Much of the calcareous center of the nerve head lesion has been fragmented and lost in sectioning. ×13.

3. Nasal half of disk is partly obscured by overhanging edge of lesion. The irregularly rounded calcareous deposits have formed within the hamartomatous mass of large glial cells. ×70. Same case.

giant drusen are believed to represent a special variant of the optic nerve head glioma and are completely unrelated to the small drusen of the disk. The two lesions differ also in their precise location since the small drusen typically are located deep in the substance of the nerve head, often just anterior to the lamina cribrosa, while the giant drusen are located more superficially in the papilla and adjacent retina.

Hemangiomas. Hemangiomas and arteriovenous aneurysms of the optic disk and adjacent retina are extremely rare. Some angiomatous tumors are associated with other components of Lindau-von Hippel disease (Fig. 460, 541) or Wyburn-Mason syndrome. A cavernous hemangioma, occurring as an isolated hamartoma of the optic nerve or disk, is an extreme rarity (Fig. 541–1).

Melanocytomas. Melanotic tumors arising in the optic disk present several distinguishing characteristics which serve to separate them from uveal melanomas, even though the cells from which they arise probably are closely related. The melanocytomas

of the nerve head are always very small and deeply pigmented (Figs. 542, 543, 544), while those of the uveal tract vary enormously in size and color. Rarely do melanocytomas become larger than the nerve head itself and they seldom protrude forward more than 1 mm. Often they are situated eccentrically and spill over from the nerve head into the adjacent retina (Fig. 543), usually in the lower temporal quadrant. Every cell in the melanocytoma is uniformly and heavily laden with melanin (Figs. 542, 543, 544). The pigment granules morphologically appear to be uveal rather than retinal. Melanocytomas also appear remarkably uniform in their other cytologic characteristics, and they do not present the many variations of spindle and epithelioid cells observed in uveal melanomas. They are composed of tightly packed, moderately plump ovoid to polyhedral cells which often become compressed and distorted by the nerve fibers, lamina cribrosa, and other anatomical structures of the nerve head. Their nuclei are generally small, uniform, round, moderately chromatic structures which contain only small, inconspicuous nucleoli (Fig. 544–2). Superficially these cells resemble macrophages, but their contained melanin granules do not reveal the great variations characteristic of degenerating phagocytosed pigment. They are indistinguishable from those observed to thicken the uvea so diffusely and to involve the nerve head in melanosis oculi (Fig. 67).

In addition to having a benign cytology, melanocytomas appear to be benign clinically. They have never been reported to metastasize or even to extend out of the ocular tissues into the orbit. On the other hand they seem to be locally invasive. They do infiltrate the retina and they extend into the nerve posterior to the lamina cribrosa where they have been observed to invade the walls of the central retinal vessels and the pial sheath of the nerve (Fig. 544–1). Several patients with typical optic nerve head melanomas have been studied for long periods without enucleation, and in these cases there has been no significant change in the ophthalmoscopic appearance of the tumors or in the patient's vision. The most striking of these is a patient with such a tumor who has been observed for almost 30 years (Bruce) and has not lost vision

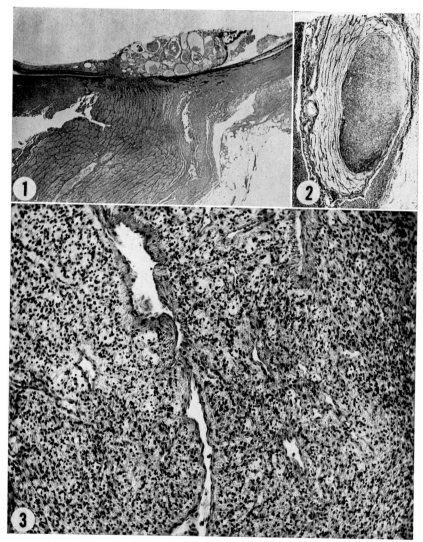

Figure 541. Angiomatous Tumors of the Optic Disk and Nerve

1. Cavernous hemangioma of optic disk and retina. (Case reported by Davies and Thumin, 1956.) ×15. AFIP Acc. 219953.

2 and 3. Hemangioendothelioma of optic nerve in a patient who had a similar tumor of the cerebellum (Lindau's disease). ×10 and ×115, respectively. AFIP Acc. 847731.

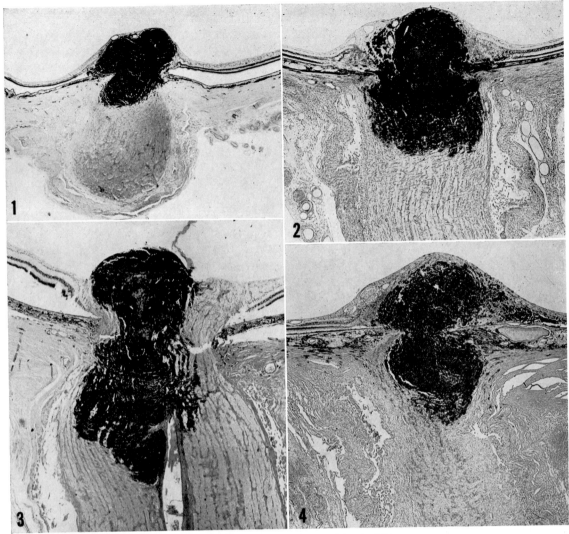

Figure 542. Melanocytoma of Optic Disk

1. 56 year old colored man. ×12. AFIP Acc. 749631.
2. 29 year old colored woman. ×19. AFIP Acc. 507852.
3. 65 year old colored man. Autopsy specimen. No evidence of metastasis found at autopsy. ×14. AFIP Acc. 262946.
4. 51 year old white woman. ×25. AFIP Acc. 683403.

or the eye. Still another observation which sets these melanocytomas apart from malignant melanomas of other tissues is their relatively frequent occurrence in non-Caucasians. Fewer than one half of the known cases have involved Caucasian patients and in these the patients have generally been of very dark complexion and often of Mediterranean or Jewish lineage.

The validity of separating optic disk melanomas from those of the uvea had been critically questioned by deVeer (1954), who pointed out that a uveal origin has rarely been adequately excluded. In fact, some of these tumors do exhibit continuations into the peripapillary choroid and it is impossible to determine whether the tumor has extended into the choroid from the disk or vice versa. This, however, is probably not of paramount importance since the cells from which these tumors arise, whether in the disk or in the peripapillary choroid, are undoubtedly identical. The important considerations which justify segregating these disk melanomas are those clinical, racial, cytologic, and prognostic features which have already been enumerated.

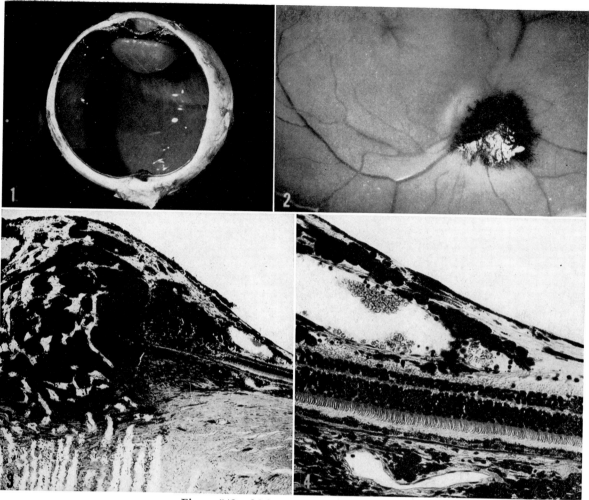

Figure 543. Melanocytoma of Optic Disk

1. Small eccentric heavily pigmented tumor of optic nerve head. AFIP Acc. 624158.
2. Same case. Tumor occupies nasal two-thirds of disk and spreads out into adjacent retina. ×9.
3 and 4. Same case. Infiltration of retina mainly along nerve fibers and blood vessels. ×50 and ×210, respectively

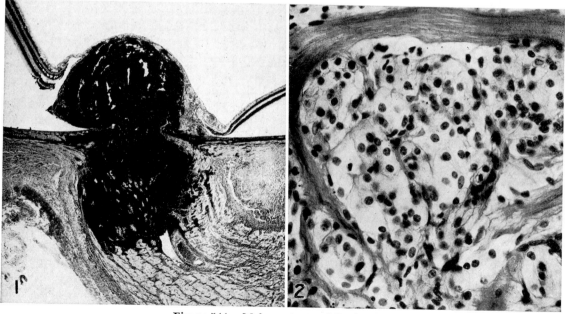

Figure 544. Melanocytoma of Optic Disk

1. Tumor cells are present in wall of central vein. ×24. AFIP Acc. 279875.
2. Bleached section of same case. Tumor cells in intertrabecular spaces. ×200. AFIP Acc. 279875.

611

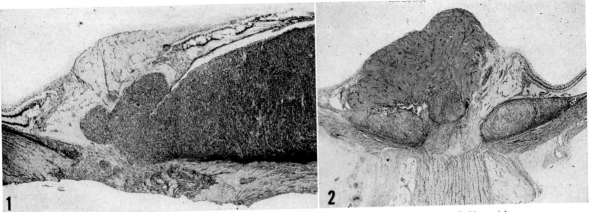

Figure 545. Invasion of Disk by Juxtapapillary Malignant Melanoma of Choroid

1. ×22. AFIP Acc. 606632.
2. ×9. AFIP Acc. 514792.

Secondary and metastatic tumors. Secondary neoplasms of the optic nerve include those which have spread into or onto the disk from adjacent structures and those which have metastasized from distant primaries. The former not only are more common than the latter, but they occur more frequently than primary optic nerve tumors. Two important examples are malignant melanomas of the choroid and retinoblastomas. Rarely gliomas and meningiomas of the orbital segment of the optic nerve may extend forward to involve the disk. Hematogenous metastases to the disk are exceedingly rare.

Malignant melanoma. Choroidal melanomas involving the disk (Fig. 545), in contrast with the primary melanocytomas of the nerve head, exhibit all of the expected variations in size, shape, degree of pigmentation and cytologic characteristics that are observed in

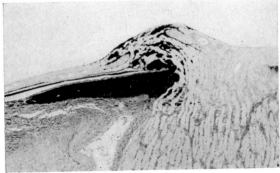

Figure 546. Pigmentation of optic disk secondary to small juxtapapillary malignant melanoma of choroid. ×18. AFIP Acc. 302230.

other uveal melanomas. The type of choroidal tumor which is most likely to present difficulties in differential diagnosis is the diffuse, nonelevated malignant melanoma which does not cause much retinal detachment or great visual disturbance until a late stage (Fig. 546). This type of choroidal melanoma may extend around the termination of Bruch's membrane at the disk margin and infiltrate the nerve head. Having lost the restraining effect of Bruch's membrane, the tumor grows more luxuriantly, forming a mass in and on the disk. Continued observation of this type of tumor (in contrast with the primary melanoma) reveals progressive enlargement, often associated with progressive visual disturbance, retinal detachment, hemorrhages or evidence of extrachoroidal extension.

Retinoblastoma. Retinoblastoma may arise in the juxtapapillary retina and form a bulky mass overlying the nerve head (Fig. 547). The importance of these tumors is not related to difficulties in clinical diagnosis but to their prognostic significance. Such tumors are likely to have infiltrated the nerve head beyond the lamina cribrosa. Extension in the nerve continues to the point of departure of the central vessels from the nerve, and beyond this point backward spread also occurs via the subarachnoid space. Therefore, every effort must be made at the time of enucleation to obtain a long orbital segment of the optic nerve with the globe.

Carcinoma. Carcinomas metastatic to the optic disk and nerve (Fig. 548) are uncom-

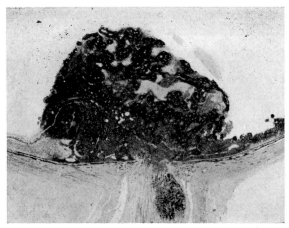

Figure 547. Retinoblastoma

The retinal tumor has formed a mass centered over the optic disk and there is also invasion of the optic nerve. AFIP Acc. 85270.

mon and most have been associated with other intraocular metastases. Primary lesions in the breast and lung provide most of the ocular and optic nerve metastases.

"Pseudotumors." Non-neoplastic masses simulating primary tumors of the optic disk rarely are observed. Most of these "pseudotumors" are the result of congenital malformations (Fig. 514) or represent a reactive proliferation due to inflammation, hemorrhage, or trauma (Fig. 549).

Gliomas of the nerve. Primary optic nerve tumors arising behind the eye are of two main types: gliomas and meningiomas. Gliomas of the optic nerve are relatively rare, slow-growing tumors which usually arise in the orbital segment of the nerve (Fig. 550). It is the interstitial cells, the astroglia and oligodendroglia, which give rise to these neoplasms. Since they have not yet been subclassified satisfactorily they are simply called "gliomas." Considerable cytologic variation is observed, not only from case to case but also in different portions of a given tumor. It is not surprising, therefore, that various authors have subclassified these gliomas as astrocytomas, spongioblastomas, oligodendrogliomas, and astroblastomas. Since no meaningful classification of a large series of cases has been reported, these tumors are simply lumped together under the general heading of "glioma."

As Verhoeff pointed out many years ago, microscopic examination often reveals three different types of tumor tissue, even within any one specimen. There are areas, particularly in the transitional zone where the tumor merges with normal nerve, wherein the proliferation of glia may be impossible to differentiate from reactive gliosis. In such areas the glial cell nuclei may simply appear to be more

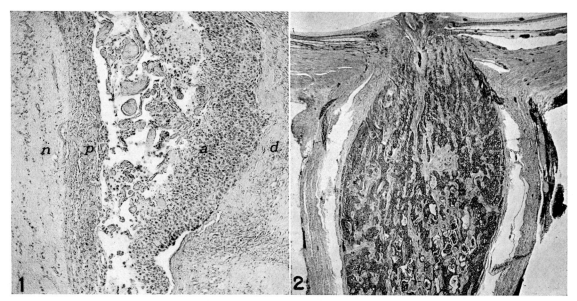

Figure 548. Metastatic Carcinoma

1. Metastatic carcinoma in arachnoid, a; nerve, n; pia, p; dura, d. ×75. AFIP Acc. 682589.
2. Massive infiltration of optic nerve by breast carcinoma. ×9. AFIP Acc. 57689.

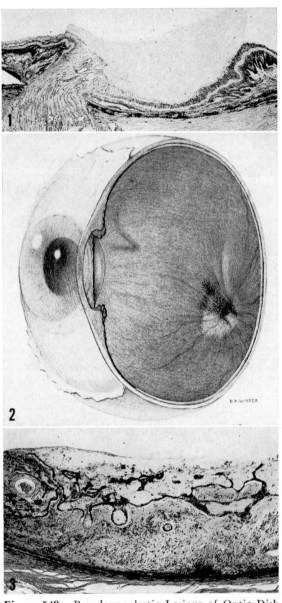

Figure 549. Pseudoneoplastic Lesions of Optic Disk

1. Fibrous plaque arising from nerve head and adjacent retina in a 6 year old child. Enucleation was performed because the lesion clinically was considered a probable glioma. ×21. AFIP Acc. 690481.

2. Proliferated retinal pigment epithelium in papilla and adjacent retina in a 49 year old man. Enucleation was performed because malignant melanoma could not be excluded. AFIP Acc. 291045.

3. Marked gliosis and architectural disorganization of the disk and retina are present in the same areas containing the proliferated pigment epithelium shown in 2. ×56.

numerous and less orderly in arrangement than in the normal nerve (Fig. 551). Each nerve bundle may appear considerably enlarged by the uniform increase in glial cells. The disappearance of nerve fibers from these nerve bundles and the absence of significant production of glial fibers by the tumor cells may give the affected nerve a finely reticulated microscopic appearance (Fig. 550–2). The second type is an exaggeration of the first, resulting in the formation of coarsely reticulated myxomatous and cystic areas (Fig. 552). An abundance of acid mucopolysaccharide, a variable proportion of which is sensitive to hyaluronidase, may be found in such myxomatous areas. Russell and Rubinstein are convinced that the mucinous parts of gliomas are formed by oligodendroglia, but they doubt that pure oligodendrogliomas occur in the optic nerve. The third type of tumor tissue found in optic nerve gliomas is characterized by the presence of plump spindle-shaped cells and coarse fibers of astrocytic derivation (Fig. 553). In such areas, large globoid eosinophilic structures resembling the cytoid bodies of retinal "cotton-wool exudates" may be found, sometimes in great numbers (Fig. 553). These "Rosenthal fibers" occur in other fibrillary astrocytomas, particularly those of the third ventricle and cerebellum, and also in areas of severe reactive gliosis about other brain lesions. They are also observed in areas where optic nerve gliomas have invaded the meninges. Hence they are believed to represent degenerative changes occurring within astrocytic fibers (Russell and Rubinstein, 1959), and are therefore different from retinal cytoid bodies (see Chapter VIII).

As gliomas increase in size, they tend to form a bulbous enlargement of the nerve (Fig. 554). They also extend along the nerve peripherally toward the eye and centrally toward the brain. In so doing they often produce great enlargement of the optic canal, an important diagnostic sign for the radiologist. In such cases the optic nerve fibers are likely to be completely destroyed and the optic disk typically presents the ophthalmoscopic characteristics of primary optic atrophy. The less common tumors arising close to the globe may cause papilledema or they may actually

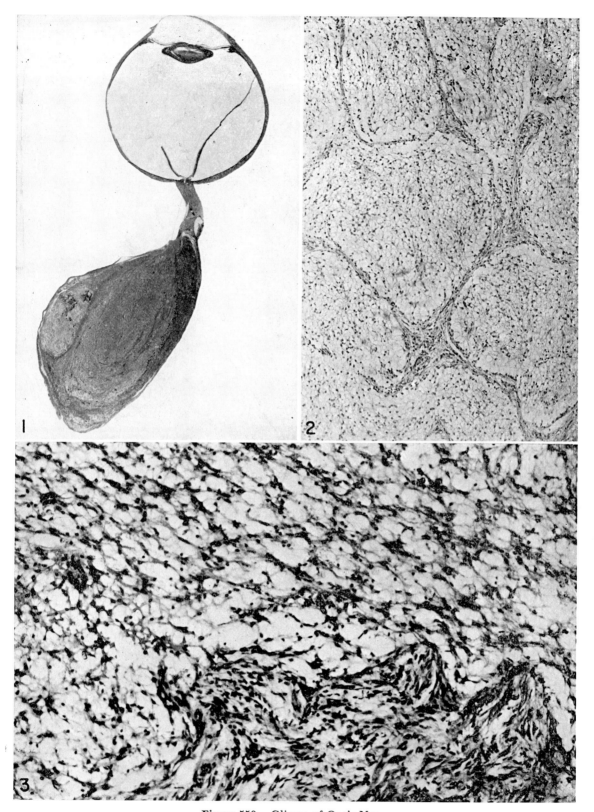

Figure 550. Glioma of Optic Nerve

1. Glioma of optic nerve forming ovoid mass behind globe. AFIP Acc. 29397.
2. Proliferated glia in intertrabecular spaces. Small vacuoles in cytoplasm, and fine fibers. ×9. AFIP Acc. 36001
3. Tumor cells showing small dark nuclei, vacuolated cytoplasm and coarse fibers. ×175. AFIP Acc. 29397.

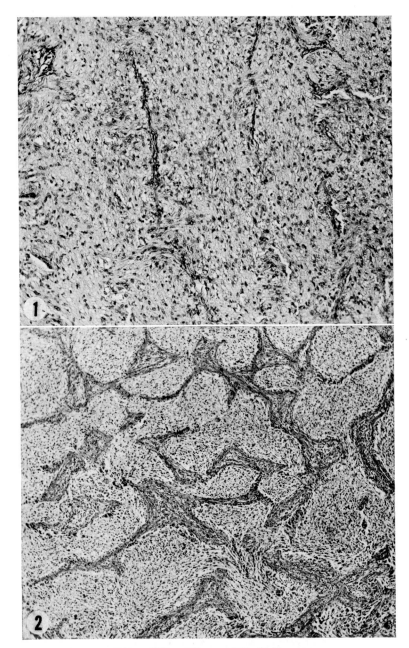

Figure 551. Glioma of Optic Nerve

1. Transitional area between involved and uninvolved portions of nerve; general architecture is preserved but there is an increased number of glial cells. ×115. AFIP Acc. 842777.

2. More pronounced proliferation of glial cells and thickening of septums. ×50. AFIP Acc. 936826.

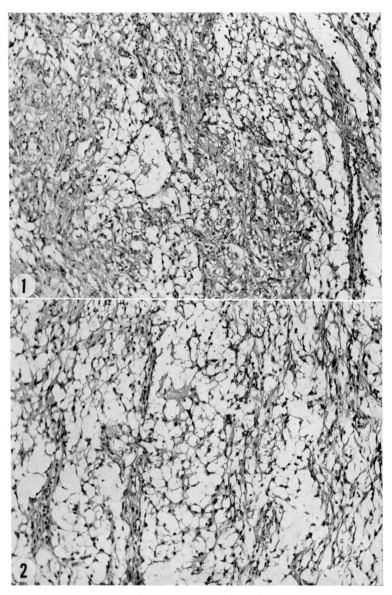

Figure 552.   Myxomatous Glioma of Optic Nerve

1 and 2. Between the stellate cells there is an abundance of acid mucopolysaccharide which is only partially sensitive to hyaluronidase. ×115. AFIP Acc. 842777.

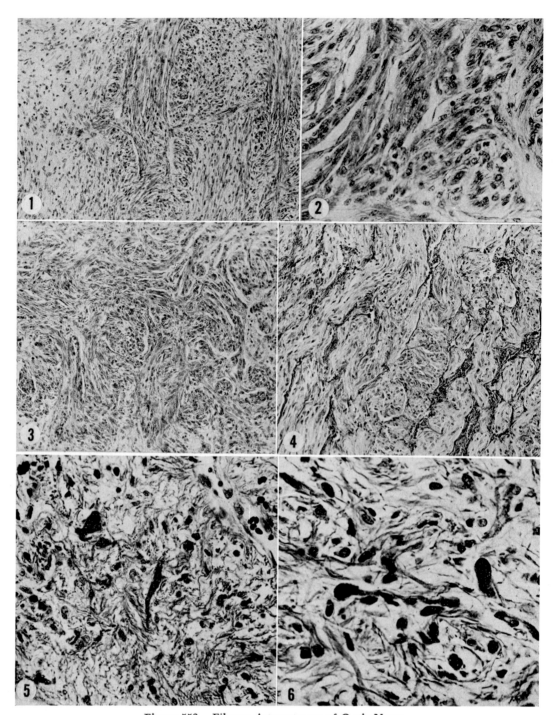

Figure 553. Fibrous Astrocytomas of Optic Nerve

1 to 3. Varying degrees of cellularity and spindle cell formation in different portions of same tumor. ×115, ×305, and ×115, respectively. AFIP Acc. 269268.

4. ×115. AFIP Acc. 524289.

5 and 6. Rosenthal fibers ("cytoid bodies" of Verhoeff). ×380 and ×600, respectively. AFIP Acc. 896490.

infiltrate the nerve head. Compression or thrombosis of the central retinal vein may be an early or late complication. Ischemic infarcts develop as a consequence of obliteration of the vascular supply to the tumor. Occasionally the degree of necrosis is such that viable neoplastic cells may be difficult to demonstrate and the diagnosis of glioma may be difficult to establish. Rarely does the tumor first make itself evident by intracranial extension and chiasmal involvement.

Another typical growth pattern exhibited by a majority of optic nerve gliomas is that of infiltration through the pia (Figs. 550-1, 555). This leads to great thickening of the arachnoid. This is partly the result of more exuberant growth of the tumor cells once they have reached the arachnoid, but equally important is the reactive proliferation of arachnoidal cells which may even create difficulties in the differential diagnosis between glioma and meningioma. Although massive arachnoidal infiltration is very typical of these tumors, extension rarely occurs through the dura. Infiltration of the orbital tissues is virtually unknown, even where there is good reason to believe excision of the uninvolved optic nerve has been incomplete. In such cases, however, intracranial extension may take place slowly over a period of many years. Metastasis does not occur via the blood stream.

Optic nerve gliomas typically make their presence known during the first decade of life. According to Davis, there is a distinct association of these optic nerve tumors with von Recklinghausen's disease. In such cases the affected patient generally presents only minor peripheral features of the disease, but bilaterality of the optic nerve involvement is more likely than in cases with no evidence of von Recklinghausen's disease.

Meningiomas. Meningiomas of the orbit may arise from the meninges of the optic nerve (Figs. 556, 557), but more often they represent orbital extensions of intracranial meningiomas. In many cases it is impossible to establish with certainty the site of origin of these slowly progressive neoplasms. In general, however, the site of origin and the position of the main tumor mass accounts for differences in the resultant clinical picture.

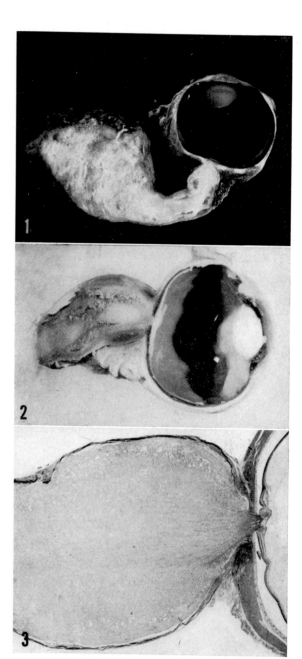

Figure 554. Glioma of Optic Nerve

1. Unusually large firm fibrous glioma arising in posterior part of orbit. AFIP Acc. 842777.

2. Extremely necrotic glioma extending forward to globe; areas of hemorrhagic necrosis in the markedly thickened meninges. AFIP Acc. 703858.

3. The architecture of the nerve is obliterated by the tumor which has also invaded and markedly thickened the arachnoid. AFIP Acc. 269268.

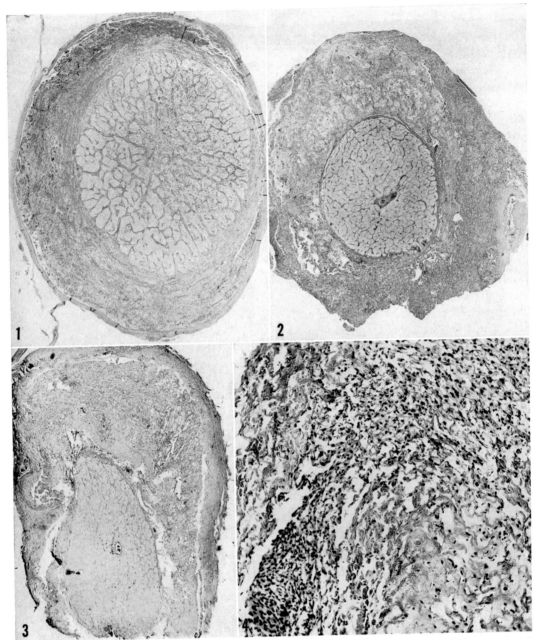

Figure 555. Meningeal Thickening by Gliomas of Optic Nerve

1. At this plane of section very little of the nerve proper is involved, but the arachnoid is markedly thickened. ×8. AFIP Acc. 936826.

2. Another case illustrating a plane of section in which there is marked arachnoidal invasion and proliferation but no involvement of the nerve itself. ×11. AFIP Acc. 939387.

3 and 4. Exuberant proliferation of arachnoid resulting from infiltration by glioma of optic nerve. ×11 and ×115, respectively. AFIP Acc. 487244.

Figure 556. Meningioma of Optic Nerve

1. The arachnoid is markedly thickened and there is severe compression atrophy of the nerve; an island of infiltrating tumor is present in the nerve head (arrow). ×22. AFIP Acc. 55939.

2. Optic atrophy has led to complete degeneration of nerve fiber and ganglion cell layers of retina. Same eye. ×175.

Figure 557. Meningioma of Optic Nerve Sheath

1. Tumor arising in arachnoid sheath and surrounding optic nerve, causing atrophy. AFIP Acc. 32097.

2. Corpora arenacea (psammoma bodies) in meningioma. ×55. AFIP Acc. 43409.

3. Whorls of arachnoid cells similar to those in normal arachnoid sheath, but exaggerated. Whorls surrounded by fibrous trabeculas. ×175. AFIP Acc. 27932.

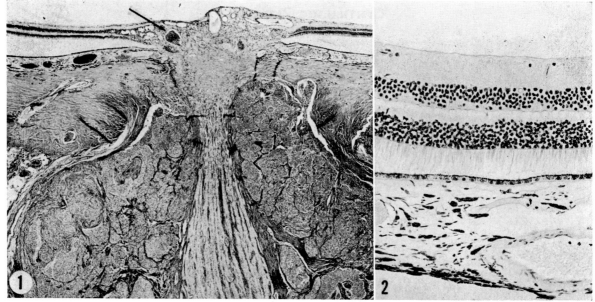

Figure 556.   Meningioma of Optic Nerve (See opposite page for legend.)

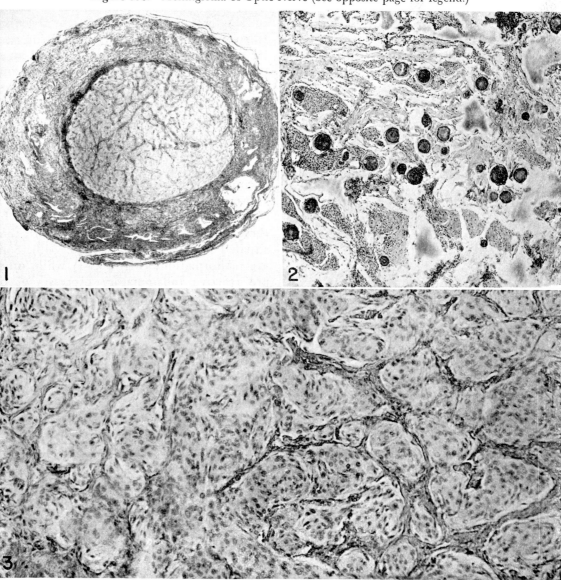

1. There is ac
The "cupping"
the latter is not
2. Cross sectic

nerve fiber
affected.
Ascending
in the retina
nerve fiber l
generation o
secutive" or
may be a ge
ganglion cell
most commor
and occlusio
When ascenc
a discrete ret
the correspo
are affected
Descendin
optic atroph

Figure 557.   Meningioma of the Optic Nerve Sheath (See opposite page for legend.)

the re
with
nerve
little
obser
the p
ically
the d
whetl
disea
orbit
gene

n

I

Manifestations. Amer. J. Ophthal. *37*:784–786, 1954.

Carroll, F. D., et al.: Symposium: Diseases of the Optic Nerve. Trans. Amer. Acad. Ophthal. Otolaryng. *60*:7–96, 1956.

Carroll, F. D.: Nutritional Retrobulbar Neuritis. Amer. J. Ophthal. *30*:172–176, 1947.

Cone, W., and MacMillan, J. A.: The Optic Nerve and Papilla. In Penfield, W.: Cytology and Cellular Pathology of the Nervous System. New York, Paul B. Hoeber, Inc., 1932, Vol. 2, Section 17, pp. 839–901.

Davies, W., and Thumin, M.: Cavernous Hemangioma of Optic Disc and Retina. Trans. Amer. Acad. Ophthal. Otolaryng. *60*:217–218, 1956.

Davis, F. A.: Primary Tumors of the Optic Nerve (a Phenomenon of Recklinghausen's Disease): A Clinical and Pathologic Study With a Report of Five Cases and a Review of the Literature. A.M.A. Arch. Ophthal. *23*:735–821; 957–1022, 1940.

Davison, C.: Diffuse Sclerosis and Other Unusual Demyelinating Processes. Proceedings of the Association for Research in Nervous and Mental Diseases. *28*:313–340, 1950.

Dennis, R. H., and Calkins, L.: Optic Neuroencephalomyelopathy (Devic's Disease): Report of a Case. A.M.A. Arch. Ophthal. *42*:768–775, 1949.

deVeer, J. A.: Juxtapapillary Malignant Melanoma of the Choroid and So-Called Malignant Melanoma of the Optic Disc. A.M.A. Arch. Ophthal. *51*:147–160, 1954.

deVeer, J. A.: Melanotic Tumors of the Optic Nerve Head. A.M.A. Arch. Ophthal. *65*:536–541, 1961.

Duke-Elder, W. S.: Text-Book of Ophthalmology. St. Louis, C. V. Mosby Co., 1949, Vol. 3, Chap. 37, pp. 2929–3101.

Finley, K. H.: The Pathology and Pathogenesis of Encephalomyelitis Associated With Vaccination and the Exanthemas. Proceedings of the Association for Research in Nervous and Mental Diseases. *28*:341–356, 1950.

Fisher, M.: Residual Neuropathological Changes in Canadians Held Prisoners of War by the Japanese. Canadian Services M. J. *11*:157–203, 1955.

François, J., and Neetens, A.: Vascularization of the Optic Pathway. I. Lamina Cribrosa and Optic Nerve. Brit. J. Ophthal. *38*:472–488, 1954.

Fry, W. E.: Variations in the Intraneural Course of the Central Vein of the Retina. A.M.A. Arch. Ophthal. *4*:180–187, 1930.

Greear, J. N.: Pits, or Crater-Like Holes, in the Optic Disk. A.M.A. Arch. Ophthal. *28*:467–483, 1942.

Guist, G.: Coincident Ophthalmoscopy and Histology of the Optic Nerve. Vienna, Maudrich, 1934.

Henderson, J. W.: In Carroll, 1956.

Hollenhorst, R. W.: Ocular Manifestations of Insufficiency or Thrombosis of the Internal Carotid Artery. Amer. J. Ophthal. *47*:753–767, 1959.

Magitot, A.: Contribution a l'étude de La Circulation Artérielle et Lymphatique du nerf Optique et du Chiasma. Thèsé de Paris, 1908.

Marshall, D.: Glioma of the Optic Nerve as a Manifestation of von Recklinghausen's Disease. Trans. Amer. Ophthal. Soc. *51*:117–155, 1953.

McLean, J. M.: Glial Tumors of Retina in Relation to Tuberous Sclerosis. Amer. J. Ophthal. *41*:428–432, 1956.

Mosher, H. A.: The Prognosis in Temporal Arteritis. A.M.A. Arch. Ophthal. *62*:641–644, 1959.

Paton, L., and Holmes, G.: The Pathology of Papilloedema: A Histological Study of Sixty Eyes. Brain, *33*:389–432, 1910.

Pinkham, R. A.: The Ocular Manifestations of the Pulseless Syndrome. Acta of the XVII International Congress of Ophthalmology, Toronto, Univ. of Toronto Press, 1955, Vol. 1, pp. 348–366.

Reese, A. B.: Relation of Drusen of the Optic Nerve to Tuberous Sclerosis. A.M.A. Arch. Ophthal. *24*:187–205, 1940.

Reese, A. B.: Tumors of the Eye. New York, Paul B. Hoeber, 1951.

Ross, R. S., and McKusick, V. A.: Aortic Arch Syndromes; Diminished or Absent Pulses in Arteries Arising from Arch of Aorta. A.M.A. Arch. Intern. Med. *92*:701–740, 1953.

Rucker, C. W.: Defects in Visual Fields Produced by Hyaline Bodies in Optic Disks. A.M.A. Arch. Ophthal. *32*:56–59, 1944.

Russell, D. S., and Rubinstein, L. J.: Pathology of Tumors of the Nervous System, London, Edward Arnold, 1959, p. 318.

Salzmann, M.: The Anatomy and Histology of the Human Eyeball in the Normal State, English Translation by Brown, E. V. L., Chicago, Photopress, Inc., 1912.

Spalter, H. F.: Ophthalmodynamometry and Carotid Artery Thrombosis. Amer. J. Ophthal. *47*:453–467, 1959.

Spencer, W. H., and Hoyt, W. S.: A Fatal Case of Giant Cell Arteritis (Temporal or Cranial Arteritis) with Ocular Involvement. A.M.A. Arch. Ophthal. *64*:862–867, 1960.

Tour, R. L., and Hoyt, W. F.: The Syndrome of the Aortic Arch; Ocular Manifestations of "Pulseless Disease" and a Report of a Surgically Treated Case. Amer. J. Ophthal. *47*:35–48, Part II, 1959.

Verhoeff, F. H.: Tumors of the Optic Nerve. In Penfield, W.: Cytology and Cellular Pathology of the Nervous System. New York, Paul B. Hoeber, 1932, Vol. 3, pp. 1029–1039.

Wagener, H. P., and Hollenhorst, R. W.: The Ocular Lesions of Temporal Arteritis. Amer. J. Ophthal. *45*:617–630, 1958.

Walsh, Frank B.: Clinical Neuro-Ophthalmology. Baltimore, Williams and Wilkins Company, Ed. 2, 1957.

Wolff, E.: The Anatomy of the Eye and Orbit. Ed. 4, London, Lewis and Co., 1954.

Wolter, J. R.: Reactions of the Elements of Retina and Optic Nerve in Common Morbid Entities of the Human Eye. Amer. J. Ophthal. *42*:10–26, Part II, 1956.

Wolter, J. R.: The Human Optic Papilla: A Demonstration of New Anatomic and Pathologic Findings. Amer. J. Ophthal. *44*:48–65, Part II, 1957.

Wolter, J. R., and Butler, R. G.: Pathology of Papilledema in the Human Eye. Klin. Mbl. f. Augenheilk. *130*:154–163, 1957.

Wolter, J. R., and Liss, L.: Efferent (Antidromic) Nerve

Fibers in the Optic Nerve. Graefe Arch. Ophthal. *158*:1–7, 1956.

Wolter, J. R., and Liss, L.: The Evolution of Hyaline Corpuscles (Cytoid Bodies) in the Human Optic Nerve. Amer. J. Ophthal. *43*:885–892, 1957.

Wolter, J. R., and Liss, L.: Hyaline Bodies of the Human Optic Nerve; Histopathologic Study of a Case of Advanced Syphilitic Optic Atrophy. A.M.A. Arch. Ophthal. *61*:780–788, 1959.

Wybar, Kenneth C.: Anastomoses between the Uveal and Retinal Circulations, and Their Significance in Vascular Occlusion. Acta of the XVII International Congress of Ophthalmology, Toronto, Univ. of Toronto Press, 1955, Vol. 1, pp. 294–302.

Wyburn-Mason, R.: Arteriovenous Aneurysm of Mid-brain and Retina, Facial Naevi and Mental Changes. Brain, *66*:163–203, 1943.

Zimmerman, H. M., and Netsky, M. G.: The Pathology of Multiple Sclerosis. Proceedings of the Association for Research in Nervous and Mental Diseases. *28*:271–312, 1950.

Zimmerman, L. E.: Applications of Histochemical Methods for the Demonstration of Acid Mucopolysaccharides to Ophthalmic Pathology. Trans. Amer. Acad. Ophthal. *62*:697–701, 1958.

Zimmerman, L. E.: In Carroll, 1956.

Zimmerman, L. E., and Walsh, F. B.: Clinical Pathologic Conference. Amer. J. Ophthal. *42*:737–747. 1956.

Chapter X

Vitreous

ANATOMY AND HISTOLOGY

The vitreous or hyaloid body is a transparent gel which fills the globe behind the lens. It conforms generally to the topography of the surrounding structures. The posterior half is spheroidal. The anterior surface has a concavity (the patellar fossa) corresponding to the convex posterior surface of the lens. The anterolateral surface adjacent to the posterior half of the corona ciliaris receives the radial impressions of the ciliary processes.

Attachments. Normally the vitreous is attached to the disk, the retina, and the ciliary body. The attachment is strongest along the peripheral retina and pars plana (Fig. 565), where it is known as the vitreous base. The anterior extension of this attachment is about 1.5 mm. in front of the ora serrata. The attachment here is so firm that the retina will separate and the ciliary epithelium will tear apart when traction is applied to the vitreous base. Delicate vitreous attachments continue forward along the pars plana to the ciliary processes. The vitreous body adheres to the posterior capsule of the lens along a ring-like zone 8 to 9 mm. in diameter, the ligamentum hyaloideocapsulare (Figs. 565, 566). Within this ring the vitreous is less firmly applied to the posterior surface of the lens, and is demonstrable clinically when exudate or blood accumulates behind the lens. The adherence

of the lens to the vitreous body may be excessively firm either because of anatomic variation or as a result of pathologic processes.

Hyaloid canal. The vitreous body is traversed sagittally from the optic disk to the patellar fossa by the canal of Cloquet, the walls of which are formed by the condensation between the primary and secondary vitreous. This tubular space contains the remnants of the primary vitreous. It is optically clearer than the surrounding vitreous, and its fibrils form micellae that are comparatively sparse and thin. Generally, in the adult, it lies below the horizontal plane. However, when the hyaloid vessels (which traverse it in embryonic life) fail to regress, the canal may extend axially from the optic disk to the lens (persistence of the hyaloid vessels) (Fig. 567). Clinically, free blood may appear in this canal without spreading into the surrounding vitreous body.

With ordinary light microscopy the fibrils within the vitreous cortex appear to pass into the internal limiting membrane of the retina (Fig. 399). Electron microscopy reveals the inner surface of the retina to be covered by a basement membrane into which the very fine collagen filaments of the vitreous are inserted (Fig. 398). The so-called posterior hyaloid

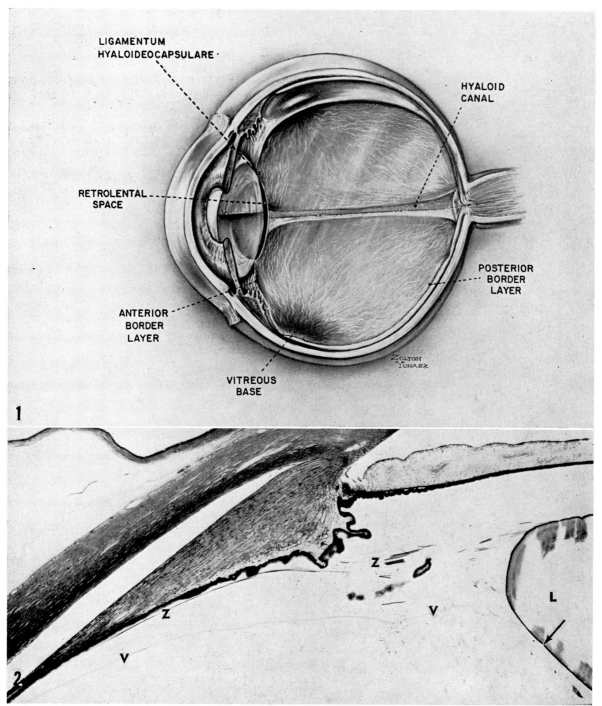

Figure 565. The Vitreous Body

1. Semischematic drawing.

2. Photomicrograph of normal human eye: Z, zonular fibers; V, anterior surface of vitreous body; L, lens; arrow, attachment of vitreous to posterior lens capsule (ligamentum hyaloideocapsulare). ×28. AFIP Acc. 630832.

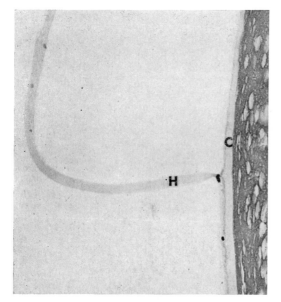

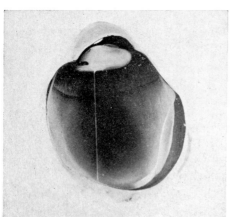

Figure 566. Adherence of anterior hyaloid "membrane" (H) to posterior lens capsule (C). ×305. AFIP Acc. 772617.

membrane in the normal eye appears to be nothing more than a condensation of vitreous filaments at their attachment to this basement membrane on the inner surface of the retina (Fine and Tousimis, 1961). In pathologic states, however, detachment of the vitreous may be associated with the formation of a cellular membrane on its posterior surface (Fig. 568).

Hyaloid membranes. About 2 mm. anterior to the ora serrata a condensation of vitreous fibers appears, the anterior border layer (the anterior hyaloid membrane). This separates the vitreous from the lens and posterior chamber. It is thicker, more prominent, and more sharply demarcated from the main body of the vitreous than is the posterior border layer (Fig. 565). The anterior border layer is largely separated from the ciliary processes by the posterior chamber. However, delicate vitreous processes do extend forward and outward from the periphery of the anterior border layer, intermingle with the zonular fibers, and terminate in the internal limiting membrane of the ciliary body. Some

Figure 567. Persistence of hyaloid vessels. AFIP Acc. 721733.

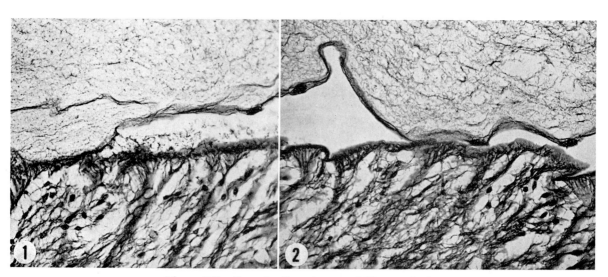

Figure 568. Posterior Detachment of Vitreous Body

1. Edge of detached vitreous body. ×220. AFIP Acc. 833505.
2. A cellular membrane has formed on the posterior surface of the detached vitreous body. ×305. AFIP Acc. 833505.

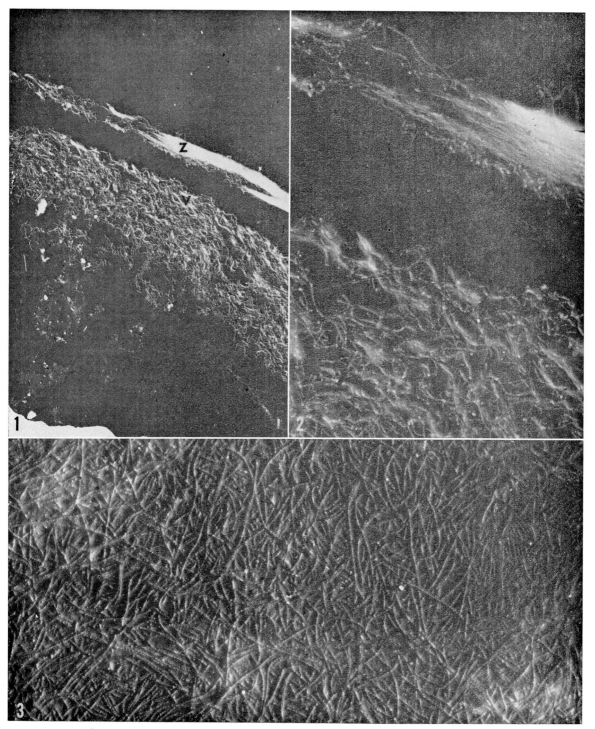

Figure 569. Electron Micrographs of Shadowcast Sections of Zonule and Vitreous

The filamentous structures contained in the zonules and in all portions of the vitreous are similar in width (200A).

1. Zonular fibers (Z) and anterior vitreous (V). Human infant eye. ×2,580.
2. Same as 1. ×11,850.
3. Cortical vitreous near equator. Human eye. ×15,800.

(From Fine and Tousimis, 1961.)

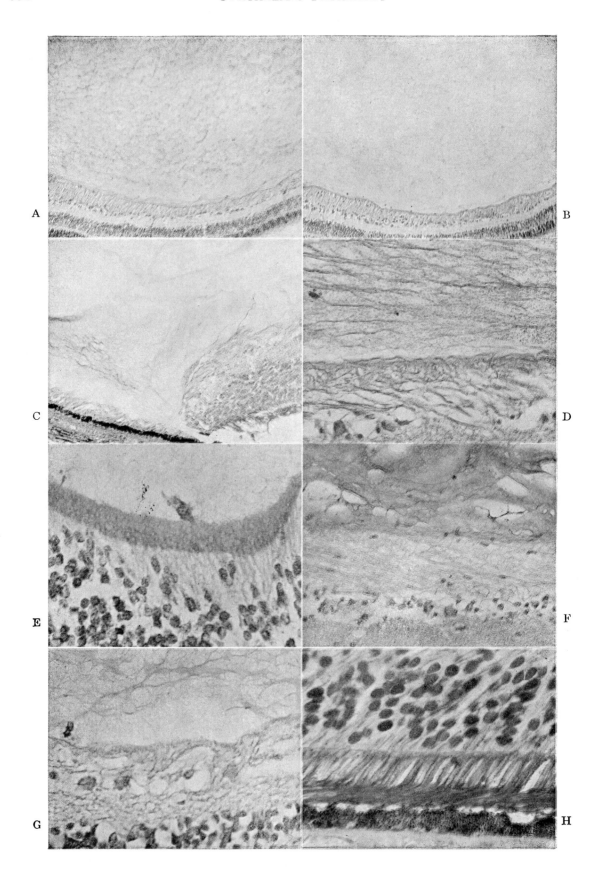

vitreous extensions terminate in the valleys between the ciliary processes of the corona ciliaris. Although the anterior border layer is rather sharply defined, and often is called the "anterior hyaloid membrane," it is neither a cellular structure nor a true glass membrane. The fibrils of the vitreous are more dense at its base than elsewhere. The majority of these fibrils fan out from the base into the body of the vitreous.

Vitreous cells. There are a few large, flat cells on the outer surface and within the most superficial cortical layers of the vitreous. These are observed especially along the peripheral retina and near retinal vessels (Fig. 399). While the function of these cells is not known, it has been suggested that they might be phagocytic. Their occurrence in that part of the vitreous which has the highest hyaluronic acid content has led to the speculation that their function may be related to production of hyaluronic acid (Szirmai and Balazs).

Fibrous structure. Study of the vitreous utilizing a variety of biomicroscopic and histologic methods, including electron microscopy, reveals the vitreous structure to be formed by minute, virtually acellular sheets composed of extremely delicate collagen filaments. The sheets are interconnecting and arranged in an irregularly laminated pattern roughly concentric with the vitreous surface. The collagenous filaments comprising these sheets are peculiar in that they appear to be similar to the "immature" type with a periodicity of about 200A. "Mature" collagen characterized by a 640A average periodicity does not seem to be present (Fine and Tousimis, 1961). Individual collagen filaments are so fine that they cannot be visualized by light microscopy, and even when aggregated into sheets they are difficult to demonstrate by ordinary histologic methods. Filling up all the spaces between the vitreous filaments and sheets are very abundant highly hydrated mucoproteins. Though sometimes detectable because of its very faint grayish-blue staining reaction, the presence of hyaluronic acid in the vitreous body is usually not appreciated in ordinary histologic preparations. With the aid of special stains for acid mucopolysaccharides and with the use of bovine testicular or streptococcal hyaluronidases, the presence of an abundance of acid mucopolysaccharide sensitive to hyaluronidase can be demonstrated very satisfactorily (Color Plate III).

EMBRYOLOGY

Primary vitreous. Formation of the primary vitreous is complete by the 13 mm. stage of embryonic development. It is derived from three sources: the surface ectoderm in the region of the lens plate, the adjacent neural ectoderm, and mesodermal tissue from the hyaloid vascular system. As the surface ectoderm and the adjacent neural ectoderm of the inner layer of the optic cup separate, protoplasmic processes, or fibrils, are formed between them. These fibrils blend with and are indistinguishable from cellular processes developing from the stellate cells of mesodermal tissue entering through the fetal

Plate III. A. The vitreous is stained by Alcian blue. Pretreatment with heat-inactivated streptococcal hyaluronidase had no effect on subsequent staining of vitreous. ×50. AFIP Acc. 833082. B, The vitreous is not stained by Alcian blue because the section has been pretreated with active streptococcal hyaluronidase. ×50. AFIP Acc. 833082. C, Attachments of vitreous base to ciliary epithelium of pars plana and to peripheral retina. (Rinehart-Abul-Haj method.) ×45. AFIP Acc. 754690. D, Attachments of posterior vitreous to retina. (Rinehart-Abul-Haj method.) ×220. AFIP Acc. 787115. E, Junction of vitreous and retina in a 5-week human embryo. (Alcian blue, nuclear fast red.) ×540. AFIP Neg. No. 57–18053. F, Junction of retina and vitreous in a 12-month-old child. (Alcian blue, nuclear-fast red.) ×220. AFIP Acc. 821550. G, Degeneration of peripheral cortical layers of vitreous has led to the formation of a pocket of liquefied vitreous next to the retina. (Alcian blue, nuclear-fast red.) ×380. AFIP Acc. 822982. H, Coating the visual cells, particularly abundant about their outer segments, is an interstitial substance which gives intensely positive staining reactions (blue) for acidmucopolysaccharide. (Alcian blue, nuclear-fast red.) ×540. AFIP Acc. 759804. (Zimmerman, L. E., and Straatsma, B. R.: *In* Importance of the Vitreous Body in Retina Surgery, edited by C. L. Schepens, C. V. Mosby Co., 1960.)

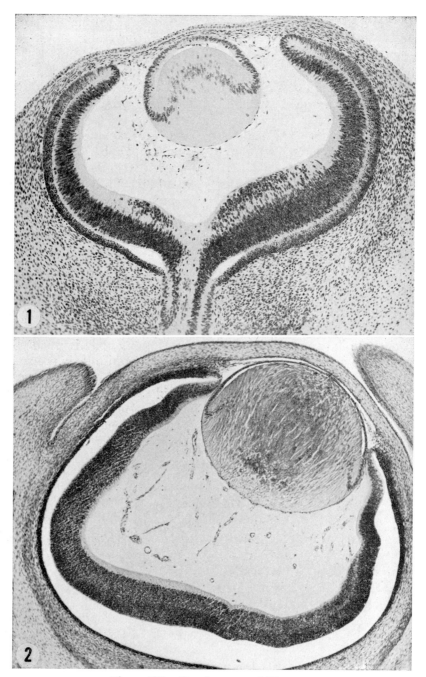

Figure 570. Development of Vitreous

1. 12 mm. human embryo. ×115. AFIP Neg. 60–4414.
2. 25 mm. human embryo. ×50. AFIP Neg. 60–4408.

cleft. The development of the primary vitreous terminates with the formation of the lens capsule.

Secondary vitreous. The secondary vitreous develops between the 13 and 65 mm. stage. After the lens capsule has formed, the cells of the lens vesicle no longer can con-

tribute to the developing vitreous. Protoplasmic processes continue to project into the vitreous from the retina (Figs. 570, 571, 572). The outermost fibrils of the secondary vitreous remain in intimate contact with processes of the retinal glial cells (Color Plate III–E). The fetal hyaloid vascular system continues

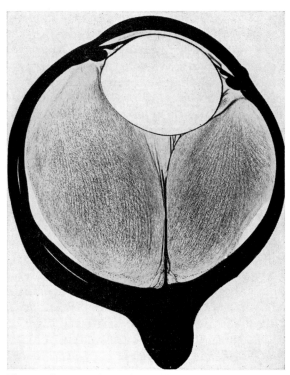

Figure 571. Horizontal meridional section through the eye of a 180 mm. human fetus. (Jokl.)

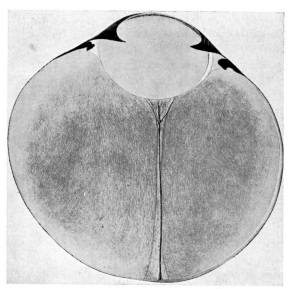

Figure 572. Horizontal meridional section through the eye of a 390 mm. human fetus. (Jokl.)

to grow, and its cells form fibrils which contribute to the formation of the secondary vitreous. Shortly after the 40 mm. stage, the hyaloid vessels within the vitreous begin to atrophy. As avascular vitreous continues to be formed by the retina, the vascular mesodermal portion ceases to grow and becomes limited to a cone-shaped region extending sagittally through the center of the eye, its base encasing the posterior lens and its truncated apex terminating at the margin of the optic disk.

Tertiary vitreous. The tertiary vitreous is concerned with the development of the zonular fibers, a process that is first seen at the 65 mm. stage and becomes fully developed by the 110 mm. stage. Anteriorly, in the region of the lens, the vitreous processes lie parallel to the lens and become radially arranged. The latest formed become larger, and attach to the lens capsule, forming the suspensory ligament.

BIOCHEMISTRY AND PHYSIOLOGY

Because of its peculiar structural, chemical, and biophysical properties, the vitreous exhibits pathologic changes which often are different from those observed in other tissues. For example, the vitreous body may simply liquefy and become detached from the retina, factors which are important in retinal detachment. Liquefaction also permits rapid dispersion of toxins, allergens, infectious agents, and inflammatory cells.

More than 99 per cent of the vitreous body is water. Inorganic salts and organic compounds of low molecular weight account for all but 0.1 per cent of the solids. The high molecular weight compounds—soluble plasma proteins, hyaluronic acid, and the insoluble residual protein—make up the very small remainder. The liquid portion of the vitreous contains the soluble components and is termed the vitreous humor; the insoluble part is called the residual protein.

The low molecular weight components apparently are similar in kind and concentration to those found in the plasma, with the possible exception of a higher content of ascorbic acid in the vitreous humor. The plasma proteins, albumin and globulins, are present in very low concentration.

Low in concentration but high in significance is the hyaluronic acid which is a high molecular weight (between one-half and one million) polymer of two simple glucose derivations, glucosamine and glucuronic acid. Hyaluronic acid is present in a concentration of 20 to 30 mgm. per cent. It has the property of binding many hundred times its weight of water. When hydrated it is a large molecule which may be 100 millimicrons in length. The concentration and degree of polymerization are low enough that the viscosity of vitreous humor is only twice that of water, and it does not show any thixotropy, a property which is characteristic of long, chain-like entangled molecules.

The residual protein is the insoluble protein remaining after the vitreous humor has been separated by filtration, high speed centrifugation or self-dialysis. There is less than 0.5 mg. of this residue in a human eye. It has been classed as a collagen by x-ray diffraction analysis and by its conversion to a gel by heating to 120° centigrade in water. Chemically it is similar to tendon collagen except for its slightly greater polysaccharide content. The fibers do not show the typical 640A banding seen in electron micrographs of collagen. Enzymatically it is partially resistant to trypsin, but is hydrolyzed by collagenase. This evidence suggests that the residual protein is a collagen, but is not identical with other collagen found in animal tissues.

Friedenwald demonstrated that when the vitreous humor was washed out and replaced by water after prolonged immersion (a process called self-dialysis), the globular shape of the vitreous was retained. In order for the trace amount of residual protein to convey gel-like properties to water, it must be in a highly organized state, probably in the form of a fine network of fibers. The diameter of these fibers is less than can be resolved by light microscopy so that their true arrangement in the vitreous can be determined only by electron microscopy.

Whether the vitreous humor interacts with the residual protein and imparts additional properties to those accounted for by its viscosity is unknown.

The vitreous then is a dilute solution of salts, plasma proteins, and hyaluronic acid contained in a fine meshwork of insoluble residual protein collagen. A multicompartmented gel is formed that is elastic and is maximally turgid. Its fibrillar structure provides continuity and cohesiveness, and attracts tremendous amounts of water with small amounts of water-binding substance.

There is no bulk flow of liquid in or out of the vitreous. The small molecules are in diffusional exchange with the retina and the aqueous humor. The presence of hyaluronic acid in constant amount may be explained by synthesis from either the ciliary body or the peripheral cells, or both. The residual protein is formed during growth of the eye, and in the adult state the turnover is little, if any. Liquefaction of the vitreous in older eyes or in pathologic conditions suggests that there may be a mechanism for hydrolysis or shrinkage of the network fibers.

GROWTH AND AGING

In the very young the vitreous is intimately united with the retina throughout its circumference. Very little is known of the increase in volume of the vitreous, or the nature of the changes during early growth. The volume of the eye increases 3.25 times from birth to adult life, and after the first year the greatest change is in the posterior segment. Therefore, it must be assumed that the fluid, the soluble and the insoluble components, increases after birth. Boyer et al. have shown there is increase in those components in the bovine eye after birth.

With increasing age the vitreoretinal attachments weaken, and posterior detachment from the retina may occur, following which the vitreous shrinks toward its base (Figs. 568, 573). The border layers of the vitreous thicken and become more condensed with age, especially in the anterior region. Such changes in themselves may have no adverse effect on the general health of the eye. How-

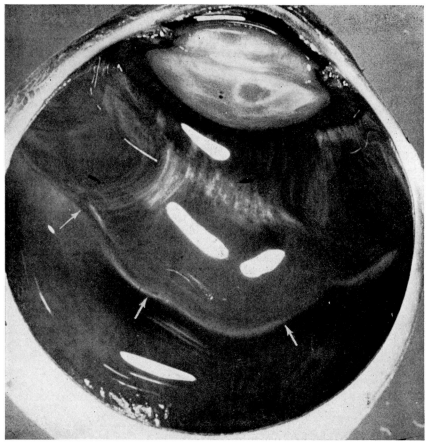

Figure 573. Posterior Detachment and Shrinkage of Vitreous
Arrows indicate posterior surface of shrunken vitreous.

ever, some degenerative changes associated with senescence may result in serious complications, i.e., retinal detachment (see Chapter VIII).

Liquefaction (more accurately syneresis) of the vitreous increases with age and is common after 45. It usually starts near the center and extends anteriorly and posteriorly but may vary in location and degree. However, the anterior and peripheral parts usually are least involved. The upper central and posterior vitreous usually liquefies first, presumably because of the effect of gravity, and results in separation of the vitreous from the retina. The spaces created within the vitreous and between it and the retina become filled with a fluid which resembles aqueous. While the vitreous attachment to the optic nerve may persist (Fig. 574) the entire posterior vitreous often becomes detached and clear fluid collects behind it (Fig. 573). Detachment from the optic disk may be ophthalmos-copically apparent as a circular or oval dehiscence on the posterior surface of the vitreous in the midpart of the eye.

As a result of pathologic processes, such as chorioretinitis, firm adhesions may form between the vitreous and retina; these usually persist despite liquefaction of the adjacent vitreous. This causes traction on the retina and may lead to hole formation. Simple detachment and shrinkage of the vitreous occur in about 75 per cent of eyes after the age of 65 years, and while frequently they are not associated with other lesions, it is apparent that such alterations may be important in provoking serious retinal disease. Posterior detachment and liquefaction of the vitreous are common in myopia and undoubtedly related to the greater incidence of retinal detachments occurring in near-sighted individuals.

In the absence of previous ocular disease, shrinkage of the vitreous may cause no dam-

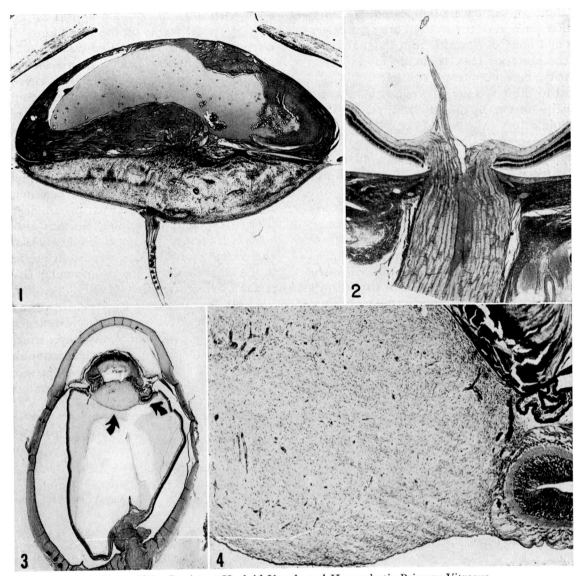

Figure 576. Persistent Hyaloid Vessels and Hyperplastic Primary Vitreous

1. Insertion of hyaloid vessels into retrolental mass of hyperplastic primary vitreous; invasion of the lens by the PHV with formation of hypermature cataract. ×20. AFIP Acc. 79594.

2. Origin of hyaloid vessels from optic disk. ×20. AFIP Acc. 79594.

3. Ciliary processes and peripheral retina are drawn into the retrolental mass; area indicated by arrows shown in 4. ×6. AFIP Acc. 744398.

4. A ciliary process is wedged between the lens equator and the retinal fold on the right. ×57.

occurs in a microphthalmic eye (Figs. 575, 576), though the degree of microphthalmia may be minimal. The anterior chamber usually is shallow and the iridocorneal angle often is incompletely developed (see Chapter XII). Iris processes extend from the iris root to the trabecular area, and the iris vessels may be abnormally large. Anomalous vessels may extend to the lens surface or around the pupil.

A significant finding in many cases of PHV is a dehiscence in the posterior lens capsule. Fibrous tissue and blood vessels extend through this capsular defect into the cortex (Fig. 576–1). Liquefaction of the cortical fibers is seen. The time at which the posterior capsular defect appears is not known. A possibility is that the lens capsule never forms posteriorly and that the lens fails to separate from the primary vitreous, allowing ingrowth of the posterior tunica vasculosa lentis into the primary lens fibers. On the other hand, the fact that the lens is usually clear at birth, becoming cataractous later suggests that the dissolution of the posterior capsule develops postnatally.

A dense fibrovascular tissue which is thicker centrally than peripherally forms behind the lens. It often extends laterally to the equator, especially on the nasal side, and occupies the circumlental space. Elongated ciliary processes, enmeshed in this tissue, often are visible ophthalmoscopically through a widely dilated pupil. This is a characteristic clinical finding which aids greatly in the differential diagnosis from retinoblastoma. Remnants of the hyaloid artery are present within this tissue near the posterior pole of the lens.

The retrolental membrane most often is continuous with the peripheral retina and pulls it forward in a loop over the pars plana of the ciliary body. The retinal tissues, however, usually are normal.

Glaucoma is a common complication of PHV. It may be due to malformation of the chamber angle or to intumescence of the lens, which produces either a pupillary block or peripheral anterior synechias. The lens often becomes increasingly cataractous, and the liquefied elements may undergo absorption.

Spontaneous intraocular hemorrhage may occur at approximately four months of age. As a result, blood or its products are seen within the lens capsule, in the iris, the retrolental membrane of the vitreous cavity. Such hemorrhages may organize and cause retinal detachment.

Retinal dysplasia is associated with many features of persistent hyperplastic vitreous and the two conditions may be related (see Chapter VIII). While Mann suggests that failure of the secondary vitreous to form may lead to abnormal changes in the retina with development of folds or septums, it seems just as logical to suspect that the dysplastic retina fails to produce a normal secondary vitreous. Consequently, hyperplastic primary vitreous frequently adheres to the fold of dysplastic retina, and often there is an atypical displacement of Cloquet's canal toward the septums. Branches of the retinal vessels may be malplaced and are included in the folds.

Malformation of the tertiary vitreous fibrils usually is associated with abnormalities of the lens and zonular fibers, and is discussed in Chapter XI. Colobomas of the ciliary body often produce zonular defects and colobomas of the lens.

INFLAMMATION

General considerations. The metabolic activity of the vitreous is slight compared with that of other tissues, therefore its pathologic reactions are largely passive and usually are characterized by liquefaction, opacification and shrinkage. The colloidal structure of the vitreous is delicately balanced, and is disturbed easily by abnormal concentrations of carbon dioxide, salts, toxins, and inflammatory products. Its avascularity and relative acellularity provide little protection and account for its susceptibility to infection.

The vitreous appears to be an excellent culture medium in vivo, and some organisms which are introduced into it multiply and disseminate rapidly, producing severe inflammation in neighboring tissues (Figs. 72, 75, 78) (see Chapter II). Abscess formation is common. Even organisms of low pathogenicity, such as a nonhemolytic Staphylococcus which, under other conditions, might be saprophytic, can grow rapidly and produce extensive changes in the vitreous and adjacent tissues. The anterior hyaloid layers tend to restrict the extension of inflammation either anteriorly or posteriorly.

Acute inflammatory exudates rapidly become necrotic in the vitreous, and the polymorphonuclear leukocytes appear as peculiar globoid, variably staining, degenerative cells. Often they greatly exceed normal size and lose their usual nuclear characteristics. These cells infiltrate the vitreous in columns between its collagenous sheets (Fig. 577). Peripherally adjacent to the retina and ciliary body, which are the source of these cells, the typical polymorphonuclear configuration is more apparent.

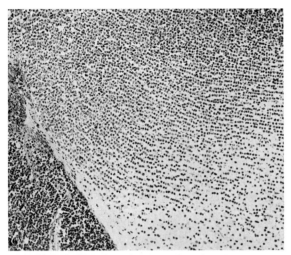

Figure 577. Purulent Exudate in Vitreous

The polymorphonuclear leukocytes appear in single file arrangement because their migratory activity is curbed by the collagenous vitreous sheets. ×115. AFIP Acc. 765628.

In the early stages of an acute inflammatory process within the vitreous all the cells appear to be polymorphonuclear leukocytes. Subsequently, large mononuclear phagocytes become increasingly numerous and fibroblastic proliferation is observed. These cells may lay down an encapsulating wall of fibrous connecting tissue about discrete abscesses or diffusely invade the vitreous in the case of more widespread inflammation. Varying degrees of capillary proliferation are observed and associated with the formation of blood vessels is the appearance of lymphocytes and plasma cells. After the acute phase, polymorphonuclear leukocytes may virtually disappear but mononuclear inflammatory cells often persist for very long periods.

Cyclitic membrane. A succession of serious changes often is observed with organization of inflammatory exudates in the vitreous. The volume of the vitreous is reduced by the connective tissue contraction and loss of water. Traction of this tissue upon the retina and choroid usually produces a detachment of these structures (Figs. 75, 79, 80, 81). The eye atrophies and its outer tunics become thickened. A cyclitic membrane may be formed by the proliferation of connective tissue from the ciliary body and by proliferation and metaplasia of the ciliary epithelial layers. This membrane most often extends across the vitreous face behind the lens. Quite often it forms a dish-like structure with its concavity directed anteriorly. The retina very often is totally detached and is intimately connected with retrolental connective tissue.

Infections of the vitreous. In addition to the common bacteria found in suppurative conditions of the eye (see Chapter II), saprophytic fungi such as Aspergillus and Cephalosporium have been observed in vitreous abscesses. Mycotic infections of the vitreous may not appear until many months after the initial infection. They progress more slowly and tend to remain localized much longer than do bacterial infections which characteristically spread rapidly (Fine and Zimmerman, 1959) (Fig. 76).

Parasitic. Parasitic infections of the eye are not uncommon. The larvae of insects, Cysticercus, and microfilaria have been demonstrated. Alive, they incite little inflammation, but when dead and disintegrating they cause an intense inflammatory reaction associated with eosinophilia (Fig. 26). Echinococcus cysts are known to form in the vitreous, and filariae have been observed clinically and their presence confirmed by microscopic examination.

Nematode. Nematode infections, most of which are apparently caused by larvae of Toxocara canis, usually produce the appearance of a pseudoglioma (Fig. 27) (Wilder; Beaver; deBuen). The natural hosts of these worms are dogs (T. canis) and cats (T. cati), and the infection is acquired by ingestion of eggs from contaminated pets, clothes, soil, etc. The larvae do not complete their life cycle within the human host but are capable of invading human viscera, where they may survive for many months. After the ova are ingested they hatch in the stomach and intestine, migrate through the walls of these organs, and are disseminated via the blood, lymphatics and tissue spaces.

In humans, T. canis infestation occurs almost exclusively in children of preschool or early school age. There is often a history of dirt-eating (geophagia), or close contact with dogs. Although fever, general debility, and pulmonary and hepatic involvement are frequently present in disseminated worm infections, the ocular cases have been peculiar in that there has been no history of such generalized symptomatology. Eosinophilia is typical, and in some cases exceeds 50 per cent. This finding, together with general symptoms, has been often attributed to other intestinal helminths. Infections from T. canis probably are more prevalent than supposed. Recent reports (Ashton) of macular retinal and choroidal involvement by a nematode indicate the widespread distribution of this infectious agent as well as the varied pattern of the ocular disease. The severity of clinical symptoms and the degree of eosinophilia may be proportional to the number of ova ingested.

The possibility of ocular T. canis infestation in children should be suspected from the clinical history and the physical findings. The diagnosis is confirmed by serial sections of tissues harboring the larva or fragments thereof. Due to the failure of the larva to complete its life cycle in the human, stool examinations are noncontributory.

The nematodes usually gain access to the eye either by the ciliary vessels to the choroid or by the retinal vessels to the retina and vitreous. In the eye the wandering nematode larvae are usually found in the vitreous, between folds of the detached retina or, rarely, in chorioretinal lesions. There is an early diffuse polymorphonuclear reaction in which eosinophils predominate. As the larvae die and disintegrate (Fig. 27), focal granulomas form. There is a diffuse plasma cell reaction about the granulomas and often diffusely through the vitreous. This subacute endophthalmitis rarely produces noteworthy symptoms of a uveitis. Almost inevitably the reaction in the vitreous leads to massive retinal detachment.

THE PATHOLOGY OF SURGICAL AND TRAUMATIC RUPTURE OF THE VITREOUS FACE

Excessive fibrosis. Many delayed complications of surgery and trauma result from a fibrocytic reaction which disturbs the normal architecture of intraocular tissues. When fibrosis, the final stage of repair, involves tissues adjacent to the site of injury, its beneficial effect is lost, and ocular function may suffer. Foreign body reactions and traumatic alteration or displacement of tissues often provoke excessive fibrosis, and in this sense the lens and vitreous commonly act as contributory agents. A damaged lens may be removed or allowed to absorb. The restoration of normal architecture rarely occurs when disruption of the vitreous occurs. When disorganized, the vitreous becomes more fluid but is not miscible with aqueous. Its preservation and confinement to the posterior segment is essential to normal ocular physiology. The postsurgical or traumatic influx of vitreous anteriorly not only interferes with the normal dynamics of aqueous flow, but often produces structural changes in the tissues of the anterior segment (Fig. 578). The irritative effect of vitreous upon traumatized tissues often stimulates connective tissue formation which may have widespread intraocular extensions. This complication results more commonly following accidental trauma, but it is also seen after operative procedures. Vitreous may adhere to the posterior iris surface following cataract extraction, effecting pupillary block (Fig. 579), iris bombé, and closure of the filtration angle. Its adherence to the wound, and the fibrous tissue induced by its presence may impede aqueous flow. Secondary glaucoma, then, may result from any of the vitreal changes noted above and can occur directly by the gel blocking the trabeculas, inducing fibrosis and closing the angle.

Vitreous loss during cataract surgery. Prior to the use of sutures, vitreous loss during cataract surgery often initiated complications resulting in loss of the eye. Although serious, disruption of the vitreous need not be catastrophic providing reasonably normal architecture of the intraocular tissue is restored.

Following rupture of the anterior hyaloid, the vitreous tends to envelop the adjacent structures. Because of its viscosity, it carries the iris toward the chamber angle as it escapes. The flexible iris tends to fold within the viscid fluid and often becomes massed at the chamber angle, adherent to the posterior cornea, or incarcerated in the wound. De-

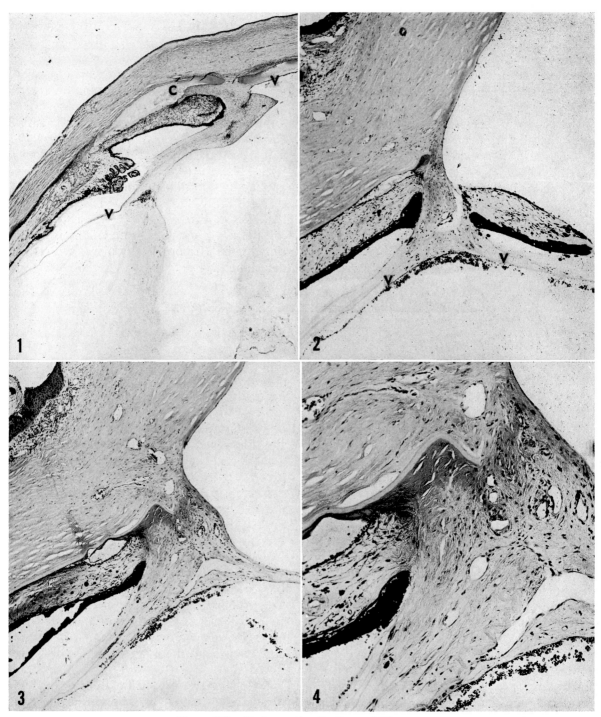

Figure 578. Postoperative Prolapse of Vitreous

1. A band of dense connective tissue binds the prolapsed vitreous (V) to the cornea and iris. The very shallow anterior chamber (C) contains serous exudate. ×12. AFIP Acc. 924896.

2 to 4. Dense connective tissue fills a coloboma of the iris, binding the prolapsed vitreous to the cornea at the site of cataract extraction. ×50. ×50, ×115, respectively. AFIP Acc. 822983.

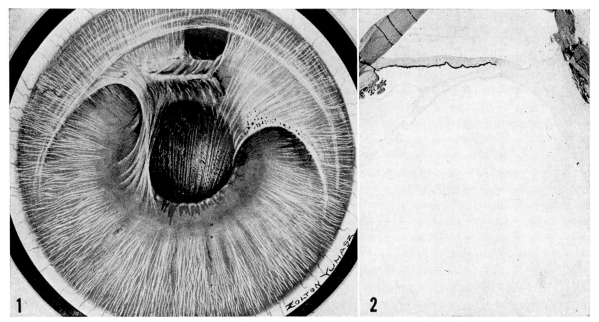

Figure 579. Postoperative Prolapse of Vitreous

1. Vitreous has prolapsed through pupil and through iris coloboma against the cornea.
2. Vitreous adheres to the pupillary margin and to the corneal scar (upper right corner). ×9. AFIP Acc. 741354.

spite attempted replacement, the iris, lacking support of an intact anterior hyaloid layer, usually assumes an abnormal position. The immediate effect may be a hammock pupil, or this may occur later from contraction of organized vitreous strands extending from the wound to the lower pupillary margin. In such cases, the filtration angle in the region of the wound is usually occluded by iris, condensed vitreous, or connective tissue. The consequences of allowing the vitreous and iris to remain in contact with the wound far outweigh the hazard of any additional vitreous loss that may occur in re-establishing a more normal arrangement of the ocular tissues. The more solid, tenacious peripheral vitreous, particularly that comprising the base, is retained longest within the eye, but when displaced anteriorly it is particularly irritating, and excites fibrosis more readily than does the less viscid central vitreous. Fluid vitreous is comparatively nonirritating, is not conducive to the development of traction bands, and often is lost without causing any of the complications discussed above.

The vitreous face often thickens after cataract surgery and may reform after rupture. This is enhanced by inflammation. In the latter case, either the pupil may be secluded without pathologically demonstrable poste-rior synechias, or fibrous tissue may form a dense pupillary membrane.

Delayed rupture of vitreous. Delayed rupture of the vitreous face may occur at any time after uncomplicated intracapsular cataract extraction. Whereas this usually creates no problem other than a transitory blurring of vision, occasionally secondary glaucoma can ensue either because of pupillary block or possibly because of the impermeable vitreous which occludes the angle recess. Vitreous may attach to the posterior corneal wound and form annoying traction bands many months after surgery (Fig. 580). At times, the attachment of the vitreous to the corneal endothelium causes local corneal edema and opacification. The apposition of vitreous to cornea probably does not cause abnormal hydration in the presence of normal endothelium.

Retinal detachment. The incidence of retinal detachment following vitreous loss is greater than that following uncomplicated extractions. Fibrous bands may extend to the retina from the wound, the iris, or from cataractous remnants. Contraction of these bands ultimately leads to retinal detachments that are difficult to repair. When lost vitreous is replaced by aqueous, the incidence of retinal detachment is greater because of

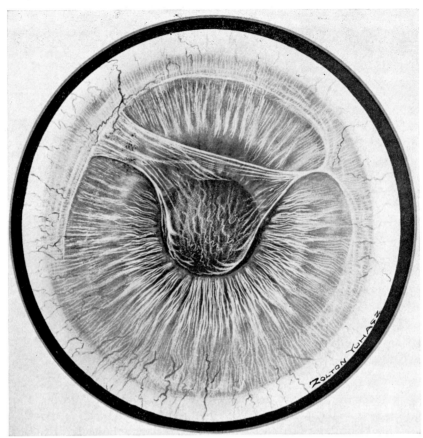

Figure 580. Delayed rupture of vitreous face following uncomplicated cataract extraction with adhesions to the cornea.

syneresis of the remaining vitreous with consequent traction upon the retina.

When the lens and vitreous have been disrupted, danger of fibrosis is greatly increased because both are not only irritants, but serve as framework for the intraocular extension of traction bands originating from the wound and iris. They frequently envelop lens remnants and the adjacent iris, forming dense pupillary membranes that are amenable only to excision.

Disruption of vitreous during filtering operations is usually followed by a rise in intraocular pressure. Vitreous within the surgical dehiscence prohibits the escape of aqueous and its presence within the posterior chamber may block the chamber angle by displacing the iris root anteriorly. Vitreal contact with the wound often incites fibrosis in the filtering scar.

Vitreous damage in traumatic injuries. When foreign bodies penetrate the eye and lodge in the orbit, fibrosis arising at the point of exit is not unusual. Such penetrating wounds often are associated with vitreous loss. As a result of this and the coincident hemorrhage, fibrous proliferation may be marked. The same reaction occurs at times after posterior extraction of intraocular foreign bodies, by the penetrating diathermy treatment used for repair of retinal detachment, and less commonly by excessive surface diathermy.

THE ROLE OF THE VITREOUS IN ANGLE CLOSURE AND MALIGNANT GLAUCOMA

The vitreous may play an important role in the pathogenesis of angle closure and malignant glaucoma. In malignant glaucoma there is a shallow anterior chamber, a large lens, and a small intercalary space. In such an eye after paracentesis, iridectomy, or filtering operations, the lens-iris diaphragm is anteriorly displaced, and the tension remains elevated. Sometimes following lens extraction the hyaloid extends anteriorly and may produce a physiologic pupillary block. It has been postulated that the vitreous gel, and particularly its hyaluronic acid component, is capable of binding large amounts of water, and it is conceivable that this condition could lead to turgescence, thereby producing the events outlined above. This subject was investigated by Duke-Elder who found that dehydrated vitreous imbibes water and swells when exposed to a moist atmosphere. The total swelling, however, is but a small fraction of the original volume, and his experiments indicate that normal vitreous is fully hydrated. Von Sallmann found that the vitreous, if carefully dissected out of the eye, exudes fluid and collapses, but if the vitreous with attached zonules, lens, and retina is placed in hypertonic or isotonic saline solutions small imbibitions of water can be measured. Whether the water is imbibed by the vitreous or by the other attached structures is not clear, and therefore it is thought un-

likely that swelling of the vitreous is ever responsible for angle closure glaucoma. However, there is some evidence to indicate that, with detachment and anterior dislocation of the vitreous face, the preferential flow of aqueous is posteriorly where it pools in the vitreous, causing the more solid peripheral and basal portion to become dislocated. These conditions are usually enhanced by posterior superior detachments of the vitreous, which permit the more solid portions to become dislocated anteriorly against the lens. When fluorescein is injected intravenously in such instances, it may be recovered through a posterior sclerotomy, indicating that the passage of aqueous has been posterior rather than anterior. The vitreous may infiltrate between the zonular fibers and fill the circumlental space. Whether it actually turgesces, or whether aqueous lakes occur within the vitreous pushing it forward is therefore debatable. Clinically, the latter thesis is supported by the relief of intraocular pressure and deepening of the anterior chamber when the thickened anterior hyaloid is incised or when solid vitreous is purposely removed through a posterior sclerotomy.

VITREOUS OPACITIES

Mononuclear phagocytes. In addition to the cells of acute and chronic inflammation, mononuclear phagocytes infiltrate the vitreous in a variety of conditions. They engulf the nuclear debris of inflammatory exudates, red cells in hemorrhagic extravasations, pigment liberated from the retina, the uvea, and tumors. They are the principal inflammatory cells in phacolytic glaucoma where they are seen throughout the vitreous and around the hypermature cataractous lens, particularly on the posterior surface where the capsule is thinned or nonexistent. Their cytoplasm is swollen, with acidophilic liquefied lens cortex producing cells of such size as to block the trabeculas and to impede aqueous outflow. Most of these cells are washed out in preparing histologic sections, but some may still be seen where the vitreous is solid, especially at its base and in clusters along the surface of the posterior retina. Ophthalmoscopically,

they produce vitreous opacities which disappear slowly after cataract extraction (see Chapter XI).

Blood. Vitreous hemorrhage usually comes from the retina, and may be preretinal, in Cloquet's canal, confined to a vitreous compartment, or widely dispersed. Occasionally it is seen as a thin layer immediately behind the lens. The blood corpuscles may remain well preserved and bright red for many months. Massive hemorrhages are quite impermeable to light, and may reduce vision to light perception. Their outcome varies, but frequently they may be absorbed without fibroblastic organization. If little or no absorption occurs hemorrhages frequently stimulate invasion of fibroblasts, ultimately leading to retinal detachment. Vitreous hemorrhage may be followed by proliferation of blood vessels forming thin sheets extending from the retina and into the vitreous. They

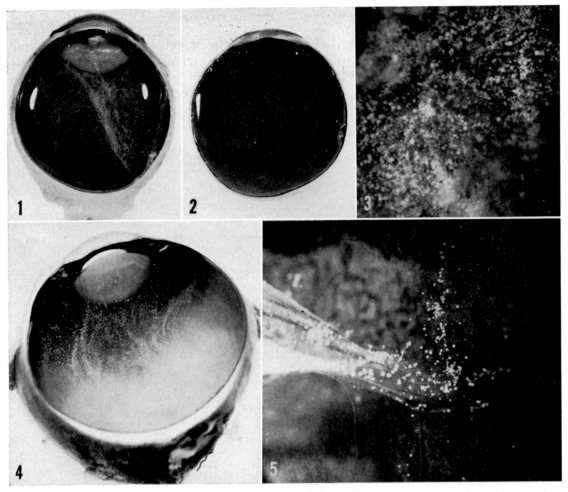

Figure 581.   Asteroid Hyalosis

1 and 2. The vitreous opacities resemble a galaxy of stars. ×2. AFIP Acc. 523342.
3. Same specimen. ×40.
4 and 5. Another case, AFIP Acc. 583036. ×3 and ×40, respectively.

usually arise from the disk, but may, as in retrolental fibroplasia, originate from other parts of the retina. The contraction of blood clots may cause the vitreous and/or retina to become detached. They often are surrounded by an endothelial membrane consisting of a single or laminated cell layer derived from the inner layer of the retina. Vascularization may be represented by a single vessel coiled back on itself; more often there is an intricate arrangement of delicate vessels forming an anastomosing network known as rete mirabile. This mass of vessels is held together by a delicate sheet of connective tissue which may thicken because of fibroblastic and neuroglial proliferation, may regress, or disappear completely.

Epithelial cells. Epithelial cells from the ciliary body may also invade the vitreous. Usually they are fragmented and their pigment granules are often engulfed by macrophages, sometimes making it difficult to differentiate them from the latter. Spherical cellular elements may be seen free in the vitreous or attached to the retina or nerve head by a pedicle. They may represent proliferations of glial cells, or if they contain pigment granules, may be derived from the pigment epithelium.

Tumor cells. Tumor cells are commonly seen floating free in the vitreous or lying on the retina in retinoblastoma. They are rarely seen in malignant melanoma and metastatic carcinoma.

Asteroid hyalosis. The occurrence of spherical or disk-shaped white bodies, sometimes referred to as "snow-ball" opacities, Scintillatio Albescens or Nivea, is a rare phenomenon which is known best, though inappropriately, under the designation of asteroid hyalitis (Fig. 581). It is unilateral in 75 per cent of the cases, is twice as frequent in men as in women, and is found in patients with an average age of sixty. The opacities typically occur in vitreous that appears otherwise normal. The etiology is unknown, and the condition is clinically innocuous.

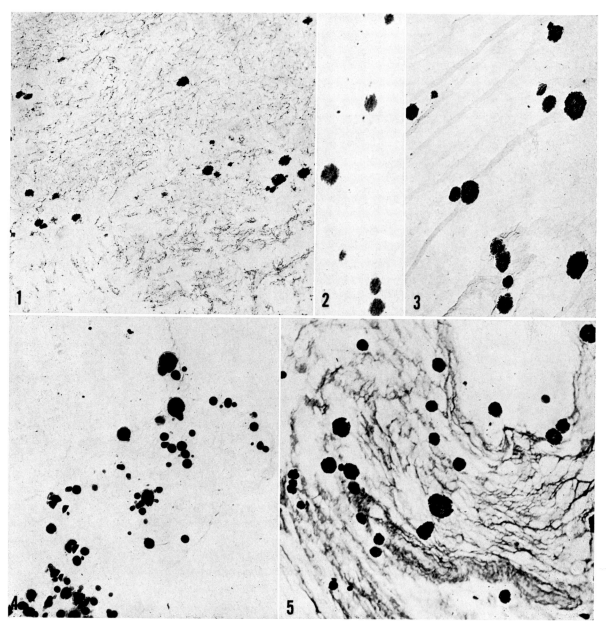

Figure 582. Asteroid Hyalosis

1. In this case the opacities within the vitreous are stained more deeply than usual. H and E, ×80. AFIP Acc. 906582.

2. Positive staining with oil red O. ×160. AFIP Acc. 330261.

3. Positive staining with Sudan black B. ×160. AFIP Acc. 523342.

4. Positive staining with alizarin red after microincineration. ×105. AFIP Acc. 715044.

5. Positive staining with colloidal iron reaction for acid mucopolysaccharides. ×95. AFIP Acc. 523342.

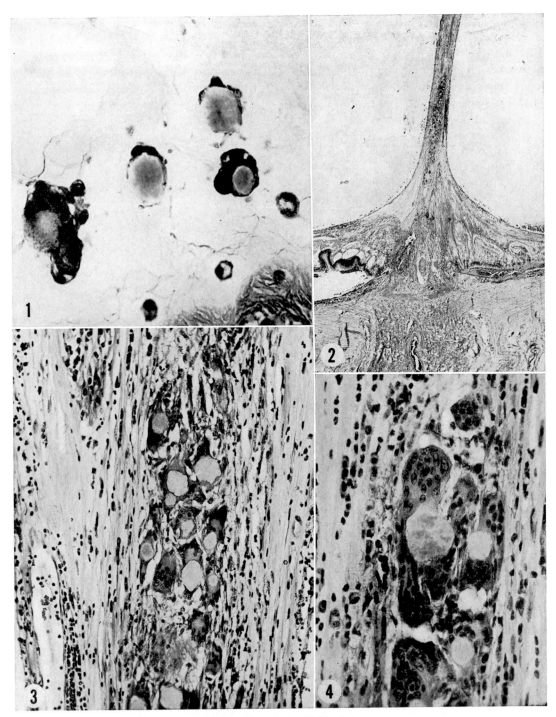

Figure 583. Asteroid Hyalitis

1. The vitreous opacities are similar to those shown in Figure 582 except that they are surrounded by foreign body giant cells. ×530. AFIP Acc. 269271.

2. Projecting from the optic disk is a mass of shrunken vitreous containing similar lesions shown at greater magnification in 3 and 4. ×14. AFIP Acc. 955663.

3 and 4. These deposits have special staining and histochemical reactions similar to those of the vitreous opacities in ordinary cases of asteroid hyalosis but here they have provoked a foreign body giant cell reaction. ×180 and ×305, respectively.

The vitreous opacities of asteroid hyalosis have such characteristic histologic features that they can be recognized readily in routine preparations (Fig. 582). They are roughly spherical bodies, .01 to 0.1 mm. in diameter, which usually are stained only weakly with hematoxylin and eosin. When examined with polarized light the asteroid bodies appear to be composed of crystalline particles. Although they resist the usual fat solvents, they are nevertheless stained by the ordinary lipid stains (e.g., Oil red O, Sudan black B, Scharlach R, Nile blue sulfate, etc.). When stained with Alcian blue or the colloidal iron method for acid mucopolysaccharides, they give reactions that are much more intensely positive than the remaining vitreous and this staining reaction is not affected by hyaluronidase. Current histochemical studies (Rodman et al.) have provided additional evidence in support of Verhoeff's suggestion, made about 40 years ago, that these vitreous opaci-

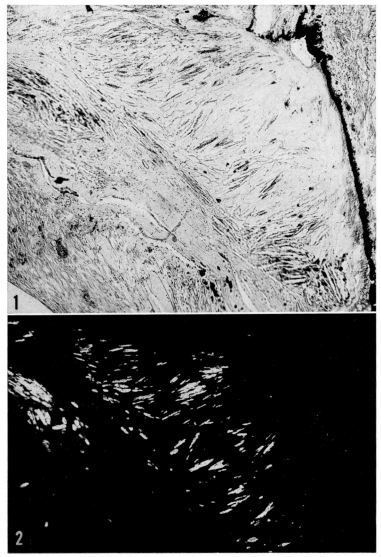

Figure 584.   Cholesterolosis Bulbi

1. The innumerable slit-like spaces contained in the organized vitreous exudate represent the sites of cholesterol crystal deposition. ×50. AFIP Acc. 929200.

2. The cholesterol crystals are birefringent when examined with polarized light. Frozen section, ×50. AFIP Acc. 929200.

ties consist chiefly of calcium soap.

Typically these vitreous opacities do not stimulate any cellular reaction. Recently, however, deposits which by their general microscopic appearance, special staining characteristics, and histochemical reactions cannot be distinguished from those observed in asteroid hyalosis have been found in association with a foreign body type of response (Rodman et al.). In some cases the individual deposits are surrounded by a few macrophages and giant cells (Fig. 583–1), while in other examples a large group of these bodies is contained in a foreign body granuloma (Fig. 583–2, 3, 4).

Synchysis scintillans. Synchysis scintillans occurs more often in patients under thirty-five years of age, is usually bilateral, is associated with a fluid vitreous, and is often the consequence of another important pathologic process. The flat, roughly rectangular crystalline deposits are composed primarily of cholesterol, although tyrosine and margarine needles have been noted. This condition, also appropriately called cholesterolosis bulbi, occurs after other ocular disease, such as chronic degenerations, trauma, hemorrhage, or inflammation (Fig. 584).

Protein coagula. Proteinaceous coagula may produce opacities as the vitreous gel is liquefied. Protein may also enter the vitreous from the ciliary body and retina when their vessels are engorged as a result of inflammation. Such plasmoid vitreous may reduce vision.

REFERENCES

Ashton, N.: Larval Granulomatosis of the Retina Due to Toxocara. Brit. J. Ophthal. *44:*129–148, 1960.

Beaver, P. C.: Larva Migrans. Exp. Parasit. *5:*587–621, 1956.

Berliner, M.: Biomicroscopy of the Eye. New York, P. B. Hoeber, Vol. I, 1943; Vol. II, 1949.

Boyer, H. K., Suran, A. A., Hogan, M. J., McEwen, W. K.: Increase of Residual Protein of Bovine Vitreous During Growth of the Eye. A.M.A. Arch. Ophthal. *56:*861–864, 1956.

de Buen, S., Zimmerman, L. E., and Foerster, H. C.: Inflamaciones Oculares Granulomatosas Consecutivas a Infecciones Endogenas. An. Soc. Mex. Oftal. *29:*39–69, 1956.

Duke-Elder, W. S.: Nature of the Vitreous Body. Brit. J. Ophthal., Supp. *4:*1–72, 1930.

Fine, B. S., and Tousimis, A. J.: The Structure of the Vitreous Body and the Suspensory Ligament of the Lens. A.M.A. Arch. Ophthal. *65:*95–110, 1961.

Fine, B. S., and Zimmerman, L. E.: Exogenous Intraocular Fungus Infections: with Particular Reference to Complications of Intraocular Surgery. Amer. J. Ophthal. *48:*151–165, (Aug.) 1959.

Friedenwald, J. S., and Stiehler, R.: Structure of the Vitreous. A.M.A. Arch. Ophthal. *14:*789–808, 1935.

Irvine, S. R.: A Newly Defined Vitreous Syndrome Following Cataract Surgery Interpreted According to Recent Concepts of the Structure of the Vitreous. Amer. J. Ophthal. *36:*599–619, (May) 1953.

Jokl, A.: Comparative Researches on the Structure and Development of the Vitreous and Its Contents in Vertebrates and Man. Uppsala, Sweden, Almquist and Wirksells, 1927.

Mann, I. C.: Developmental Abnormalities of the Eye. London, Cambridge University Press, 1937.

Mann, I. C.: The Development of the Human Eye. 2d ed. New York, Grune and Stratton, 1950.

Moore, R. F.: Subjective "Lightning Streaks." Brit. J Ophthal. *19:*545–547, 1935.

Parsons, J. H.: The Pathology of the Eye. Hodder and Stoughton, London, 1904–1908.

Reese, A. B.: Persistent Hyperplastic Primary Vitreous. Amer. J. Ophthal. *40:*317–331, (Sept.) 1955.

Rodman, H. I., Johnson, F. B., and Zimmerman, L. E.: New Histopathological and Histochemical Observations Concerning Asteroid Hyalitis. A.M.A. Arch. Ophthal. *66:*552–563, 1961.

Salzmann, M.: The Anatomy and Histology of the Human Eyeball in the Normal State. Trans. by E. V. L. Brown, Chicago, University of Chicago Press, 1912.

Schepens, C. L.: Clinical Aspects of Pathologic Changes in the Vitreous Body. Amer. J. Ophthal. *38:*8–21, 1954.

Szirmai, J. A., and Balazs, E. A.: Studies on the Structure of the Vitreous Body. III. Cells in the Cortical Layer. A.M.A. Arch. Ophthal. *59:*34–48, (Jan.) 1958.

Vail, D.: The Zonule of Zinn and Ligament of Wieger; Their Importance in the Mechanics of the Intracapsular Extraction of Cataract. Trans. Amer. Ophthal. Soc. *77:*441–499, 1957.

Verhoeff, F. H.: Microscopic Findings in a Case of Asteroid Hyalitis. Amer. J. Ophthal. *4:*155–160, 1921.

von Sallmann, L.: Expansion Tendency of the Vitreous and Its pH Volume Curve. A.M.A. Arch. Ophthal. *25:*243–254, 1941.

von Sallmann, L.: Experimental Studies on Vitreous Detachment. Amer. J. Ophthal. *24:*1349–1353, 1941.

Wadsworth, J. A. C.: The Vitreous. Gross and Microscopic Observations Seen in Age and Disease, with Special Emphasis on the Role of Vitreous in Detachment of the Retina. A.M.A. Arch. Ophthal. *58:*725–734, (Nov.) 1957.

Wilder, H. C.: Nematode Endophthalmitis. Trans. Amer. Acad. Ophthal. Otolaryng. *55:*99–109, 1950.

Chapter **XI**

Diseases of the Lens

EMBRYOLOGY

A knowledge of the embryology and anatomy of the lens is essential in order to understand its function, growth, nutrition and diseases. The lens is an epithelial structure, derived from the surface ectoderm overlying the optic vesicle. The first evidence of its development in the embryo is at the 4.5 mm. stage when a thickening of the surface ectoderm occurs to form the lens plate. The plate consists of tall cylindrical cells, which are so closely packed that the nuclei are forced to occupy different levels, giving it a multilayered appearance. A small depression, the lens pit, develops in the center of the lens plate. The pit deepens and invagination proceeds until a vesicle is formed. This vesicle completely separates from the surface ectoderm by the 12 mm. stage (Fig. 570–1). At this time the lens assumes an almost spherical form.

The anterior cells of the vesicle increase in number to keep pace with the growth of the lens. However, important changes take place in the cells forming the posterior half of the lens. They elongate and completely fill the lens vesicle at about the 20 mm. stage (Fig. 570–2). These are the primary lens fibers. At the 12 mm. stage a hyaline capsule begins to form posteriorly; by the 70 mm. stage it is well developed and surrounds the whole lens.

Anteriorly the capsule covers the lens epithelium whereas posteriorly it is in direct contact with the lens fibers. Subsequent fibers develop from lens cells at the equatorial region. They elongate and extend anteriorly and posteriorly to form the secondary lens fibers, which surround the original primary fibers. Continued formation and growth of fibers produce multiple layers. The cells at the equator are responsible for the continued growth of the lens throughout life.

The terminations of the lens fibers anteriorly and posteriorly form lines of contact with each other which are known as the lens sutures. The secondary fibers of the fetal lens meet anteriorly to form the erect, and posteriorly to form the inverted Y sutures. These sutures delineate the fetal nucleus of the lens and lie beneath the capsule at term. Those fibers which form subsequent to development of the fetal nucleus form more complicated suture lines with many branchings. The fibers which form the adult nucleus grow during childhood and adolescence. The lens cortex surrounds this nucleus and continues to develop throughout life.

In the case of skin, hair and nails, exfoliation of the older cells makes way for younger cells. However, this is not possible in the

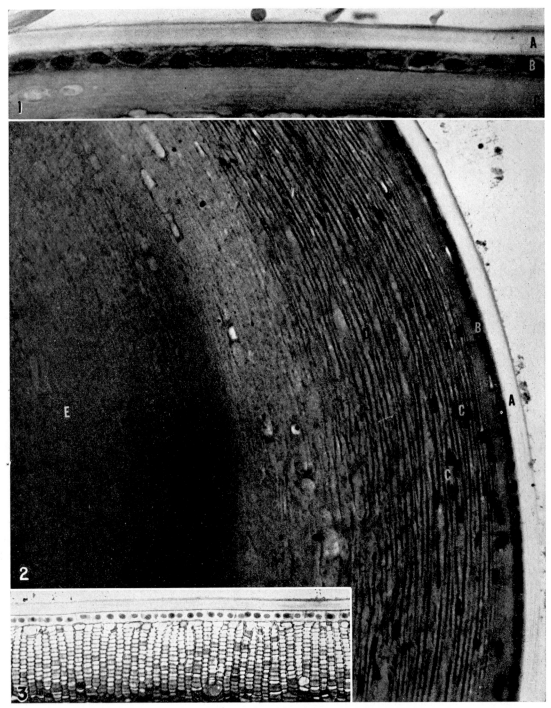

Figure 585. Normal Lens

1. A, capsule. B, anterior subcapsular epithelium. C, cortical lens cells. ×1000. AFIP Acc. 59755.

2. Equator. A, capsule. B, subcapsular epithelium. C, nuclei of nuclear bow. D, cortical cells. E, nucleus. ×330. AFIP Acc. 50846.

3. Cross section of cortical cells reveals their hexagonal outline. Occasional irregularity is caused by early degenerative change. ×260. AFIP Acc. 132413.

lens, so the younger cells merely surround and compress those which are older. This growth accounts, at least in part, for the increase in both the density and the volume of the lens.

The lens is held in position by the zonules, which are formed from the tertiary vitreous. As the margin of the optic cup moves forward, forming the ciliary body at about the third month of fetal life, the vitreous, which is produced by the neuroepithelium, assumes a backward direction. This anterior part of the secondary vitreous is called the marginal bundle. A little later newly formed fibers from the ciliary region, the tertiary vitreous or zonules, grow forward through the marginal bundle, causing it to atrophy. This leaves the zonules as a complex system of fibers running from the ciliary body to the lens (Figs. 301, 565).

The fetal lens is nourished by the tunica vasculosa lentis. The hyaloid artery, after entering the eye through the posterior end of the fetal fissure at the 7 mm. stage, passes anteriorly to reach the posterior pole of the lens vesicle. A net of capillaries spreads out on the lens to form the posterior part of the tunica vasculosa lentis. This net then sends branches to anastomose with the annular vessel to form the lateral portion of the vascular network around the lens. Finally, at about the 17 mm. stage, buds from the annular vessel run along the anterior surface of the lens to complete the anterior portion of the tunica vasculosa lentis. At about the end of the third month the hyaloid system has reached its greatest development. From this time on it atrophies, and usually has disappeared by the time of birth.

ANATOMY AND HISTOLOGY

The lens is a soft, elastic, nonvascular, transparent, highly refractive, biconvex structure. Three different portions can be demonstrated: the lens capsule, epithelium, and cells.

The lens *capsule,* as seen by ordinary light microscopy, is a structureless membrane (Fig. 585). It is highly resistant to chemical and toxic influences. If it is lacerated, the wound borders gape and have a tendency to roll outward. The capsule helps the lens utilize nutrients from the aqueous, provides insertions for the zonular fibers, and plays an important part in molding the shape of the lens in ac-

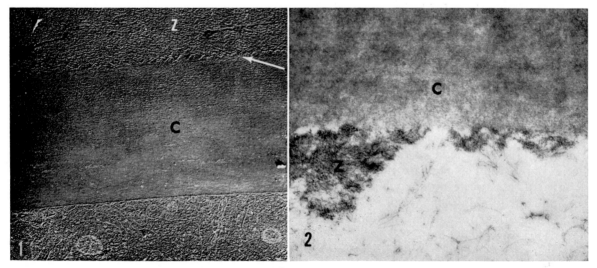

Figure 586.

1. The specimen has been shadow cast with uranium and the micrograph enlarged photographically to ×2,600. The capsule (C) has a laminated appearance. The undulated line (arrow) marks the zone of continuity of the anterior zonular filaments (Z) with the capsule. Epithelial cells are seen at the bottom of the field.

2. This section has been treated with uranyl acetate and the micrograph enlarged photographically to ×14,400. Zonular filaments (Z) are attached to the finely laminated posterior lens capsule (C). Courtesy Dr. B. S. Fine.

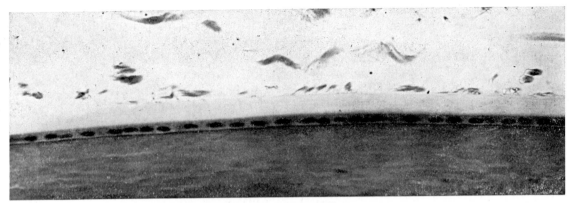

Figure 587. Normal Lens

Zonular fibers are shown at their insertions into the lens capsule. ×435. AFIP Acc. 181211.

commodation. Although it appears to be homogeneous, the capsule has a laminated appearance when studied with special stains or in the electron microscope (Fig. 586). According to Bahr, this method shows the capsule to have a lamellar arrangement and the lamellas appear to have an amorphous material adherent to their surfaces.

A thin superficial lamella can be shown at the zonular attachment to the capsule (Fig. 587). The capsule is thickest anteriorly over the lens epithelial cells and in the equatorial zone, where it measures from 13 to 15 microns, and is thinnest posteriorly.

The lens capsule is intensely periodic acid-Schiff positive and probably is composed of an insoluble protein combined with a polysaccharide. Dische and Borenfreund found the capsule to contain galactose and glucose in the ratio of 3 to 2. Gifford has shown that the zonular lamella stains differently, being positive with the Rinehart and Abul Haj modification of the colloidal iron stain, which is more specific for acid mucopolysaccharides. The capsule is important for the integrity of the lens and seems to regulate the transport of nutrients and waste products between the lens and aqueous. Maintenance of its permeability is important for normal metabolism of the various parts of the lens.

A layer of *epithelial cells* lies immediately beneath the anterior lens capsule. These cells are large and cuboidal, with large spherical nuclei (Fig. 585). Nearer the anterior periphery they are smaller and more cylindrical, with spherical nuclei. At the equator they be-

come more columnar and their nuclei increase in height and stain more intensely. In flat preparations of very fresh tissue studied with the phase contrast microscope, the normal form of the epithelial cells is irregularly polygonal with slightly curved angles and sides. Cell borders are hardly visible. Van den Heuvel was not able to detect syncytial connections or tonofibrils mentioned by older investigators. By electron microscopy Wanko and Gavin observed numerous cytoplasmic processes to interdigitate with those of neighboring cells (Fig. 586). A Golgi complex, endoplasmic reticulum, mitochondria and a small vesicular structure peculiar to lens epithelium were seen by these workers in the cytoplasm of the cells.

The nuclei of lens epithelial cells are oval in the lenses of cattle and round in the human lens, with a smooth regular nuclear membrane. Within the nucleus several condensations of irregular slightly angular form are noted. One of these is probably the nucleolus.

Near the equator of the lens the axis of the epithelial cells becomes more oblique, and at the equator itself they have rotated 90 degrees to their position under the anterior capsule. Here the cells elongate to form new lens fibers (Fig. 588). As new fibers form under the capsule they displace the most recently formed fibers centrally. The fibers which are crowded more deeply into the lens substance have their nuclei displaced slightly forward to form a nuclear zone in the shape

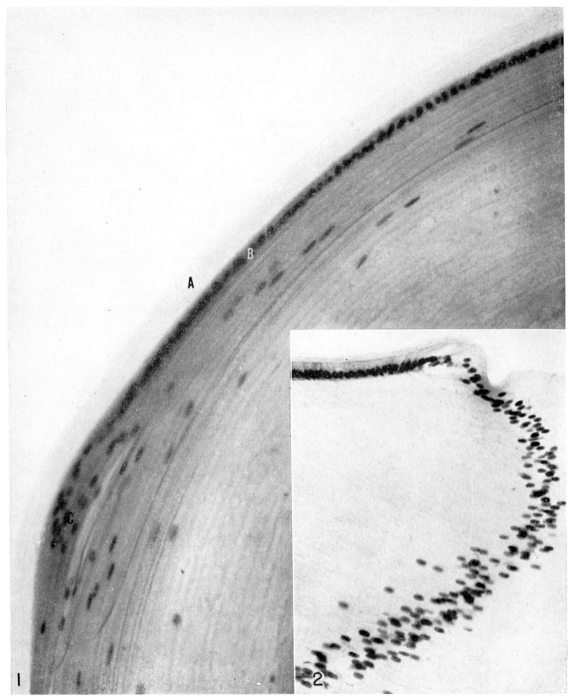

Figure 588. Normal Lens

1. Equator. A, capsule. B, subcapsular epithelium. C, nuclear bow. ×425. AFIP Acc. 35023.
2. Nuclear bow. ×330. AFIP Acc. 58670.

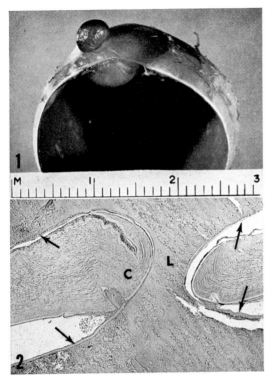

Figure 589. Partial Herniation of Lens through Corneal Wound

1. Specimen opened after formalin-fixation. AFIP Acc. 728663.

2. Arrows indicate intact capsule of lens (L) adjacent to the edges of the defect in the cornea (C). Same case. ×50.

of a bow (Fig. 588–2). Posteriorly the lens capsule is in direct contact with the lens cells. The epithelium is the only tissue in the lens which is capable of regeneration; it may proliferate when stimulated by injury, such as inflammation in neighboring tissues.

The *lens substance* is composed of lens cells (or fibers) arranged in layers called lamellas (Figs. 585, 588). The outer colorless cells form the cortex; the deeper yellowish central zone is designated the nucleus. In cross section the long ribbon-like superficial cells are hexagonal prisms; one row of cells fits neatly into the sawtooth-like edge of another (Fig. 585–3). In the center of the lens the arrangement becomes more irregular. The young cells have a smooth border and a large oval nucleus; the older ones have finely serrated edges, and have lost their nuclei. The soft pliable nature of the normal cortical cells coupled with the relatively tough quality of the capsule permits molding of the

lens by tumor masses, and herniation through corneal wounds or ulcers (Fig. 589).

The conversion of the soft lens fibers in the cortex into the compact structure of the nucleus is a process that goes on steadily throughout life. There is a slow but steady increase in nuclear volume, the nuclear fibers losing water and becoming compressed, producing sclerosis or hardening.

Friedenwald and Small have shown that the younger cells of the cortex have a lipid membrane stainable with heavy metals and that this membrane is absent in the deeper cortex and nucleus. Van den Heuvel also found faint but clear staining with Sudan black and Sudan red on the boundaries of the epithelial cells and in the fibers of the transitional layer near the nucleus. He believed lipids in the cell boundary to be a strong argument in favor of the existence of a cell membrane.

Loss of the cell membrane, diminution in size of the fibers and the loss of nuclei would suggest that the inner lens cells are dead. Studies by Merriam and Kinsey, however, have shown that these cells still have metabolic activity.

The *suspensory ligament* helps hold the lens in place through its attachment to the ciliary body. Additional support is gained through the hyaloid ligament, which forms a weak attachment of the lens to the vitreous. In cross section the area of attachment of the zonular fibers to the lens forms a funnel. The apex of the funnel encompasses the equator and extends over the anterior and posterior lens surface a short distance. The lenticular endings of the zonular fibers are quite different from those at the ciliary body. At the lens the fibers are inserted rather at a tangent to the capsule. As they insert into the capsule they subdivide into divergent fibrils, which are firmly united with the outer layer of the lens capsule. The middle or equatorial fibers, few in number and more delicate, insert practically at right angles into the capsule in the immediate neighborhood of the equator.

At the ciliary body the zonular fibers unite directly with the epithelial cells, either in the ciliary valleys or on the lateral surfaces of the ciliary processes, but never with those at the summit of the processes. Pappas and Smelser have shown by electron microscopy that an internal membrane lines the apical surfaces of the epithelial cells of the ciliary body, facing the posterior chamber. Zonular fibrils enter this membrane and contribute to its formation. From the pars plana there is a continuous union of zonular fibrils to form bundles of fibers. These pass toward the lens to join other fibers prior to their insertion into the capsule.

The transparency of the normal lens is a manifestation of its relative optical homogeneity. Since the protein content of the lens fibers is very high, the refractive index of these fibers is correspondingly high and differs widely from that of extracellular fluid or aqueous. It follows that in the normal lens there must be little, if any, extracellular fluid

or that fluid must be of a high refractive index in order that light be not refracted upon passing from extracellular to intracellular media. The mechanism of transparency of the lens is probably not the same as occurs in the cornea. The lens fibers themselves, if viewed under the dark field microscope, are relatively devoid of the cytoplasmic granules seen in most other cell types. In this respect the cytoplasm of the lens cells resembles that of the red blood cells. Indeed there are many analogies between these two cell types. Both have a low respiratory activity, a high protein content, a homogeneous cytoplasm, and a capacity to survive for long periods without a nucleus.

BIOCHEMISTRY OF THE NORMAL AND CATARACTOUS LENS

The lens has a relatively simple composition and morphologic structure. It is a particularly favorable tissue for the study of the chemistry and metabolism of one type of cell at all stages of growth. The older methods of separating the proteins from lens extracts by precipitation at different degrees of acidity yield soluble fractions called α-crystallin and β-crystallin. These account for 85 per cent of the total protein nitrogen present. An insoluble protein called albuminoid accounts for 12.5 per cent of the protein nitrogen and another soluble protein albumin (gamma crystallin) is present in a small amount (1 to 2 per cent). Traces of mucoprotein, nucleoprotein and phosphoprotein have also been reported. The dry weight of the lens is about 35 per cent of its wet weight. The lens, therefore, has an unusually high protein content, one that compares with that of hair and nails.

Electrophoretic analysis of lens extracts has provided new and interesting data. The work of François and Rabaey suggests a much more complicated schema of protein composition than has heretofore been realized. The crystallins appear to be mixtures of proteins and there may be as many as ten different components of lens protein. Also there probably is a third soluble protein formed only in embryonic life and perhaps for a few months after birth.

Electrophoretic patterns in the young human lens show four easily separated components which are called Fraction I, II, III and IV. These cannot be demonstrated in the adult lens because the entire protein complex of the lens tends to migrate in bulk. In fact, it is difficult to demonstrate the four components beyond the age of ten years, suggesting a fairly rapid aging change in the human lens, and a chemical alteration in the proteins during early life. When various parts of the lens are investigated, Fraction I remains constant throughout various layers of the young lens; Fraction II predominates in the cortex and Fraction III predominates in the nucleus. Fraction IV is not synthesized at all after infancy, and in the adult is localized in the nucleus. This suggests that Fraction IV is that protein in the human lens which corresponds to the embryonal protein isolated by François and associates from beef lenses. Fraction I resembles α-crystallin on the basis of its mobility and other properties. Fractions II, III and IV have not been identified.

Lens proteins are unique; they show a certain uniformity throughout different species and they are immunologically tissue specific as well as species specific (Ulenhuth, 1903; Hektoen and Schulhof, 1924; Woods and Burky, 1927). Woods et al. showed that α-crystallin is the main organ specific protein.

cataract formation are amino acid and vitamin deficiencies. Among the essential amino acids, the lack of tryptophan has been most often implicated. Riboflavin deficiency is the only vitamin deficiency which produces cataracts consistently. The cataracts usually develop after the animals have been on the deficient diet for from six to ten weeks. They first appear as flaky irregular opacities scattered in the lens cortex.

Associated with the onset of nutritional cataract, there is vascularization and ulceration of the cornea, conjunctivitis, dermatitis with areas of baldness, irregularities in the teeth, and gonadal atrophy.

Buschke has suggested that the metabolic systems of the tissues which sustain similar damage in these deficiency states probably require both riboflavin and tryptophan for normal functioning. He indicated that there is a group of endogenous cataracts in humans with associated lesions of the cornea, conjunctiva, skin, teeth, and gonads, producing a disease pattern similar to that seen in experimental riboflavin cataract. The resemblance is most striking in cataracts complicating atopic eczema, but it also exists in those associated with scleroderma, myotonia, and mongolian idiocy. Most of these conditions are hereditary and congenital. They perhaps represent an endogenous disturbance of the same metabolic pathways that are affected by riboflavin or tryptophan deficiency.

A calcium to phosphate ratio, lowered to the point of tetany, may be considered in this deficiency mechanism of cataract formation. The tetany can be elicited by parathyroidectomy or by dietary deficiency in association with rickets. The lenticular lesion appears in the form of flaky subcapsular opacities. If the tetany is cured the existing opacities do not clear; with normal growth, new clear cortex is laid down outside the zone of opacities. Repeated intermittent production of tetany can lead to the development of successive zones of opacity in the lens, separated from each other by clear normal cortex. There would appear to be little doubt that this form of experimental cataract is related to that associated with tetany in humans.

Some general poisons will produce cataract in susceptible animals. Belonging to this group are dinitrophenol, naphthalene, thallium and ergot. A new compound *Myleran* used in the treatment of myeloid leukemia has produced lens opacities. The earliest pathologic change in the lens is a marked increase in the number of mitoses in the lens epithelium which suggests that Myleran acts as a radiomimetic drug. The method by which these substances produce degenerative changes in the lens is not known. *Dinitrophenol* formerly was used therapeutically for obesity and when it was available for this purpose many cataract cases were reported. The cataracts usually were bilateral. Vacuoles were noted early in the posterior subscapular region, resembling a secondary cataract. The evolution of the degenerative process was rapid, until the whole lens became opaque. Cogan and Cogan, recalling that dinitrophenol apparently increases the cellular metabolism above the level which can be supplied by the usual means of oxidation, explained the cause of the cataract on the basis of anoxia.

The feeding of *naphthalene* has been used for many years to produce experimental cataracts. A number of related compounds also are effective as cataractogenic agents. Naphthalene cataract has been attributed to the conjugation of naphthalene with the cysteine of lens glutathione. In some way too, there is marked derangement of carbohydrate metabolism. According to Pirie and van Heyningen there is a large increase in the lactic acid content of the lens; organic phosphate decreases; glucose consumption is higher than normal before there are any lens changes, and is normal by the time the first opacities are visible. As opacification increases glucose consumption falls below the normal level.

An interesting explanation for the production of cataracts by naphthalene was offered by Ogino and Ichihara. These authors suggest that naphthalene, dinitrophenol and senile cataracts are caused by the formation of certain quinones which are cataractogenic.

The biochemical changes which accompany the experimental cataracts follow the same pattern. There is a cessation of those processes which require metabolic energy: protein and glutathione synthesis, cell division, and active transport of sodium and water out and potassium in. Hence there is loss of protein, glutathione, potassium, sodium and water. This is accompanied by an initial increase of weight followed by a decrease. All of these effects point to a disturbance in the formation of high energy phosphate bands. Because of the particular prominence of oxidation-reduction couples in the lens (β-crystallin, glutathione and ascorbic acid), it is tempting to attribute the formation of some cataracts to interference with the oxidation-reduction potential of the lens.

GROWTH AND AGING

During fetal life the lens is almost spherical; the anterior-posterior diameter increases until the seventh month, following which it remains stationary, while the equatorial diameter gradually increases. The latter change continues into adult life as the lens gains in density and volume. In this way the lens loses its approximate globular shape in the infant and assumes the typical lenticular shape in the adult. The normal lens remains perfectly clear until maturity. After this, the signs of senescence appear. These aging changes must be considered physiological until they interfere with the function of the lens. They depend on hereditary factors, constitution, and the ordinary stresses of life.

The entire lens capsule normally increases in thickness with age. Evidence was presented by Clapp that there must be postnatal growth to account for this. Undoubtedly submicroscopic changes take place in the structure of the capsule throughout life. These may account for its decreasing permeability with age.

According to Callahan and Klien, the capsule in older patients may form coarse single lamellas which exfoliate or split from the surface of the lens. This picture of capsular exfoliation also follows prolonged exposure to high concentrations of heat. Some confusion exists between this true exfoliation of the lens capsule, in which an anterior layer of capsule separates and rolls up in scroll-fashion in the pupillary zone, and a condition known as pseudoexfoliation. The latter condition has been discussed in Chapter II.

As the lens ages the epithelial cells become flatter and the nuclei take a lighter stain. Vacuoles may appear in their cytoplasm; some of the cells may show lipoidal degeneration. At times gaps are found, and an occasional cell may enlarge.

The aging of lens cells is similar to that seen in epithelial cells of the skin. Unlike the skin, however, these older cells cannot be desquamated; they are compressed and forced toward the center of the lens by the continuous formation of new fibers. In this way a hard central nuclear core forms in the lens. The conversion of the soft, gelatinous lens fibers in the cortex into the compact structure of the nucleus is a process that goes on throughout life. It leads to a slow but steady increase in volume in the nucleus, and the lens becomes progressively larger. Over a period of years the whole lens becomes less pliable. For this reason the relation of sclerosis to the diminishing accommodative range in presbyopia is well established. Excessive sclerosis of the lens nucleus brings with it loss of transparency, irregular refracting surfaces and usually a yellow to brownish tint. This is the sclerotic form of senile cataract.

In the normal lens one can trace the aging processes in the lens fibers by comparing successively deeper layers. The youngest fibers near the surface of the equator still have their nuclei. They evidently are continually growing in length since each successive layer from outside inward is longer. As one proceeds inward the nuclei become pale and disappear. Fibers located beneath the nucleated area are longer, but they also are more slender, so that their volume may not be increased significantly. The edges of the non-nucleated fibers appear serrated; the lipoid membrane demonstrable in the younger fibers no longer is evident in the deeper cortex and lens nucleus, and so the lens becomes sclerotic. Nuclear cataract may be regarded as an early exaggerated local senile manifestation.

GENERAL PATHOLOGY OF CATARACT

The types of change which may occur in the lens as a result of disease are:

A. Alterations in the lens substance
1. Degeneration
2. Sclerosis
B. Alterations in the epithelium
1. Degeneration
2. Proliferation
C. Alterations in the capsule
1. Thickening
2. Thinning
3. Spontaneous rupture

Changes in the Lens Substance

A. Incomplete cortical liquefaction
1. Acidification
2. Loss of water
3. Breakdown of lens cell into soluble and insoluble proteins and water
4. Liberation of cell contents into open spaces, forming water clefts (riders; spokes) between cells. The water clefts contain water, soluble and insoluble proteins, lipids, calcium salts, and small round fragments of lens (Morgagni's globules).
5. Occasional intumescence due to absorption of water as a result of increased osmotic pressure
6. Posterior subcapsular degeneration of fibers may occur alone or in conjunction with cortical water clefts or spokes (cupuliform cataract).
B. Complete cortical liquefaction
1. Hypermature cataract
   a. Loss of water and soluble products of the fibers through the intact capsule
   b. Diminution in size of the lens with wrinkling of the capsule
2. Morgagnian cataract
   a. Retention of broken down lens debris and water
   b. Nucleus becomes freely movable in the liquefied cortex

C. Nuclear sclerosis (Discussed in detail under Growth and Aging.)

Epithelial Changes

A. Degeneration
1. Cloudy swelling due to the toxic effects of inflammation or injury
2. Cytoplasmic vacuolation
3. Pyknosis and cell death
B. Proliferation
1. Beneath the posterior capsule as a single layer during liquefaction of the cortex
2. Beneath the anterior capsule as a fibrous mass, due to metaplasia of the cells (congenital disease; injury; iridocyclitis)

Capsular Changes

A. Thickening occurs in some senile cataracts
B. Thinning occurs in intumescent and morgagnian cataracts
C. Spontaneous rupture occurs rarely in morgagnian or very mature (intumescent) cataracts

Cortical Cataract

Once lens changes are initiated they may assume many clinical forms such as spokes, fissures, lamellar separation, dot-like opacities, wedge-shaped opacities, rosettes, etc. Histologically, however, the process is not so varied. Inflammation as we know it elsewhere does not take place as long as the capsule remains unbroken because the lens is lacking in blood vessels and a connective tissue framework. The pathology of cataract, therefore, is relatively simple and the changes which may take place are limited.

Nuclear sclerosis may occur by itself but often is associated with cortical cataract (Fig. 590). The cortical fibers ordinarily suffer rapid death, with autolysis (Fig. 591). The

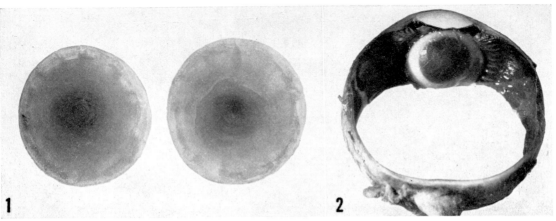

Figure 590. Nuclear Sclerosis

1. Deep amber sclerotic nucleus of a mature senile cataract. AFIP Acc. 506688.
2. Deep amber sclerotic nucleus of a morgagnian cataract; cortical material is a milky fluid. AFIP Acc. 646924.

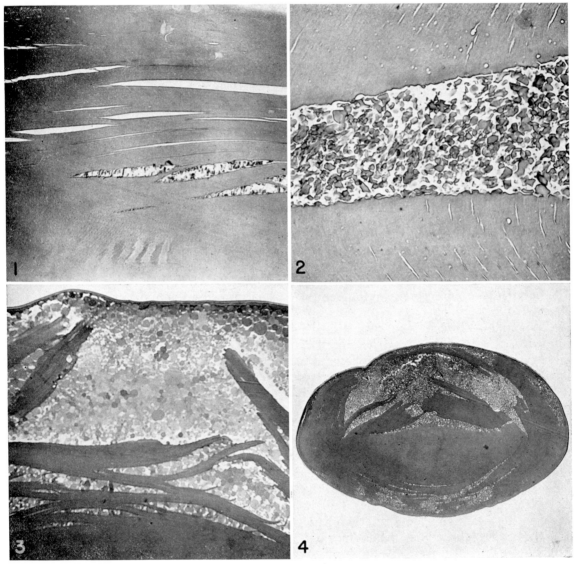

Figure 591. Cataract

1. Clefts containing degenerated lens substance. Empty clefts between lens fibers, possible result of technical shrinkage. ×70. AFIP Acc. 51149.
2. Morgagnian globules. ×145. AFIP Acc. 262207.
3. Fragmented lens fibers and morgagnian globules. ×48. AFIP Acc. 69523.
4. Mature cataract involving cortex and nucleus. ×27. AFIP Acc. 47676.

667

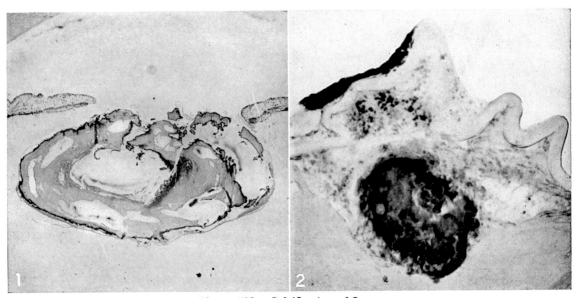

Figure 592. Calcification of Lens

1. Calcareous cataract. ×30. AFIP Acc. 82461.
2. Calcium in anterior subcapsular cataract. ×73. AFIP Acc. 21481.

older, tougher nuclear fibers are more re-sistant to change. The degenerative changes about to be described are those seen in cor-tical type of cataract. Without regard to eti-ology the general changes in cataract are es-sentially the same, and they are relatively simple.

The initial change in the cortical lens cells during cataract formation is acidification. This probably is due to the accumulation of products of a slowed or altered metabolism. The fibers lose fluid. shrink, and the fluid collects in the resulting clefts or vacuoles (Fig. 591–1). This is seen, for instance, in the incipient stage of senile cortical cataract. These early changes are difficult to recognize histologically, because similar artifacts often are produced in normal lenses by technical procedures.

Coagulation of the proteins in the cells then occurs, and permanent lens opacities form. The clinical picture is determined by the nature and position of these opacities. They seldom appear simultaneously throughout the whole lens cortex. Sometimes they remain stationary for a long time, and interfere little with vision. At other times, when they are associated with considerable imbibition of fluid into the cortex, complete opacification may be rapid. Degeneration of all the cor-

tical cells then may occur, with rapid lique-faction of the fibers. Microscopically they become edematous and the cell walls dis-integrate. Vacuoles form which coalesce to form larger spaces; eventually the fibers break down into morgagnian globules (Fig. 591). As the fragments of the lens disintegrate, the intercellular fluid becomes albuminous and takes a pale pink stain. If the lens epithe-lium has proliferated beneath the posterior capsule the contents often are retained and malformed fibers appear at the posterior pole.

In young individuals especially, dystrophic calcification of the degenerated lens (Fig. 592) may be marked. On the other hand, in elderly patients complete liquefaction necrosis of the lens fibers is more often observed (Fig. 593). Disintegration of the cortex proceeds much more rapidly than does autolysis of the scle-rotic nucleus. In these hypermature cataracts the nuclear remains may be freely movable in the milky cortical fluid in which it is sus-pended. Such cataracts typically appear shrunken because varying amounts of the liquid cortex are absorbed. Rarely, all of the lens tissue may escape, even though the cap-sule remains intact (Fig. 594).

As the hypermature lens cortex escapes through the capsule into the posterior cham-ber it provokes a macrophagic response (Fig.

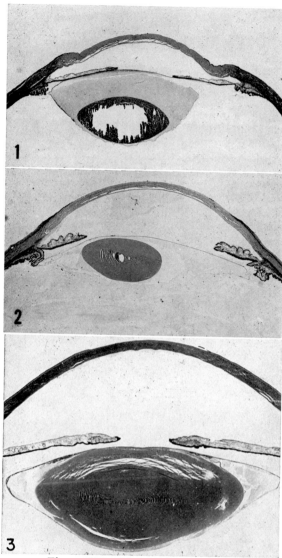

Figure 593. Morgagnian Cataracts

The lens cortex has been converted into homogeneous pink-staining fluid in which the sclerotic nucleus is suspended.

1. ×6. AFIP Acc. 609920.
2. ×7. AFIP Acc. 57055.
3. ×14. AFIP Acc. 67652.

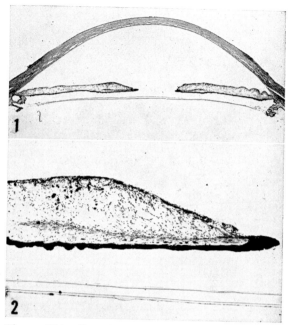

Figure 594. Complete Absorption of Hypermature Cataract

Only the lens capsule remains. ×8 and ×50, respectively. AFIP Acc. 235329.

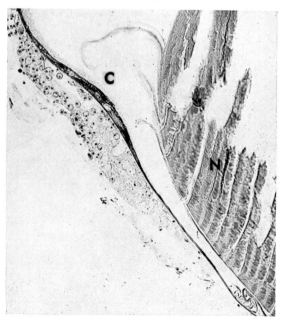

Figure 595. Phacolytic Glaucoma

Hypermature lens cortex has escaped into the posterior chamber where macrophages have been attracted. The posterior lens capsule is covered by macrophages and precipitated lens protein. C, liquefied cortex; N, sclerotic nucleus (fragmentation is artifactitious). ×70. AFIP Acc. 197063. (From Flocks et al., 1955.)

595). In histologic sections the escaped liquefied cortical material appears as faintly stained, finely granular precipitated protein. The macrophages which this material attracts contain similar fine pink granules in their cytoplasm. The flow of aqueous carries both the cells and the free cortical fluid into the anterior chamber. There it becomes concentrated in the iris crypts, in the angle and in the intertrabecular spaces (Fig. 596).

This sequence of events usually produces a

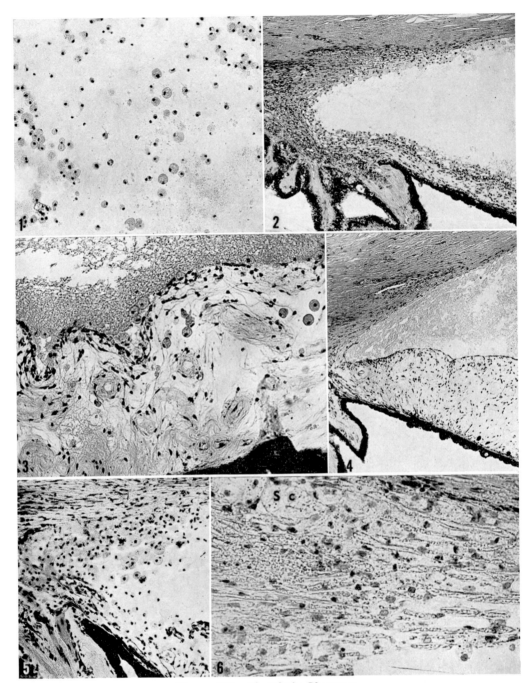

Figure 596. Phacolytic Glaucoma

1. Lens protein (finely granular particles) and macrophages in anterior chamber. ×165. AFIP Acc. 305232.

2. Macrophages are concentrated along the surface of the iris and in the chamber angle. ×75. AFIP Acc. 612178.

3. Macrophages in the iris crypts and in the iris stroma. ×165. AFIP Acc. 643703.

4. Large amount of escaped lens protein with very few macrophages. ×75. AFIP Acc. 618132.

5. Macrophages packed in chamber angle. ×150. AFIP Acc. 57055.

6. Macrophages fill the intertrabecular spaces and Schlemm's canal (S.c.). Anterior chamber is seen at lower right. ×385. AFIP Acc. 168726.

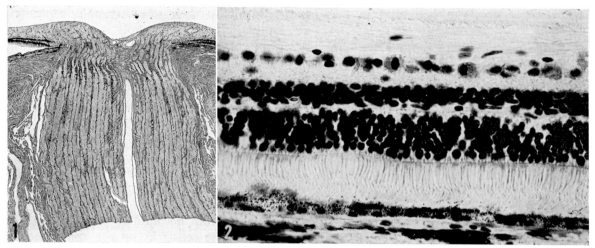

Figure 597. Acute Phacolytic Glaucoma

1. There is no evidence of optic atrophy or glaucomatous cupping. ×19. AFIP Acc. 232645.
2. The retinal architecture is well preserved and there is no loss of ganglion cells. ×410. AFIP Acc. 207298.
(From Flocks et al., 1955.)

sudden obstruction to aqueous outflow, a syndrome for which the name phacolytic glaucoma has been suggested by Flocks, Littwin, and Zimmerman (1955). (See Chapter XII.) The sudden appearance of symptoms of acute congestive glaucoma in an eye that has long been "blind" as a result of cataract should always suggest phacolytic glaucoma, particularly if the patient is elderly. Examination reveals a deep anterior chamber containing cells and exhibiting a marked aqueous flare, features which serve to differentiate this type of acute glaucoma from angle-closure glaucoma. The cells may become packed in the chamber angle but they characteristically do not adhere to the cornea or form agglutinated masses such as those which are so typical of granulomatous uveitis. As the Irvines have described, the aqueous does not clot upon removal, suggesting that the aqueous flare is produced by the escaped morgagnian fluid rather than by blood proteins.

In many of the cases studied by Flocks, Littwin and Zimmerman, enucleation was performed within a week of the onset of acute ocular pain. Examination of the retina and optic nerve in these early cases of phacolytic glaucoma often revealed little or no evidence of damage to the retina or optic nerve (Fig. 597), suggesting that not only could the glaucoma have been prevented, but it might have been successfully treated by cataract extraction.

Nuclear Cataract (Sclerosis)

Continuous changes take place in the cortical and nuclear fibers throughout life. The nuclear fibers become more and more compressed, lose their nuclei, contain less water and soluble proteins, and the refractive index increases. This process may go on very slowly, without effect on the vision; however, if the sclerosis is excessive or proceeds unevenly vision is altered. The lens contains a yellow pigment identified as urochrome which is probably formed from the metabolic degradation products of proteins. In the child it is present in such small amounts as to be colorless. The concentration increases with age, causing the lenses of elderly people to be distinctively yellow.

In some lenses a dusky brown or black color appears in severe sclerosis (brunescent cataract). The origin of the color in brunescent cataract has caused considerable speculation. It is most probable that the color is mainly due to an excessive amount of urochrome.

Sclerosis is extremely gradual. There is no sharp line of demarcation between living and dead cells (Fig. 598–1). It even can happen that a nucleus which is clearly abnormal on clinical examination shows no characteristic change when it is examined microscopically. The most that is seen is a dense, uniform, homogeneous appearance of the affected area. The hardened and compressed fibers show

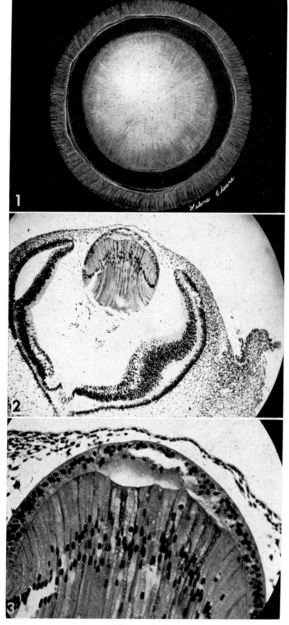

Figure 604.

1. Rubella cataract—diffuse type. (Courtesy of Dr. F. C. Cordes.)

2. Section through 7–8 weeks old embryo; history of rubella during the 6th week. Both Theodore Terry and Ida Mann examined the sections and agreed the posterior portion of the eye was that of a 26 mm. embryo while the lens vesicle corresponded in size to that of a 17 mm. embryo. Both noted there were abnormal changes in the anterior lens vesicle. ×164. (From Cordes and Barber, 1946.)

3. Same as section 2. ×500.

processes in the mother are known to produce cataracts in the fetus. Zonular cataract frequently is associated with imperfect calcification of the enamel organs of the permanent teeth; or it may be seen in infantile tetany. The whole endocrine system is in a state of heightened activity during pregnancy. It is possible that a parathyroid deficiency with a disturbance in the calcium metabolism in the mother may lead to cataracts in the fetus.

Knowledge of the development of the lens provides information concerning the gestation period when the lens is damaged. A small central area of opacification less than a millimeter in diameter corresponding to the region of the embryonal nucleus, indicates an injury during the first two months of gestation (embryonal nuclear cataract). Opacities which lie at the level of and internal to the anterior and posterior Y sutures indicate damage at about the third fetal month (fetal nuclear cataract). Following formation of the fetal nucleus, further development of the lens takes place at a progressively slower rate, so that assignment of the time of injury becomes progressively less and less exact for the more peripheral opacities. At times the history of a maternal illness agrees fairly closely with the estimated time of injury to the lens. This is especially true in the cases of congenital cataract in the offspring of mothers with rubella or other infectious diseases in early pregnancy.

In embryos *rubella* produces general retardation of development. The cataracts are bilateral and may show a dense white central opacity surrounded by some clear cortex. The cardiovascular and central nervous systems particularly are affected. The eye participates in this disturbance in a number of ways. There may be bilateral incomplete or mature cataracts, ocular deviations of various types, and a pigmentary type of degeneration of the retina. The primary lens fibers are degenerated and are separated from the capsule by new fibers (Fig. 604). The damage occurs to the lens fibers which are being formed during the period of injury, usually in the first trimester. Cordes has suggested that the protection afforded by the cornea and lids may explain why no cases of rubella cataract have

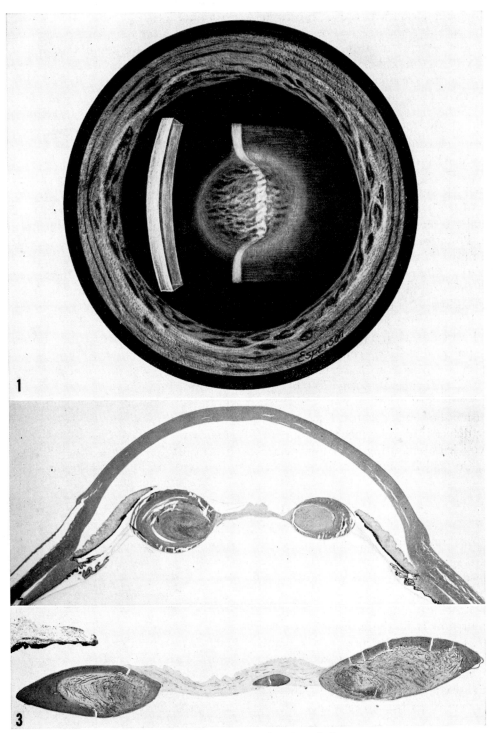

Figure 605. Congenital Disk-Shaped Cataract

1. Artist's drawing of slit-lamp appearance. (Courtesy of Dr. F. C. Cordes.)
2. Configuration is that of a Soemmerring-ring type cataract. (Courtesy of Dr. F. C. Cordes.)
3. In this case the patient was a Mongolian idiot with acute keratoconus. ×22. AFIP Acc. 991726.

been reported after the third month of pregnancy.

Most congenital cataracts are of the zonular type because the causative factor acts over a period of time and injures a number of generations of developing lens fibers. Many lenses show arcuate or spoke-shaped opacities in the otherwise clear zone outside the lamellar opacity. These presumably represent local regions in which the equatorial epithelium did not recover completely from the injury which produced the lamellar lesion.

Lens opacities associated with the vascular network which surrounds the lens in early embryonal life already have been mentioned. They usually occur at the anterior or posterior pole. Posterior polar opacities may vary from a minute white spot, which indicates the site of union of the posterior tunica vasculosa lentis and the hyaloid system, to a larger disk-shaped posterior polar opacity, which is due to marked persistence and proliferation of retrolental vascular tissue (see Chapter X). Anterior polar opacities, commonly disk-shaped, also are frequent. They may be related to a disturbance in formation of the embryonal pupillary capillary net. This type of cataract more often is due to a fetal inflammation or defect in development at the time the lens vesicle is separating from the surface ectoderm. Corneal inflammation in the fetus

may result in anterior lens damage and an anterior polar cataract. Such cataracts are less common than those which are posterior. They rarely are seen in association with persistent pupillary membranes. The opacities are subcapsular in location and are due to proliferation and metaplasia of the subcapsular epithelium. This is essentially identical with that seen in the anterior subcapsular cataracts of the adult (Figs. 599 to 601).

Rarely the cells from the back of the embryonic lens fail to form the primary lens fibers, producing defective development of the lens vesicle. The fibers arising from cells at the equator continue to grow but do not have the fetal nucleus to grow around. In this way a dumbbell-shaped lens or ring cataract results (Fig. 605).

The histology of most developmental cataracts is unknown because so few have been obtained for pathological study. In many the opacities are minute and assume shapes which cannot be correlated with a normal arrangement of lens fibers. Zonular cataracts in which a large segment of the central lens is opaque show an area which is composed of granular hyaline material. It is not known whether this represents degenerated lens elements which have failed to develop into lens fibers, or lens fibers which have undergone degeneration after development.

INFLAMMATIONS

Except for the epithelium the lens reacts passively to surrounding inflammatory processes. The normal metabolism of the lens is affected by inflammation, leading to degeneration and opacification. As we have seen, if the inflammation is in the anterior segment of the eye, the lens epithelium may respond by proliferation, but if it is severe there is degeneration.

Inflammatory processes in the posterior segment of the eye often lead to cataracts. These have been called "complicated cataracts" although it is better to use the term "secondary" if the disease process is known. This type of cataract can proceed to complete opacification. In its earlier stages it is distinctive in appearance, with clefts, vacuoles and disintegrated fibers in the posterior subcapsular cortex. The process may extend from this area in all directions. The nucleus, however, remains uninvolved for a long time. The capsule may become thickened, and there is active proliferation of the epithelium to line the whole capsule. Other diseases such as retinitis pigmentosa, myopia, intraocular tumors, glaucoma, and retinal detachment may cause this type of cataract. The cataract seems to be produced either by the toxins which are associated with the disease or by those resulting from the degeneration of adjacent tissues. The posterior pole seems to be more vulnerable because of the thinness of its capsule, and quite often, this part of the lens is nearest the focus of disease; also the protection afforded by the lens epithelium in the anterior lens is lacking.

The lens may be involved in and may even excite severe inflammation in the eye. These reactions most often are associated with rupture of the lens capsule. Lens material may escape into the eye following traumatic or spontaneous rupture of the capsule. Interesting and important inflammatory reactions may be set up by the liberated lens substance. These have been considered in Chapter III. Lens cortex may remain as an apparently inert substance, causing little or no reaction whether the absorption is slow or rapid. The time required for absorption of lens cortex often is prolonged after discission of a congenital or secondary cataract.

Liquid cortex may act as a chemical irritant and produce a bland macrophagic reaction, as already described. Lens products can also act as antigens and cause a phaco-anaphylactic endophthalmitis. This reaction occurs most often after accidental or surgical injuries to the lens, rarely spontaneously; it is centered about the injured lens. Large numbers of polymorphonuclear leukocytes and large mononuclear macrophages are seen surrounding and invading lens substance. Lymphocytes and plasma cells predominate in the iris and ciliary body but at times eosinophils and giant cells are present (Figs. 29, 100).

Large precipitates form on the corneal endothelium. The posterior segment is less involved but polymorphonuclear leukocytes and clusters of macrophages may be seen in the vitreous and on the inner retina. Usually there is a perivascular infiltration of lymphocytes in the retina, choroid and optic disk. The presence of polymorphonuclear leukocytes and giant cells distinguishes this group of cases.

INJURIES AND THEIR EFFECT ON THE LENS

Contusions without rupture of the lens capsule result in cataract. The damage probably is sufficient to destroy the normal semipermeability of the capsule and allow the entrance of fluid. Moreover, the shock not only is transmitted to the lens as a whole but to the capsular epithelium and to each lens cell; this affects the continuity and structure of the cells. These disturbances, depending on their severity, may lead to reversible or permanent changes in the lens substance. Reversible opacities usually are seen immediately after the contusion and probably are due to edema. Irreversible opacities frequently form a stellate figure outlining the anterior or posterior suture pattern. These are due to a derangement or distortion of the lens cells. Both experimentally and clinically the opacities start in the cortical layers close to the lens capsule. The opaque areas show fluid clefts and vacuoles due to fragmentation of lens fibers. As time goes on, and new lens fibers form, the opacities come to lie deeper in the lens.

A ring of pigment (Vossius ring) on the anterior capsule of the lens, corresponding to the pupillary aperture, may be seen after contusions of the eye. A small subcapsular cortical opacity may be associated with this pigmented ring. The pigment comes from the iris epithelium and probably is imprinted on the lens at the time of injury. As time goes on it tends to absorb.

The lens may be displaced from its normal position after an injury or contusion, and this often is a serious complication (Figs. 94, 95). If the lens remains in the pupillary aperture it is said to be subluxated; if it is completely displaced from the pupil it is dislocated or luxated. The dislocation of the lens may be anterior or posterior. It may lie in the anterior chamber, or be displaced into the vitreous. In anterior dislocations there is a mechanical obstruction of the angle which often produces glaucoma. Posterior dislocations into the vitreous are better tolerated. Glaucoma, however, may be caused by the irritation produced by the constant trauma of the lens to the ciliary body. Peripheral anterior synechias form because of the irritation. The lens may remain clear for a period of time, but before long it becomes swollen and opaque.

The elastic lens capsule normally is under some tension from the pull of the zonular fibers. When the capsule is lacerated the wound edges roll outward. Lens substance protrudes through the wound, imbibes aque-

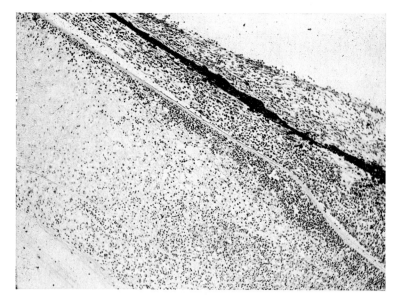

Figure 606. Lens Abscess

Bacterial infection may convert the lens into a bag of pus and even the relatively resistant capsule may be digested by leukocytic proteolytic enzymes. ×75. AFIP Acc. 502856.

ous, and swells. The aqueous soon causes dissolution of the exposed cells. This allows more fibers to come in contact with the aqueous, until eventually the entire lens may become opaque.

The ultimate changes in the lens depend to a large extent on the age of the patient and the severity of the injury. A small penetrating injury may be sealed by contact with the iris or by proliferating lens epithelium. A small opacity results at the site of the injury in such cases. More severe injuries, especially in the young, may produce complete absorption of the lens substance, leaving only the clear lens capsule. Such a happy event rarely occurs in the adult lens, because the nucleus resists enzymatic action.

The lens is an exceedingly rich culture medium and bacteria implanted in it, even if of relatively low virulence, tend to gain a foothold before wandering cells can enter and participate in its defense. Very soon an abscess forms, with marked destruction of the lens material (Fig. 606). This may be the start of a purulent panophthalmitis. If the organism is of low virulence, however, a mild and self-limited inflammation results.

Following discission, extracapsular extraction of the lens and trauma, the capsule, some cortex, and epithelium may remain. The epithelium may proliferate to produce abortive lens fibers (Fig. 607). These take the form of large globules in the pupil (Elschnig's pearls). Clinically they appear in the pupil as a nest resembling a cluster of fish eggs. After lens surgery or injury the anterior capsule may come in contact with the posterior capsule, trapping varying amounts of lens substance

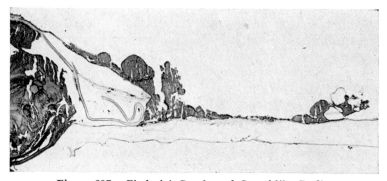

Figure 607. Elschnig's Pearls and Crumblike Bodies

Solid and cystic formations on the lens capsule after a penetrating wound with almost complete resorption of lens substance. ×50. AFIP Acc. 987420.

peripherally. This remaining lens may take the form of a doughnut-shaped ring behind the pupil (Soemmerring's ring) (Fig. 608).

Thickening of the posterior capsule in the pupillary region, plus proliferation of lens fibers and fibroblasts, produces a pupillary membrane which affects vision. This is known as a "postoperative after-cataract," and is distinguished from secondary cataract (p. 678).

Siderosis and Chalcosis

Metallic intraocular foreign bodies may damage the lens directly during their passage. They also may cause cataract even without direct mechanical injury to the lens. Alloys of iron and copper are the most common types of intraocular foreign bodies; they are quite toxic. Gold, platinum, tantalum and aluminum are inert; they cause little damage when retained in the eye. Lead also is inert and may remain in the eye without causing undue reaction.

Alloys of copper which are retained in the eye cause a striking clinical picture. A grayish-green to brownish-red discoloration of the pupillary area is noted. Radiation spokes in the lens give the opacity a flower-like arrangement, thus the name "sunflower cataract." The copper is deposited in the deep layers of the lens capsule and between it and the epithelial cells.

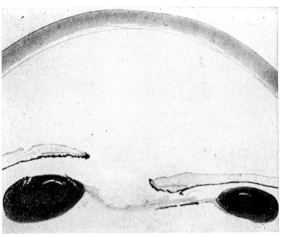

Figure 608. Soemmerring's ring cataract. ×12. AFIP Acc. 131271.

The cataract of siderosis is unique and begins as minute brownish dots over the anterior surface just beneath the lens capsule. The whole lens takes on a characteristic yellow tint; it finally becomes densely opaque. Histologic examination shows that the subcapsular epithelium picks up the metal which gives a positive Prussian blue reaction (Fig. 104–5). As degeneration occurs a homogeneous light blue staining material and dark granules appear just beneath the capsule. Later the cortical fibers may also show a positive reaction for iron. Eventually the epithelium almost completely disappears and the lens fibers degenerate.

EFFECTS OF RADIATION

Not all the radiant energy in the electromagnetic spectrum produces pathologic effects. Duke-Elder states that only radiations which are absorbed by a tissue can cause harm. As far as the eye is concerned, all radiations, if intense enough, may damage ocular tissues. As for the lens in particular, visible and ultraviolet light seldom cause damage as the lens is transparent to the visible spectrum and the cornea absorbs much of the ultraviolet.

All electromagnetic wavelength radiations outside of the visible spectrum can cause cataracts in experimental animals provided there is sufficient energy absorbed.

The cornea transmits short infrared rays. Infrared radiations, therefore, if severe enough, can cause a thermal burn. If the

energy is large in amount, and acts over a short period of time, a flash burn develops, with few serious consequences to the eye. A smaller concentration of energy over a longer period of time leads to cumulative effects, and the lens or retina may suffer serious damage.

Experimentally, cataracts are easy to produce with large doses of infrared rays. If the dose is sufficient a dense white cataract occurs. Lesser amounts cause opacities to appear earliest and most rapidly in the pupillary zone. A ring of pigment resembling the ring of Vossius may be deposited on the lens capsule. If the dosage is less intense and particularly if it is repeated, a delayed opacity in the posterior cortex may appear after a considerable interval (16 to 37 days).

Heat cataract is rare but it has been known

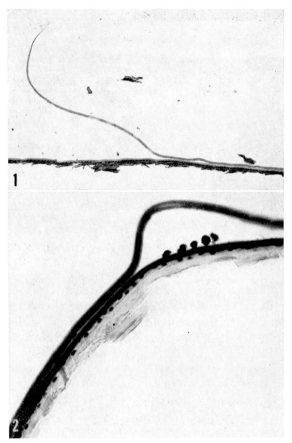

Figure 609. True Thermal Exfoliation of Lens Capsule

The outer half of the greatly thickened lens capsule is broken and partially peeled away from the intact inner half of the lens capsule. (Case reported by Callahan and Klien, 1958.)

1. H and E, ×80. AFIP Acc. 279665.
2. PAS, ×305. AFIP Acc. 279665.

for many years that cataracts occur early among glass blowers, steel puddlers, and other workers exposed to high temperatures for long periods of time. The acute lens lesions of experimental animals do not occur but an opacity in the posterior cortex greatly resembling delayed opacity in experimental animals occurs. The clinical appearance is typical. A cobweb-like opacity is noted early in the outer layers of the posterior cortex; this later develops into a sharply defined saucer-shaped disk with an irregular outline. Progress may be slow but eventually the entire lens becomes involved. Most evidence points to the indirect thermal effect of the heat absorbed by the iris and transmitted to the lens as the cause of the cataracts. Gold-

man investigated this possibility in great detail and concluded that on exposure to hot glowing surfaces, such as are met with in industry, a measurable heating of the iris occurred, with production of secondary effects on the lens. Absorption by the lens itself of that portion of the spectrum transmitted by the cornea is relatively feeble, but since the lens possesses no blood supply, any heat produced within it is dissipated very slowly.

Changes in the lens capsule may also be noted. Linear splits may appear in the zonular lamella in the pupillary aperture followed by sheet-like stripping of this layer of the capsule. Among workers exposed to high concentration of heat only a few develop exfoliation of the lens capsule. Callahan and Klien have shown by histochemical tests that there is damage to the interfibrillary cement substance of the outer layers of the lens capsule (Fig. 609).

Much of the ultraviolet below the 3,900 A band of the spectrum is absorbed by the cornea so that under ordinary circumstances the shorter biologically effective rays fail to injure the lens. Even under experimental conditions the dose has to be massive to produce lens damage. Those lenses which are damaged show degeneration of the superficial cortical fibers. In the capsular epithelium there is complete absence of mitosis, fragmentation of the nuclei and eventual disintegration of the cells in the pupillary area. At the edge of this area just under the margin of the pupil there may be heaping up of the epithelial cells due to proliferation. These lesions could be produced with exposures to ultraviolet irradiation 100 times that which produced severe actinic keratitis. The clinical observation that senile cataracts are much more common and mature earlier in tropical countries has caused considerable speculation about the role of ultraviolet irradiation in production of senile cataract.

The vast number of people exposed to ionizing radiation in this atomic age has stimulated interest in its biologic effects. The lens is very susceptible to ionizing radiation and may show evidence of cataractous changes even though the rest of the eye escapes injury.

Early workers in the field were not aware of the lens changes probably because of the long latent period for their clinical development. Scattered reports of cataracts in radiation workers led to studies on the use of x-rays and gamma rays for the production of experimental cataracts; before long the nature of this type of cataract was well known. There is considerable correlation between experimental and clinical radiation cataract. The younger the subject the more susceptible the lens is to radiation and the shorter is the latent period. Information is available on x-ray cataracts in humans to indicate that the cataractogenic dose of x-rays of 100 kv. energy or greater is somewhere between 500 r and 1000 r. Cogan and Donaldson have shown that it takes 250 r to produce cataracts in rabbits. The larger the dose, however, the shorter is the latent period. The dose need not be given all at one time to produce the cataract for there is a cumulative effect. Without a doubt the epithelium, especially at the equator, is the most susceptible part of the lens. Damage to these cells leads to the opacities seen clinically at a later date.

Clinically lens changes in the form of a few discrete dots are noted in the cortex near the posterior pole. These spread and later a clear area in the center develops producing a doughnut appearance. About this time opacities and granules are noted in the anterior subcapsular zone in the pupillary area. Later a dense disk-shaped central opacity occupies the region of the posterior cortex, and, depending on the amount of damage done, mature cataracts with liquefaction of the cortex can develop; the lesion need not be progressive and arrest may occur at any stage, depending on the dose. Kandori and Masuda showed that most of the survivors of the atomic bombs of Hiroshima and Nagasaki escaped with good vision. Their lesions stopped at the disk-shaped posterior subcapsular stage.

Current studies on animals have shed some light on the course of the disease. Von Sallmann has shown that in rabbits there are visible opacities at the lens equator as early as four weeks after irradiation. Histologic studies show cells in pathologic mitosis with nuclear fragmentation as early as ten days after irradiation. These cells disintegrate and disappear, but it seems possible that toxic products liberated from these cells may initiate the cataractous process. The latent period before the abnormal mitosis and disintegration represents in rabbits the duration of mitotic inhibition following irradiation. This suggests that cells may recover from this inhibition before showing evidence of more irreversible damage.

Cogan and Donaldson have found approximately one month after irradiation that cells from the capsular epithelium near the equator migrate along the inner surface of the capsule toward the posterior pole (Fig. 610). It is possible that these migrated cells subsequently may undergo the same type of mitotic death described by von Sallmann. They may account for the ring-shaped opacity which develops at the posterior pole in human beings. In any case the extremely long latent period noted clinically in man is probably merely an expression of the inaccessibility of the lens equator to clinical observation. Postmortem studies on atomic bomb casualties indicate that lesions in the equatorial cortex may be present in man as early as a month after irradiation.

After a latent period characteristic changes take place in lenses of survivors of electrical injuries. Voltages as low as 500 and as high as many million may produce a lesion. There is no definite relation to the strength of the current. The first changes are noted in the capsule and the underlying cortex in the form of grayish-white punctate opacities which give the lens a hazy appearance. The opacities in the posterior cortex resemble a secondary cataract. Immediately beneath the capsule are numerous vacuoles. Rarely these changes may clear but more often maturation slowly occurs over a period averaging six months. Their cause is unknown. The passage of the current through the lens fibers probably initiates effects which lead to coagulation of protein.

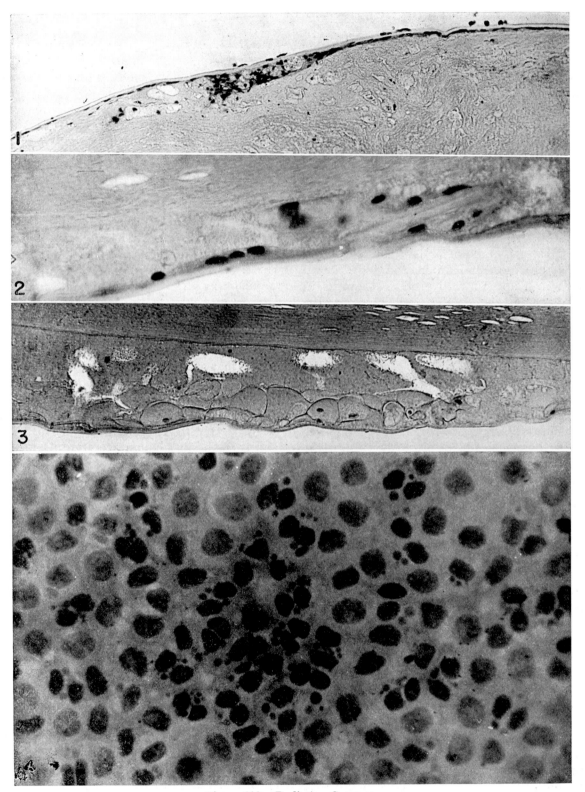

Figure 610. Radiation Cataract

1. Piling up of epithelial cells at equator following radiation exposure of eye several years previously in course of treatment for carcinoma. (Figs. 1, 2, 3: Cogan, D. G., Donaldson, D. D., and Reese, A. B.: Arch. Ophth. *47*:55–70, 1952.)

2. Aberrant epithelial cells beneath posterior capsule.

3. Bladder cells beneath posterior capsule.

4. Nuclear fragmentation. Flat preparation of lens epithelium of rabbit's eye, exposed 150 days previously to 2,000 r. (Cogan, D. G., and Donaldson, D. D.: Arch. Ophth. *45*:508–522, 1951.)

CATARACTS DUE TO SYSTEMIC DISEASES

Cataracts associated with various disease states in man are in some ways analogous to experimental cataracts in that a similar etiology applies. Diabetic cataract, endocrine cataracts, and those associated with mongolian idiocy and certain skin disorders are to be considered.

It has long been known that cataracts are very prone to develop in diabetic persons. Most often the cataract differs in no way from that senile cataract met with in old age, except that it comes earlier in life and tends to progress more rapidly to maturity. Rarely a cataract may develop in a very young diabetic, and it is characterized early by rather typical snowflake opacities and vacuoles in the subcapsular cortex, with rapid progression to maturity. The condition usually is bilateral. Histologically the degenerative changes are most marked just beneath the capsule and in many instances the nucleus remains unchanged until a late date. In the early stages, before the denaturation of the proteins occurs, control of the diabetes may halt further progress of the cataract and even result in a disappearance of opacities. The cause of this true diabetic cataract still is not settled, although much experimental work has been done. Many believe it is due to the high blood sugar levels. However, Farkas and Patterson have shown that reduction of the blood supply to an eye of an alloxon diabetic rat does not diminish the rate of cataract formation in that type. This makes it possible that it is the lack of insulin which upsets the lens rather than the excess of sugar. Clinically those diabetic patients with marked hyperglycemia may have clear lenses, while patients with a relatively low blood sugar display opacities.

Postoperative or idiopathic *tetany* often is associated with rather typical lens changes in the form of punctate and flaky subcapsular opacities. These are most marked in the posterior cortex and are separated by a clear zone from the capsule. Even if the tetany is controlled the opacities remain. Repeated attacks may cause zonular opacities, which result from the clear lens fibers which are laid down between attacks. That the low concentration of calcium in the blood and aqueous has something to do with the development of the cataracts seems to be undoubted from experimental work. The defect in the lens metabolism which is produced by the deficiency remains unsolved.

Early lens changes associated with cretinism, myotonic dystrophy, mongolian idiocy and certain skin disorders are characterized by punctate and flaky opacities in the cortex. These are separated from the capsule by a clear zone. These changes are bilateral and are similar to those occurring in other endocrine diseases. Histologically, these opacities are produced by the degeneration of lens fibers which either are deeply staining, light staining and homogeneous, or granular. Experimental studies have done more to elucidate pathogenesis of the above type of cataracts than of senile cataracts.

DEGENERATIONS OF THE LENS

The changes in senile cataract are found in many types of cataract, and are considered to be the prototype of all cataracts, because of their frequency. The cortical changes most often are discovered to be wedge- or spoke-like opacities at the equator of the lens extending into the anterior and posterior cortex. Microscopically, the breakdown is noted to appear as a pink-staining granular material which eventually becomes liquid. This process may be slow or it can progress rapidly, so that within a year the lens cortex may be quite white and milky.

Posterior subcapsular senile cataract is the

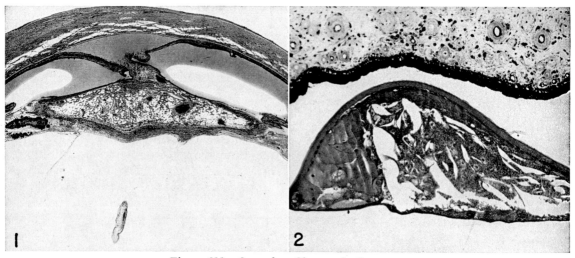

Figure 611. Secondary Changes in Cataracts

1. Fatty metaplasia of connective tissue in congenital cataract. ×15. AFIP Acc. 96585.
2. Cholesterol clefts in degenerated cortex of traumatic cataract. ×125. AFIP Acc. 282711.

second most common type. Granular flaky opacities are seen, which gradually spread toward the periphery. This change differs from that seen in secondary cataract (erroneously called complicated cataract) in that in senile cataract the opacity remains confined to the zone immediately beneath the capsule, whereas in most secondary cataracts the new-formed lens fibers from the equator gradually crowd the posterior opacity forward so that it lies within the cortex. In congenital and traumatic cataracts, the lens may be invaded by mesenchymal cells and replaced to varying degrees by connective tissue, mineral deposits, or lipids (Figs. 592, 611).

REFERENCES

Bahr, G. F.: Investigation of the Lamellar Structure of the Lens Capsule by Electron Microscopy. Graefe Arch. Ophthal. *155*:635–638, 1954.

Bellows, J. G.: Cataract and Anomalies of the Lens. St. Louis, C. V. Mosby Co., 1944.

Bellows, J. G., and Rosner, L.: Studies on Galactose Cataract. Amer. J. Ophthal. *20*:1109–1114, 1937.

Burky, E. L.: Experimental Endophthalmitis Phacoanaphylactica in Rabbits. A.M.A. Arch. Ophthal. *12*:536–546, 1934.

Buschke, W.: Dystrophic Cataracts and Their Relations to Other Metabolic Cataracts. A.M.A. Arch. Ophthal. *30*:751–762, 1943.

Callahan, A., and Klien, B. A.: Thermal Detachment of the Anterior Lamella of the Anterior Lens Capsule. A Clinical and Histopathologic Study. A.M.A. Arch. Ophthal. *59*:73–80, 1958.

Clapp, C. A.: Alterations in the Capsular Epithelium in Immature Cataracts. Amer. J. Ophthal. *25*:437–445, 1942.

Cogan, D. G., and Cogan, F. C.: Cataracts and Dinitrophenol. New Eng. J. Med. *213*:854–856, 1935.

Cogan, D. G., and Donaldson, D. D.: Experimental Radiation Cataracts. I. Cataracts in the Rabbit following Single X-ray Exposure. A.M.A. Arch. Ophthal. *45*:508–522, 1951.

Cordes, F. C.: Types of Congenital and Juvenile Cataracts. In Haik, G. M.: Symposium on Diseases and Surgery of the Lens. St. Louis, C. V. Mosby Co., 1957, pp. 43–63.

Cordes, F. C., and Barber, A.: Changes in Lens of Embryo after Rubella. A.M.A. Arch. Ophthal. *36*:135–140, 1946.

Dische, Z., and Borenfreund, E.: Composition of the Polysaccharide of the Lens Capsule and Its Topical Distribution. Amer. J. Ophthal. *38*:165–173, 1954.

Dische, Z., Borenfreund, E., and Zelmenis, G.: Changes in Lens Proteins of Rats during Aging. A.M.A. Arch. Ophthal. *55*:471–483, 1956.

Duke-Elder, S.: Textbook of Ophthalmology. Vol. 6. St. Louis, C. V. Mosby Co., 1954, p. 6455.

Farkas, T. G., and Patterson, J. W.: Insulin and the Lens. Amer. J. Ophthal. *44*:341–346, 1957.

Flocks, M., Littwin, C. S., and Zimmerman, L. E.: Phacolytic Glaucoma; a Clinicopathologic Study of One Hundred Thirty-eight Cases of Glaucoma Associated with Hypermature Cataract. A.M.A. Arch. Ophthal. *54*:37–45, 1955.

Franceschetti, A., and Rickli, H.: Posterior (Eccentric) Lenticonus. Report of First Case with Clinical and Histological Findings. A.M.A. Arch. Ophthal. *51*:499–508, 1954.

François, J., and Rabaey, M.: The Protein Composition of the Human Lens. Amer. J. Ophthal. *44*:347–357, 1957.

François, J., Rabaey, M., Wieme, R. J., and Kaminski, M.: Study of the Antigens of the Crystalline

Lens by Immunochemical Methods of Protein Fractionation. Amer. J. Ophthal. *42:*577–584, 1956.

Friedenwald, J. S., and Small, M. L.: A New Stain for Cell Surfaces. Bull. Johns Hopkins Hosp. *48:*104, 1931.

Gifford, H.: A Clinical and Pathologic Study of Exfoliation of the Lens Capsule. Amer. J. Ophthal. *46:*508–524, 1958.

Goldman, H.: Genesis of Heat Cataract. A.M.A. Arch. Ophthal. *9:*314, 1933.

Haik, G. M.: Symposium on Diseases and Surgery of the Lens. St. Louis, C. V. Mosby Co., 1957.

Harris, J. E., and Gehrsitz, L. B.: Significance of Changes in Potassium and Sodium Content of the Lens. Amer. J. Ophthal. *34:*131–138, 1951.

Harris, J. E., and Nordquist, L. T.: Factors Effecting the Cation and Water Balance of the Lens. Acta of the XVII International Congress of Ophthalmology, Toronto, Univ. of Toronto Press, 1955, Vol. II, pp. 1002–1014.

Hektoen, L., and Schulhof, K.: Further Observations on Lens Precipitins. Antigenic Properties of Alpha and Beta Crystallins. J. Infect. Dis. *34:*433–439, 1924.

Irvine, S. R., and Irvine, A. R., Jr.: Lens-Induced Uveitis and Glaucoma. Part I. Endophthalmitis Phaco-anaphylactica. Amer. J. Ophthal. *35:*177–186, 1952.

Irvine, S. R., and Irvine, A. R., Jr.: Lens-Induced Uveitis and Glaucoma. Part II. The "Phacotoxic" Reaction. Amer. J. Ophthal. *35:*370–375, 1952.

Irvine, S. R., and Irvine, A. R., Jr.: Lens-Induced Uveitis and Glaucoma. Part III. "Phacogenetic Glaucoma"; Lens Induced Glaucoma; Mature or Hypermature Cataract; Open Iridocorneal Angle. Amer. J. Ophthal. *35:*489–499, 1952.

Kandori, F., and Masuda, Y.: Statistical Observations of Atom-Bomb Cataracts. Amer. J. Ophthal. *42:*212–214, 1956.

Kinoshita, J. H.: Carbohydrate Metabolism of Lens. A.M.A. Arch. Ophthal. *54:*360–368, 1955.

McGavic, J. S.: Monocular and Binocular Reactions of the Lens. Acta of the XVII International Congress of Ophthalmology, Toronto, Univ. of Toronto Press, 1955, Vol. II, pp. 1088–1100.

Makley, T. A., Jr.: Posterior Lenticonus. Report of a Case with Histological Findings. Amer. J. Ophthal. *39:*308–312, 1955.

Mann, I.: Developmental Abnormalities of the Eye London, Cambridge University Press, 1937, Chapter VIII, The Lens.

Merriam, F. C., and Kinsey, V. E.: Studies on the Crystalline Lens. I. Technic for in Vitro Culture of Crystalline Lenses and Observations on Metabolism of the Lens. A.M.A. Arch. Ophthal. *43:*979–988, 1950.

Ogino, S., and Ichihara, T.: Biochemical Studies on Cataract. V. Biochemical Genesis of Senile Cataract. Amer. J. Ophthal. *43:*754–764, 1957.

Pappas, G. D., and Smelser, G. K.: Studies on the Ciliary Epithelium and the Zonule. Amer. J. Ophthal. *46:*299–318, 1958.

Patterson, J. W.: The Effect of High Carbohydrate Levels on the Lens. Acta of the XVII International Congress of Ophthalmology, Toronto, Univ. of Toronto Press, 1955, Vol. II, pp. 992–1001.

Pirie, A., and van Heyningen, R. V.: Biochemistry of the Eye. Oxford, Blackwell Scientific Publications, 1956, p. 115 and p. 128.

Ulenhuth, P. P.: Zur Lehre von der Unterscheidung verschiedener Eiweissarten mit Hilfe spezifischer Sera. Festschr. z. 60. Geburtst. v. Robert Koch, Jena, 1903, pp. 49–74.

Van den Heuvel, J. E. A.: Cytological Aspects of the Crystalline Lens. A Critical Review and an Outlook on Future Developments. Adv. Ophth. *5:*54–182. Basel and New York, S. Karger, 1956.

Van Heyningen, R. V., and Pirie, A.: Reduction of Glutathione Coupled with Oxidative Decarboxylation of Malate in Cattle Lens. Biochem. J. *53:*436–444, 1953.

Verhoeff, F. H., and Lemoine, A. N.: Endophthalmitis Phacoanaphylactica. Amer. J. Ophthal. *5:*737–745, 1922.

von Sallmann, L.: Experimental Studies on Early Lens Changes after Roentgen Irradiation. I. Morphological and Cytochemical Changes. A.M.A. Arch. Ophthal. *45:*149–164, 1951.

Wanko, T., and Gavin, M. A.: The Fine Structure of the Lens Epithelium An Electron Microscopic Study. A.M.A. Arch. Ophthal. *60:*858–879, 1958.

Woods, A. C., and Burky, E. L.: Lens Protein and Its Fractions. Preparation and Immunologic and Chemical Properties. J.A.M.A. *89:*102–110, 1927.

Zimmerman, L. E.: Personal Communication.

Chapter **XII**

Glaucoma

Glaucoma is characterized by an elevation of the intraocular pressure. The increased pressure almost always is due to tissue changes which reduce the normal outflow of aqueous humor from the eye. The reduction in outflow may result from a considerable number of different pathologic mechanisms. Glaucoma. therefore, is a complex of diseases which have as a common feature an abnormal elevation of the intraocular pressure. Clinically this is expressed as the ocular tension, which is the means by which the intraocular pressure usually is estimated. Considering the differences induced by variations in the ocular rigidity the measured tension and the intraocular pressure usually are comparable.

Although the clinical findings in glaucoma usually are characteristic, slight rises in tension are often difficult to evaluate. Provocative tests and tonography may be helpful, but at times, in early borderline cases, the presence of glaucoma may be almost impossible to diagnose, because it is difficult to establish a "normal" tension for a particular eye. At times the eye with an apparently normal tension develops definite glaucomatous changes, while another continues to function normally with a tension definitely above the usual level. Therefore, glaucomatous pressure is that which is incompatible with the continued health and function of the eye.

In the normal state there is a constant outflow of aqueous through the structures at the chamber angle and this outflow may be measured by tonography. It is well recognized that, with the exception of the rare hypersecretion glaucomas, in all glaucomas there is a reduction in the outflow of aqueous from the eye. This reduction in "facility of outflow" of aqueous from the glaucomatous eye also may be considered as an accentuation of the normal resistance to outflow of aqueous. This may be due to an increase in the resistance at the same sites as seen in the normal eye or by additional obstructive factors elsewhere. These normal and pathologic sites of resistance to outflow are located in the region of the trabecular meshwork and canal of Schlemm. From a physiologic standpoint, therefore, glaucoma can be said to be due to a reduction in the facility of outflow of aqueous from the eye as a result of obstruction in the region of the anterior chamber angle.

From the functional or visual standpoint the most important aspect of the pathology of glaucoma includes the various changes induced in the intraocular tissues by the continued elevation of the intraocular pressure. Irrespective of the mechanism causing the increased intraocular pressure, these changes induced in the tissues usually are characteristic.

Although in both the normal and the glaucomatous eye the outflow may be influenced by extraocular, neural, and humoral forces, in glaucoma the reduced outflow is produced as a result of a block by some pathologic process. This block in aqueous outflow may be a complication of a recognized disease, in which case the glaucoma is known as secondary. If the elevation of pressure, or the block of aqueous outflow, occurs spontaneously without antecedent ocular disease it is classified as primary. There are two distinct types of acquired primary glaucoma, the angle closure type, and the open angle type. Both usually are bilateral. In certain eyes the anterior chamber is shallow, particularly at the periphery where the iris root lies close to the trabecular meshwork. This type of eye is susceptible to the classic acute glaucomatous attack produced by approximation of the iris root to the trabecular area, but occasionally the course may be slowly progressive.

Open angle glaucoma is characterized by an anatomically open angle by gonioscopy, but the pressure nevertheless rises insidiously over a long period. In this type the block to outflow is thought to be in the trabecular meshwork near the canal of Schlemm.

Glaucoma appearing in infancy or during early years of life, as a consequence of some developmental malformation of the eye is so different that it is considered as a separate entity, congenital glaucoma.

From the preceding discussion it is evident that all glaucomas may be classified both clinically and pathologically in one of these four large categories: (1) primary angle closure, (2) primary open angle, (3) congenital and (4) secondary.

Employing these fundamental concepts the pathology of glaucoma most logically can be presented as follows: First, a discussion of the normal anatomy and physiology, particularly in relation to aqueous formation and outflow; second, a consideration of the pathologic changes that cause the block to aqueous outflow in primary angle closure, primary open angle, congenital glaucoma, and the various kinds of secondary glaucoma; third, a description of the changes induced in the various ocular tissues by the increased intraocular pressure. To conclude this chapter there will be a discussion of reduced intraocular pressure or hypotony.

ANATOMY OF STRUCTURES INVOLVED

Stimulated by such advances in clinical and laboratory investigation as tonography, gonioscopy and electron microscopy, the anatomy of the anterior chamber angle structures and adjacent tissues has been of exceptional interest during recent years. Rapid progress has been made in the understanding of the form and function of the structures about to be described.

The principal exit pathway for aqueous humor is through the trabecular meshwork, Schlemm's canal, the external collector channels, and the anterior ciliary veins. The trabecular meshwork and the canal of Schlemm lie in a corneoscleral groove (the internal scleral sulcus) at the deeper aspect of the limbus in the region of the anterior chamber angle. If the human eye is divided just anterior to the equator, the lens removed, and the iris is torn loose, the trabecular area can be seen as a narrow lighter gray zone just anterior to the attachment of the ciliary body at the scleral spur. This tissue can be removed by teasing, leaving the overlying sclera and its inner sulcus exposed.

The Trabecular Meshwork

This meshwork is composed of (1) the uveal meshwork, and (2) the corneoscleral meshwork (Figs. 232, 233, 612). It is somewhat triangular in meridional sections, with its base at the scleral spur and apex at Schwalbe's line. At the base it contains approximately 12 layers of trabecular bands, while at the apex there are only 2 to 3. The corneoscleral meshwork is composed of sheets, the course of which is principally circumferential (concentric with the limbus), while those of the uveal meshwork are mainly meridional. The corneoscleral meshwork blends with the scleral spur and longitudinal portion of the ciliary muscle posteriorly and with Schwalbe's line and cornea anteriorly.

The bands forming the *uveal meshwork* extend from the region of Schwalbe's line

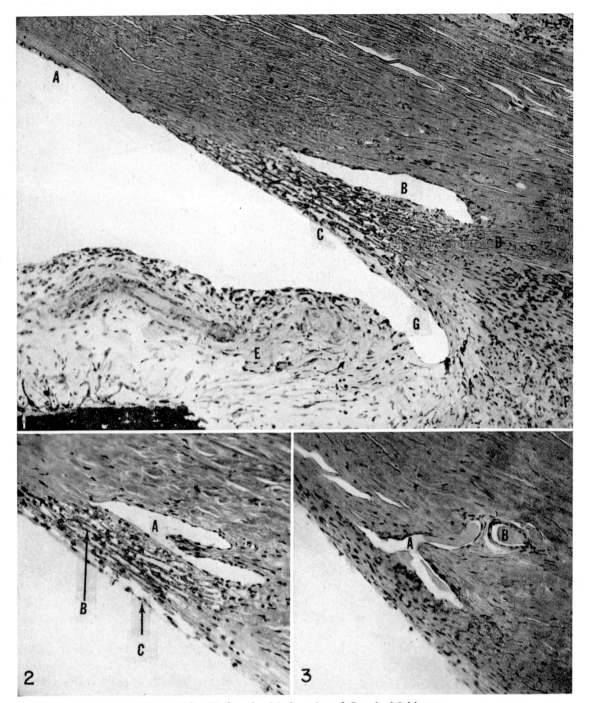

Figure 612. Trabecular Meshwork and Canal of Schlemm

1. A, Descemet's membrane. B, Schlemm's canal. C, trabeculas. D, scleral spur. E, iris. F, ciliary body. G, anterior chamber angle. ×150. AFIP Acc. 55063.

2. A, coalescing lumina of Schlemm's canal. B, corneoscleral trabeculas. C, uveal trabeculas. ×180. AFIP Acc. 61823.

3. A, Schlemm's canal. B, vein of intrascleral plexus. ×145. AFIP Acc. 271074.

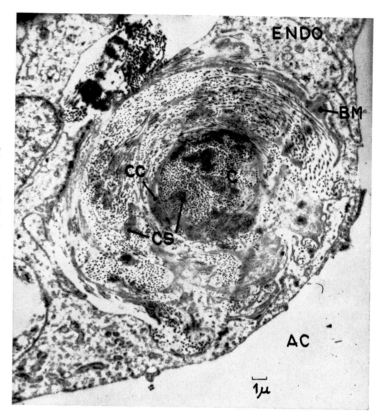

Figure 613. Electron Micrograph, of Uveal Trabecular Fiber

AC, anterior chamber; C, collagen fibers cut in cross section; CS, amorphous cement substance; CC, irregular clumps of 1000 A-banded material; ENDO, endothelium; BM, basement membrane. Section was treated with uranium acetate. ×5000. (From Garron and Feeney, 1959.)

backward around the angle of the anterior chamber to become continuous with the stroma of the ciliary body and iris (Fig. 612). The collagen and elastic fibers of these bands mainly have a meridional course. As a result, cross sections of this meshwork have an oval appearance. Each uveal band has a central collagen core, the bundles of which are surrounded by an amorphous ground substance (Fig. 613). Surrounding these are more obliquely disposed collagen fibers which are likewise embedded in ground substance. The outer surface of each uveal band is surrounded by an endothelium not unlike that of the corneoscleral meshwork. The uveal portion of the meshwork is not so highly organized as the corneoscleral.

The *corneoscleral meshwork* is formed of wide sheets or bands which run circumferentially around the eye (Fig. 614). Anteriorly, they are attached at the anterior border ring (line of Schwalbe) while posteriorly they unite with the sclera at the posterior border ring (scleral spur) and blend with the tendinous insertion of meridional and radial ciliary muscle fibers (Fig. 615). Early histo-

logic investigations, using conventional techniques, showed the trabecular bands to be composed of a central collagenous core which was surrounded by a thin layer, staining like elastic tissue. A third layer, resembling Descemet's membrane, surrounded the latter zone and in turn was covered by a delicate layer of endothelium.

Recent studies by Garron et al., utilizing light and electron microscopy, show that the central core of the trabecular band is composed of bundles of tightly packed collagen fibrils with a periodicity of 640 Å (Fig. 616). Surrounding this core is a homogeneous matrix (ground substance) containing loosely arranged fibers having a periodicity of 1000 Å. A definite layer of elastic fibers was not seen. The layer formerly believed to represent an extension of Descemet's membrane is composed of a homogeneous matrix of light density in which are fine fibrils and an irregular tortuous material having a periodicity in the order of 1000 Å. The aggregates of this material appear in a variety of configurations, oval, crescentic, round, or rod-shaped. A basement membrane is found beneath the endo-

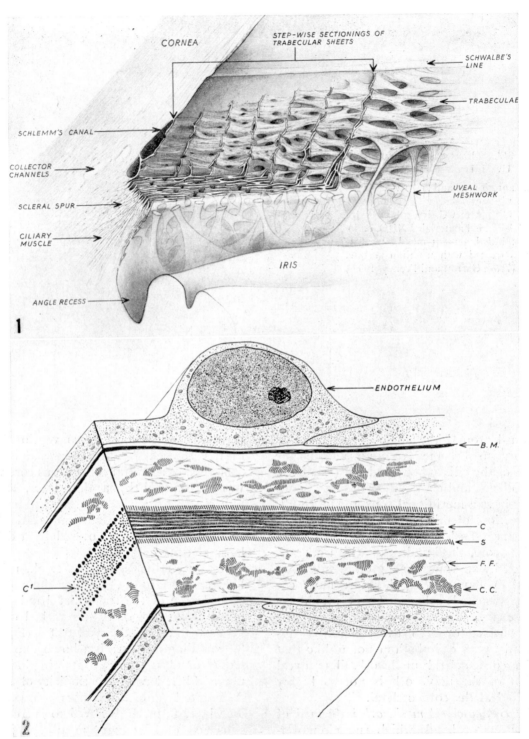

Figure 614.

1. Diagrammatic representation of the trabecular area. The trabecular meshwork is cut away at progressively deeper levels to show the size of the openings and disposition of the layer. Note the large openings in the uveal meshwork, and the progressive diminution of this size as Schlemm's canal is approached.

2. Tilted frontal and meridional representation (see Fig. 615) of a corneoscleral trabecular sheet. C, central collagenous tissue; S, sheath of thick fibers with 1000 A periodicity; F.F. and C.C., zone of ground substance containing irregular clumps of 1000 A material and very fine fibrils; B. M., basement membrane.

(From Garron and Feeney, 1959.)

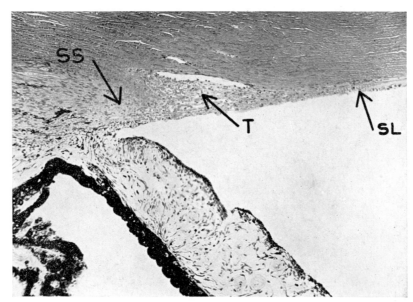

Figure 615. Normal corneoscleral trabecular meshwork. T, trabecular meshwork; SS, scleral spur; SL, Schwalbe's line.

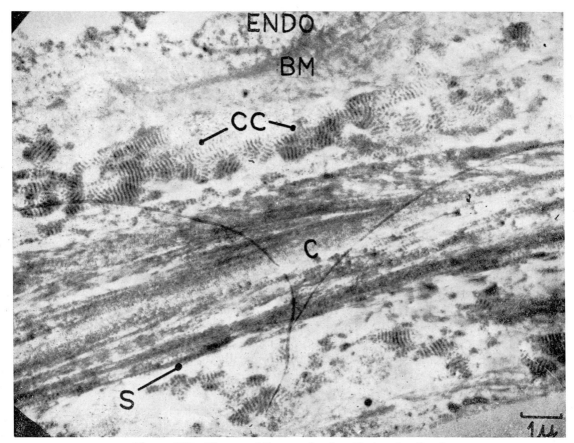

Figure 616. Electron Micrograph of a Trabecular Band

C, central connective tissue core; S, sheath of denser 1000 Å material; CC, clumps of 1000 Å banded material in a light dense matrix; BM, basement membrane; Endo., endothelial cell cytoplasm and wall.

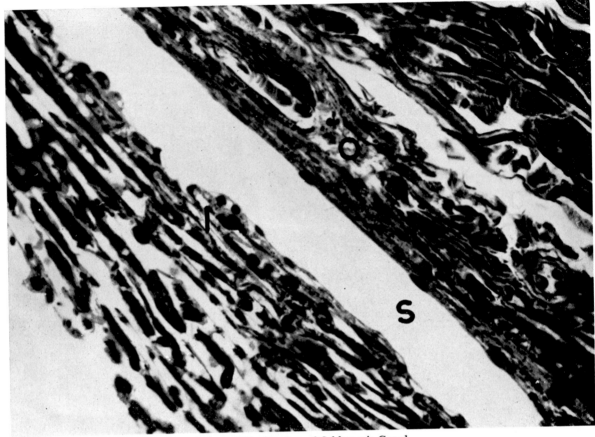

Figure 617. Region of Schlemm's Canal

Outer wall has a thin layer of endothelium. Inner wall of vacuolated endothelial cells. Inner trabeculas show fewer spaces. S, Schlemm's canal; O, outer wall; I, inner wall.

thelium, but is so thin that it is doubtful if it could be seen by light microscopy. The endothelial cells, except for the finer details observed with electron microscopy, are much as observed by light microscopy and form a complete covering layer over the trabecular bands.

These circumferentially disposed trabecular bands interconnect with each other at different levels, and contain many perforations, mostly oval, which are so disposed in succeeding layers that the openings connect by tortuous pathways almost to the level of Schlemm's canal. It is agreed by most observers that the long axis of these openings is oriented circumferentially, and that the apertures become smaller as Schlemm's canal is approached.

There is good evidence, based on perfusion studies, that communications exist between the trabecular spaces and Schlemm's canal. Particulate matter measuring less than 2 microns in diameter passes readily from the anterior chamber into Schlemm's canal, while particles of 2 to 3 microns size pass with slight difficulty. Particles larger than this are retarded in the trabecular meshes.

Relatively large passages lined by endothelium (Sondermann's canals) have been described by a number of investigators, especially Theobald, as communications between the intertrabecular spaces and the canal of Schlemm but it seems these large passages must be considerably modified both anatomically and functionally *in vivo*.

Recent histologic studies have focused attention on structural differences in that part of the trabecular area immediately adjacent to Schlemm's canal. The tissue in this region appears more cellular and less fibrous (Fig. 617). By electron microscopy the trabecular bands close to Schlemm's canal have been found to be devoid of the central collagen core that characterizes most of the trabecular bands. Garron and Feeney, and Holmberg, have shown that the large endothelial cells which line the inner (trabecular) wall of Schlemm's canal appear to be vacuolated and do not possess a basement membrane (Fig. 618). With the aid of serial sections these "vacuoles" have been found by Holmberg to be a system of intercommunicating passages, measuring about 1 micron in diameter, which tunnel through the walls of endothelial cells to enter Schlemm's canal. These, then, may represent some of the pathways by which aqueous is removed from the eye and which produce part of the normal resistance to out-flow of aqueous humor from the anterior chamber.

The intertrabecular spaces adjacent to Schlemm's canal contain an acid mucopoly-saccharide that is sensitive to hyaluronidase (Zimmerman, 1957). It is possible that this corresponds to the hyaluronidase-sensitive substance that Bárány found responsible for half of the normal resistance to aqueous out-flow in several species of experimental animals.

The Canal of Schlemm

This outpost of the venous system follows a tortuous course around the circumference of the eye in the most posterior part of the internal scleral sulcus. It is rather large, but the size is variable. It either appears as a single channel, or is divided into two or three

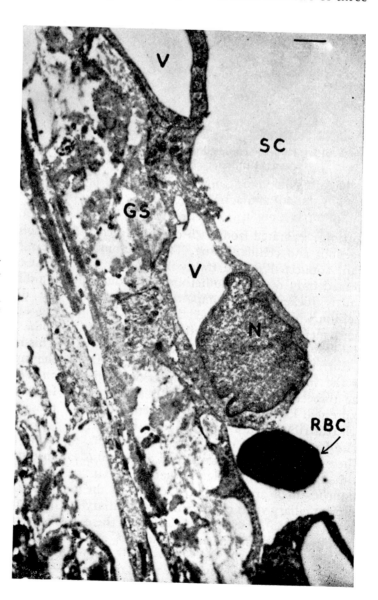

Figure 618. Electron micrograph of inner wall of Schlemm's canal showing "vacuoles" in endothelium. SC, Schlemm's canal; V, "vacuoles"; GS, ground substance; N, nucleus of endothelial cell; RBC. portion of red blood cell in canal. ×11,000. (From Garron and Feeney, 1959.)

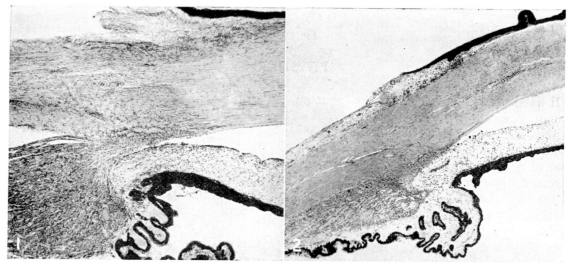

Figure 620. Angle Closure Glaucoma

1. Trabecular meshwork is partially blocked by apposition of iris root. ×40. AFIP Acc. 28249.
2. Trabecular meshwork is completely covered by iris root. ×45. AFIP Acc. 183941.

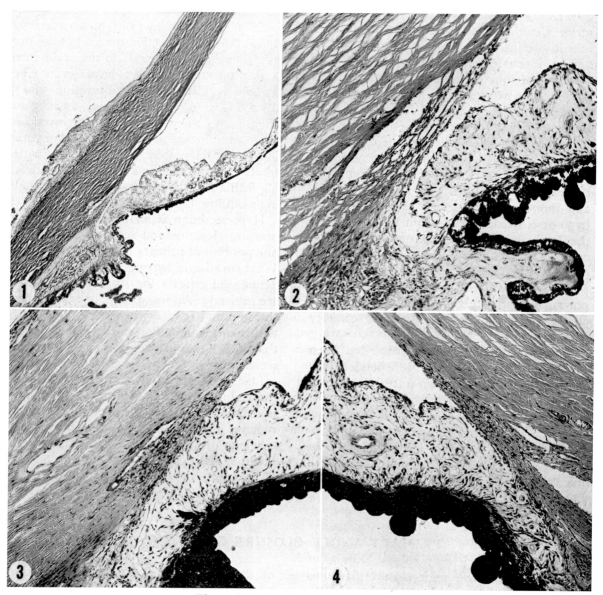

Figure 621. Angle Closure Glaucoma

1 and 2. The chamber angle is exceedingly shallow but open. Enucleation performed 5 days after onset of angle closure glaucoma. ×26 and ×115, respectively. AFIP Acc. 687300.

3 and 4. Chamber angle on both sides is occluded by apposition of the iris root. Enucleation performed 6 days after onset of angle closure glaucoma. ×115 (both). AFIP Acc. 570376.

cornea. The attack is accompanied by pain, headache, nausea, vomiting, and reduction of vision. Milder attacks may occur in which there is transient discomfort, and halos, which are produced by corneal edema. These symptoms and findings are produced not only by the marked elevation of pressure, but also by the rapidity with which it develops. In primary simple glaucoma which develops insidiously there may be very high tensions which persist over long periods of time, without the classic signs and symptoms.

A fundamental characteristic of angle closure glaucoma is that, at least during the early stages, the process is entirely reversible. Between attacks there may be no evidence of glaucoma, and the facility of outflow, tension, and clinical appearance are normal, except for the shallow chamber and narrow anterior chamber angle. However, with repeated attacks, iris-trabecular adhesions form, angle closure becomes more permanent and the glaucomatous state becomes irreversible. Permanent angle closure is seen not only in this type of primary glaucoma, but also in a number of types of secondary glaucoma, as will be discussed later.

Pathologic Anatomy

The essential anatomic finding of acute angle closure glaucoma is the contact of the peripheral iris with the inner surface of the trabecular meshwork (Fig. 620). Originally this contact simply may be a juxtaposition without actual adhesion (Fig. 621). With proper treatment at this stage the angle usually reopens and the aqueous outflow and pressure return to normal. More prolonged contact of iris and trabecular meshwork leads to the formation of true adhesions (peripheral anterior synechias). In a severe attack, the contact between these two structures may be so extensive as to completely block the trabecular channels. In cases with less severe attacks which recur, the adhesions gradually extend and encroach on the angle. The meshwork to which iris is adherent undergoes progressive fibrosis and degeneration. Schlemm's canal becomes compressed and eventually is obliterated (Fig. 622). Aqueous outflow from the eye gradually is reduced as the formation of peripheral anterior synechias progresses, and by the time the adhesion becomes complete it approaches zero. The tissue changes of acute angle closure glaucoma occur sooner and are more marked than in most other glaucomas. They primarily occur in the anterior segment, involving the cornea, iris, trabecular area and ciliary body.

The corneal stroma and epithelium become edematous. A sudden attack of acute glaucoma often produces small to large areas of necrosis of the iris stroma (Fig. 622–2) due

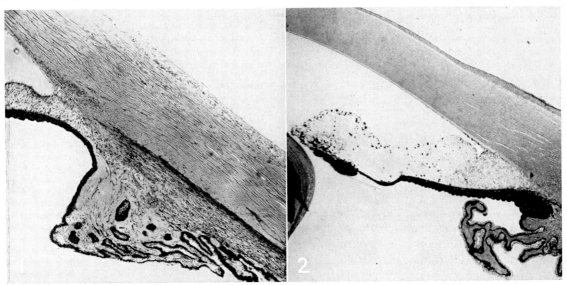

Figure 622. Chronic and Acute Angle Closure Glaucoma

1. Atrophy of iris root, compression of trabecular meshwork, and obliteration of Schlemm's canal in chronic glaucoma. ×45. AFIP Acc. 193988.

2. More severe atrophy of iris root, trabeculas, and Schlemm's canal; ischemic necrosis of pupillary zone in acute glaucoma. ×48. AFIP Acc. 88968.

to interference with its blood supply during apposition of the iris root to the trabecular meshwork. The necrosis affects both the stroma and pigment epithelium and usually is most severe in the pupillary zone, where the sphincter is affected. As a result the pupil becomes enlarged and eccentric. The ciliary body shows edema of the processes and congestion of the vessels. A moderate inflammatory reaction occurs, with passage of a few inflammatory cells, mainly lymphocytes, into the posterior and anterior chambers.

Over a longer period of time changes occur in the optic nerve and retina. These will be discussed in detail later.

Pathogenesis

Primary angle closure glaucoma essentially is dependent on an anatomically narrow angle which can be appreciated clinically by gonioscopic examination (Figs. 623, 624). This narrow angle is probably developmental and may be hereditary. Hypermetropic eyes are especially prone to develop acute angle closure glaucoma. This is not due primarily to the hyperopia but to an associated shallow anterior chamber. It has been well shown that acute angle closure glaucoma is not only associated with a shallow anterior chamber but the shallower the anterior chamber the more likely the glaucoma is to occur. One of the earliest theories of glaucoma (Priestly Smith) was based on the disproportion of the size of the structures in the anterior segment, particularly the lens, causing an angle block in an eye with a small anterior segment.

Although the fundamental background of this type of glaucoma is the narrow angle, there must be some factor which precipitates the acute attack. We have mentioned the work of Priestly Smith, who was the first to demonstrate the relationship between hyperopia, shallow anterior chamber, and acute glaucoma. He showed the *disproportion* which may exist in the anterior segment of some hyperopic eyes between the lens and other structures. Recently Tornquist has shown that the anterior chamber actually does lose depth with increasing age, possibly due to increase in size of the lens. In this country it is believed by many that mydriasis produces acute glaucoma in a predisposed eye by creating a physiologic block between the lens and iris. If such a block occurs, aqueous is retained in the posterior chamber, and displaces the relaxed iris forward into the angle, obstructing outflow of aqueous. Not only does pharmacologic mydriasis produce this effect, but the dilatation which occurs in the dark (darkroom test), and in emotional shock have the same effect. The mechanism by which emotional shock produces the attacks is not well understood, and some have postulated that a vasomotor crisis can produce swelling of the ciliary processes, which in turn displace the iris forward. It seems certain that swelling of the vitreous does not produce such attacks. As von Sallmann has shown, the vitreous is not capable of swelling sufficiently that it could displace the lens and iris forward to produce acute glaucoma. A factor of importance, and which furnishes fairly clear proof of the physiologic pupillary block mechanism, is the curative effect of a peripheral iridectomy, which causes prompt deepening of the anterior chamber, widening of the angle, and prevents further attacks in most eyes.

PRIMARY OPEN ANGLE GLAUCOMA

Open angle glaucoma (chronic simple glaucoma) is a chronic, slowly progressive disease in which the anterior chamber angle as seen with the gonioscope is open even though the pressure is elevated (Figs. 625, 626). The width of the chamber angle varies from extremely wide to moderately narrow. In the early stages the rises of intraocular pressure may be intermittent; following this for a considerable period the pressure may be only slightly elevated. However, a decrease in aqueous outflow may be demonstrated by tonography even in the very early stages of the disease. At times the decreased outflow is greater than would be anticipated in view of the tension. It is possible in these cases that there is a compensatory decrease in aqueous formation which keeps the pressure from rising excessively. The dramatic fluctuations of intraocular pressure which characterize angle

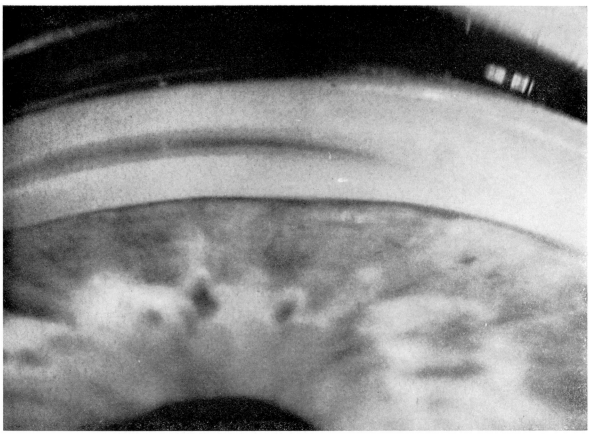

Figure 623. Gonioscopic view of extremely narrow angle. (From Shaffer, 1960.)

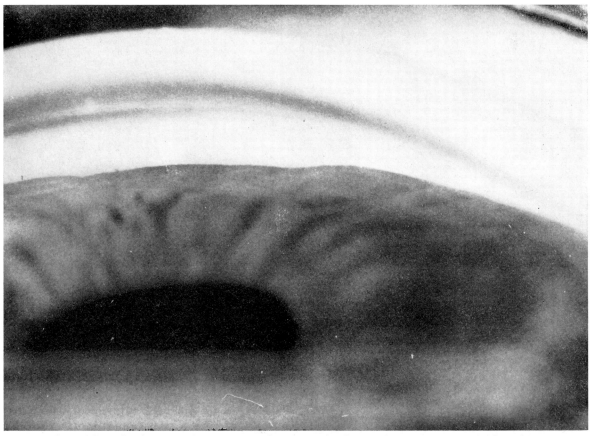

Figure 624. Gonioscopic view (preoperative) in angle closure glaucoma. (From Shaffer, 1960.)

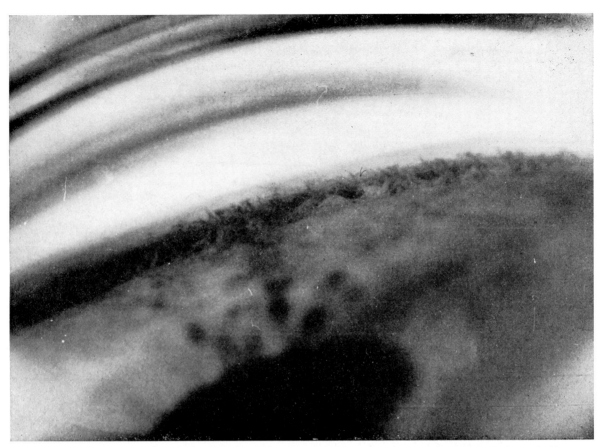

Figure 625. Gonioscopic view of wide open angle, blood in Schlemm's canal. (From Shaffer, 1960.)

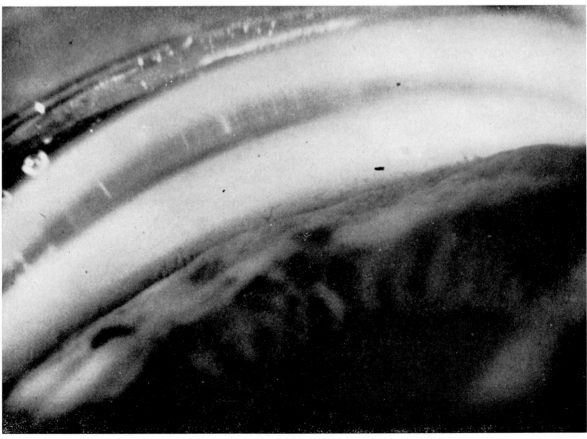

Figure 626. Gonioscopic view of moderately narrow angle. Patient's father had acute glaucoma. (From Shaffer, 1960.)

Figure 627.

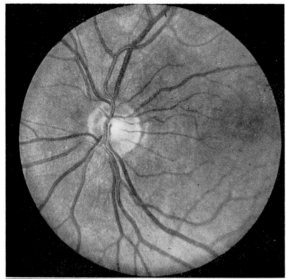

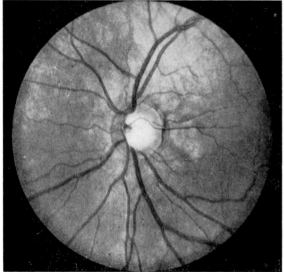

Figure 628.

Figure 627. Ophthalmoscopic Appearance of Normal Optic Disk. (Courtesy of Dr. R. N. Shaffer.)

Figure 628. Ophthalmoscopic Appearance of Early Glaucomatous Cupping. (Courtesy of Dr. R. N. Shaffer.)

closure glaucoma are absent, as are the acute attacks of pain, congestion, and corneal edema. However, the most characteristic signs of progression of open angle glaucoma are those which occur in the visual field and optic disc (Figs. 627, 628, 629). These will be discussed later.

Inasmuch as the anterior chamber depth and angle configuration in open angle glaucoma are clinically normal, the outflow passages from the chamber angle have been postulated as the site where increased resistance to aqueous outflow occurs. Trabecular sclerosis as the cause of this type of glaucoma has been considered for many years. There is increasing evidence that the principal pathologic changes which produce most cases of open angle glaucoma occur in the trabecular area. It has been recognized that open angle glaucoma not only is bilateral, but also increases in frequency and in severity with advancing age. This suggests that connective tissue changes, particularly swelling and sclerosis, might be responsible for the obstruction to outflow of aqueous humor. Microdissection and perfusion studies by Grant have demonstrated that in normal human eyes 75 per cent of the outflow resistance is in the trabecular meshwork; also that the increased resistance to outflow of aqueous in cases of open angle glaucoma is in the trabecular area. There is increasing evidence that heredity is important in open angle glaucoma. Becker has found a remarkably high incidence of impaired facility of outflow in the younger family members of patients with established glaucoma.

The chief obstacle to determination of the early pathologic changes occurring in the eye in chronic open angle glaucoma has been the lack of adequate histologic material from established cases. In fact, even in relatively far

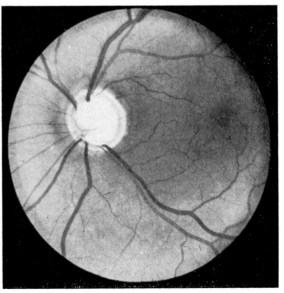

Figure 629. Ophthalmoscopic Appearance of Severely Cupped Disk. (From Shaffer, 1960.)

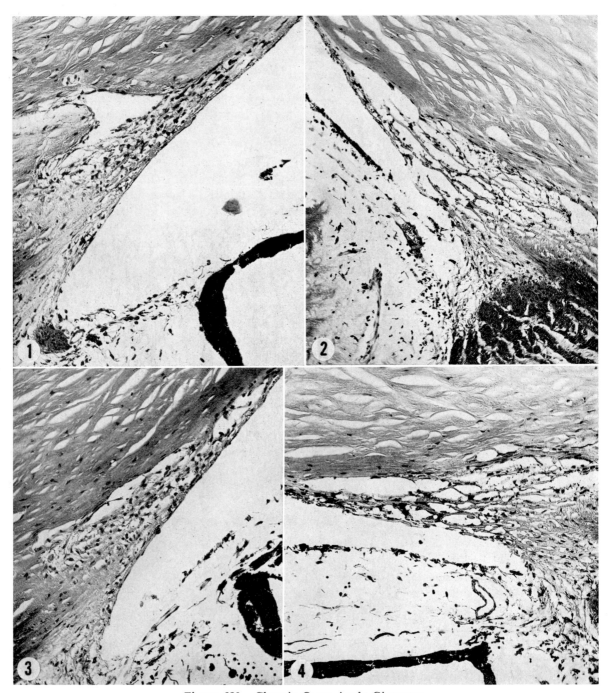

Figure 630. Chronic Open Angle Glaucoma

1 to 4. All fields are from different portions of the trabecular meshwork and Schlemm's canal of the same eye obtained at autopsy in the case of a patient with primary open angle glaucoma. Very subtle degenerative changes are observed in the "pore tissue" forming the inner wall of Schlemm's canal. In places the canal is partially obliterated, apparently by adhesions of the cells of the inner wall to the outer wall. The trabecular sheets are thickened and the intertrabecular spaces narrowed. ×180, ×115, ×145, and ×145, respectively. AFIP Acc. 850088.

advanced cases there is a distinct paucity of histopathologic material because in the absence of complications, these eyes are not painful and there is no indication for enucleation. Those advanced cases of open angle glaucoma that have been enucleated most often have extensive anterior segment changes due to congestion of the eye, with bullous keratopathy, corneal ulceration, and changes produced by surgical procedures. The intratrabecular changes found in studies of autopsy cases of early open angle glaucoma have provided the most valuable information. The changes occurring in the trabecular meshwork in these cases are extremely subtle and are difficult to interpret and recognize.

In his critical appraisal of the observations published to the present time, Ashton concluded that no microscopic studies have been made which are sufficiently free of artifact to provide completely reliable evidence as to what constitutes the early pathologic anatomy of this disease. The trabecular sclerosis, obliteration of Schlemm's canal and its outlets, and the increased trabecular cellularity that have been described by Teng et al., Theobald and Kirk, and Kornsweig and associates may all be early changes resulting from the elevated intraocular pressure rather than primary pathologic changes. On the other hand, Becker has reported that degenerative changes of the type described by Teng and his associates are found more frequently in patients with established glaucoma and that the degree of severity roughly parallels the diminution in facility of outflow. These changes occur in the trabecular fibers adjacent to Schlemm's canal and probably consist chiefly of degeneration and swelling of the collagen fibers with proliferation of endothelium. At times the endothelium proliferates into Schlemm's canal (Fig. 630). These changes produce narrowing and closure of the intertrabecular spaces adjacent to Schlemm's canal. It also is probable that the channels leading from the trabecular area to the canal of Schlemm also are narrowed or closed.

As mentioned previously the presence of acid mucopolysaccharides in the intertrabecular spaces has been demonstrated histochemically. Some evidence exists that alteration of this material by enzyme action might influence the facility of outflow.

Although it is probable that the primary mechanism of open angle glaucoma is a degenerative change in the trabecular meshwork, it is also possible that this is not necessarily the resistance site in all eyes with open angle glaucoma. It is theoretically possible that the collector channels and episcleral veins could be a site of resistance to outflow.

CONGENITAL GLAUCOMA

Congenital glaucoma and hydrophthalmia are terms which apply to a disorder resulting from defective development of structures in and around the anterior chamber angle. Congenital glaucoma is much less common than adult glaucoma. In a large series of cases compiled by Scheie, about half were recognized at birth and almost 90 per cent were diagnosed by the end of the first year. In over 10 per cent symptoms of the disorder were not apparent until the child was one to six or more years of age. Two-thirds of the cases have bilateral involvement. When congenital glaucoma is transmitted as a hereditary disorder it probably occurs as a simple recessive, therefore glaucoma will not develop unless two carriers of the condition marry, in which case 25 per cent of the children will be affected. Of the unaffected members two out of three will, in turn, be carriers. Consanguinity of the parents is found in about 10 per cent of cases. Congenital glaucoma may be associated with other developmental disorders, particularly neurofibromatosis, the Sturge-Weber syndrome, aniridia, Axenfeld's syndrome, and persistent hyperplastic primary vitreous, but these are considered in other chapters. The most important type of congenital glaucoma is that which is unassociated with other ocular malformations.

Any child under the age of two years who has constant sensitivity to light, blepharospasm and epiphora should be suspected of having glaucoma. In more advanced cases the cornea becomes diffusely hazy or completely

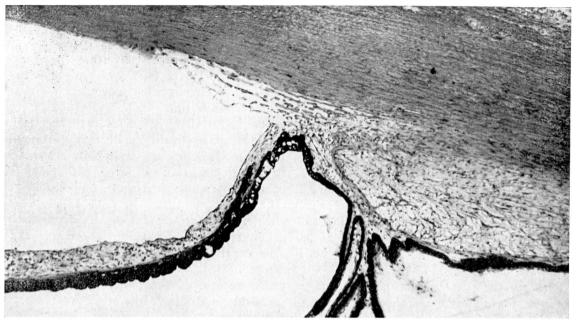

Figure 631. Congenital Glaucoma

Incomplete separation of iris root from trabecular meshwork. ×130. AFIP Acc. 101285.

cloudy due to edema. Occasionally the cornea is so edematous it resembles white porcelain.

Early examination shows a deep anterior chamber and, possibly, an increase in the size of the cornea. The tension is found to be elevated. More advanced cases show definite enlargement of the anterior segment and cornea, a deep anterior chamber, and an atrophic iris. Cupping of the disk occurs very late.

Barkan and other observers have described characteristic gonioscopic changes in the angle, consisting of an ill-defined membranous tissue covering the trabecular zone. According to Scheie and to Maumenee, however, the diagnosis of congenital glaucoma usually cannot be established on the basis of the gonioscopic appearance of the angle alone even though structural alterations in the angle are responsible for the disorder.

Pathologic Anatomy

Several recent histologic descriptions (Burian et al.; Allen et al.; Shaffer; Maumenee, 1958) of the pathology of congenital glaucoma have emphasized that the most consistent finding is an anterior insertion of the iris on the trabecular meshwork (Fig. 631). The absence of Schlemm's canal is rarely, if ever, the essential feature and there is no evidence to sup-

port the early clinical impression by some observers that an abnormal membrane covers the angle tissues to produce the glaucoma. The most recent and extensive study is that of Maumenee. His observations suggest that the abnormality which produces the glaucoma consists of an abnormal anterior insertion of the longitudinal fibers of the ciliary muscle Fig. 632). Many of the fibers insert directly into the trabecular bands whereas normally

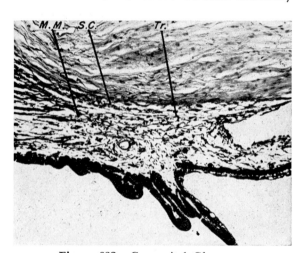

Figure 632. Congenital Glaucoma

Anterior insertion of meridional fibers of ciliary muscle (M.M.). Iris root and some ciliary body stroma remain attached to trabecular meshwork (Tr.). Canal of Schlemm (S.C.) is present but is only a slit-like space. (From Maumenee, 1958.)

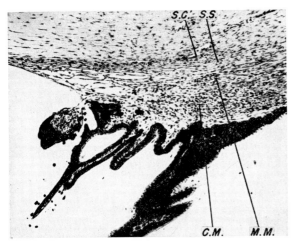

Figure 633. Congenital Glaucoma

The circular (C.M.) and meridional (M.M.) fibers of the ciliary muscle are located far forward in relation to Schlemm's canal (S.C.) and the scleral spur (S.S.). (From Maumenee, 1958.)

they insert into the scleral spur. Associated with this anomaly, the circular bundles of the ciliary muscle and the iris root are located farther forward and inward than normally (Fig. 633).

Eyes enucleated late in the course of the disease typically are enlarged in all dimensions. At times they are enormous (Fig. 634). Such massive enlargement is due to the relative ease with which the ocular coats can be stretched during infancy. It is not restricted to congenital glaucoma but may be seen in any type of secondary glaucoma which develops early in life (Fig. 635). These latter cases typically have greatly enlarged, thinned, flattened corneas and marked ectasia of the limbal area. Here the scleral thickness may be reduced to 0.20 to 0.24 mm. Anderson has shown that the anterior segment presents a characteristic configuration and becomes enlarged out of proportion to the remainder of the eye. The corneal epithelium is edematous and there are tears in Descemet's membrane.

In congenital glaucoma the interior chamber is deep and the angle is unusually wide, except after unsuccessful surgical procedures complicated by the formation of synechias. The iris root and trabecular band in these advanced cases are extremely degenerated and thinned, and the canal of Schlemm may have

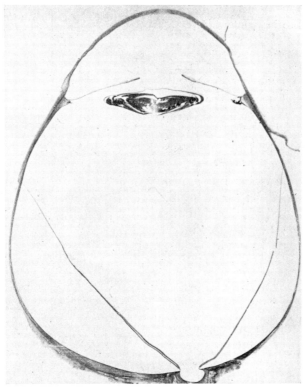

Figure 634. Congenital Glaucoma

Enlargement of whole eye and of corneal diameter, deepening of anterior chamber, cupping of nerve head. AFIP Acc. 38269.

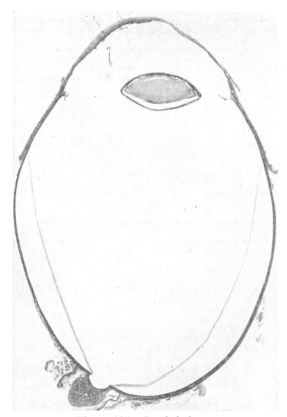

Figure 635. Buphthalmos

Glaucoma secondary to old perforated corneal ulcer; great enlargement of cornea and whole eye. AFIP Acc. 35681.

completely disappeared. The ciliary body is extremely atrophic and flattened except for some ciliary processes which are drawn inward by a taut zonule. Degenerative changes in the zonule may lead to subluxation of the lens. Marked degenerative changes are observed in the retina but most often there is less cupping of the nerve head than might be expected. It is believed that the early stretching of the sclera, particularly at the limbus, protects the nerve head.

Pathogenesis

In order to understand the pathologic anatomy of the chamber angle in congenital glaucoma it is necessary to review the normal embryologic development of the tissues involved. The eye of a 45 to 55 mm. embryo (10 to 12 weeks) has the beginning of an anterior chamber but the trabecular meshwork

is not clearly defined (Fig. 636). At the periphery of Descemet's mesothelium a condensation of dark staining, radially arranged cells is seen. These end more peripherally in the sclera, and are the anlage of the trabecular meshwork. Even at this stage, the cells can be differentiated from the adjacent looser mesodermal tissue which is beginning to form the ciliary body and iris. The ciliary muscle and scleral spur are not yet formed.

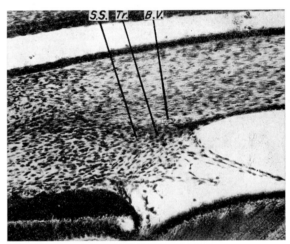

Figure 636. Embryologic Development of Anterior Chamber Angle

Normal 55 mm. human embryo. S.S., scleral spur; Tr., trabecular meshwork; B.V., blood vessel. (From Maumenee, 1958.)

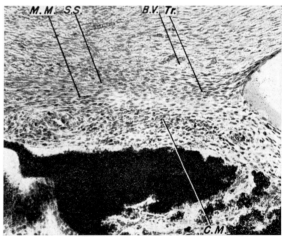

Figure 637. Embryologic Development of Anterior Chamber Angle

Normal 150 mm. embryo. M.M., meridional ciliary muscle fibers; C.M., circular fibers; S.S., scleral spur; B.V., blood vessel; Tr., trabecular meshwork. (From Maumenee, 1958.)

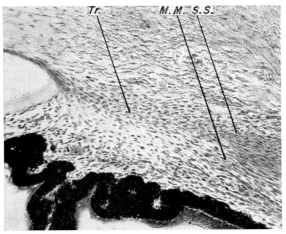

Figure 638. Embryologic Development of Anterior Chamber Angle

Normal 220 mm. human embryo. (From Maumenee, 1958.)

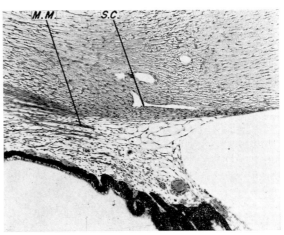

Figure 639. Embryologic Development of Anterior Chamber Angle

The iris root in this normal 7 month old fetus has not yet separated from the trabecular meshwork. (From Maumenee, 1958.)

During the 75 to 85 mm. stage (14 weeks), a distinct cleavage plane forms between the meshwork and the ciliary body. The scleral spur and the longitudinal portion of the ciliary muscle appear. By the 140 to 160 mm. stage (20 weeks), the ciliary body is partially formed, the trabecular sheets measure 0.23 mm. in length and the longitudinal part of the ciliary muscle extends forward of the anlage of the scleral spur (Fig. 637). The eye of the 220 mm. (28 weeks) embryo shows distinct ciliary processes, a scleral spur, and longitudinal fibers of the ciliary muscle (Fig. 638). The trabecular sheets measure 0.30 to 0.35 in length from Schwalbe's line to the scleral spur.

The chamber angle of fetal eyes between the sixth and ninth month opens by a process of cleavage (Fig. 639). Maumenee found only one of eight anterior chamber angles completely open in fetuses aged six and seven months. The other seven showed various degrees of attachment of ciliary body to the trabecular area. Eight of thirteen eyes of eight months fetuses had normal open angles, but in five the angles were incompletely developed. Fifteen eyes of fetuses at nine months gestation all had open angles but occasional fine iris processes or pectinate ligaments connecting with Schwalbe's ring were seen.

Allen, Burian and Braley, in an excellent series of papers, demonstrated that a process of cleavage occurs between two clearly defined groups of cells which are the anlage of the trabecular fibers on one hand and the root of the iris on the other. This cleavage forms the anterior chamber angle. The cleavage process is determined by a differential growth rate between the external and internal tissues of the anterior segment, resulting in altered tissue relationships. These authors also described two cases of congenital glaucoma and demonstrated that incomplete cleavage of the iris root from the posterior part of the trabecular fibers was probably responsible for the peculiar configuration of the chamber angle.

The reason for this arrest in the normal cleavage which leads to abnormal formation of the anterior chamber angle structures is not known. It is not due to prematurity because the disease is not more common in premature infants than in those which are full-term. Most likely the condition is genetically determined. It has been observed histologically that microphakia is often present, but actual measurements are not available to support the concept that microphakia might prevent the ciliary muscle and iris root from moving backward in relation to the cornea, trabecular meshwork, and scleral spur, as they should in normal development.

SECONDARY GLAUCOMA

Secondary glaucoma may occur as a complication of a large number of intraocular and a few systemic diseases. Among these are inflammatory, traumatic, vascular, mechanical, neoplastic, and degenerative conditions, which have been described in detail in other chapters. The vast majority of cases of secondary glaucoma may be explained on the basis of mechanical obstruction to the outflow of aqueous humor. Secondary glaucoma may be considered from the standpoint of the site of block, and on the basis of the etiology of the causative condition. Although some cases of secondary glaucoma are bilateral, most are unilateral, appearing in the eye with the causative lesion.

Much like primary glaucoma, secondary glaucoma can be divided into open angle and angle closure varieties. With the exception of the pupillary block type of glaucoma, secondary glaucoma usually is caused by changes occurring in the anterior chamber angle. In the open angle variety of secondary glaucoma the change is usually within or near the trabecular meshwork.

SECONDARY ANGLE CLOSURE GLAUCOMA

Pupillary Block

The simplest cases of secondary angle closure glaucoma are those caused by pupillary block, which obstructs the flow of aqueous between the posterior and anterior chambers.

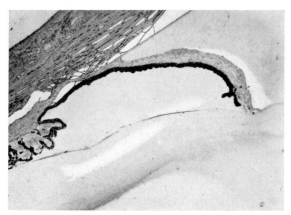

Figure 640. Iris Bombé Following Cataract Extraction

The pupillary margin of the iris is firmly adherent to the anterior hyaloid surface. ×25. Univ. of Cal. Acc. 49–99

In certain types of iritis, annular adhesions develop between the lens and the pupillary part of the iris, causing seclusion of the pupil (Fig. 36). As the pressure rises in the posterior chamber the iris is pushed forward producing an iris bombé (Fig. 36). If an iridectomy is done to establish continuity between the anterior and posterior chambers the tension may become normal. However, this must be done before peripheral anterior synechias form. If there is an inadequate iridectomy opening following a cataract extraction, the vitreous face may become adherent to the pupil, producing iris bombé and a flat chamber due to pupillary block (Fig. 640).

In certain cases a partially dislocated lens may also block the pupil.

Peripheral Anterior Synechias

Glaucoma may follow a flattening of the anterior chamber due to cataract or glaucoma surgery. Peripheral anterior synechias develop during the period the chamber is absent and are due to inflammation at the site of contact between iris and trabecular meshwork.

Peripheral anterior synechias also occur in cases of recurrent acute and chronic iridocyclitis. At times these are localized, and result from large conglomerate precipitates, which cause adhesions of iris to the trabecular meshwork. At other times they result from iris swelling, congestion of the iris vessels, exudation into the angle, and organization of the exudate by capillaries and fibroblasts. It is uncommon for glaucoma to result from peripheral anterior synechias in iridocyclitis, but at times they become so extensive as to obstruct the angle.

Trauma frequently produces peripheral anterior synechias, especially if the anterior chamber has been opened by a lacerated wound. The hemorrhage which results from contusions also causes early and late glaucoma. This has been discussed in Chapter III.

Vascular diseases of the posterior eye, especially the retina, such as diabetes, central retinal vein occlusion, central retinal artery occlusion, Eales's disease, and retinal vasculitis, often result in development of peripheral anterior synechias and secondary glaucoma. The mechanism by which these diseases produce synechias is obscure, but it is known from gonioscopic observations that new-vessel formation occurs in the anterior ciliary body and the trabecular area, with extensions into the angle itself, and that these gradually lead to progressive adhesion of the peripheral iris and trabecular tissues. At the same time a layer of newly formed vascular tissue forms on the iris surface. A clinically important aspect of glaucoma secondary to occlusion of the central vein is its relationship to chronic simple glaucoma. In many eyes in which there is a glaucoma secondary to this condition the fellow eye is found to have chronic open angle glaucoma. This relationship has been recognized for years and has been attributed to the fact that in eyes with chronic open angle glaucoma, sclerotic changes are more likely to be severe in the central retinal vessels in the optic nerve. It is also possible that in those eyes with chronic open angle glaucoma which develop central vein occlusions, a severe secondary glaucoma is more likely to occur because the trabecular tissues are already somewhat damaged. Central artery occlusion also may produce secondary glaucoma for the same reason as that in central vein occlusion.

Intraocular tumors may produce peripheral anterior synechias by displacing the iris forward against the trabecular meshwork, or by producing iridocyclitis. Iris and ciliary body tumors may invade and obstruct the angle to produce glaucoma (Figs. 351, 352).

Essential atrophy of the iris produces glaucoma by gradual development of peripheral anterior synechias. Initially the iris atrophy results in displacement of the iris tissues toward the angle on the side opposite the affected zone. Hole formation then is accompanied by further displacement with formation of extensive synechias which block the outflow of aqueous (Fig. 388).

SECONDARY OPEN ANGLE GLAUCOMA

Although most of the cases of secondary glaucoma are due to peripheral anterior synechias and a resulting block in aqueous outflow, there are a number of types of open angle secondary glaucoma in which the patho-logic process directly involves the trabecular meshwork. In these cases the block usually is by particulate matter such as the debris of inflammation, hemorrhage, or other material.

This type of secondary glaucoma often is associated with acute *anterior uveitis*. It is more likely to occur, however, in the long-standing, chronic forms of uveitis. Patients with acute iridocyclitis frequently show a markedly reduced aqueous outflow, but do not develop glaucoma because there is a simultaneous reduction of aqueous production. In either case the glaucoma may be caused by a block of the intertrabecular spaces with inflammatory cells and debris (Figs. 33, 35–1, 336–2). The exudate thus forms a mechanical barrier to passage of fluid. If the iris and ciliary body inflammation is continuous to the trabecular area a certain amount of trabeculitis occurs, with swelling of the trabecular bands and endothelium, further blocking the trabecular spaces.

The more prolonged the intraocular disease the more severe is the scarring and organization of the trabeculas. Eventually large areas are seen in which the intertrabecular spaces are obliterated, and the trabecular bands are matted together by connective tissue. The canal of Schlemm may be much reduced in caliber, or obliterated (Fig. 641).

The pathology of the trabecular region in the condition known as glaucomato-cyclitic crisis is not known.

Phacolytic glaucoma is another type of open angle secondary glaucoma associated with a hypermature cataract (Flocks et al., 1955). The glaucoma in this condition is due to obstruction of the intertrabecular spaces by macrophages containing lens material (Figs. 595, 596, 597). In the early stages the inflammation often is so subtle that, except for a few keratic precipitates, the presence of inflammation is not suspected. Later, as the process becomes more severe, congestion, pain, a hazy cornea, and markedly elevated tension are present. The liquefied lens material diffuses through the capsule where it produces an unusually bland type of inflammation characterized by a large pale phagocytic type of cell which engulfs the lens material. These cells infiltrate the angle and trabecular spaces, iris stroma and crypts (Fig.

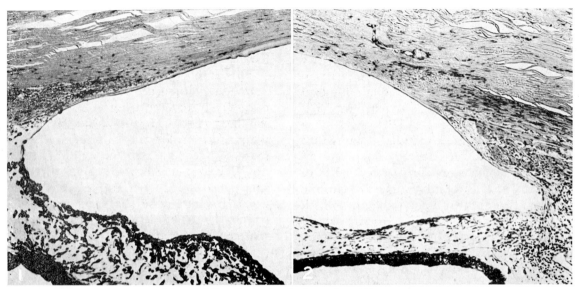

Figure 641. Open Angle Secondary Glaucoma

1. The degenerated, heavily pigmented trabecular meshwork is covered by an extension of endothelium and Descemet's membrane; Schlemm's canal is obliterated. ×75. AFIP Acc. 68554.

2. Advanced degeneration of trabecular meshwork; obliteration of intertrabecular spaces and of Schlemm's canal; extension of Descemet's membrane into chamber angle. Deeply recessed angle suggests glaucoma secondary to old contusion (see also Fig. 91). ×100. AFIP Acc. 193113.

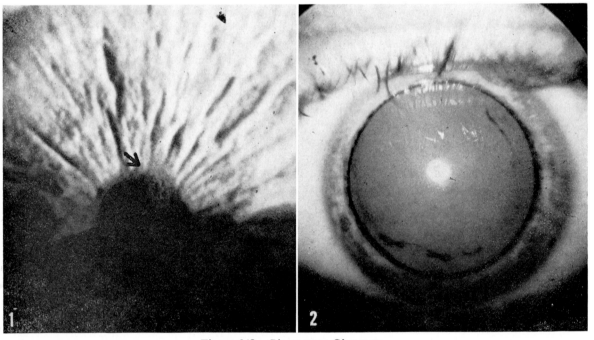

Figure 642. Pigmentary Glaucoma

1. Krukenberg spindle on inner surface of cornea (arrow).
2. Deposits of pigment on posterior surface of lens.

596). If the lens is removed the inflammatory reaction disappears and normal aqueous drainage is re-established.

Pseudoexfoliation of the lens capsule often is associated with open angle secondary glau-coma. This condition is associated with widespread lesions in the anterior segment and has been considered in Chapter II, page 117.

Pigmentary glaucoma is a rare but characteristic type of open angle secondary glaucoma of unknown etiology. It usually occurs in both eyes of young people who are myopic. It may be discovered at a time when the tension and the facility of outflow are normal. This state may persist for some time before glaucoma ensues. On examination there usually is a Krukenberg spindle (Fig. 642–1), depigmentation of the epithelium of the iris, circulating pigment granules in the aqueous humor and pigment deposition on the posterior lens (Fig. 642–2), iris surface, trabeculas, and lower retina. Gonioscopy shows heavy pigmentation of the trabecular meshwork (Fig. 643).

Although many patients show some pigmentation of the trabeculas without glaucoma, those with pigmentary glaucoma have an extreme degree of pigmentation.

Trauma is an important cause of open angle secondary glaucoma. The elevated pressure may arise from a number of different mechanisms. Severe contusions may produce a recurrent massive anterior chamber hemorrhage, of the so-called "eight ball" type. The clotted blood frequently obstructs the outflow channels by filling the angle (Figs. 89–1, 344–1). In less severe hemorrhage, red cells themselves may infiltrate the trabecular spaces and produce a temporary mechanical block. If the blood is slow to absorb it induces degenerative and sclerotic changes in the trabecular fibers which are irreversible. Organization of the clot by fibrous tissue may

induce changes which produce either pupillary or angle block (Fig. 90).

Open angle glaucoma secondary to trauma and inflammation also may occur when tissue proliferates over the angle, blocking ingress of aqueous to the trabecular spaces (see also p. 143 and Fig. 91). This occurs typically in epithelialization of the anterior chamber following perforating injuries and surgery (Fig. 102). The epithelium may form a sheet which spreads over the angle and onto the iris. Eventually sufficient trabecular area is blocked to produce a severe glaucoma. At times the epithelium forms a cyst, which gradually enlarges and obstructs the angle. Traumatic inflammation, and iridocyclitis, may cause formation of a hyaline membrane due to endothelial proliferation which eventually covers the trabecular area and results in open angle secondary glaucoma (Fig. 641). The majority of cases of traumatic glaucoma, however, are due to angle closure produced by synechias, organization of hemorrhage, or lens cortex (Fig. 89). Other cases are caused by the mechanical involvement of the iris in the traumatized area. This latter mechanism is characteristically seen in ruptured corneal ulcers with the subsequent development of an anterior staphyloma (Fig. 258).

The loosely adherent cells of diffuse *iris melanomas* may be shed into the anterior chamber, and deposited in the trabecular

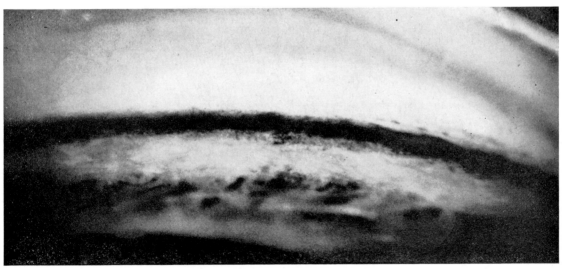

Figure 643. Pigmentary Glaucoma

Gonioscopic view of heavily pigmented anterior chamber angle. Most of the pigment is deposited in the trabecular meshwork. (Courtesy of Dr. R. N. Shaffer.)

spaces to result in an obstruction to outflow. Such tumors may be poorly pigmented. Often they produce early inflammation, which obscures the true disease process. Lymphomatous tumors and juvenile xanthogranuloma (Fig. 378) may behave in a similar manner.

Choroidal tumors may, somehow, affect the outflow of aqueous humor from the eye. Becker finds that 40 per cent of eyes with choroidal melanomas have relatively flat tonographic tracings, without glaucoma. This may be of significance in connection with development of glaucoma in those patients with small choroidal tumors and an open anterior chamber angle.

Increased venous pressure due to carotid-cavernous communication and lesions which obstruct the venous return from the eye (orbital tumors, orbital thrombophlebitis, etc.) may produce open angle secondary glaucoma.

THE TISSUE EFFECTS OF ELEVATED INTRAOCULAR PRESSURE

In longstanding glaucoma almost every tissue in the eye shows some alteration. Marked characteristic changes may be seen in the cornea, sclera, uveal tract, retina, optic nerve and in the angle of the anterior chamber.

From the point of view of visual impairment, the most important damage to the ocular structures from excessive pressure is at the *optic disk*. Clinically the disk gradually becomes excavated. Histologically the excavated disk is characterized at first by fusion and compression of its tissues, followed by backward bowing of the cribriform lamellas, and loss of substance due to atrophy of the nerve fibers and supporting cells (Figs. 564, 644). The ectasia of the cribriform plate often extends beyond the level of the sclera. Occasionally in some forms of secondary glaucoma, particularly those due to occlusion of the central retinal vein, fibrosis may occur. In the majority of the optic nerves in which there is marked cupping, the nerve shows a typical atrophy of the columnar gliosis type (Fig. 562). However, in a few cases in which the glaucoma probably is slowly progressive, an optic atrophy of the cavernous type develops (Fig. 564). In this type there are large cystoid spaces involving part of the nerve in which essentially no replacement gliosis occurs. The cavernous spaces are filled with a mucoid material that is sensitive to hyaluronidase (Zimmerman, 1958).

The mechanism of the damage to the visual fibers in glaucoma is not entirely clear. It probably is due to stretching, compression and increased angulation as the fibers cross the disk and enter the cribriform plate. The characteristic progressive field changes of

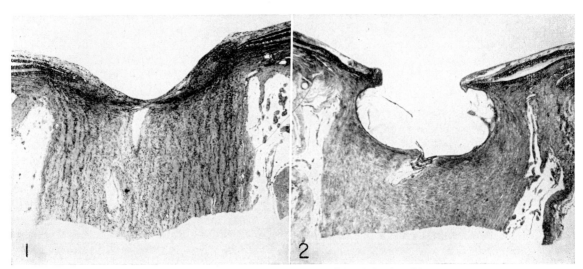

Figure 644. Glaucomatous Cupping of Optic Disk

1. Moderate. AFIP Acc. 80713.
2. Advanced. AFIP Acc. 28712.

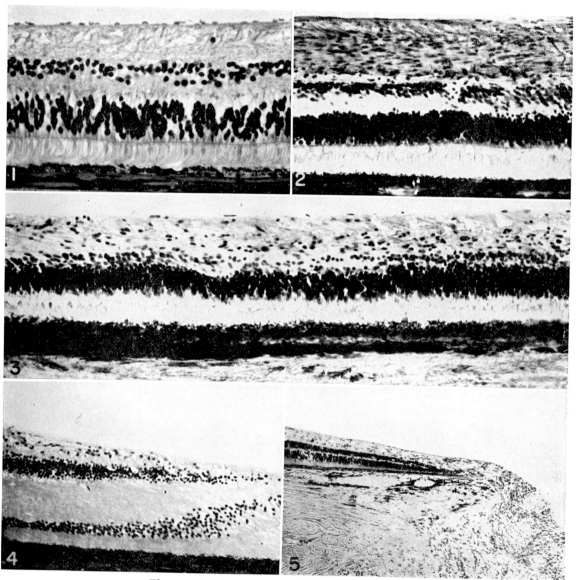

Figure 645. Glaucomatous Degeneration of Retina

1. Disappearance of retinal ganglion cells. Loss of nuclei from inner nuclear layer. ×230. AFIP Acc. 149729.
2. Loss of retinal ganglion cells. Gliosis of nerve fiber layer. ×175. AFIP Acc. 27028.
3. Disappearance of retinal ganglion cells. Almost complete loss of nuclei from inner nuclear layer. Atrophy of outer plexiform layer. Moderate gliosis of atrophic inner layers. Rods and cones and their nuclei less affected. ×175. AFIP Acc. 27028.
4. Loss of ganglion cells in macular region. ×115. AFIP Acc. 88968.
5. Atrophy of nerve fiber layer at disk margin. ×60. AFIP Acc. 193988.

glaucoma are so pathognomonic that these would seem to be based on some constant anatomic pattern at the optic disk. Because the anatomic arrangement of the nerve fibers in the disk is much more constant than the blood supply, the visual field defect seems to be due primarily to direct effect of the glaucoma on the nerve fibers. It is possible that some of the defect is due to compression in the pores of the cribriform lamellas. This type

of injury might explain the field defects. Some of the damage may result from a disturbance of the blood supply to the retinal ganglion cells, but it is difficult to determine how such a lesion might produce the typical field changes of glaucoma.

The most characteristic finding in the *retina* is degeneration of the nerve fiber and ganglion cell layer (Fig. 645). This may progress to the stage of complete absence of these

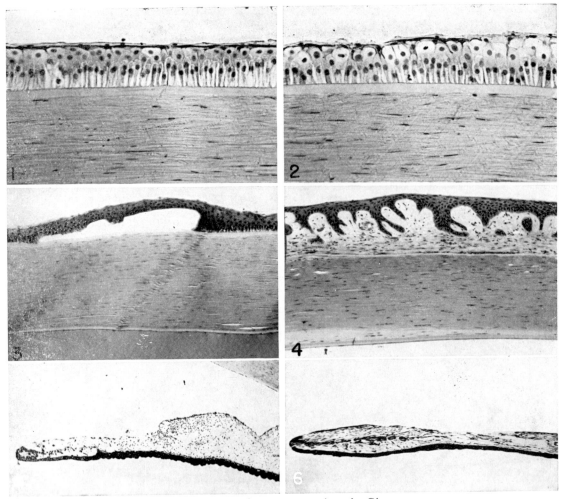

Figure 646. Secondary Degenerations in Glaucoma

1. Edema of corneal epithelium. Cells of basal layer separated by edematous fluid. ×180. AFIP Acc. 101143.
2. Intercellular and intracellular edema of corneal epithelium. ×180. AFIP Acc. 101143.
3. Bullous separation of the corneal epithelium following edema. ×75. AFIP Acc. 49729.
4. Pannus degenerativus. ×75. AFIP Acc. 161820.
5. Early atrophy of pupillary zone of iris following necrosis. ×40. AFIP Acc. 84215.
6. Fibrosis of iris following necrosis. ×41. AFIP Acc. 207027.

elements. There usually is some secondary gliosis as a result of this degeneration, but the outer neuronal layers of the retina usually remain unchanged.

The *uveal tract* may show general atrophy with some vascular sclerosis in longstanding open angle glaucoma. The iris stroma becomes atrophic and fibrotic and may show slight ectropion of the pupillary margin. Severe acute glaucoma may damage the nerve or blood supply to a segment of the iris stroma. This leads to ischemic necrosis with almost complete disappearance of the stroma and sphincter muscle (Fig. 622–2). The fixed and dilated oval pupil which follows acute

glaucomatous attacks is due to this necrosis and loss of stroma. The ciliary body, particularly the ciliary processes, in longstanding glaucoma becomes atrophic and fibrotic, similar to the changes occurring in the iris (Figs. 622–1; 646–5, 6). The processes become small and shrunken with some increased hyalinization. There also may be extensive atrophy and fibrosis of the ciliary muscle. These ciliary body changes tend to compensate for the reduced outflow in severe glaucoma by lessening the secretory ability of the ciliary body. Although difficult to evaluate, the choroid is less damaged by the intraocular pressure than are the other ocular tissues. Atrophy takes place principally in the peripapillary region, where there also may be associated hyperplasia of the overlying pigment epithelium. This leads to the peripapillary glaucomatous halo.

The *lens* does not appear to be damaged directly by the glaucomatous process, but in the advanced stages of glaucoma cataractous changes rarely are absent. Following cyclodialysis and filtering operations, cataractous changes are more common than in nonglaucomatous eyes, even though there has been no direct injury to the lens. It is possible that these lens changes are nutritive in character and are due to some alteration in the composition of the aqueous humor.

In the *cornea* epithelial edema in acute attacks of glaucoma has been mentioned (Fig. 646–1, 2, 3). In longstanding glaucoma this edema may become chronic, with the forma-tion of the epithelial bullae. Bulla-formation is particularly prone to occur over a degenerative pannus in which fibroblasts are laid down between an intact Bowman's membrane and the epithelium (Fig. 646–4). Atrophic changes have been demonstrated in the endothelium, and may cause the epithelial edema.

Under the influence of long-continued pressure, especially in young persons, *scleral staphylomas* often develop. These ectasias most commonly are seen in the equatorial region around the openings of the vortex veins (Figs. 94–3, 391). They are associated with long-continued pressure. *Intercalary* staphylomas occur at the limbus as a result of peripheral anterior synechias, long-continued glaucoma, and softening of the limbus by inflammation. *Ciliary* staphylomas occur in glaucoma due to cyclitis as a result of softening of the sclera by the inflammatory process.

HYPOTONY

Occasionally eyes are encountered which show no evidence of disease and in which the intraocular pressure as measured with the tonometer is as low as ten millimeters of mercury. In some instances the low tonometric readings are due to an extremely low ocular rigidity, and the actual intraocular pressure is higher than that obtained by tonometry. However, there remain cases with extremely low normal pressures without any evidence of ocular disease.

Aside from these instances of extreme normal variation, ocular hypotension may be secondary either to a marked increase in outflow of aqueous, or to an appreciable decrease in aqueous formation. The commonest causes of an increased outflow are a draining fistula, which may be postoperative, as for previous glaucoma, or due to an injury with delayed healing of a wound. Occasionally a massive retinal detachment or a posterior scleral rupture may produce an extremely low tension.

Injury to the ciliary body, either by trauma or by inflammatory disease, can lead to hypotony. The hypotension in such instances probably is due to reduced aqueous formation. In many such instances, as described in Chapter II, the hypotony is a pre-cursor of atrophy of the eyeball with disorganization.

Mild degrees of ocular hypotension cause little or no visual disturbance. However, if the hypotony is severe and of long standing, such as is seen following some fistulizing operations for glaucoma, permanent and marked visual loss may occur due to persistent macular and disk edema (Fig. 647).

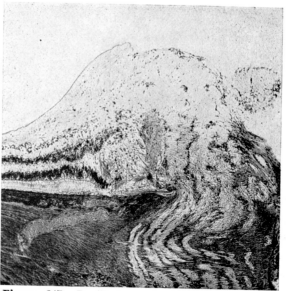

Figure 647. Papilledema due to hypotony. ×48 AFIP Acc. 283414.

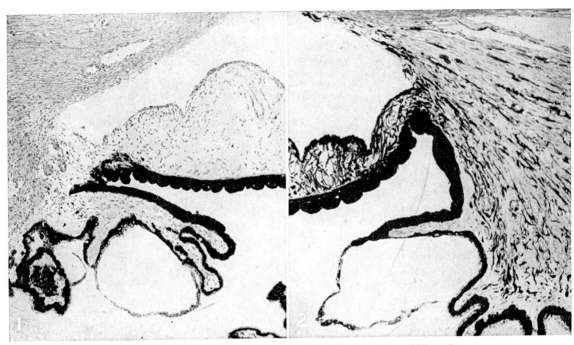

Figure 648.   Cystoid Separation of Pars Ciliaris Retinae Over Ciliary Processes

1. ×75. AFIP Acc. 152059.
2. ×105. AFIP Acc. 158930.

Hypotony associated with leaking wounds is characterized by accumulation of fluid under the choroid and ciliary body and often by detachment of the retina and choroid (Figs. 86–1, 93, 101–2, 345–2, 348–4). These usually are associated with a shallow anterior chamber. The fluid usually disappears and the chamber deepens after closure of the fistula. Folds in Descemet's membrane are also characteristically present, both clinically and histologically in hypotony. Another frequent finding in hypotony is cyst formation in the epithelium of the ciliary body over the ciliary processes (Fig. 648).

REFERENCES

Allen, L., Burian, H. M., and Braley, A. E.: A New Concept of the Development of the Anterior Chamber Angle. A.M.A. Arch. Ophthal. *53:*783–798, 1955.

Allen, L., Burian, H. M., and Braley, A. E.: The Anterior Border Ring of Schwalbe and the Pectinate Ligament. A.M.A. Arch. Ophthal. *53:*799–806, 1955.

Anderson J. R.: Hydrophthalmia or Congenital Glaucoma: Its Causes, Treatment and Outlook. Cambridge, University Press, 1939.

Ascher, K. W.: Aqueous Veins. Amer. J. Ophthal. *25:* 31–38, 1942.

Ashton, Norman: Anatomical study of Schlemm's canal and aqueous veins by means of neoprene casts. Part I. Aqueous veins. Brit. J. Ophthal. *35:*291–303, 1951. Part II. Aqueous veins (continued). Brit. J. Ophthal. *36:*265–267, 1952.

Ashton, N.: The Role of the Trabecular Structure in the Genesis of Simple Glaucoma Particularly with Regard to the Significance of Mucopolysaccharides. In Newell, F. W.: Trans. Fourth Conference on Glaucoma. New York, Josiah Macy, Jr. Foundation, 1959, p. 89.

Bárány, E. H.: Physiologic and Pharmacologic Factors Influencing the Resistance to Aqueous Outflow. In Newell, F. W.: Trans. First Conference on Glaucoma. New York, Josiah Macy, Jr. Foundation, 1955, pp. 123–221.

Barkan, O.: Operation for Congenital Glaucoma. Amer. J. Ophthal. *25:*552–563, 1942.

Becker, B.: In Newell, F. W.: Trans. Third Conference on Glaucoma. New York, Josiah Macy, Jr. Foundation, 1958, p. 100.

Becker, B.: In Newell, F. W.: Trans. Fourth Conference on Glaucoma. New York, Josiah Macy, Jr Foundation, 1959, p. 223.

Burian, H. M., Braley, A. E., and Allen, L.: Visibility of the Ring of Schwalbe and the Trabecular Zone. A.M.A. Arch. Ophthal. *53:*767–782, 1955.

Curran, E. J.: A New Operation for Glaucoma Involving a New Principle in the Etiology and Treatment of Chronic Primary Glaucoma. A.M.A. Arch. Ophthal. *49:*131–155, 1920.

Flocks, M., Littwin, C. S., and Zimmerman, L. E.: Phacolytic Glaucoma; a Clinicopathologic Study of 138 Cases of Glaucoma Associated with Hypermature Cataract. A.M.A. Arch. Ophthal. *54:*37–45, 1955.

Garron, L. K.: The Fine Structure of the Normal Trabecular Apparatus in Man. In Newell, F. W.: Trans. Fourth Conference on Glaucoma. New York, Josiah Macy, Jr. Foundation, 1959, pp. 11–57.

Garron, L. K., and Feeney, M. L.: Electron Microscopic Studies of the Human Eye. II. Study of the Trabeculas by Light and Electron Microscopy. A.M.A. Arch. Ophthal. 62:966–973, 1959.

Garron, L. K., Feeney, M. L., Hogan, M. H., and McEwen, W. K.: Electron Microscopic Studies of the Human Eye. I. Preliminary Investigations of the Trabeculas. Amer. J. Ophthal. 46:27–35, 1958.

Garron, L. K., Hogan, M. J., McEwen, W. K., Feeney, M. L., and Esperson, J.: Electron Microscopy of Ocular Tissue. A.M.A. Arch. Ophthal. 61:647–653, 1959.

Goldmann, H.: Abfluss des Kammerwassers beim Menschen. Ophthalmologica 111:146–152, Feb.-Mar. 1946.

Goldmann, H.: Weitere Mitteilung über den Abfluss des Kammerwassers beim Menschen. Ophthalmologica 112:344–49, Dec. 1946.

Grant, W. M.: Further Studies on the Facility of Flow through the Trabecular Meshwork. A.M.A. Arch. Ophthal. 60:523–533, 1958.

Holland, M. G., von Sallman, L., and Collins, E. M.: A Study of the Innervation of the Chamber Angle. Part I. Amer. J. Ophthal. 42:148–161, 1956.

Holland, M. G., von Sallman, L., and Collins, E. M.: A Study of the Innervation of the Chamber Angle. Part II. Amer. J. Ophthal. 44:206–221, 1957.

Holmberg, A.: Ultrastructure of the Normal Trabecular Apparatus in Man. In Newell, F. W.: Trans. Fourth Conference on Glaucoma. New York, Josiah Macy, Jr. Foundation, 1959. pp. 59–87.

Karg, S. J., Garron, L. K., Feeney, M. L., and McEwen, W. K.: Perfusion of Human Eyes with Latex Microspheres. A.M.A. Arch Ophthal. 61:68–71, 1959.

Kornsweig, A. L., Feldstein, M. D., and Schneider, J.: Pathology of the Angle of the Anterior Chamber in Primary Glaucoma. Amer. J. Ophthal. 46:311–327, 1958.

Maumenee, A. E.: Classification of Glaucoma. In Clark, W. B.: Symposium on Glaucoma. St. Louis, C. V. Mosby Co., 1959, pp. 98–107.

Maumenee, A. E.: The Pathogenesis of Congenital Glaucoma: A New Theory. Trans. Amer. Ophthal. Soc. 56:507–570, 1958.

Maumenee, A. E.: Surgery for Congenital Glaucoma.

In Clark, W. B.: Symposium on Glaucoma. St. Louis, C. V. Mosby Co., 1959, pp. 209–226.

Scheie, H. G.: Symposium: Congenital Glaucoma-Diagnosis, Clinical Course, and Treatment Other Than Goniotomy. Trans. Amer. Acad. Ophthal. Otolaryng. 59:309–321, 1955.

Shaffer, R. N.: The Role of Vitreous Detachment in Aphakic and Malignant Glaucoma. Trans. Amer. Acad. Ophthal. and Otolaryng. 58:217–231, Suppl. 1954.

Shaffer, R. N.: Pathogenesis of Congenital Glaucoma: Gonioscopic and Microscopic Anatomy. Trans. Amer. Acad. Ophthal. and Otolaryng. 59:297–308, 1955.

Shaffer, R. N.: Symposium: Primary Glaucomas: III. Gonioscopy, Ophthalmoscopy and Perimetry. Trans. Amer. Acad. Ophthal. and Otolaryng. 64:112–127, 1960.

Teng, C. C., Katzin, H. M., and Chi, H. H.: Primary Degeneration in the Vicinity of the Chamber Angle. As an Etiologic Factor in Wide-angle Glaucoma. Part II. Amer. J. Ophthal. 43:193–203, 1957.

Teng, C. C., Paton, R. T., and Katzin, H. M.: Primary Degeneration in the Vicinity of the Chamber Angle. As an Etiologic Factor in Wide-angle Glaucoma. Amer. J. Ophthal. 40:619–631, 1955.

Theobald, G. D.: Further Studies on the Canal of Schlemm: Its Anastomoses and Anatomic Relations. Amer. J. Ophthal. 39:65–89, 1955.

Theobald, G. D.: Histology of Tissues Surrounding the Angle of the Anterior Chamber. In Clark, W. B.: Symposium on Glaucoma. St. Louis, C. V. Mosby Co., 1959, pp. 21–25.

Theobald, G. D., and Kirk, H. Q.: Aqueous Pathways in Some Cases of Glaucoma. Amer. J. Ophthal. 41:11–21, 1956.

Tornquist, R.: Chamber Depth in Primary Acute Glaucoma. Brit. J. Ophthal. 40:421–429, 1956.

Wolter, J. R.: The Trabecular Endothelium: Its Degeneration in Closure of the Chamber Angle. A.M.A. Arch. Ophthal. 61:928–938, 1959.

Zimmerman, L. E.: Demonstration of Hyaluronidase-Sensitive Acid Mucopolysaccharide. In Trabecula and Iris in Routine Paraffin Sections of Adult Human Eyes. Amer. J. Ophthal. 44:1–4, 1957.

Zimmerman, L. E.: Application of Histochemical Methods for the Demonstration of Acid Mucopolysaccharides to Ophthalmic Pathology. Trans. Amer. Acad. Ophthal. and Otolaryng. 62:697–701, 1958.

Chapter XIII

The Orbit

ANATOMIC CONSIDERATIONS

The orbit is the cavity, or socket, containing the eye and its adjacent structures. It is a four-sided pyramidal space whose apex is directed backward and medially and whose base is directed forward and laterally. The bones of the face, nose and cranium participate in the formation of the walls of the pyramid. These bones are covered by periosteum (the periorbita) which is continuous with the dura. The periorbita is adherent to the bones along the sutures, at the various fissures and foramina, and at the trochlear fossa where it binds down the cartilaginous trochlea of the superior oblique muscle. Elsewhere, the periorbita is loosely attached to the orbital bones and it may be elevated by pathologic processes. The periorbita becomes continuous with the periosteum of the facial bones at the orbital margin where it is densely adherent and forms a ridge to which the orbital septum is attached. The orbital margin and the orbital septum form the base of the orbital pyramid. The orbital septum is a thin membrane of fibrous and elastic connective tissue which has numerous attachments to the orbicularis oculi and levator palpebrae superioris muscles and to the tarsal plates. The aperture left in the center of the base of the orbital pyramid is occupied by the anterior aspect of the globe and its fascia (Tenon's capsule). Thus,

except for the various foramina, fissures and apertures which transmit blood vessels and nerves, the orbital cavity is a closed space. Traditionally, the eye itself is excluded in discussions of diseases of the orbit. Therefore, except for those which secondarily involve the orbit, diseases of the eye will not be discussed in this chapter.

There remains a wide variety of soft tissue structures in the orbit: large amounts of adipose tissue, elastic and fibrous connective tissue septums, blood vessels, nerves, sympathetic ganglia, skeletal muscles, smooth muscle, and cartilage. The lacrimal gland is the only epithelial structure normally present in the orbit.

The trochlea of the superior oblique muscle is the only cartilaginous structure normally present in the orbit. It is frequently stated that the orbit contains no lymph vessels. However, this question has not been settled to everyone's satisfaction. The occurrence of lymphangiomas in the orbit and the observation of perivascular and perineural infiltration of certain tumors suggest the presence of lymphatic channels. The optic nerve and its meninges may be considered to be orbital structures, but diseases of these structures are discussed in Chapter IX.

DISEASES OF THE ORBIT

The orbital tissues may be involved in congenital, inflammatory, traumatic, vascular, metabolic or neoplastic diseases. Diseases of the orbit may be grouped into four broad categories: primary, secondary, metastatic, and systemic.

Primary disease. Neoplasms, hamartomas, and certain inflammatory "pseudotumors" constitute the most important and the most frequent primary orbital lesions.

Secondary disease. The orbit may be involved by the direct extension of pathologic processes arising in adjacent structures (e.g., meningiomas from the cranial cavity, melanomas and retinoblastomas from the eye, carcinomas from the eyelids or conjunctiva, inflammatory or neoplastic lesions from the paranasal sinuses and the nasolacrimal apparatus). Moreover, since the orbit is traversed by blood vessels connecting with the face, the pterygoid plexus of veins and the cavernous sinus, inflammatory diseases of these structures may secondarily involve the orbit. In many instances, the orbit appears to be the primary site of a disease, and the secondary nature is appreciated only after careful study.

Metastatic disease. Lesions metastatic to the orbit from distant sites, whether neoplastic or not, are relatively rare. Usually, the primary disease is apparent, or soon becomes apparent, when the orbital lesion develops. However, some cases require exhaustive search before the primary disease is demonstrated. Metastatic neoplasms may be so undifferentiated that the histologic features provide no clue as to their origin.

Systemic disease. Orbital involvement is characteristic of certain systemic diseases. Hyperthyroidism and Hand-Schüller-Christian disease are examples. In many other diseases, such as leukemia, orbital involvement is observed only occasionally.

GENERAL CLINICAL MANIFESTATIONS OF ORBITAL DISEASE

Exophthalmos. Since all but the anterior aspect of the orbit is delimited by bone, exophthalmos, or proptosis, is the outstanding manifestation of orbital disease. The degree of exophthalmos may vary greatly from case to case. Sometimes careful measurements are required to demonstrate it. At the other extreme, the eye occasionally is prolapsed in front of the lids. The proptosis may develop insidiously or with alarming rapidity. It is usually unilateral, but may be bilateral, as in most cases of "endocrine exophthalmos."

The direction of proptosis may be of diagnostic importance, since the proptosis is usually in a direction opposite the location of the lesion. Thus, lesions of the optic nerve and orbital meninges usually cause a straight forward proptosis. Lesions of the lacrimal gland push the eye downward and nasally. Embryonal rhabdomyosarcomas, because they usually arise in the upper inner quadrant of the orbit, displace the eye downward and temporally. Finally, lesions of the paranasal sinuses, which secondarily involve the orbit, generally produce proptosis in an upward or temporal direction.

Enophthalmos. Atrophy, scarring or surgical removal of orbital tissues may result in backward displacement of the globe. Defects in the bony walls due to injury ("blow-out" fracture of the orbital floor) or congenital malformation may also result in enophthalmos. It also is seen after subsidence of inflammation in inflammatory pseudotumors.

Palpable mass. The character of a mass will depend, in part, on its size, consistency and location. Sometimes an orbital mass appears beneath the bulbar or palpebral conjunctiva and is erroneously interpreted as arising from the conjunctiva or eyelid.

Limitation of motion. The motions of the eye may be limited by mechanical interference, by direct extraocular muscle involvement, or by interference with the nerve supply of the muscles. Mechanical interference may result from orbital edema or a space-occupying lesion. Scar tissue may bind the extraocular muscles to adjacent structures, thus impeding the eye movements. The muscles may be weakened or destroyed by degenerative, inflammatory, neoplastic or other disease. Limitation of motion due to loss of nerve supply in orbital diseases must be differentiated from innervational defects due to primary diseases of the eye or cranial cavity.

Edema of the eyelids and conjunctiva. Edema tends to develop in inflammatory and neoplastic diseases. Acute inflammation causes swelling more commonly than chronic inflammation. Rapidly expanding neoplasms produce edema more readily than slowly growing lesions. Venous obstruction also produces edema.

Visual disturbance. Orbital disease, by limiting ocular motility, may be responsible for diplopia. In addition, orbital lesions, by exerting pressure, may change the shape of the globe or interfere with the circulation in the eye or optic nerve. Another cause for visual loss is exposure keratitis, a most dreaded complication of exophthalmos. With exophthalmos the exposed cornea may become dried, infected, scarred, and opacified. Ultimately, it may rupture spontaneously. Keratitis may also develop when corneal sensation is lost due to destruction of its sensory modalities.

Ophthalmoscopic changes. Many of the ophthalmoscopic changes are produced by pressure on the globe or optic nerve. Pressure on the optic nerve may lead either to hyperemia or pallor of the optic disk or to papilledema. By interfering with circulation, the pressure may be responsible for retinal edema or hemorrhage. Pressure on the globe may cause retinal folding (striae) or detachment. The tough scleral tunic seems to provide a barrier to the spread of orbital neoplasms into the eye. Therefore, orbital neoplasms seldom invade the globe. Much more frequently, primary intraocular malignancies (i.e., melanoma and retinoblastoma) spread to the orbit, usually through the emissary canals.

These clinical manifestations are found in varying combinations and degrees in most orbital lesions. Hence, with the exception of some of the systemic diseases which involve the orbit, an etiologic diagnosis based on clinical manifestations alone usually is impossible. A diagnosis based on laboratory examination of representative material is, therefore, of great importance in orbital disease. On the other hand, knowledge of the pertinent clinical manifestations may be of great value to the ophthalmic pathologist.

DEVELOPMENTAL ABNORMALITIES

Bony orbit. Developmental abnormalities of the bony orbit usually are associated with deformities of the skull such as microcephaly, tower skull or hypertelorism. The size and shape of the orbit at birth do not depend on the condition of the eye. Even when the eye is absent (anophthalmos) the orbit is well formed and only slightly smaller than normal. Failure of the ectodermal portions of the eye to develop does not prevent the development of adjacent mesodermal structures. Total absence of the orbit apparently has not been reported (Mann). The congenital anomalies of the skull which affect the eye and orbit have been summarized by Blodi.

Microphthalmos with cyst. With incomplete closure of the fetal cleft, neuroectodermal tissue may herniate or proliferate into the orbit (see Chapter II). This condition is invariably associated with microphthalmos (Figs. 61–2, 62). The eye may be fairly well developed or it may be vestigial. Since the cyst extends into orbit, it may be mistaken for a primary orbital tumor. Occasionally, the cyst loses its attachment to the globe. Sclera usually forms the outer wall. The cyst contains neuroectodermal elements which rarely are well differentiated but usually are dysplastic. Proliferated glial and fibrous connective tissues are common components. Occasionally these lesions are more solid than cystic and, even after biopsy, an erroneous diagnosis of neurinoma or sarcoma is made (Fig. 649). This anomaly frequently is designated simply as "orbital cyst." "Microphthalmos with cyst" is a more precise term.

Cephaloceles. Depending on the composition, a herniation of cranial contents into the orbit is classified as meningocele, encephalocele (Fig. 650) or hydroencephalocele. The cranial contents may herniate through one of the natural foramina or fissures or

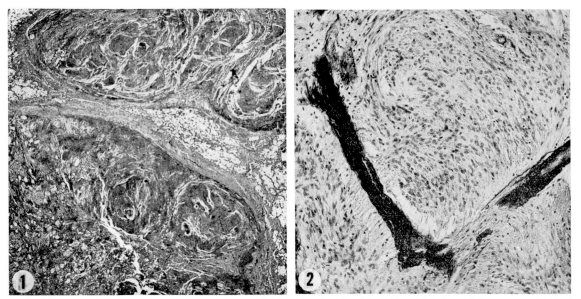

Figure 649. Pseudogliomatous Proliferation in Orbit Associated with Bilateral Microphthalmos and Ocular Colobomas

1. Encapsulated tumor lobules in orbital fat. ×8. AFIP Acc. 963785.
2. Benign proliferation of glial tissue accounts for most of the tumor. Van Gieson. ×115.

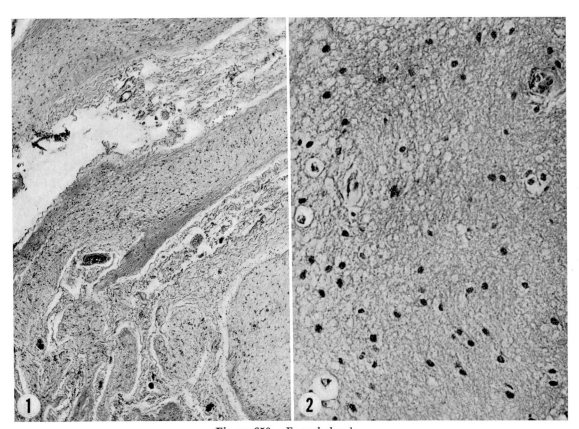

Figure 650. Encephalocele

1 and 2. A large, firm, encapsulated tumor within the muscle cone, surrounding the optic nerve, and extending from the apex of the orbit to the globe, had produced proptosis since birth. Optic nerve was considered normal. Tissue resembles cerebral white matter. AFIP Acc. 220081. ×50 and ×350, respectively. (Courtesy Dr. A. B. Reese.)

through a developmental defect in the bony orbit. Anterior cephaloceles usually appear at the inner angle of the orbit or at the root of the nose. From these locations the cystic structure may displace the globe temporally or it may elevate the skin in the region of the inner canthus. These structures are fluctuant and they may be partly reducible. Most of them are attached to the cranial contents by a small pedicle. The less common posterior cephalocele may produce a gradual downward displacement of the globe.

Ectopic tissue. Ectopic cartilage and bone may be seen in the orbit in the absence of other misplaced tissues. Choristomas (dermoid cysts, teratomas) and hamartomas (angiomas) are conveniently considered with the neoplastic diseases.

ORBITAL INFLAMMATION

As was pointed out in Chapter I, the terms inflammation and infection are not synonymous. Infectious diseases, whether due to bacteria, viruses or fungi, are seldom primary in the orbit. Usually, they reach the orbit by extension from adjacent structures or by hematogenous spread from remote lesions. The etiology and pathogenesis of most noninfectious orbital inflammatory diseases remain uncertain. It is convenient to discuss orbital inflammation under the following headings:

    I. Acute
        A. nonsuppurative
        B. suppurative
    II. Chronic
        A. nongranulomatous
        B. granulomatous

I. *Acute inflammation.* The paranasal sinuses, particularly, are likely to be a source of acute orbital inflammation. Less frequent sources of infection are the globe, teeth, middle ear, face and cranial cavity. Such systemic diseases as subacute bacterial endocarditis, influenza and scarlet fever also have been associated with acute orbital inflammation. Sometimes foreign bodies carried into the orbit at the time of an injury produce acute inflammation.

A. NON-SUPPURATIVE. Orbital cellulitis is characterized clinically by pain, fever, leukocytosis, lid edema, chemosis, proptosis and limitation of ocular movement. The orbital tissues are edematous and infiltrated by polymorphonuclear leukocytes. The cellulitis may subside spontaneously or with the aid of antibiotics. Sometimes surgical decompression is necessary to prevent ocular complications. Finally, the cellulitis may become either a suppurative or a chronic inflammatory process.

B. SUPPURATIVE. This type of inflammation is characterized by necrosis of orbital tissues and formation of pus. The necrotizing process may not be confined to the orbit. Destruction of the orbital septum with forward extension into the conjunctiva and lids occurs early. Posterior extension may produce cavernous sinus inflammation and thrombosis, meningitis, or even suppurative intracranial disease. Frequently, the necrotizing process is walled-off by local tissue responses with or without the aid of antibiotics. Such an abscess may subside spontaneously. More commonly, however, spontaneous rupture occurs or surgical drainage is carried out. Healing may be accompanied by excessive scarring, restriction of eye movements and enophthalmos.

A specific example of acute orbital infection that has been recognized with increasing frequency during recent years is mucormycosis. This is an acute, frequently fulminating fungus disease which often is characterized clinically by involvement of the orbit. Several species of ubiquitous saprophytic "bread molds" (the Mucoraceae) have been implicated. These cannot be differentiated further histopathologically, and in most of the reported cases the fungus has not been identified by mycologic methods. The fungi are easily recognized in tissue sections because of the large caliber and nonseptate character of their hyphae (Fig. 651) and because the organism (unlike many other fungi) is usually stained intensely by hematoxylin. Although generally non-pathogenic, the Mucoraceae may produce a rapidly progressive acute nec-

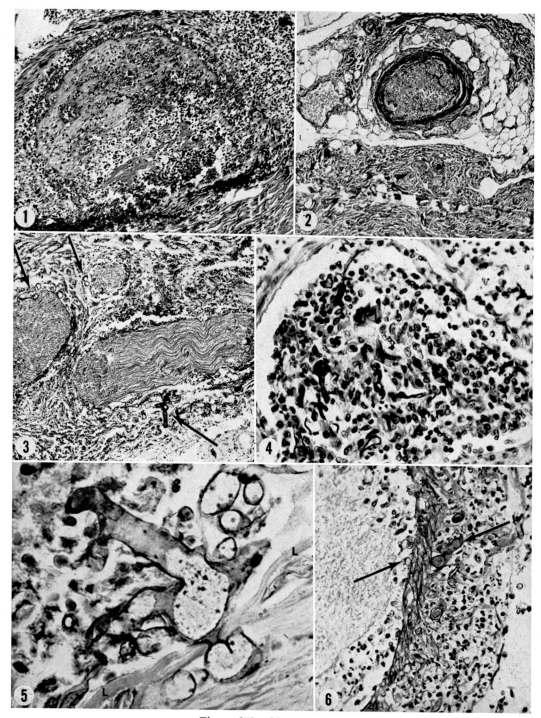

Figure 651. Mucormycosis

1. Orbital cellulitis with septic thrombosis of arteriole. ×125. AFIP Acc. 854692.
2. Thrombosed ciliary vessel in orbital fat adjacent to optic nerve. ×60. AFIP Acc. 794560.
3. Orbital cellulitis with invasion of ciliary nerves by fungi (arrows). ×145. AFIP Acc. 794560.
4. Septic thrombosis of cerebral arteriole; purulent exudate containing many mycelial structures fills lumen of vessel. ×365. AFIP Acc. 854692.
5. The Mucoraceae are characterized by their large size, lack of cross-walls (septums), their affinity for hematoxylin and their tendency to invade arteries along the internal elastic lamina (L-L). ×820. AFIP Acc. 694863.
6. Purulent meningitis; extensive invasion of vessel wall by fungi. ×305. AFIP Acc. 694863.

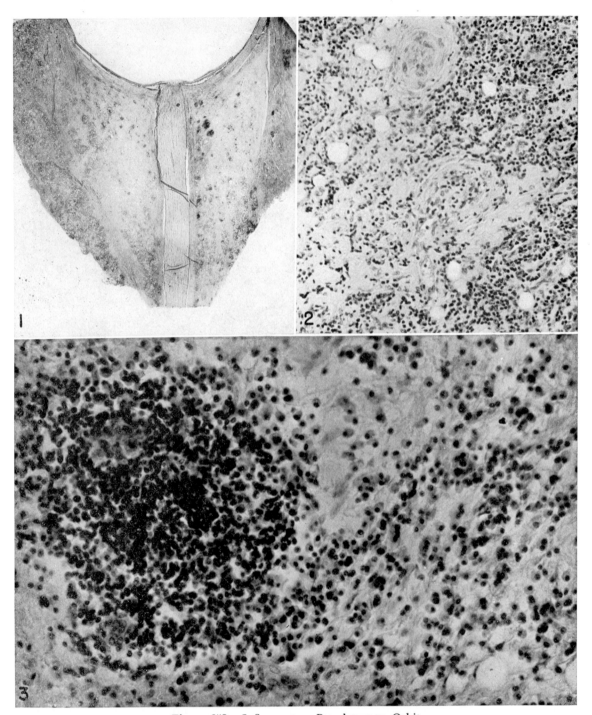

Figure 652. Inflammatory Pseudotumor, Orbit

1. Perivascular lymphocytic infiltration in large fibrous orbital mass surrounding optic nerve. ×3. AFIP Acc. 493954.

2. Lymphocytic infiltration around, and endothelial proliferation in, blood vessels. ×165. AFIP Acc. 185517.

3. Perivascular lymphocytic infiltration and diffuse plasma cell infiltration, orbit. ×330. AFIP Acc. 22054.

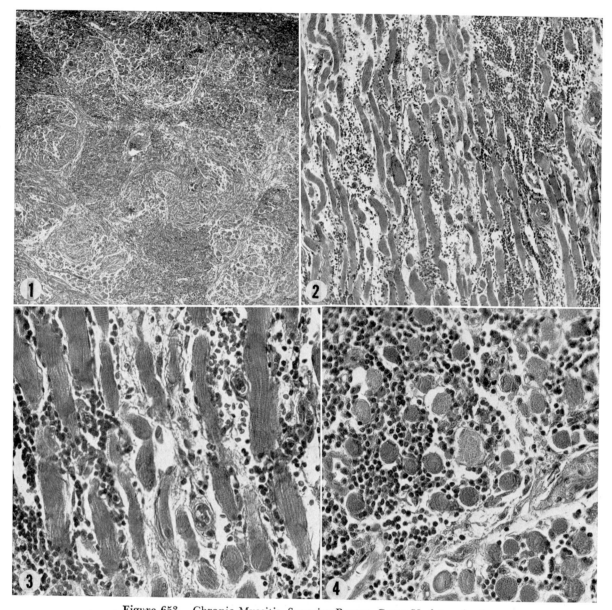

Figure 653. Chronic Myositis, Superior Rectus, Cause Undetermined

The muscle bundles are atrophic and widely separated by an infiltrate of chronic inflammatory cells, chiefly lymphocytes. AFIP Acc. 859063.　　1. ×50.　　2. ×115.　　3. ×305.　　4. ×305.

rotizing inflammatory process in certain highly susceptible individuals. Patients in acidosis (diabetic, renal, diarrheal, etc.) and those being treated for leukemia or lymphoma seem to be the most susceptible. The orbit usually is involved as a result of spread from the nose or paranasal sinuses often with vascular invasion. Characteristically the affected vessels are acutely inflamed and the organisms are observed in all layers. Frequently, however, the fungi appear to spread

along the internal elastic lamina. Thrombosis is a very common complication (Fig. 651). The initial ocular manifestations may be a consequence of cavernous sinus thrombosis or occlusion of the ophthalmic artery or one of its branches. Optic neuritis (Fig. 519–1), infarction of the retina, and panophthalmitis commonly accompany the orbital cellulitis.

II. *Chronic inflammation.* Most of the chronic inflammatory lesions of the orbit are of unknown etiology (Figs. 652, 653). Some

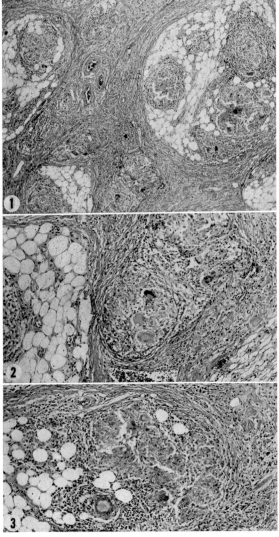

Figure 654. Granuloma of Orbit

1 to 3. The presence of many tubercles composed of epithelioid cells and giant cells without necrosis and with a paucity of other inflammatory cells is highly suggestive of sarcoidosis. ×50, ×115, and ×115, respectively. AFIP Acc. 799705.

writers lump these lesions under the term "orbital granuloma." Use of this term to cover both granulomatous and nongranulomatous lesions is confusing and unfortunate. Since the extraocular muscles may be involved, the term "orbital myositis" also has been used (Fig. 653). Clinically, these chronic inflammatory processes often are mistaken for neoplasms, hence the terms, orbital pseudotumor and inflammatory pseudotumor.

A. NONGRANULOMATOUS. Most chronic inflammatory diseases of the orbit are non-granulomatous. The etiology is obscure in the majority of cases. The clinical manifestations and course vary extremely. The lesions usually develop insidiously and may persist for months or years. Sometimes, though, they develop rapidly. They may be unilateral or bilateral, and often appear in one orbit months or years before involving the fellow orbit. The inflammatory process may be diffuse or localized. In the latter case, tumefaction may lead to confusion with neoplasia (inflammatory pseudotumor) (Fig. 652). These chronic nongranulomatous masses often contain many round cells (lymphocytes, plasma cells, large mononuclears). Because of this, they may also be misinterpreted histologically as lymphomas or plasmacytomas. Since they are of such importance in differential diagnosis, the histologic features of inflammatory pseudotumors will be discussed with neoplasms (p. 763).

B. GRANULOMATOUS. The orbit is rarely involved by truly granulomatous inflammatory processes.

Tuberculosis of the orbit is rare. The infection may reach the orbit by metastasis from a distant site or by extension from adjacent structures. *Sarcoidosis* of the orbit is also rare (Fig. 654). Winter found only 11 reported cases. Stein and Henderson encountered only two examples over a 15 year interval at the Mayo Clinic. *Syphilis* of the orbit, particularly since the advent of antibiotics, is exceedingly rare (Fig. 655). When it does involve the orbit, periosteitis often is the salient feature.

Mycoses. Certain fungi, especially species of Aspergillus, produce granulomatous lesions in the orbit (Fig. 656). Typically these appear to be foreign body reactions in which multinucleated giant cells are conspicuous. With routine stains the fungi may be impossible to detect even though they are found to be numerous with special staining methods. Microscopically, the hyphae are much narrower than those of Mucor. Several examples of orbital actinomycosis have been reported (Viers and Davis). Various saprophytic fungi may be introduced into the orbit with penetrating injuries.

Parasites infesting the orbit produce inflammation which may be granulomatous. Cysticercosis, echinococcosis, onchocerciasis,

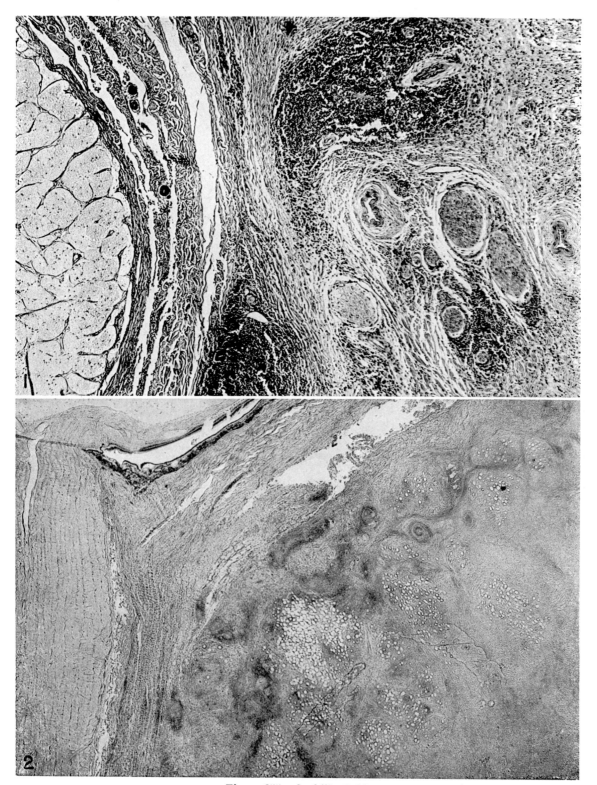

Figure 655. Syphilis, Orbit

1. Perivascular lymphocytic infiltration and fibrosis, orbit, adjacent to optic nerve. ×60. AFIP Acc. 35691.
2. Gumma of orbit around optic nerve. ×15. AFIP Acc. 22532.

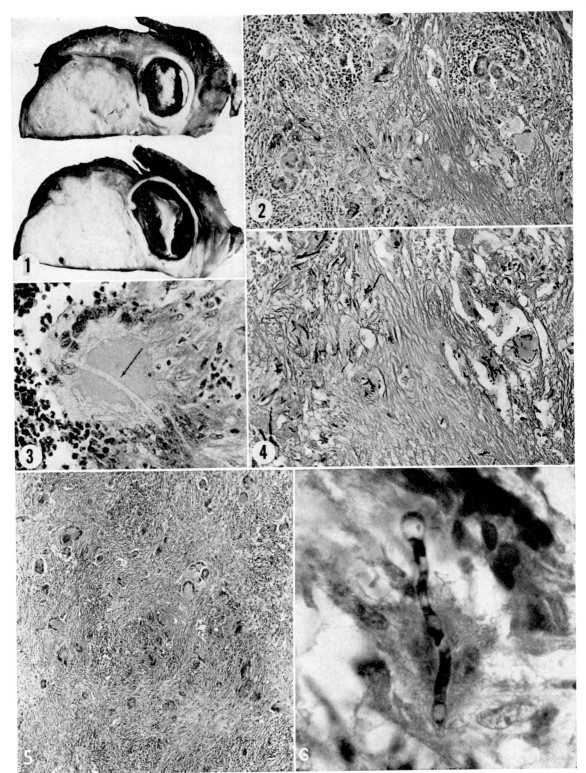

Figure 656.   Mycotic Granulomas of Orbit

1. Dense tumor-like mass behind globe. AFIP Acc. 792989. Photomicrographs from this lesion are shown in 2, 3 and 4.

2. The tissue reaction is of a foreign body type with many multinucleated giant cells and much fibrosis. ×100

3. The causative fungi (arrow) of lesions of this type (probably Aspergillus species) are rarely found in hema toxylin-eosin-stained sections. ×305.

4. With special stains for fungi, myriad hyphae are found. Gomori's methenamine silver stain of area adjacent to that shown in 2. ×145.

5. Similar reaction in another case. ×75. AFIP Acc. 79394.

6. Hypha in giant cell in still another case. ×1360. AFIP Acc. 77204.

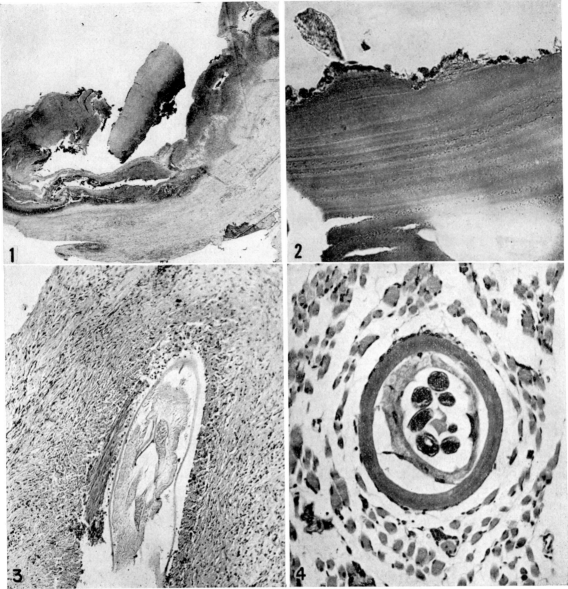

Figure 657. Parasitic Infections of Orbit

1. Echinococcosis. Acute necrotizing and granulomatous inflammation about wall of cyst. ×7. AFIP Acc. 949196.
2. Laminated hyaline wall of cyst; same case. ×350.
3. Tangential section of adult nematode in eosinophilic abscess surrounded by granulomatous mass. ×125. AFIP Acc. 100082.
4. Encysted trichina in orbital muscle. ×175. AFIP Neg. 47486

and trichiniasis are examples. Cysticercosis is produced when the embryo of *Taenia solium* (pork tapeworm) becomes encysted. While intraocular lesions are common, cysticercosis rarely affects the orbit. As long as the larva is alive there is little more than slight lymphocytic infiltration. After the cysticercus dies, the cyst becomes surrounded by an intense granulomatous reaction which contains many eosinophils. Ultimately, the cystic area is re-placed by fibrous tissue or undergoes calcification. Echinococcosis is widespread throughout the world, but it is rare in the United States. There are only three examples of orbital echinococcosis (hydatid disease) in the Registry of Ophthalmic Pathology (Fig. 657–1, 2). Onchocerciasis, while a most important cause of blindness in certain areas of the world, seldom involves the orbit.

Trichiniasis (trichinosis) often affects the

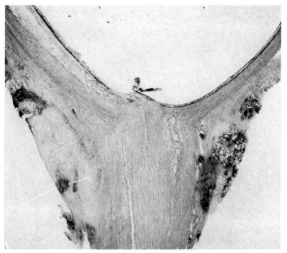

Figure 658. Orbital Involvement in Wegener's Granulomatosis

There is extensive necrosis and nonspecific acute and chronic granulomatous inflammation in the orbital fat. Ischemic necrosis of the optic nerve, retina, and choroid are secondary. (Case reported by Cutler and Blatt, 1956.) ×7.5. AFIP Acc. 684869.

extraocular muscles. It is estimated that each year in the United States 350,000 people are infected with *Trichinella spiralis;* 16,000 develop symptoms; and 800 die of their infection (Greenstein and Steinberg). Clinically, there is pain and tenderness on movement of the eye, ophthalmoplegia, and edema of the lids and conjunctiva. The larvae are encysted in the extraocular muscles (Fig. 657–4). The degenerating muscle may be surrounded and infiltrated by variable numbers of lymphocytes, eosinophils and polymorphonuclear leukocytes. After a few weeks, the larvae become calcified.

Wegener's granulomatosis is a rapidly fatal disease of obscure etiology. According to Straatsma, this disorder has three characteristic pathologic features: necrotizing granulomatous lesions in the respiratory tract, widespread focal arteritis, and necrotizing thrombotic glomerulitis. The orbit is involved by direct extension from diseased upper respiratory passages. Histologically, tissues from the upper respiratory passages and orbit reveal extensive ulceration, necrosis and edema (Fig. 658). Some areas of necrosis are surrounded by epithelioid and giant cells. Focal vasculitis frequently is a prominent feature.

Midline lethal granuloma is another granulomatous inflammatory disease or group of diseases of unknown etiology involving the upper respiratory passages. It is characterized by progressive destruction of the nose and facial area and it may involve the orbit. Forty-two per cent of the 100 cases reviewed by Cutler and Blatt had orbital or ocular involvement. Straatsma indicated that some patients also have vascular, renal and pulmonary lesions at autopsy. This raises the question of the possible relationship between midline lethal granuloma and Wegener's granulomatosis. At the present time, most writers distinguish between the two conditions; others use the terms interchangeably. Until more is known about both conditions, these questions will remain in dispute.

INJURIES

Penetrating wounds are important, not only because of their direct damage to specific orbital structures, but also because of their complications. Hemorrhage usually is stopped by compression of the hematoma between the orbital wall and globe. Absorption of the hematoma may be slow and a "blood cyst" may develop. Alternatively, a foreign body reaction may develop around hemosiderin deposits, cholesterol crystals, and other components of disintegrating erythrocytes. Ultimately, scarring may lead to decreased ocular motility. If pyogenic organisms are introduced into the wound, a suppurative inflammatory process may supervene. Foreign bodies, including cilia and fungi, may be carried into the wound and produce a granulomatous reaction (Fig. 659). However, some relatively inert foreign bodies may remain in the orbit for a long time without producing significant inflammation.

Fractures of the orbit and surrounding regions of the skull are common. Frequently, more serious intracranial damage overshadows the local injuries to the orbit. Bone fragments may damage such important orbital structures as the eye, optic nerve, muscles, or lacrimal apparatus. Fractures also may be re-

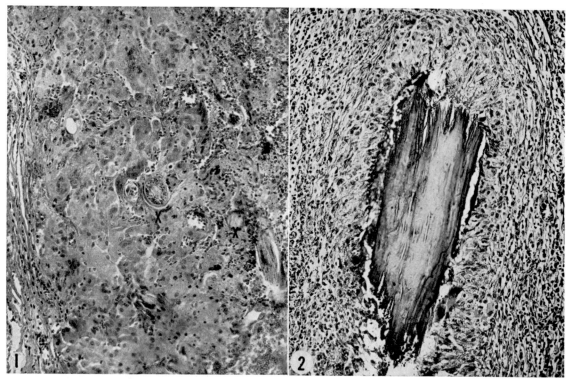

Figure 659.   Postoperative Foreign Body Granulomas in Orbit

1. Epithelioid cell proliferation about cilia (X). ×165. AFIP Acc. 487978.
2. Reaction to catgut suture material. ×130. AFIP Acc. 982629.

sponsible for orbital hemorrhage, emphysema and infection. Fracture deformity of the orbit may permit displacement of the eye. On occasion, a fragment of bone lying in the orbit serves as a nidus for an inflammatory or benign proliferative mass long after the initial injury has been forgotten by the patient. Such a mass may be mistaken for a neoplasm.

VASCULAR DISEASE

In the orbit, as in many other tissues, vascular lesions are rarely primary. The blood vessels are involved in a wide range of inflammatory and degenerative diseases. Occasionally such lesions appear to develop primarily in the orbital vessels.

Orbital thrombophlebitis, which once was a relatively common condition, is characterized by acute fulminating infection associated with great toxicity, sepsis, and such grave complications as orbital cellulitis, cavernous sinus thrombophlebitis and meningitis. As with other orbital infections, most cases develop by spread from adjacent structures. Less common causes include penetrating wounds and hematogenous spread from dis-

tant sites of suppuration. Rarely a chronic orbital thrombophlebitis of obscure etiology may simulate an orbital neoplasm (Fig. 660) (Zimmerman and Rogers).

Aneurysms in the orbit are rare. Traumatic or spontaneous intracranial arteriovenous aneurysms are of much greater importance. Most of these are formed by traumatic rupture of the carotid artery into the cavernous sinus. The cardinal signs are "pulsating exophthalmos" associated with bruit and thrill.

Orbital varices have received attention far out of proportion to their frequency. This probably is due to their dramatic clinical picture of transient proptosis which may be increased by stooping, straining or pressure on

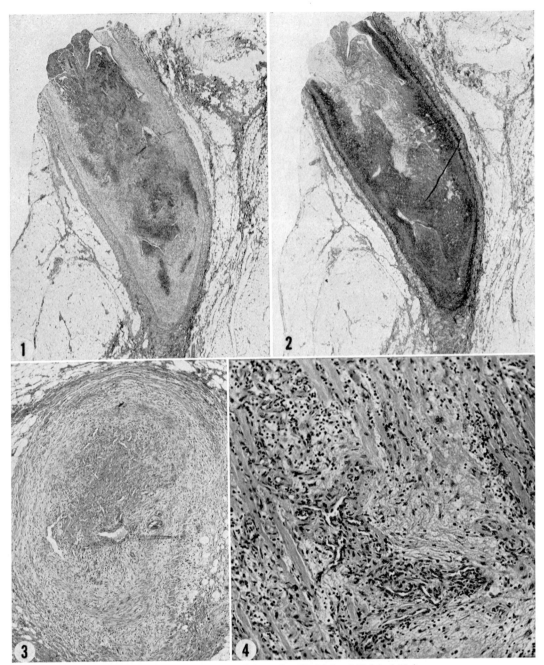

Figure 660. Idiopathic Thrombophlebitis of Orbital Veins

Unilateral proptosis associated with marked pain and congestion in a 69 year old woman was believed due to an orbital neoplasm. AFIP Acc. 737987. (Case reported by Zimmerman and Rogers, 1957.)

1. Longitudinal section of a large vein with greatly thickened tunics reveals lumen to be occluded by an organized thrombus. H and E, ×13.

2. Same vessel shown in 1, stained for elastic tissue in order to demonstrate that the vessel is a vein rather than an artery. ×13.

3. Transverse section of another thrombosed vein. H and E, ×45.

4. Degenerated extraocular muscle contains a great increase in interstitial connective tissue and ground substance and many new capillaries. ×125.

the jugular veins. Although there may be a congenital structural predisposition, most varices become evident and the calcified areas (phleboliths) may be demonstrated roentgenographically.

OCULAR MUSCLE INVOLVEMENT IN SYSTEMIC DISEASES

Endocrine exophthalmos. In goiter associated with thyrotoxicosis the lid retraction rarely is accompanied by significant amounts of proptosis. Numerous theories have been advanced to explain the various manifestations of endocrine exophthalmos. The popular dualistic school championed by Mulvany divides endocrine exophthalmos into the thyrotoxic and thyrotropic forms. The thyrotoxic form is believed to be due directly to the hyperthyroidism and is relieved or arrested after thyroidectomy or other therapy. The thyrotropic form seemingly is due to the action of the anterior pituitary hormone upon the orbital tissues, and may follow therapy for thyrotoxicosis or appear spontaneously.

Normal thyrotropins (TSH), which are secreted by the pituitary in response to low thyroid hormone levels and are suppressed by high hormone levels, do not show a tendency to produce exophthalmos. Thyroid administration may not always inhibit thyrotropin production and all cases of malignant exophthalmos do not show increased thyrotropin production. In most cases excess thyrotropin in the blood does not lead to malignant exophthalmos.

Adams and Purves state that by sensitive assay methods a form of thyrotropin can be demonstrated in the blood of patients suffering from hyperthyroidism or exophthalmos, or a combination of hyperthyroidism and exophthalmos, which differs from the normal thyrotropin in not being suppressed by excess thyroid hormone levels. This substance may be an abnormal form of thyrotropin which is responsible both for exophthalmos and hyperthyroidism, or it may be a manifestation of an abnormality of pituitary secretion which involves more than one factor.

The primary causes of hyperthyroidism and the exophthalmos frequently associated with it are unknown. The dualistic concept of thyrotoxic and thyrotropic exophthalmos generally has been replaced by a unitarian view which maintains that there is but one pathologic mechanism and that differences in the clinical picture are quantitative rather than qualitative.

Except for the lid signs and occasional papilledema the eyes rarely are affected in thyrotoxicosis. In those instances where the orbit is affected the changes are seen in the extraocular muscles. They are normal in size and consistency, but microscopically there is generalized muscle degeneration characterized by atrophy of the muscle fibers with loss of striation, fibrillation, amorphous granulation of the sarcoplasm forming clumps resembling giant cells, and duplication of sarcolemmal nuclei. The muscles show lipomatosis with rows of fat cells infiltrating between the muscle bundles and between individual muscle fibers. The orbit shows an increased amount of fat. In a group of 17 patients with thyrotoxicosis, Rundle and Pochin found the fat in the eye muscles to be double the normal amount.

In the nerves there is also granulation in the neuroplasm and diffuse proliferation of the neurilemmal nuclei. This reaction is scattered throughout the orbit and may result in foci of degeneration. The orbital fat may be slightly increased. There is absence of edema, fibrosis, or extensive lymphocytic infiltration, although a few perivascular accumulations of lymphocytes may be present. The exophthalmos often is more apparent than real due to widening of the lid fissure, the lids otherwise being unaffected.

Malignant exophthalmos also is known as hyperophthalmopathic Graves' disease, progressive or postoperative exophthalmos, exophthalmic ophthalmoplegia, thyrotropic exophthalmos, and ophthalmopathic form of Graves' disease. Henderson has shown that it occurs in three clinical states: (1) as part of Graves' disease in addition to the thyrotoxic signs, (2) after thyroidectomy when the picture of thyrotoxicosis has been ameliorated,

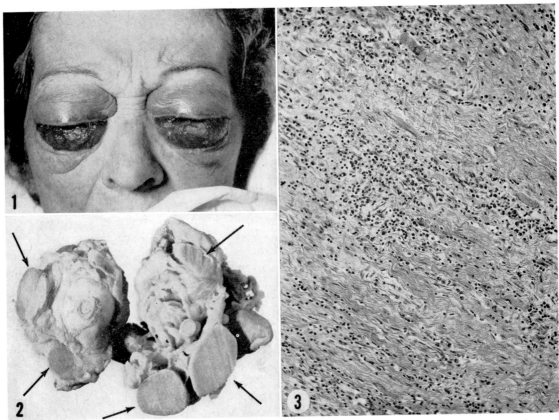

Figure 661. Malignant Endocrinopathic Exophthalmos

1. A 65 year old white woman who had had malignant exophthalmos of about 10 months' duration finally died in congestive heart failure. AFIP Acc. 692463.

2. At autopsy the extraocular muscles (arrows) were found to be massively thickened.

3. Varying degrees of fibrous connective tissue replacement of degenerated skeletal muscle fibers, accumulation of ground substance, and infiltration by chronic inflammatory cells are evident in extraocular muscles. ×145.

and (3) in patients without goiter or preceding thyrotoxicosis.

Malignant exophthalmos may appear in various grades of severity. In the most fulminating form, there is progressive edema of the lids, chemosis of the conjunctiva, exophthalmos developing to such severity that there may be an exposure keratitis, immobility of the globe, visual field changes, glaucoma, and panophthalmitis (Fig. 661–1).

Malignant exophthalmos often occurs in older individuals and is more common in males. It is usually, though not invariably, bilateral, but may be asymmetric and may be associated with a hyperthyroid, hypothyroid, or euthyroid state.

The alterations occurring in the orbit in malignant exophthalmos are: (1) edema of the orbital tissues, (2) lymphocytic infiltration, (3) increase in the mucin content, (4) fibrosis and (5) severe degeneration and inflammation of extraocular muscles (Fig. 661–3). An increased size of the muscles often occurs and they are pale and rubbery (Fig. 661–2). Orbital myositis may be a prominent feature of progressive exophthalmos (Fig. 662). At times the hypertrophy of the extraocular muscles is so great they can be seen as large cords through the conjunctiva. François exenterated the orbits of three patients for suspected neoplasms and on histologic examination found a myositis of one or more ocular muscles. Lymphocytic follicles were found in the muscles, associated with degeneration of the muscle bundles. The surrounding orbital tissues were only slightly involved. Only one of the three cases had a history of thyrotoxicosis.

The orbital edema in malignant exophthalmos is not evenly distributed and is more

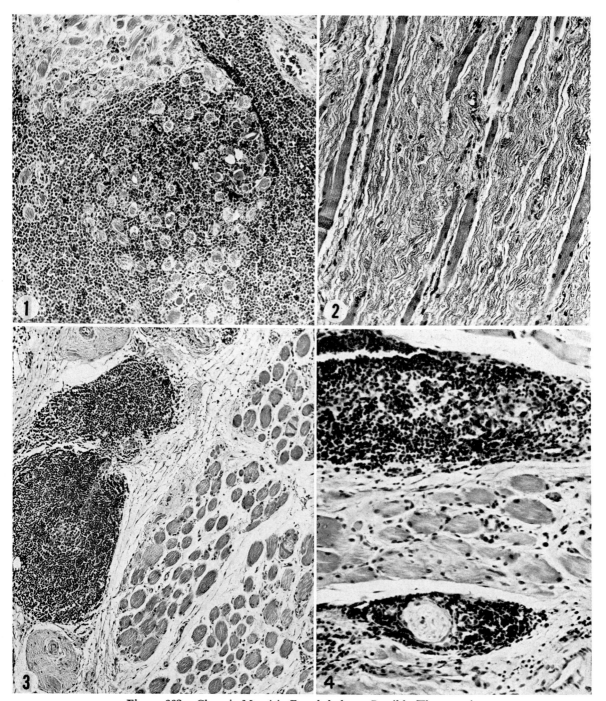

Figure 662. Chronic Myositic Exophthalmos, Possibly Thyrotropic

1. Intense lymphocytic infiltration in degenerating inferior rectus muscle. ×130. AFIP Acc. 824224.

2. Marked fibrous tissue replacement of extraocular muscle. ×130. AFIP Acc. 861748.

3 and 4. Perivascular lymphoid nodules in edematous interstitial connective tissue of levator palpebrae. ×90 and ×280, respectively. AFIP Acc. 36675.

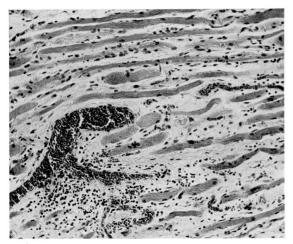

Figure 663. Myasthenia Gravis

There is an increased amount of interstitial connective tissue which is lightly but diffusely infiltrated by chronic inflammatory cells. Perivascular infiltrates are somewhat more dense. ×168. AFIP Acc. 677734.

marked in the orbital fat than in the extraocular muscles. The mechanism by which orbital edema develops has not been clearly elucidated. The increased deposition of mucopolysaccharide which has a strong property of binding water may be an important factor. In advanced cases, venous obstruction may play a part; however, orbital edema may occur even if the eye has been enucleated.

Excessive amounts of mucin have been found within the orbital tissues in experimental exophthalmos as shown by increased hexosamine content and by increased amounts of metachromatic ground substance.

The fibrosis involves all of the orbital tissues. The involvement of the extraocular muscles accounts for subsequent restriction of movement. It may be so extreme that there is no decrease of the exophthalmos after the subsidence of the acute phase. The fibrotic changes within the muscles are not uniform so that a single biopsy may not be representative of the true pathologic picture. In malignant exophthalmos there is an abundant lymphocytic infiltration of the muscles and the adjacent soft tissue. These cells are highly radiosensitive, which may be a factor in the improvement of exophthalmos which sometimes occurs following radiation of the orbit.

Myasthenia gravis. Presumably, in myasthenia gravis there is a chemical defect in which circulating cholinesterases affect the function of acetylcholine at the myoneural junction. The extraocular muscles, particularly the levator, are affected, and minimal histologic changes may be found in the muscles. Lymphocytic infiltrations may be found in the muscles, especially around blood vessels (Fig. 663). Adams and co-workers state that the muscle fibers, however, show no alterations, even in the region of the lymphocytic infiltrations.

Myotonia congenita. In myotonia congenita there is widespread disease of striated muscle, which appears early in life, and often is associated with mental deficiency. The muscles show hypertrophy, but the reason for this change is not known.

Myotonic dystrophy. This heredofamilial disease is characterized by myotonia, baldness, gonadal atrophy, premature senility and mental deficiency. There is a selective atrophy of the muscles, and the eye signs consist of cataracts and ptosis.

Primary ocular myopathy. Ptosis, followed by limitation of eye movements which progresses to complete immovability of the eyes, characterizes this disease. The pupil usually has normal reactions. Retinitis pigmentosa may be associated. At autopsy the nuclei supplying the muscles are fairly normal. The extraocular muscles show changes compatible with a dystrophic myopathy. Senita and Fisher have described two typical cases which followed trauma. Biopsy of the muscles showed atrophy of the muscle bundles and fatty and fibrous replacement. The sarcolemmal nuclei showed focal areas of hyperplasia. There was an absence of myofibrils and crossstriations in occasional fibers.

Dermatomyositis. According to Walsh, the skin and muscles or nerves and muscles may be inflamed in dermatomyositis, and the extraocular muscles may be affected so as to produce oculomotor palsies. Conjunctivitis, iritis, and retinitis also have been reported to occur. The skin of the brow and lids may become reddened so that the diagnosis of erysipelas is suggested. A pale thickening may occur in the skin of the brow, described as "marble brow." If eosinophilia occurs the diagnosis of trichiniasis is suspected. The affected skin and muscles show infiltrations with lymphocytes, plasma cells and edema fluid. Secondary degeneration occurs, with fibrous replacement. The etiology of this condition is unknown, but it is classified with the "connective tissue" diseases.

Cranial arteritis. The extraocular muscles may be affected in a small percentage of cases. Wagener and Hollenhorst studied 122 persons affected with temporal arteritis, and found diplopia in 12 patients, but the extraocular muscles were affected only in three patients. The characteristic lesion is a giant cell arteritis, which may affect any of the orbital vessels (Figs. 46–3, 4, 534) including those to the muscles.

NEOPLASMS

Neoplasms and other tumefactions of the orbit, although they are not rare, are still not so common that any single institution can collect and systematically study a large series of representative cases. Therefore, it is extremely difficult to state categorically the relative frequency of the numerous lesions we must consider here. In making statements regarding the frequency of various lesions, such variables as the nature of one's material and practice and the patient's age and general state of health always must be kept in mind. For example, mucocele may be the most frequently encountered orbital tumor in the practice of radiology, yet the pathologist rarely sees these lesions. In the discussions to follow, such statements as "most common," or "rare" are based largely on impressions gained from study of material on file in the Registry of Ophthalmic Pathology and on statements in the literature.

CLASSIFICATION OF ORBITAL TUMORS

For discussion purposes, tumors of the orbit may be classified as follows:

PRIMARY IN ORBIT

A. Choristomatous: dermoid cyst; epidermal cyst; teratoma
B. Hamartomatous: hemangioma; lymphangioma; neurofibroma
C. Mesenchymal:
   Adipose: lipoma; liposarcoma
   Fibrous: fibroma; fibrosarcoma
   Myomatous: leiomyoma; leiomyosarcoma; rhabdomyoma; rhabdomyosarcoma
   Cartilaginous: chondroma; chondrosarcoma
   Osseous: osteoma; osteosarcoma
D. Neural: neuroma; neurofibroma; neurilemoma; "neurogenic sarcoma;" meningioma of orbital portion of optic nerve; glioma of optic nerve; granular cell myoblastoma; non-chromaffin paraganglioma
E. Epithelial: lacrimal gland tumors
F. Inflammatory (pseudotumors): lymphoid, chronic sclerosing, plasmacytoid, granulomatous, lipogranulomatous, fibromatous

SECONDARY IN ORBIT FROM ADJACENT STRUCTURES

A. Intraocular: malignant melanoma; retinoblastoma
B. Cornea and conjunctiva: malignant melanoma; epidermoid carcinoma
C. Eyelids and face: basal cell carcinoma; meibomian gland carcinoma; epidermoid carcinoma; malignant melanoma
D. Upper respiratory tract: carcinoma of upper respiratory epithelium; sarcoma; mucocele
E. Cranial cavity: meningioma; other intracranial neoplasms

METASTATIC FROM DISTANT SITES

A. Carcinoma
B. Sarcoma
C. Neuroblastoma

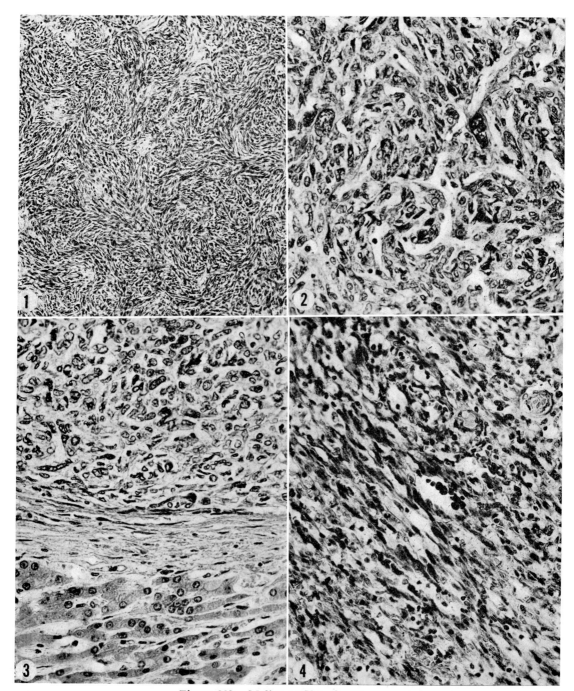

Figure 669.   Malignant Vascular Tumors

1 to 3. Hemangiopericytoma of orbit with metastasis to liver. Upper half of field in 3 shows metastatic tumor nodule while lower part shows liver parenchyma. ×115, ×305, and ×305, respectively. AFIP Acc. 725795.
    4. Kaposi's sarcoma ("malignant granulation tissue"). ×305. AFIP Acc. 943024.

hemorrhage, inflammation and scarring, the vascular nature of these tumors may be obscured. Some vascular tumors are composed of channels which have walls of smooth muscle. These have been referred to as venous hemangiomas.

Malignant vascular tumors (angiosarcomas) are very rare (Fig. 668). Ordinarily they do not develop from pre-existing benign vascular tumors but appear to arise *de novo*, mainly in older individuals. They are highly cellular and are often difficult to differentiate from other sarcomas. Malignant hemangiopericytoma (Fig. 669) and Kaposi's sclerosing angiosarcoma (sometimes called malignant granulation tissue) are the specific types of malignant vascular tumors that have been recognized most often in the orbit, but it should be emphasized that all are exceedingly rare.

Lymphangioma. This type of tumor is much less common than hemangioma. Most lymphangiomas involving the orbit arise in the lids or conjunctiva. These tumors consist of congeries of small, thin-walled channels lined by endothelium. The channels typically contain no erythrocytes, and when hemorrhage has occurred, the tumor is likely to be mistaken for hemangioma. There are no examples of lymphangiosarcoma in the Registry of Ophthalmic Pathology.

Neurofibroma. This tumor occurs in the orbit as an apparently isolated lesion. Most recent investigators think neurofibroma is never a truly isolated lesion but is always a part of multiple neurofibromatosis (von Recklinghausen's disease). The association of multiple neurofibromatosis with café-au-lait spots, redundant skin, gliomas of the optic nerve, and secondary alteration in skeletal development is discussed in other chapters. Morphologic features of orbital neurofibromas will be discussed with the other neural tumors.

Mesenchymal Tumors

These tumors are classified according to the adult tissues they resemble or from which they may arise.

Lipoma. Many of the so-called lipomas probably represent herniations of orbital fat. Histologically, lipoma resembles adult fat (Fig. 670). The individual fat cell has a small, pyknotic, eccentric nucleus and clear cytoplasm. Groups of cells are separated from other groups by delicate fibrovascular septums. Coarser septums divide the tumor into lobules. A true lipoma has a thin fibrous capsule. Therefore, in most instances, the surgeon is better equipped than the pathologist to distinguish between true lipoma and herniated orbital fat. If fibrous tissue contributes

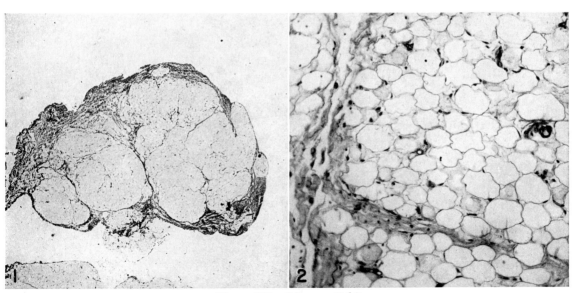

Figure 670. Lipoma, Orbit

1. ×11. AFIP Acc. 38100.
2. ×125. AFIP Acc. 316765.

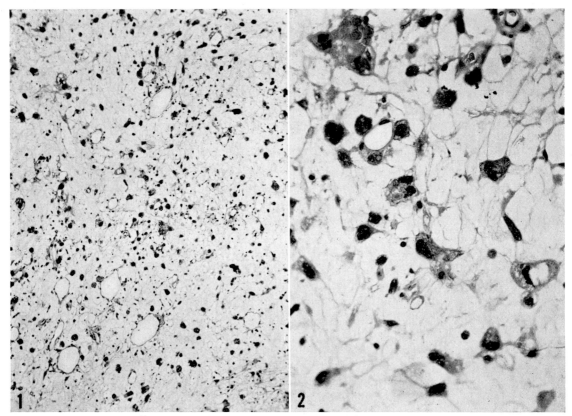

Figure 671. Liposarcoma, Orbit

This tumor developed several years after intensive radiation therapy for retinoblastoma.
1. ×80. AFIP Acc. 931254.
2. ×305. AFIP Acc. 931254.

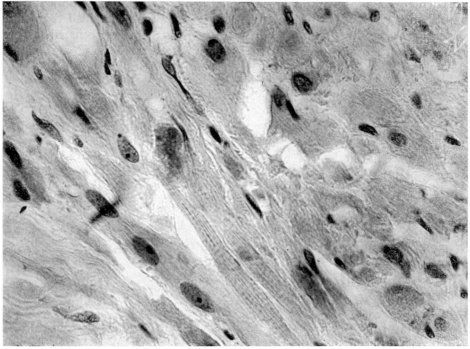

Figure 672. Possible Rhabdomyoma

This field, taken from a large orbital tumor in an 18 year old boy, shows well differentiated skeletal muscle cells. While some pathologists have interpreted the tumor as a rhabdomyoma, the consensus is to regard the lesion as a degenerative and regenerative process involving skeletal muscle. ×300. AFIP Acc. 51810.

746

significantly to the tumor's composition, the designation fibrolipoma is appropriate.

Liposarcoma. It is rare for this tumor to appear in the orbit. In the Registry there is one case of orbital liposarcoma which arose after radiation therapy for retinoblastoma (Fig. 671). Histologically, the neoplastic cells in liposarcoma may have small or large hyperchromatic nuclei and foamy or coarsely vacuolated cytoplasm. More characteristically, the cells are giant and bizarre. Some areas may appear myxomatous. Since many neoplasms, other than liposarcoma, contain fat droplets as a degenerative product, demonstration of fat in neoplastic cells does not establish the diagnosis of liposarcoma.

Fibroma and fibrosarcoma. Fibrous connective tissue seldom gives rise to neoplasms in the orbit. Thus, fibroma and fibrosarcoma in the orbit are rare. Some authorities find it difficult to decide whether there is a true benign neoplasm composed of fibroblasts (Stout). Much more important in the orbit are the benign tumor-like proliferations of fibroblasts which often are mistaken for malignancies. These proliferations may have a wide variety of inciting factors, unknown and known (infections, trauma, irradiation, etc.). Their histologic characteristics are as varied as their causes. They may have any combination of fibroblastic proliferation, capillary proliferation, chronic inflammatory cell infiltration, and fibrosis. Although the appearance of hyperplastic fibroblasts may be disturbing, these benign proliferations are not known to give rise to malignant neoplasms.

Myoma and myosarcoma. Since the orbit contains smooth muscle, it is theoretically possible for leiomyoma and leiomyosarcoma to arise in the orbit. However, we have not recognized any orbital neoplasms as of smooth muscle derivation. In the Registry, there are two lesions which some pathologists have interpreted as rhabdomyoma (Fig. 672). It is doubtful that either represents a true benign neoplasm of skeletal muscle. They probably are examples of scarred, degenerated (or regenerated) muscle. At any rate, orbital rhabdomyoma, if it exists at all, is extraordinarily rare.

Rhabdomyosarcoma, on the other hand, is the most common malignant neoplasm of mesenchymal origin in the orbit (Frayer and Enterline; Porterfield and Zimmerman). The 55 cases of orbital rhabdomyosarcoma on file in the Registry of Ophthalmic Pathology may be divided into three histologic types: embryonal, differentiated, and alveolar (Porterfield and Zimmerman). All three types occur predominantly in Caucasians in the first decade of life. The average age is about 7 years and there is slight preponderance in males. The embryonal type is the most common and is characterized by a rapidly growing, soft, fleshly, sometimes cystic mass in the upper inner quadrant of the orbit. The tumor, which usually causes proptosis in a downward and temporal direction, appears to have its origin in mesenchymal tissues outside of preformed muscle. Microscopically, embryonal rhabdomyosarcoma is characterized by poorly differentiated mesenchymal cells arranged in a syncytium (Figs. 673, 674). The cells are round, oval, elongated or stellate with nuclei which are rich in chromatin. There may be many mitotic figures. The most diagnostic cell is one with a long ribbon of eosinophilic cytoplasm. The cytoplasm, like all muscle cytoplasm, takes a deep red color with Masson's trichrome stain. It is in the cells with ribbons of eosinophilic cytoplasm that longitudinal and cross striations may be found, usually after prolonged search (Fig. 674). Convincing cross-striations are found in about two-thirds of the cases. Because it is not known how often this tumor occurs in the orbit and because the cross-striations are so often overlooked, many pathologists have mislabeled embryonal rhabdomyosarcomas "neurogenic sarcoma" (Fig. 675–1, 2). This is the same type of tumor as the sarcoma botryoides of the genitourinary tract of young girls. In the orbit it only rarely grows outward, subconjunctivally, to form a botryoid mass (Fig. 675–3). More characteristically it infiltrates deeply, often beyond the margins of excision (Fig. 675–4). Metastases to the brain and lungs are common. Although the prognosis is poor, with patients rarely surviving more than two years, it is not hopeless. Early exenteration appears to offer the best chance of cure.

The differentiated type of rhabdomyosarcoma is the least common. It differs from the embryonal type in that virtually every cell has a ribbon of eosinophilic cytoplasm and

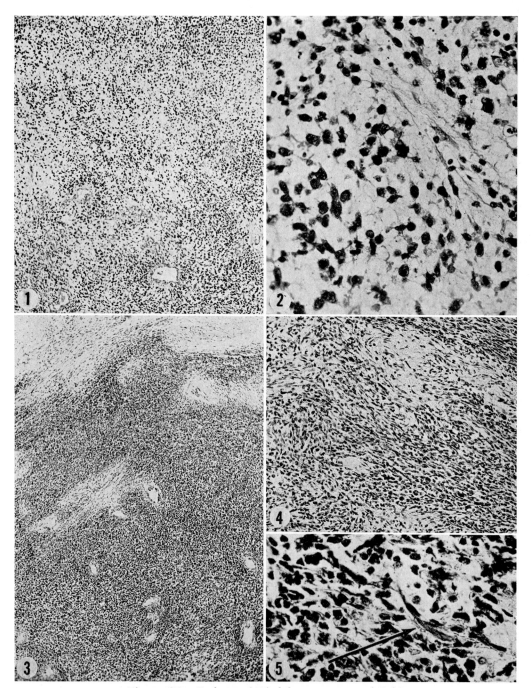

Figure 673. Embryonal Rhabdomyosarcoma of Orbit

1 and 2. Syncytial arrangement of embryonic mesenchymal cells of varying shapes. ×50 and ×305, respectively. AFIP Acc. 80857.

3 and 4. Varying degrees of cellularity are observed. ×50 and ×115, respectively. AFIP Acc. 71658.

5. Cross-striations are well developed in one of the cells containing a long ribbon of cytoplasm. Same tumor shown in 3 and 4. Phosphotungstic acid-hematoxylin stain, ×440.

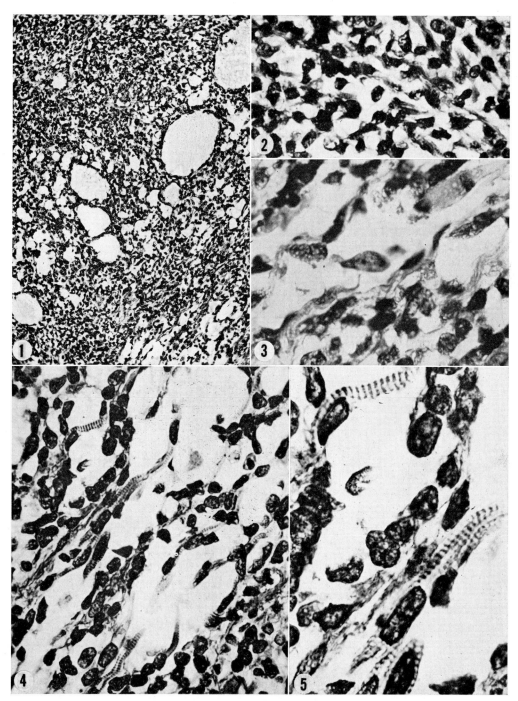

Figure 674. Embryonal Rhabdomyosarcoma of Orbit

All fields are from same tumor. The number of cells with well developed cross striations shown in 4 and 5 is most unusual for embryonal rhabdomyosarcoma. AFIP Acc. 979276.

1. Syncytial arrangement of embryonic muscle cells with numerous cystoid areas. ×115.

2. Many of the tumor cells have ribbon-shaped cytoplasmic expansions. ×525.

3. In some, but not all cells with broad cytoplasmic processess, there are cross striations. ×630.

4 and 5. Cross striations are demonstrated more effectively with Wilder's stain for reticulum. ×525 and ×1240. respectively.

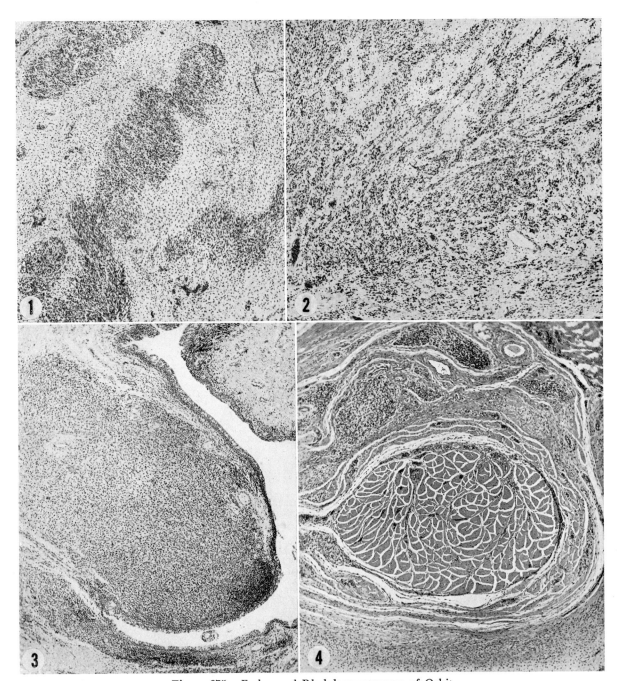

Figure 675. Embryonal Rhabdomyosarcoma of Orbit

1 and 2. Patterns such as these have led to the diagnosis of "neurogenic sarcoma" in many cases. Both ×50, AFIP Acc. 909168.

3. Pedunculated subconjunctival nodule resembling **sarcoma botryoides** of the vagina. ×136. AFIP Acc. 717260.

4. Deep diffuse infiltration about the trochlea. ×50. AFIP Acc. 798619.

cross-striations are found with relative ease (Fig. 676). The main reason for separating this type is the possibility that it may have a better prognosis than the embryonal type.

The alveolar type is slightly more common than the differentiated. It differs clinically from the other two types in that it frequently involves the lower orbit. Moreover, it appears to originate within the extraocular muscles. Histologically, the neoplastic cells are separated into "alveolar spaces" by septums (Fig. 677). Cytoplasmic processes from the neoplastic cells merge into the septums. The individual cells may be small and round or large and bizarre. Tadpole-shaped and multinucleated tumor giant cells are fairly common (Fig. 677). Longitudinal and cross striations are found with difficulty or not at all. Since the alveolar type has few features to suggest its muscle origin, the tumor usually is mistaken for neuroblastoma, angiosarcoma, reticulum cell sarcoma and even carcinoma.

However, the cells in metastases sometimes resemble skeletal muscle more closely (Fig. 678) than do those in the primary. In 3 of the 9 cases reported by Porterfield and Zimmerman, cross-striations were found in the metastases but not in the orbital tumor. This type is almost invariably fatal within a year or two.

Chondroma and chondrosarcoma. These tumors are very rare in the orbit. Chondrosarcoma is most often associated with osteosarcoma following radiation therapy for retinoblastoma. Microscopically, the neoplastic cells may have great pleomorphism, but the cartilagenous nature of the cells is evident in some areas (Fig. 679–1, 2).

Osteoma and osteosarcoma. Many of the so-called osteomas probably are exostoses, hyperostoses or hamartomas. Osteomas may have the appearance of normal or sclerotic bone. Primary osteosarcoma of the orbit is also rare. More cases following irradiation for retinoblastoma have been reported than cases

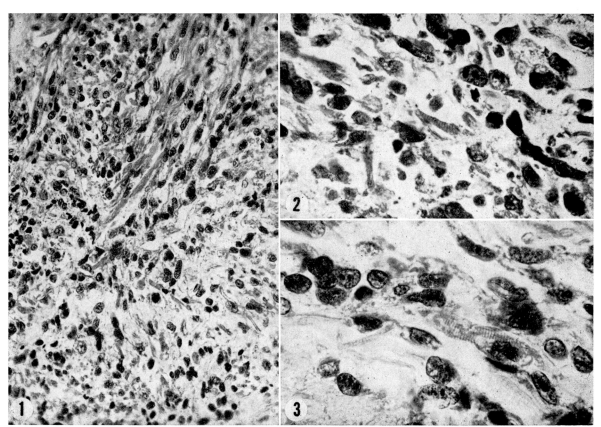

Figure 676. Differentiated Rhabdomyosarcoma of Orbit

Almost all the tumor cells have long cytoplasmic streamers and cross striations are easier to demonstrate than in the embryonal type of rhabdomyosarcoma. AFIP Acc. 773776.

1. ×305.   2. ×630.   3. ×720.

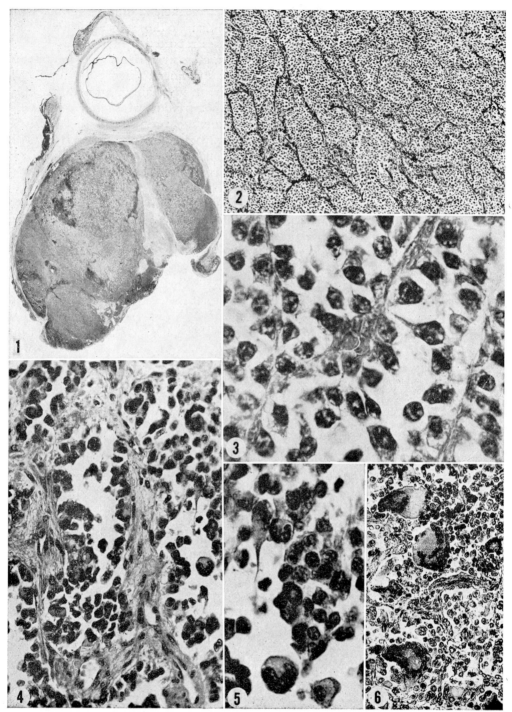

Figure 677.   Alveolar Rhabdomyosarcoma of Orbit

1. Large, rapidly growing tumor below the eye in a newborn infant. ×4. AFIP Acc. 919470.
2. The alveolar pattern is accentuated by the Wilder reticulum stain. ×80. Same case.
3. Cytoplasmic processes attach many of the cells to the connective tissue septums. ×630. Same case.
4. Often the tumor cells appear to float freely in the center of the alveolar structures. ×305. AFIP Acc. 983287.
5. Great cytologic variations are characteristic. ×615. AFIP Acc. 983287.
6. Multinucleated tumor giant cells. ×195. AFIP Acc. 191121.

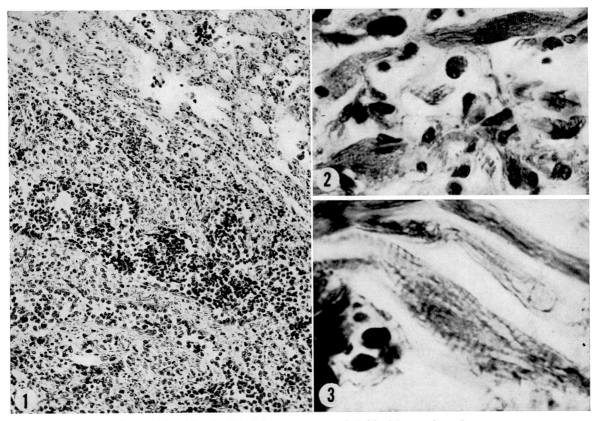

Figure 678. Alveolar Rhabdomyosarcoma of Orbit, Metastatic to Lung

1. Undifferentiated tumor cells in lung. ×130. AFIP Acc. 191121.

2 and 3. Other fields from same pulmonary metastasis show tumor cells with cross striations. ×750 and ×1750, respectively.

arising spontaneously (Cahan et al.; Tebbet and Vickery; Zimmerman and Ingalls; Forrest). Histologically, osteosarcoma varies from case to case and from one area to another in the same tumor. Some tumors following radiation have components which are indistinguishable from chondrosarcoma, liposarcoma or fibrosarcoma. The salient feature is the presence of obviously neoplastic cells forming osteoid or bone (Fig. 679–3, 4).

Neural Tumors

The peripheral nerves in the orbit contain Schwann cells which form sheaths for individual neurites. The Schwann cells are derivatives of the neural crest. As they migrate to the peripheral nerves during development, they probably carry melanoblasts with them (Masson). This may account for the presence of café-au-lait spots associated with neurofibromas and for the probable origin of some

intraocular malignant melanomas from ciliary nerves. Schwann cells cannot be distinguished with certainty from smooth muscle cells and fibrocytes in most routine hematoxylin-eosin preparations. Thus, the exact composition of tumors arising from peripheral nerves remains uncertain.

Amputation neuroma. This is not a neoplasm, but a benign proliferation of neural tissue (Fig. 680–3) following injury or severance of a peripheral nerve. When a nerve is severed, Schwann cells proliferate to form a potential sheath for axis cylinders. New axis cylinders tend to follow the potential Schwannian sheaths. If contact between the new axis cylinders and the distal nerve fragment is prevented, a bulbous enlargement develops at the end of the proximal nerve fragment. The bulbous enlargement consists of tangled neurites embedded in a matrix of proliferated Schwann cells and fibrous connective tissue. The amputation neuroma may

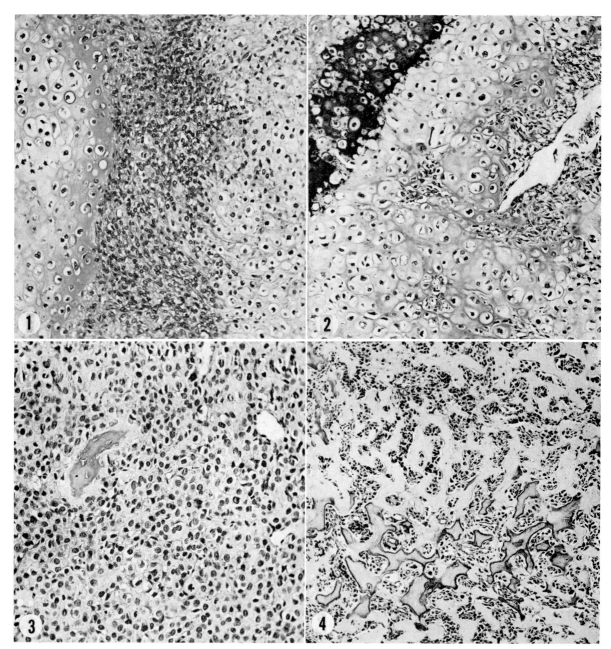

Figure 679. Post-irradiation Chondrosarcoma and Osteosarcoma of Orbit

1 and 2. Chondrosarcomatous areas in tumor. (Case reported by Skolnik et al.) AFIP Acc. 337263. Both ×115. 3 and 4. In some areas the tumor is very poorly differentiated while in others much osteoid and some bone is formed. (Case reported by Zimmerman and Ingalls.) AFIP Acc. 98729. ×160 and ×70, respectively.

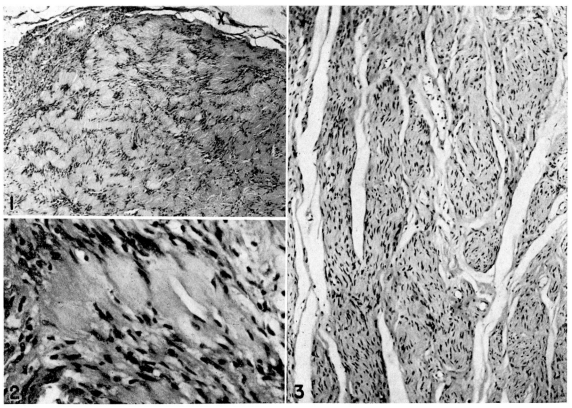

Figure 680. Peripheral Nerve Tumors

1. Neurilemoma, orbit. Antoni type A tissue. X, capsule. ×75. AFIP Acc. 59111.
2. Neurilemoma, orbit. Palisaded Schwann cells. ×280. AFIP Acc. 28907.
3. Amputation neuroma of ciliary nerve in orbit, following enucleation. Regular arrangement of Schwann cells, and of axis cylinders which are not identifiable in this hematoxylin and eosin section. This is not a true neoplasm. ×100. AFIP Acc. 80991.

be very painful. On occasion, when the eye has been enucleated for neoplasm, such an amputation neuroma has been mistaken for a recurrence of the neoplasm.

Neurofibroma. These tumors are characterized by a diffuse proliferation of Schwann cells and other connective tissue elements, often leading to gross disfiguration (Figs. 63, 64). Neurites usually run haphazardly through the tumors, but special stains often are required to demonstrate these structures. Sometimes, the proliferations occur within the nerve sheath and lead to marked enlargement and tortuosity of the nerve. This tumor, which may be visible or palpable beneath the skin as a vermiform cord, is called plexiform neurofibroma (Fig. 230).

Neurilemoma (Schwannoma). In contrast to neurofibroma, neurilemoma is almost a pure proliferation of Schwann cells within a nerve sheath. Thus, neurilemoma is encap-

sulated. A neurilemoma may have one or both of two basic patterns. In the Antoni type A, the cells are arranged in ribbons of palisaded cells alternating with relatively acellular areas (Fig. 680). Sometimes the pattern is altered to mimic tactile corpuscles (Verocay bodies). In the Antoni type B, the Schwann cells are arranged in a more haphazard fashion. Microcystoid areas often separate the cells. The cystoid areas may coalesce to form large cavernous structures in the tumor. Neurilemoma rarely, if ever, undergoes malignant change. Malignant Schwannian tumors are much more likely to arise in neurofibromatosis. "Neurogenic sarcoma" (malignant neurilemoma or malignant Schwannoma) is rare in the orbit (Fig. 681). Some of the tumors originally recorded in the Registry of Ophthalmic Pathology as "neurogenic sarcoma" are now reclassified as embryonal rhabdomyosarcoma. The latter neoplasm may have bands

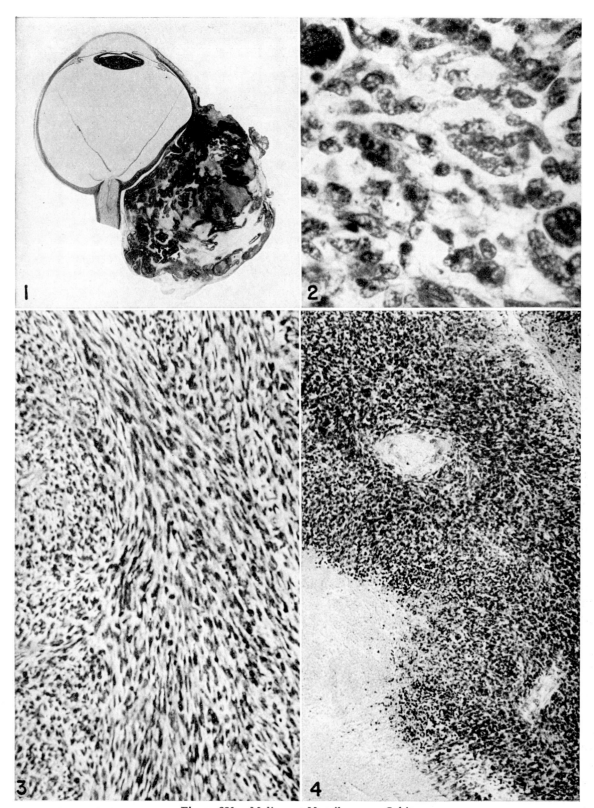

Figure 681. Malignant Neurilemoma, Orbit

1. Malignant neurilemoma of orbit, adherent to globe. AFIP Acc. 135264.

2. Pleomorphic tumor cells. Multinucleated cell in lower right quadrant. Large cell with hyperchromatic nucleus in upper left quadrant. Same case. ×750.

3. Bundles of spindle-shaped cells in longitudinal and cross section. Same case. ×235.

4. Small cells with deeply staining nuclei and scanty cytoplasm surrounding blood vessels, with adjacent areas of necrosis, simulating retinoblastoma. Same case. ×140.

of loosely arranged cells alternating with bands of closely packed cells, a pattern which superficially resembles tumors of neural origin (Fig. 675–1, 2).

Miscellaneous neurogenic tumors. Meningioma and glioma of the optic nerve are discussed in Chapter IX. There are a few examples of non-chromaffin paraganglioma in the orbit (Fig. 682–3), although normal non-chromaffin paraganglionic structures have not been demonstrated in the human orbit (Fisher and Hazard). These neoplasms are characterized by polygonal cells with small vesicular nuclei and abundant, clear or eosinophilic cytoplasm. The cells frequently contain eosinophilic granules, but chromaffin granules are absent. The cells are divided into small groups by a highly vascular network. Silver impregnation brings out the reticulin fibers in this vascular network. In contrast with granular cell myoblastoma, reticulin fibers do not extend between the individual cells (Smetana and Scott). "Granular cell myoblastoma" is a controversial tumor which rarely occurs in the orbit (Fig. 682–1, 2). The cells of this tumor do not bear the slightest resemblance to the "myoblasts" of developing skeletal muscle. In the majority of cases there is no apparent relationship to muscle. The origin of the cells in granular cell myoblastoma is in dispute. Murray, on the basis of tissue culture, concluded that the cells resemble skeletal muscle elements. Fust and Custer, on the other hand, presented evidence suggesting a neural origin. Regardless of its origin, granular cell myoblastoma has distinctive microscopic features. The cells are round, oval or polygonal with abundant, granular, eosinophilic cytoplasm and well defined cell borders. The arrangement of reticulin fibers between cells has already been described.

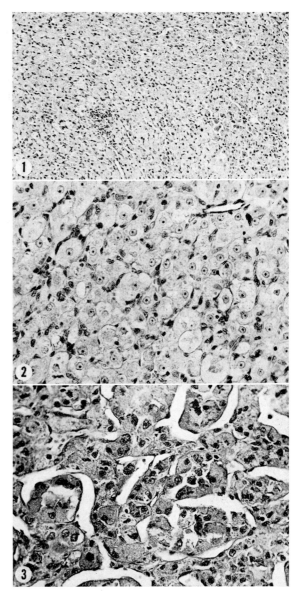

Figure 682. Alveolar Sarcomas of Orbit

1 and 2. So-called granular cell myoblastoma. ×115 and ×300, respectively. AFIP Acc. 951977.

3. Probable nonchromaffin paraganglioma. ×305. AFIP Acc. 220221.

Epithelial Tumors of the Lacrimal Gland

Tumor masses occupying the lacrimal fossa fall into three main categories: lymphomas and lymphoid hyperplasias (about 20 per cent), inflammatory pseudotumors (about 30 per cent), and epithelial tumors of the lacrimal gland (about 50 per cent) (Reese, 1956). The lymphoid tumors and inflammatory pseudotumors will be discussed later. Epithelial tumors of the lacrimal gland are very similar in type and in clinical behavior to those of the salivary glands. In the past, both the salivary and the lacrimal gland tumors were considered very difficult to classify. Estimation of their prognosis by histopathologic study was considered no better than the flipping of a coin (McFarland). As a result of this chaotic situation and because all lacrimal gland tumors were judged by the behavior of their most malignant members, many writers have recommended radical treatment regardless of histopathologic classification.

In recent years these tumors have been classified very satisfactorily and the surgical pathologist is expected to be able to predict their clinical behavior from their microscopic appearance. Forrest, utilizing the Foote and Frazell classification of salivary gland tumors, was the first to call attention to the fact that histopathologic study of these tumors was of practical importance. While it is true that lacrimal and salivary gland tumors have much in common, there are some differences. Lacrimal gland tumors are less common and the majority can be classified by the following simple schema:

Mixed tumors
    A. benign
    B. malignant
Carcinomas unrelated to mixed tumors
    A. adenoid cystic
    B. other

Mixed tumors. These account for about one-half of the epithelial tumors of the lacrimal gland (or one-fourth of all tumors in the lacrimal fossa). The great majority are benign but about one in ten shows areas of malignant change. Thus, by definition, a malignant mixed tumor is one which shows, in addition to the characteristic histologic features of benign mixed tumor, areas which appear frankly carcinomatous. Usually the malignant component is adenocarcinoma, rarely squamous carcinoma, and almost never sarcoma.

Benign mixed tumors typically are composed of a mixture of epithelial and connective tissue elements; hence such monstrous terms as fibromyxoepithelioma and myxochondrocarcinoma have been applied to them. Grossly they are single multilobulated masses which often appear encapsulated (Fig. 683). Frequently the capsule is firmly adherent to the periosteum of the lacrimal fossa. These are locally invasive tumors which may infiltrate the capsule to involve the adherent periosteum. With incomplete removal they may recur in the soft tissues or in the bony wall of the lacrimal fossa (Fig. 684). If removed piecemeal, multiple recurrences may be expected.

Microscopically, benign mixed tumors exhibit great structural variation, not only from case-to-case, but also in different portions of the same tumor (Figs. 683, 684, 685). In spite of this pleomorphism, certain features are observed with sufficient regularity that the diagnosis is made with ease. Tubular structures arranged in an irregularly anastomosing pattern and lying in a myxoid stroma are seen in almost every case. Ducts lined by a double layer of epithelium are usually present. The inner layer of epithelial cells may secrete mucus or it may undergo squamous metaplasia (Fig. 685-4). The outer layer of epithelial cells appear to give rise by metaplasia to the myxoid, fibroid, and cartilaginoid stromal tissue (Fig. 686). This basically epithelial nature of lacrimal gland mixed tumors was described by Verhoeff over half a century ago when the prevailing opinion was that they represented endothelial neoplasms.

Despite their pleomorphism and areas of great cellularity, benign mixed tumors do not exhibit either cytologic or clinical features of metastasizing neoplasms. Furthermore, even after multiple recurrences over a period of many years, the tumors tend to remain unchanged. Rarely, however, with recurrence, carcinomatous change may take place and metastasis may then occur.

Carcinoma of lacrimal gland. Carcinomas that are not associated with mixed tumors occur relatively more frequently in the lacrimal than in the salivary glands. About one-half of all epithelial tumors of the lacrimal gland are carcinomas, and of these the adenoid cystic variety (Fig. 687) is most common. This is in contrast with Foote and Frazell's observations in a series of 877 salivary gland tumors. Less than one-third were carcinomas unrelated to mixed tumors and, of these, about one in ten were adenoid cystic carcinomas.

The frequent occurrence of adenoid cystic carcinomas in the lacrimal gland is of some practical importance for two reasons: (1) In the past, this tumor has often been confused with mixed tumors; and (2) the adenoid cystic carcinoma of the lacrimal glands carries a very unfavorable prognosis. Because of certain histopathologic features that benign mixed tumors share with adenoid cystic car-

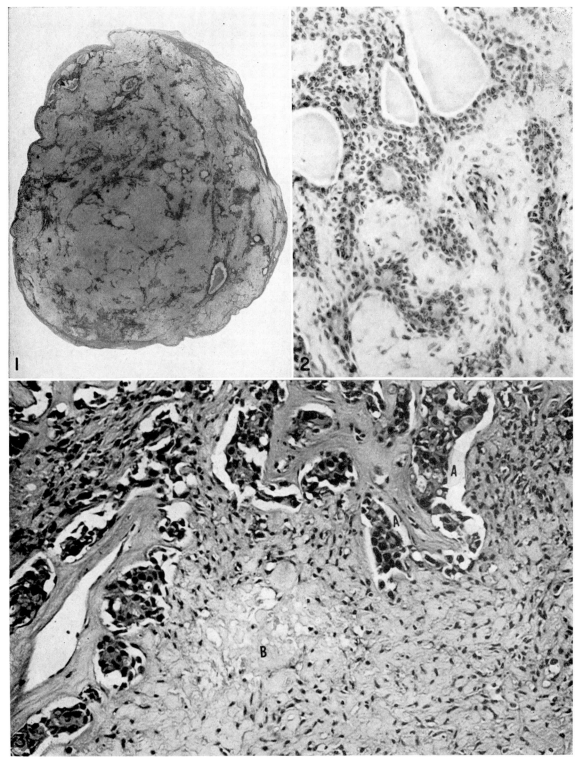

Figure 683. Benign Mixed Tumor of Lacrimal Gland

1. The encapsulation is caused by compression of the surrounding tissues. AFIP Acc. 28931.

2. Adenomatous arrangement of epithelial cells. The alveoli contain seromucinous secretion. ×330. AFIP Acc. 51727.

3. A, nests of epithelial cells. B, myxomatoid matrix. ×100. AFIP Neg. 97835.

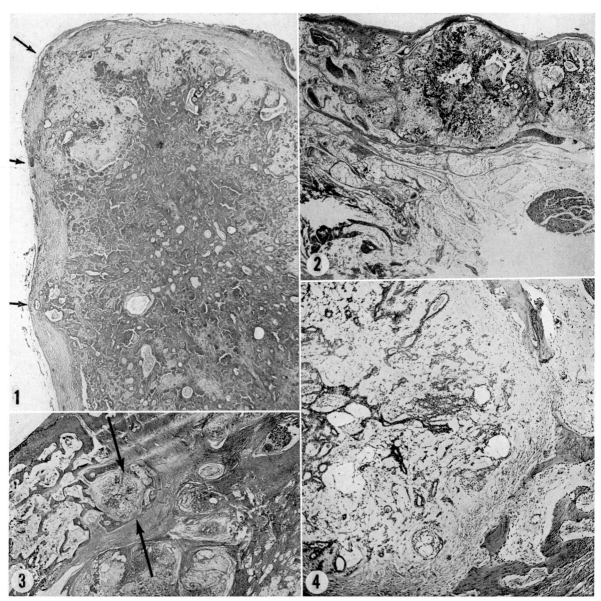

Figure 684. Infiltrative Characteristics of Benign Mixed Tumors

1. There are multiple sites of capsular invasion (arrows). ×16. AFIP Acc. 687742.

2. Invasion of orbital tissues after incomplete excision. ×8. AFIP Acc. 311948.

3 and 4. Invasion of bony wall of lacrimal fossa (same case shown in 2). ×7. Area between arrows in 3 enlarged to ×50 in 4.

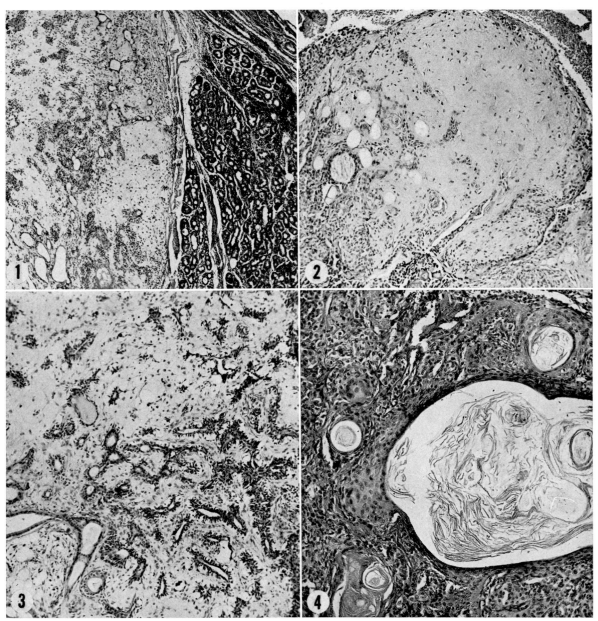

Figure 685. Benign Mixed Tumor of Lacrimal Gland

1. The tumor (on left) is separated from the uninvolved lacrimal gland (on right) by an extremely thin layer of connective tissue. ×50. AFIP Acc. 711594.

2. In this portion of same tumor the chondroid stroma predominates. ×90.

3. Anastomosing ducts, some containing seromucinous secretion. Same tumor. ×80.

4. Squamous metaplasia and formation of keratin are conspicuous in this portion of same tumor. ×115.

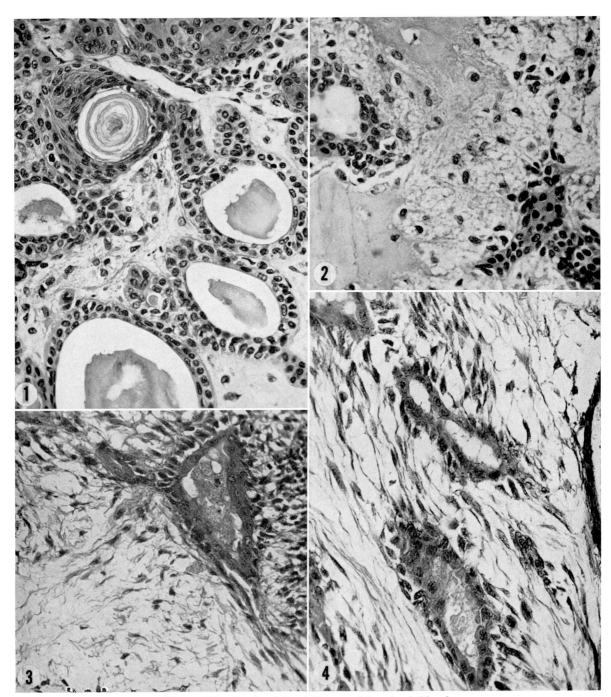

Figure 686. Benign Mixed Tumor of Lacrimal Gland

1 and 2. Different fields from same tumor. Ductal epithelium secretes seromucinous material, undergoes squamous metaplasia, and produces a variety of interstitial cells which mimic mesodermal cells. Both ×305. AFIP Acc. 616876.

3 and 4. Derivation of interstitial cells from outer layer of ductal epithelium. ×305 and ×375, respectively. AFIP Acc. 587887.

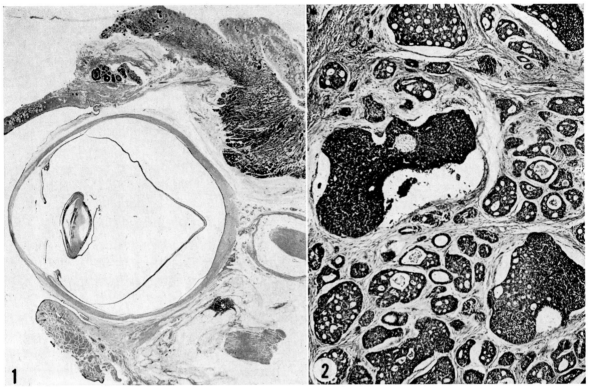

Figure 687. Adenoid Cystic Carcinoma of Lacrimal Gland

1. Extensive infiltration of orbit beyond plane of excision. ×2.5. AFIP Acc. 973493.
2. Cystic spaces within tumor lobules give rise to this typical Swiss cheese pattern. Same case. ×50.

cinomas, these two biologically different tumors were not considered separately in the ophthalmic literature of the past. Since the prognosis for adenoid cystic carcinomas is so poor, and since this tumor was usually lumped with the mixed tumors, it was only natural that the entire group of lacrimal gland tumors acquired a very bad reputation. It is very important that the two tumors be separated. The highly invasive character of the adenoid cystic carcinoma, which enables it to spread along nerves and vessels, penetrate bone, and metastasize to distant organs (Fig. 688–4), requires radical surgical management, while in the case of benign mixed tumors much more conservative excisional treatment is indicated (Reese, 1956).

Microscopically, the adenoid cystic carcinoma is characterized by aggregates of small tightly packed cells containing hyperchromatic nuclei and scanty cytoplasm (Figs. 687, 688). These aggregates which may be very small or quite large typically are sharply outlined and contain small rounded cystic foci

containing mucin. Cord-like patterns with hyalinized stroma characteristic of cylindromas (Fig. 688–3) or large sheets resembling those of certain basal cell carcinomas also may be observed.

In addition to the adenoid cystic carcinomas, other types of adenocarcinoma (Fig. 689), including occasional examples of mucinous carcinoma and mucoepidermoid carcinoma, may be encountered. All of these have a very poor prognosis and should be treated by radical surgery.

Inflammatory Pseudotumors

One of the most frequent causes of unilateral proptosis and an occasional cause of bilateral exophthalmos is a chronic sclerosing inflammatory process. While in some cases the process may be truly granulomatous, in the majority it is not. Hence the synonymous use of the terms, "inflammatory pseudotumor," and "granuloma of orbit," is inappropriate.

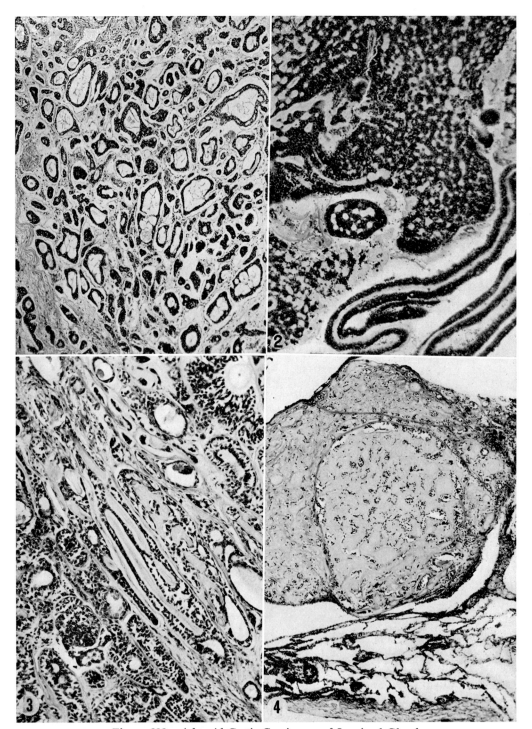

Figure 688. Adenoid Cystic Carcinoma of Lacrimal Gland

1. Typical pattern. ×61. AFIP Acc. 106106.

2. A few long cylindrical structures are present along with the more typical adenoid cystic pattern. ×73. **AFIP** Acc. 28909.

3. Cylindromatous structure accentuated by the elongated masses of hyalinized stroma between the **cords of** epithelial cells. ×140. AFIP Acc. 217304.

4. Metastatic nodule in lung reveals structure similar to that of primary tumor with much hyalinized **stroma.** ×55. AFIP Acc. 217304.

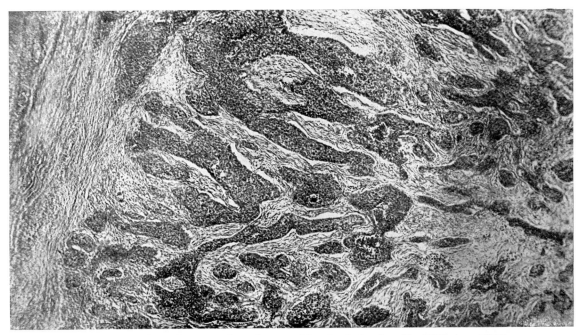

Figure 689. Undifferentiated carcinoma of lacrimal gland. ×62. AFIP Acc. 82239.

The clinical course of inflammatory pseudotumors is extremely varied. The onset may be sudden with severe diffuse congestion and edema or it may be insidious with slowly progressive infiltration of part or all of the orbit. While most often unilateral, in bilateral cases the second orbit may not be affected until several years after the first. Examination reveals edema of the lids, chemosis, restricted ocular movements, a palpable mass, proptosis, and variable degrees of congestion.

Histologically the picture is even more varied than the clinical course. While it rarely is possible to arrive at a definitive etiologic diagnosis, many of the cases fall into definite histopathologic categories. Of necessity the various lesions considered here merge with those described in other parts of this chapter.

Lymphoid pseudotumors. There is probably no aspect of ophthalmic pathology that is more difficult for both the student and the experienced practicing pathologist than the differential diagnosis of malignant lymphoma and reactive lymphoid hyperplasia (Fig. 690). At the risk of oversimplifying, lymphoid tumors of the orbit including those arising in the lacrimal gland, like those of the conjunctiva, lids, and uvea, may be placed in

three main groups with respect to the problems they present in differential diagnosis.

At one extreme there is a very small group consisting of tumors which are quite obviously malignant. The constituent cells, while typically anaplastic and poorly differentiated, all appear to belong to the same generic line. There may be cellular pleomorphism but polymorphism is conspicuously absent. Reticulum cell sarcoma and the acute leukemias are the specific types most likely to present initially as orbital tumors. In the great majority of cases, clinical, radiological, and hematological examinations will reveal confirmatory evidence of a systemic malignant disease. Most tumors of this sort are encountered in the pediatric age group and the patient generally succumbs to his disease within a year after its recognition. In adults we rarely observe malignant lymphomas or leukemia presenting first with orbital lesions. The orbit, however, may be involved later in the course of the disease but in such cases there is no serious problem in differential diagnosis.

At the opposite extreme, there is a much larger group of lymphoid tumors in which the non-neoplastic nature of the lesion should be appreciated if the constituent cells are ex-

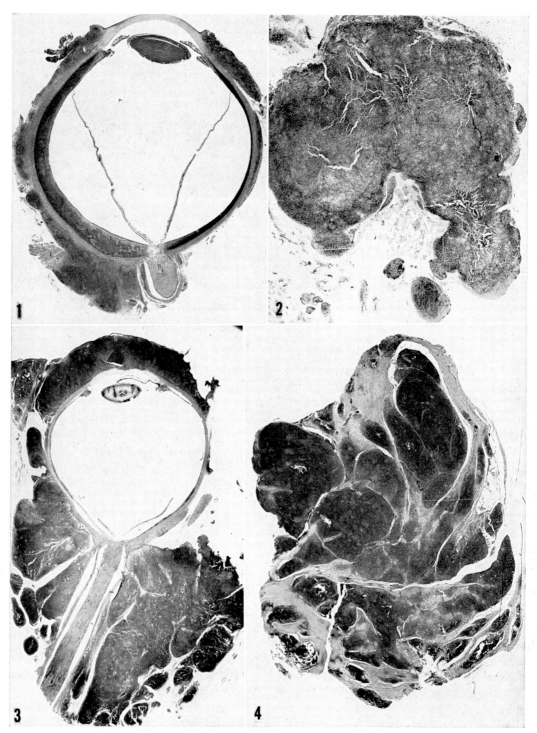

Figure 690.   Lymphoid Pseudotumors of Orbit

1. In this case the orbit is involved along with the conjunctiva and uveal tract. ×2. AFIP Acc. 947300.
2. Tissue excised from orbit. ×9. AFIP Acc. 849313.
3. Massive involvement of cornea, conjunctiva, orbit, and optic nerve. ×2. AFIP Acc. 947302.
4. Tissue excised from orbit. ×6. AFIP Acc. 690458.

amined. There are several characteristics which indicate the tumors are reactive or inflammatory rather than neoplastic. First is polymorphism. These lesions may be predominantly proliferations of lymphocytes or of reticulum cells but many other cell types participate (Figs. 691, 692). The admixture of polymorphonuclear leukocytes, eosinophils, plasma cells, and macrophages should always suggest an inflammatory basis for the lesion. Among the malignant lymphomas, polymorphism is characteristic only of Hodgkin's disease which rarely, if ever, makes its

initial appearance in the orbit. A second hallmark of these reactive lymphoid proliferations is formation of lymphoid follicles containing a central core of reticulum cells and a peripheral zone of lymphocytes. In some cases the proliferation of reticulum cells may be extremely disturbing. They may appear very large and anaplastic and mitotic figures may be numerous. Such cases have often been mistakenly interpreted as "follicular lymphoma." Fortunately, true "follicular lymphoma" rarely, if ever, begins in such nonlymphatic tissue as the orbit. The third

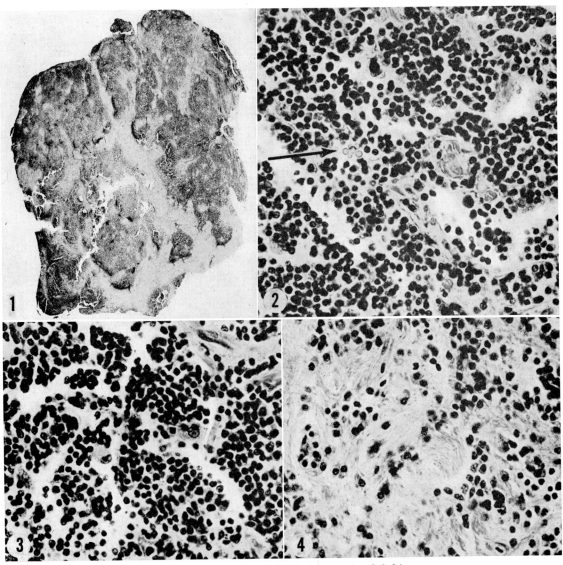

Figure 691.   Lymphoid Pseudotumor of Orbit

1. Lymphoid aggregates separated by dense collagenous connective tissue. ×5. AFIP Acc. 788125.
2. Lymphocytes predominate but there are other cell types including Russell's bodies (arrow). Same case. ×380.
3. Macrophages and plasma cells are scattered amongst the lymphocytes. Same case. ×380.
4. Plasma cells, macrophages, and fibroblasts are present in the interlobular connective tissue. Same case. ×380.

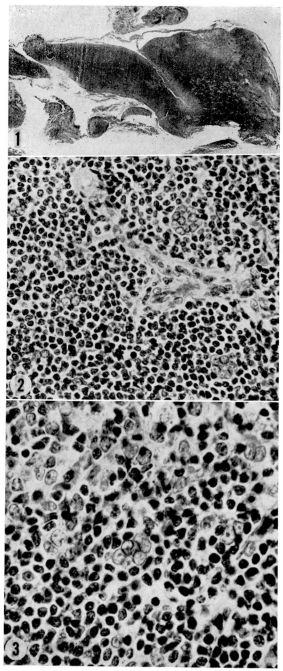

Figure 692. Lymphoid Pseudotumor of Orbit

1. Dark areas are composed mainly of lymphocytes while pale areas contain large numbers of reticulum cells. ×6. AFIP Acc. 188411.

2. Several multinucleated reticulum cells are present, and a blood vessel lined by hyperplastic endothelial cells crosses the field. Same case. ×380.

3. Many large reticulum cells are present among the lymphocytes. Same case. ×525.

characteristic of inflammatory lymphoid lesions is the presence of ancillary evidence of an inflammatory reaction. Frequently the blood vessels appear larger and more numerous than normal. Their endothelial cells are swollen and hyperplastic (Fig. 692–2). Capillaries may resemble cords of epithelial cells. The stroma often contains hyaline deposits (paramyloid).

Between the extremes of the two foregoing groups (the obviously malignant and the obviously reactive) there is another large group of lymphoid tumor masses which give trouble to even the most experienced pathologists. Most of these are relatively pure lymphocytic proliferations (Fig. 693). They lack the polymorphism of the group just described and they lack the anaplastic cytologic features of the highly malignant reticulum cell sarcomas and acute leukemias. It is possible that some of these might evolve into generalized lymphocytic lymphosarcomas, but in our experience this must be a very unusual occurrence. Follow-up studies generally fail to produce evidence of generalized disease and the lesions typically respond to small amounts of radiation.

Plasma cell pseudotumors. In this very small group, the situation is similar to that of the last group considered in the foregoing section, except that here we are dealing with relatively pure proliferations of plasma cells (Fig. 694). However, the plasma cells lack the cytologic features of neoplasia. Some of the cells may be very large and contain two or three nuclei but they are otherwise well differentiated. Most so-called plasmacytomas of the orbit are of this type. Rarely, the orbit is involved primarily in multiple myeloma. In such cases clinical and radiological studies reveal other evidence of systemic disease.

Orbital myositis. In some inflammatory pseudotumors, the process involves one or more of the extraocular muscles, almost to the exclusion of other orbital tissues (Figs. 653, 662). The reaction tends to be lymphocytic, sometimes with follicle-formation, but perivascular plasma cell proliferation is also observed. Varying degrees of degeneration of muscle fibers and accumulation of interstitial ground substance are observed. This group is distinguished from endocrinopathic exophthalmos (Fig. 661) only by clinical study since

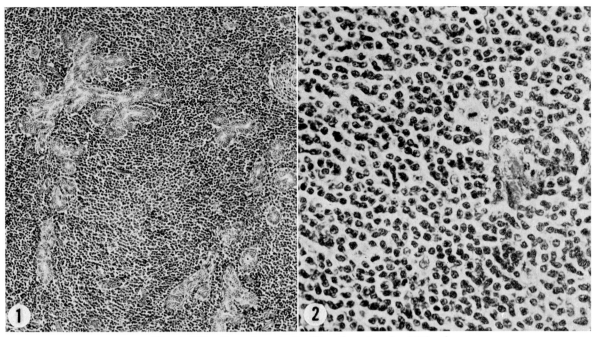

Figure 693. Lymphocytic Proliferation, Lacrimal Gland

1 and 2. The reaction consists of a disturbingly uniform proliferation of lymphocytes. While this picture is consistent with lymphocytic lymphosarcoma, most cases have a benign course. ×115 and ×450, respectively. AFIP Acc. 947303.

the tissue reaction is so similar and since the thyrotropic disease also may be unilateral.

Lipogranuloma. In some orbital pseudotumors there is widespread destruction of orbital fat. Associated with the fat necrosis is the development of a foreign body granulomatous reaction (Fig. 695). Multinucleated giant cells surround pools of lipid and these in turn are circumscribed by other inflammatory cells. In these cases the specific cause of the fat necrosis is obscure. Moreover it is not even possible to be certain that the changed orbital fat represents the seat of the disorder or merely a conspicuous feature of the final microscopic picture.

Vasculitis. A prominent perivascular distribution of the inflammatory process is observed in some cases. Small veins and capillaries are affected. Acute necrotizing angiitis, sometimes associated with a prominent eosinophilia, suggests the possibility of an allergic type of tissue damage.

Sclerosing pseudotumor. The production of interstitial connective tissue may be disproportionately great in some cases with a relative paucity of chronic inflammatory cells (Figs. 652, 696). Frequently the intersti-

tial tissue is pale staining, relatively acellular, and rich in ground substance. In other instances it may be densely collagenous or the picture may vary in different portions of the same lesion.

Dacryoadenitis. Approximately one-half

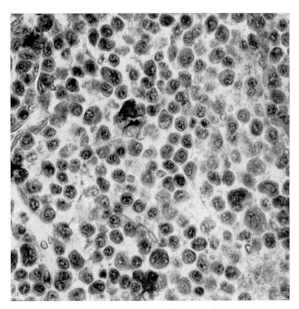

Figure 694. Plasma cell pseudotumor (benign plasmacytoma) of orbit. ×605. AFIP Acc. 80003.

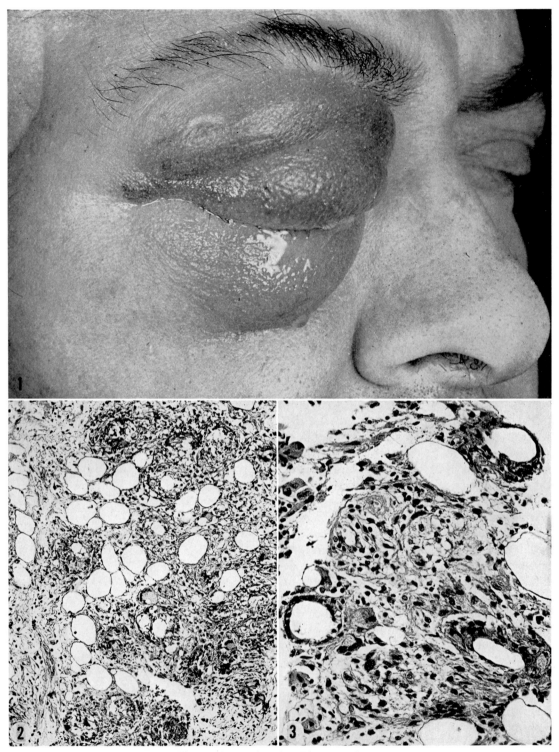

Figure 695.   Sclerosing Lipogranuloma

1. Clinical appearance of affected orbit (from Smetana and Bernhard).

2 and 3. Biopsy specimens reveal a chronic granulomatous reaction about disintegrating orbital fat. ×145 and ×305, respectively. AFIP Acc. 239826.

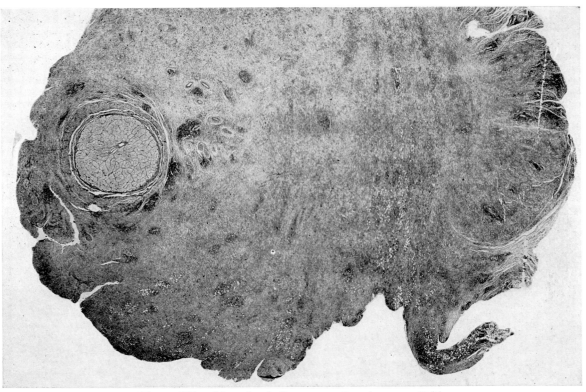

Figure 696. Sclerosing Inflammatory Pseudotumor, Orbit

The optic nerve, extraocular muscles, and all orbital structures are encased in a dense mass of connective tissue. Several foci of lymphocytic infiltration are present but the over-all cellularity is minimal. ×5. AFIP Acc. 35691.

of tumor masses presenting in the lacrimal fossa prove to be nonepithelial and, of these, the majority are pseudotumors. Some of the latter are characterized by a disturbingly uniform proliferation of lymphocytes and are often mistaken for lymphosarcoma (Fig. 693). Others are readily recognized as chronic inflammatory lesions. Some of these are nongranulomatous (Fig. 697) while others are granulomatous (Fig. 698).

Specific pseudotumors. In a minority of cases, microscopic examination provides a clue as to the specific cause of the lesion. Remnants of squamous epithelium, pieces of hair, or lobules of sebaceous glands contained in the inflammatory mass may indicate that rupture of a dermoid cyst was responsible. Strips of respiratory epithelium may point to the diagnosis of mucocele (Fig. 699). Blood filled endothelial-lined spaces together with hemosiderin-laden macrophages might suggest trauma to a deeply situated hemangioma. Foreign bodies indicate some sort of injury which may have been unsuspected or long

forgotten. The presence of innumerable discrete epithelioid cell granulomas of about the same size and shape and without necrosis suggests sarcoidosis. In other cases appropriate staining may reveal bacteria, fungi, or parasites. Very rarely the microscopic features may suggest one of the xanthogranulomatous diseases (nevoxanthoendothelioma, eosinophilic granuloma, etc.) discussed at the end of this chapter.

SECONDARY ORBITAL TUMORS

Secondary neoplasms are among the most common of all malignant tumors of the orbit. In most instances, the secondary nature of the tumor is apparent. However, there are cases in which the fact that the tumor is not primary is appreciated only after microscopic examination.

Intraocular malignant melanoma and retinoblastoma, especially when neglected, frequently invade the orbit. On rare occasions, the intraocular origin of the orbital tumor

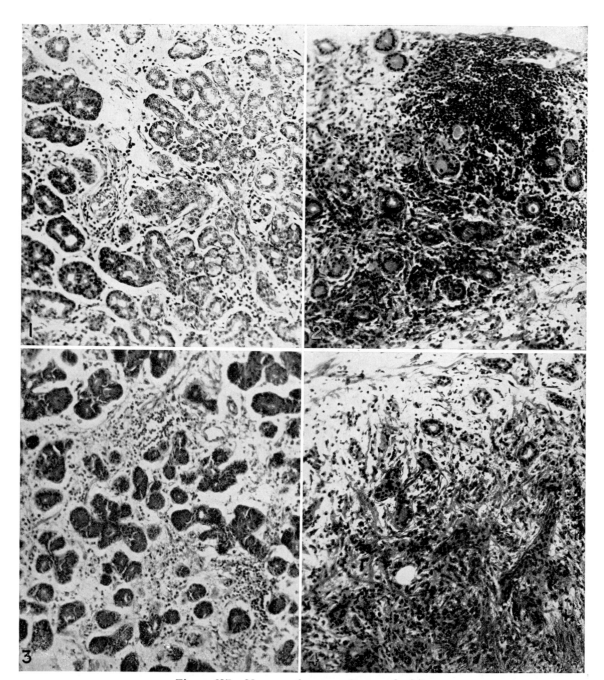

Figure 697.   Nongranulomatous Dacryoadenitis

1. Lymphocytic infiltration and moderate fibrosis of lacrimal gland in chronic dacryoadenitis. ×125. AFIP Acc. 484772.

2. Lymphocytic infiltration and fibrosis in chronic dacryóadenitis. ×145. AFIP Acc. 481234.

3. Lymphocytic infiltration, fibrosis and atrophy of tubules in chronic dacryoadenitis. ×145. AFIP Acc. 271420.

4. Replacement of lacrimal gland by inflammatory granulation tissue. Only a few tubules remain. ×145. AFIP Acc. 481234.

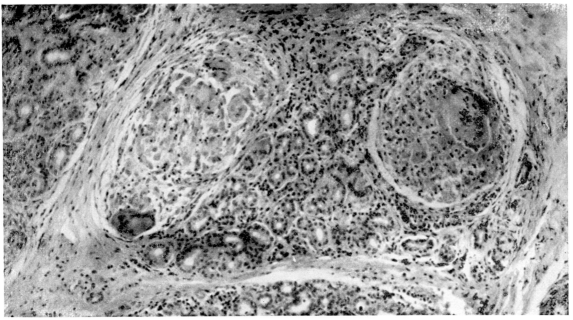

Figure 698. Granulomatous Dacryoadenitis

1. Circumscribed accumulations of epithelioid and giant cells, probably Boeck's sarcoid. ×145. AFIP Acc. 34323.

may not be suspected if the eye is phthisical. These tumors may also involve the orbit as late recurrences after the primary tumor has been removed by enucleation.

Malignant melanoma and epidermoid carcinoma of the conjunctiva are relatively rare. They occasionally invade the orbit. Basal cell carcinoma, particularly when neglected or improperly treated, is notorious for its ability to invade and destroy the orbital tissues. Although it does not metastasize by the blood stream or lymphatics, basal cell carcinoma may, nevertheless, kill the patient by infiltrating the orbit, penetrating the cranial bones, and invading the brain. Epidermoid carcinoma, malignant melanoma and meibomian gland carcinoma of the eyelids or face are much less common than basal cell carcinoma. However, the orbit may be invaded by any of these. Carcinoma arising from the upper respiratory epithelium of the nose and paranasal sinuses is relatively common (Fig.

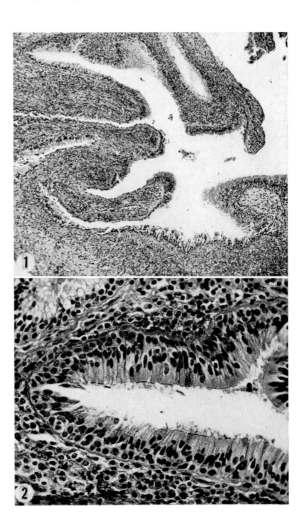

Figure 699. Mucocele, Orbit

1 and 2. Pseudostratified ciliated columnar epithelium lines a cyst, the walls of which are heavily infiltrated by chronic inflammatory cells. ×70 and ×305, respectively. AFIP Acc. 744523.

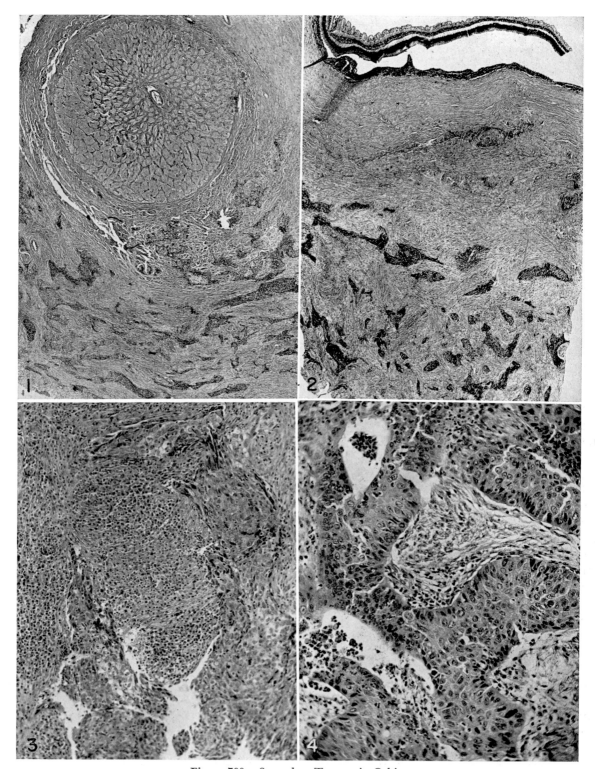

Figure 700.   Secondary Tumors in Orbit

1. Undifferentiated carcinoma from antrum, invading orbit around optic nerve. ×24. AFIP Acc. 200589.
2. Undifferentiated carcinoma from antrum, invading orbit and sclera. Same case. ×27.
3. Undifferentiated carcinoma from antrum, invading orbit. Same case. ×125.
4. Undifferentiated squamous cell carcinoma, invading orbit from nasolacrimal duct. ×160. AFIP Acc. 182546.

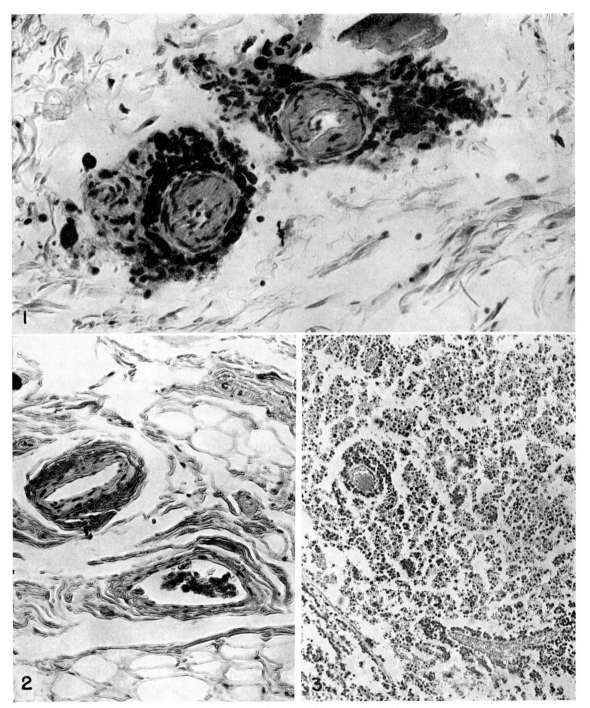

Figure 701. Metastatic Tumors in Orbit

1. Malignant melanoma, metastatic in orbit from skin. Melanoma cells around orbital arteries. ×330. AFIP Acc. 131550.

2. Same case. Melanoma cells in orbital vein. ×330. AFIP

3. Neuroblastoma (sympathicoblastoma) metastatic in orbit from adrenal. ×98. AFIP Acc. 47588.

700–1 to 3). Carcinoma arising from the naso-lacrimal drainage apparatus is somewhat rare (Fig. 700–4). Sometimes the carcinoma is well differentiated and its derivation from epithelium of the upper respiratory tract is readily recognized. Other times the tumor is so undifferentiated that its microscopic features provide no clue as to its origin. Sarcoma of these structures rarely involves the orbit.

Most meningiomas in the orbit are believed to arise in the cranial cavity. Rarely do other intracranial neoplasms, such as pituitary tumors, spread to the orbit.

Tumors Metastatic from Distant Sites

Neoplasms metastatic to the orbit are most unusual (Fig. 701). They have been reported from many different primary sites but the mammary gland and bronchial tree are responsible for most cases. The metastatic tumor which has received the most attention is neuroblastoma. Although this is said to be the most common malignant orbital tumor in children, there are very few documented cases on file in the Registry of Ophthalmic Pathology. Neuroblastoma arises in the adrenal medulla of infants and young children. Occasionally it may arise from one of the sympathetic chains. It may metastasize to the orbital bones and produce periorbital hemorrhage and proptosis. In the primary site the neoplastic cells usually have small, round or oval, vesicular nuclei. The cells may be arranged in rosettes with delicate fibrils in the center. Some of the cells may resemble ganglion cells (ganglioneuroblastoma). In metastastases, most of the cells are round or oval and somewhat nondescript. In a biopsy specimen, it may be impossible to distinguish these cells from those of retinoblastoma or lymphosarcoma.

SYSTEMIC DISEASES WITH ORBITAL MANIFESTATIONS

Hematopoietic diseases. The orbital bones and soft tissues may be affected in the leukemias and malignant lymphomas. When this occurs late in the disease, as is most often the case, there is usually no great problem in differential diagnosis and very rarely is a biopsy indicated. Occasionally, particularly in children, the development of an orbital tumor is the first indication of leukemia or malignant lymphoma. As a matter of fact, such orbital tumors are second only to rhabdomyosarcoma among the malignant orbital neoplasms of childhood (Porterfield). In most cases there is no great difficulty in recognizing histopathologically that the orbital tumor is malignant. The orbital tissues are infiltrated by large anaplastic cells which exhibit no tendency to differentiate. The cells appear to grow as individuals and do not form sheets. From biopsy specimens it is usually not possible to state anything more definite, diagnostically, than "undifferentiated malignant tumor of orbit." In every case of this sort, a thorough clinical, hematological, and radiological study is indicated. As a result it is usually evident that the patient has a very serious systemic disease of which the orbital tumor is merely the presenting manifestation.

The prognosis is characteristically very poor since it is the fulminating acute leukemias and the stem cell (undifferentiated reticulum cell) malignant lymphomas that are most likely to begin in this fashion.

Orbital tumors composed of mature lymphocytes, plasma cells, or a mixture of cell types rarely prove to be malignant. When there is a mixture of cell types, even though one cell type may predominate, it is quite certain that the lesion represents an inflammatory pseudotumor (see pp. 763 to 768). This is also true of lesions composed exclusively of rather mature plasma cells. The terms "benign plasmacytoma" and "solitary plasmacytoma" are often applied, but the lesion really is nothing more than another type of inflammatory pseudotumor. The most difficult group prognostically is rather purely lymphocytic in composition. The lymphocytes may be large or small but they do not appear undifferentiated or anaplastic. Often these lymphocytic tumors occur in older individuals but rarely is there clinical, hematological, or radiological evidence of lymphatic leukemia or lymphosarcoma. On the basis of the biopsy material alone, a definitive diagnosis cannot be established, but experience has shown that, in the great majority of such cases, the subsequent course is that of a benign reactive lesion.

Reticuloendothelioses. The reticuloendothelioses are diseases of unknown etiology. There is no incontrovertible evidence that they are true neoplasms. Most recent writers believe eosinophilic granuloma, Hand-Schüller-Christian disease and Letterer-Siwe disease are closely related disorders. All three are relatively rare. Of the three, Hand-Schüller-Christian disease most characteristically involves the orbit.

Eosinophilic granuloma is a relatively benign destructive process which usually involves a single bone in children and young adults. The lesions are soft and friable. Microscopically they are characterized by the presence of large numbers of eosinophils (Fig. 702) and reticulum cells, some of which may be lipid-laden histiocytes. In exceptional cases the orbital bones may be involved. The upper temporal portion of the orbital brim is the site of predilection.

Hand-Schüller-Christian disease is a disorder of children and young adults characterized by: (1) sharply defined roentgenographic defects in the skull, (2) unilateral or bilateral exophthalmos and (3) signs of pituitary dysfunction, particularly diabetes insipidus. Any organ may be involved in destructive lesions composed of lipid-laden histiocytes. Analysis of the lesions reveals a high content of cholesterol, cholesterol esters, and neutral fat. With increasing age, the lesions exhibit variable amounts of fibrosis and inflammatory cell infiltration. Exophthalmos develops when the lesions extend into the orbital soft tissues.

Letterer-Siwe disease (non-lipoid histiocytosis) is the most serious of the reticuloendothelioses. It affects infants and very young children and often follows a rapidly progressive downhill course. The lesions are composed essentially of large mononuclear cells containing little or no demonstrable lipid. The infiltrative lesions are widespread in bone and other tissues. In the very few cases that have had orbital involvement, there was histopathologic evidence of transition to Hand-Schüller-Christian disease (Fig. 703).

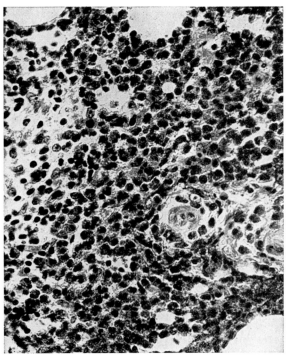

Figure 702. Eosinophilic granuloma, orbit. Nearly all the cells in this field are eosinophils. ×400. AFIP Acc. 109437.

Juvenile xanthogranuloma. This disease, also known as nevoxanthoendothelioma, has been discussed in the chapters dealing with the eyelids and uvea. Most widely recognized as a cutaneous lesion of infants, in recent years it has become increasingly apparent that such other tissues as the conjunctiva, iris, ciliary body, and orbit may also be affected. In the orbit the lesions tend to be localized around an extraocular muscle. Microscopically they are characterized by a proliferation of histiocytic cells including Touton giant cells. Eosinophils often are prominent. There is as yet no good evidence to suggest that juvenile xanthogranuloma is related etiologically to eosinophilic granuloma, Letterer-Siwe, or Hand-Schüller-Christian disease, although microscopically the four have much in common.

Other systemic diseases involving the orbit (e.g., thyrotropic exophthalmos and the phakomatoses) have already been discussed. Osseous lesions (e.g., Paget's disease) are of such little importance to the ophthalmic pathologist that they will not be considered.

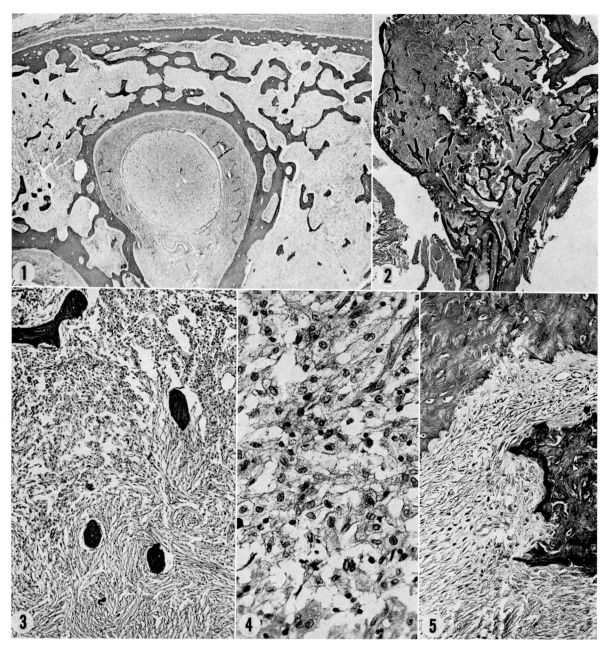

Figure 703. Letterer-Siwe and Hand-Schüller-Christian Disease

Orbital involvement in an infant with Letterer-Siwe disease. At autopsy, some of the lesions showed transition to Hand-Schüller-Christian disease. AFIP Acc. 795765.

1. Involvement of wall of optic canal. ×11.
2. Massive thickening of orbital roof with extensive destruction of bone. ×6.
3. Replacement of marrow spaces by histiocytes and fibrocytes. ×80
4. Some of the histiocytes contain fine cytoplasmic lipoidal vacuoles. ×305
5. Fibrosis of bone marrow. ×165.

REFERENCES

Adams, D. D., and Purves, H. D.: The Role of Thyrotrophin in Hyperthyroidism and Exophthalmos. Metabolism 6:26–35, 1957.

Adams, R. D., Denny-Brown, D., and Pearson, C. M.: Diseases of Muscle. A Study in Pathology. New York, Paul B. Hoeber Co., 1953.

Benedict, W. L., and Martens, T. G.: Malignant Lymphocytic Tumors of the Orbit. Surg. Clin. N. Amer. 26:871–875, 1946.

Blodi, F. C.: Developmental Anomalies of the Skull Affecting the Eye. A.M.A. Arch. Ophthal. 57:593–610, 1957.

Botar, J., and Pribek, L.: Corpuscle paraganglionnaire dans l'orbite (note préliminaire). Ann. d'anat. Path. 12:227–228, 1935.

Cahan, W. G., Woodward, H. Q., Higinbotham, N. L., Stewart, F. W., and Coley, B. L.: Sarcoma Arising in Irradiated Bone. Cancer 1:3–29, 1948.

Clarke, E.: Plasma Cell Myeloma of the Orbit. Brit. J. Ophthal. 37:543–554, 1953.

Cushing, H., and Eisenhardt, L.: Meningiomas. Their Classification, Regional Behaviour, Life History, and Surgical End Results. Springfield, Ill., Charles C Thomas, 1938.

Cutler, W. M., and Blatt, I. M.: The Ocular Manifestations of Lethal Midline Granuloma (Wegener's Granulomatosis). Amer. J. Ophthal. 42:21–35, 1956.

Dunnington, J. H.: Granular Cell Myoblastoma of the Orbit. A.M.A. Arch. Ophthal. 40:14–22, 1948.

Erdbrink, W. L., Edwards, J. E., Crowe, W. W., Johnson, H. S., Cooke, S. L., and Richmond, R. W.: Orbital Fractures. A.M.A. Arch. Ophthal. 61:55–67, 1959.

Falls, H. L., Jackson, J., Carey, J. H., Rukavina, J. G., and Block, W. D.: Ocular Manifestations of Hereditary Primary Systemic Amyloidosis. A.M.A. Arch. Ophthal. 54:660–664, 1955.

Fisher, E. R., and Hazard, J. B.: Nonchromaffin Paraganglioma of the Orbit. Cancer 5:521–524, 1952.

Foote, F. W., Jr., and Frazell, E. L.: Tumors of the Major Salivary Glands. Cancer 6:1065–1138, 1953.

Forrest, A. W.: Epithelial Lacrimal Gland Tumors: Pathology as a Guide to Prognosis. Trans. Amer. Acad. Ophthal. Otolaryng. 58:848–866, 1954.

Forrest, A. W.: Intraorbital Tumors. A.M.A. Arch. Ophthal. 41:198–232, 1949.

Forrest, A. W.: Tumors following Radiation about the Eye. Trans. Amer. Acad. Ophthal. Otolaryng. 65:694–717, 1961.

François, J.: Clinical Manifestations of Exophthalmos. Belg. tijdschr. Geneesk. 14:590–594, 1958.

Frayer, W. C., and Enterline, H. T.: Embryonal Rhabdomyosarcoma of the Orbit in Children and Young Adults. A.M.A. Arch. Ophthal. 62:203–210, 1959.

Fust, J. A., and Custer, R. P.: On the Neurogenesis of So-called Granular Cell Myoblastoma. Amer. J. Clin. Path. 19:522–535, 1949.

Gass, J. D. McI.: Ocular Manifestations of Acute Mucormycosis. A.M.A. Arch. Ophthal. 65:226–237, 1961.

Goodman, S. A.: Hemangiopericytoma of the Orbit. Amer. J. Ophthal. 40:237–243, 1955.

Gotfredsen, E.: Studies on Orbital Tumors. Nature and Incidence of Orbital Tumors over a Period of 15 Years (1932–1946) from Eye Department of Karolinska Sjukhuset. Acta Ophthal. 25:279–293, 1947.

Greenstein, N. M., and Steinberg, D.: The Prompt and Effective Response of Trichinosis to Corticotropin. J. Dis. of Child. 95:261–269, 1958.

Henderson, J. W.: Round Table Conference: Exophthalmos. Amer. J. Ophthal. 44:266–274, 1957.

Lattes, R., McDonald, J. J., and Sproul, E.: Nonchromaffin Paraganglioma of Carotid Body and Orbit. Ann. Surg. 139:382–384, 1954.

McFarland, J.: The Histopathologic Prognosis of Salivary Gland Mixed Tumors. Amer. J. Med. Sci. 203:502–519, 1942.

Mann, I.: Developmental Abnormalities of the Eye. London. Cambridge University Press. 1937.

Masson, P.: Pigment Cells in Man. In the Biology of Melanomas. New York, The New York Academy of Sciences, 1948.

Mulvany, J. H.: The Exophthalmos of Hyperthyroidism; Differentiation in Mechanism, Pathology, Symptomatology and Treatment of Two Varieties. Amer. J. Ophthal. 27:589–612, 693–712, 820–832, 1944.

Murray, M. R.: Cultural Characteristics of Three Granular Cell Myoblastomas. Cancer 4:857–865, 1951.

Newell, F. W.: Osteoma Involving the Orbit. Amer. J. Ophthal. 31:1281–1289, 1948.

Patek, P. R., and Bernick, S.: Extravascular Pathways of the Eye and Orbit. Amer. J. Ophthal. 49:135–140, 1960.

Porterfield, J. F.: Orbital Tumors in Children. Int. Ophthal. Clin. To be published, 1962.

Porterfield, J. F., and Zimmerman, L. E.: Orbital Rhabdomyosarcoma: A Clinicopathologic Study of 55 Cases. Virchows Arch. Path. Anat. To be published, 1962.

Reese, A. B.: Treatment of Expanding Lesions of the Orbit (7th Arthur J. Bedell Lecture). Amer. J. Ophthal. 41:3–11, 1956.

Reese, A. B.: Tumors of the Eye. New York, Paul B. Hoeber, 1951.

Rundle, F. F., and Pochin, E. E.: The Orbital Tissues in Thyrotoxicosis: A Quantitative Analysis Relating to Exophthalmos. Clin. Science. 5:51–74, 1944.

Senita, G. R., and Fisher, E. R.: Progressive Dystrophic External Ophthalmoplegia following Trauma. A.M.A. Arch. Ophthal. 60:422–426, 1958.

Skolnik, E. M., Fornatto, E. J., and Heydemann, J.: Osteogenic Sarcoma of the Skull following Irradiation. Ann. Otol. 65:915–936, 1956.

Smetana, H. F., and Bernhard, W.: Sclerosing Lipogranuloma. A.M.A. Arch. Path. 50:296–325, 1950.

Smetana, H. F., and Scott, W. F.: Malignant Tumors of Nonchromaffin Paraganglia. Mil. Surgeon 109:330–349, 1951.

Stein, H. A., and Henderson, J. W.: Sarcoidosis of

the Orbit. Survey of the Literature and Report of a Case. Amer. J. Ophthal. *41*:1054–1056, 1956.

Stout, A. P.: Hemangio-endothelioma: A Tumor of Blood Vessels Featuring Vascular Endothelial Cells. Ann. Surg. *118*:445–464, 1943.

Stout, A. P.: Tumors of the Soft Tissues, Atlas of Tumor Pathology, Section II, Fascicle 5, AFIP, Washington, D.C., 1953.

Straatsma, B. R.: Ocular Manifestations of Wegener's Granulomatosis. Amer. J. Ophthal. *44*:789–799, 1957.

Tebbet, R. D., and Vickery, R. D.: Osteogenic Sarcoma following Irradiation for Retinoblastoma. Amer. J. Ophthal. *35*:811–818, 1952.

Verhoeff, F. H.: The Mixed Tumors of the Lachrymal and Salivary Glands. J. Med. Research. *13*:319–340, 1905.

Viers, E. R., and Davis, T.: Fungus Infections of the Eye and Orbit. A.M.A. Arch. Ophthal. *59*:172–176, 1958.

Wagener, H. P., and Hollenhorst, R. W.: The Ocular Lesions of Temporal Arteritis. Amer. J. Ophthal. *45*:617–630, 1958.

Walsh, F. B.: Extraocular Muscles in Systemic Disease. Ophthal. Ibero Americana *21*:83–115, 1959.

Winter, F. C.: Annual Reviews, The Orbit. A.M.A. Arch. Ophthal. *62*:508–530, 1959.

Zimmerman, L. E., and Ingalls, R.: Clinical Pathologic Conference. Amer. J. Ophthal. *43*:417–426, 1957.

Zimmerman, L. E., and Rogers, J. B.: Idiopathic Thrombophlebitis of Orbital Veins Simulating Primary Tumor of Orbit. Trans. Amer. Acad. Ophthal. Otolaryng. *61*:609–613, 1957.

INDEX

Folios in **boldface type** indicate reference to illustrations.